To Ted:

Hope you enjoy this book, a gift from your friend Chuck Yesalis.

Matt Chaney

1-17-09

Spiral of denial

Muscle Doping in American Football

MATT CHANEY

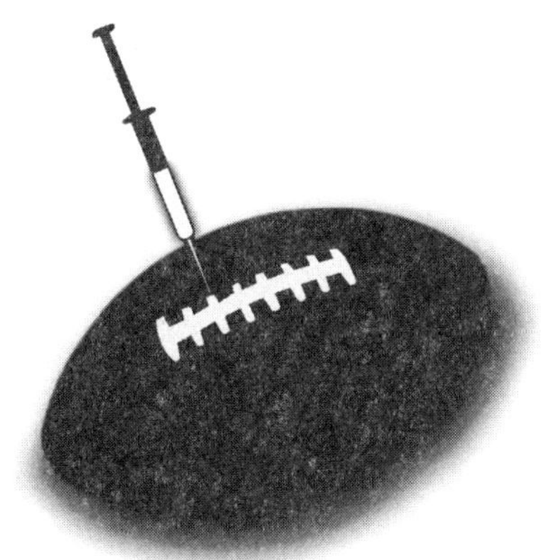

For my parents,
Louis and Lillian Chaney

Editor: Nancy Thompson
Proofreader: Tony Shaffer
Cover design, page composition: Didier Bahuaud

To order this book, or for more information, visit:
www.fourwallspublishing.com or **www.spiralofdenial.com**.

Excerpts on pages 143-144 from "Drugs in Sports: Symptoms of a Deeper Malaise," by Sandy Padwe for The Nation, September 27, 1986. Reprinted with permission from *The Nation*. For subscription information, call (800) 333-8536. Portions of each week's *Nation* magazine can be accessed at **http://www.thenation.com**.

10 9 8 7 6 5 4 3 2 1

ISBN: 978-0-9639316-4-1 (Hardcover)
978-0-9639316-5-8 (Softcover)

Contents
Spiral of Denial

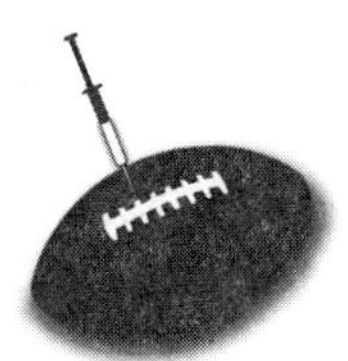

Chapter 1 [Game Problem]

Introduction

> "The spectacle is reminiscent of Ancient Rome. Instead of the gladiators and chariot races in the Circus Maximus, we have football and NASCAR and all kinds of sports on TV. People don't care how athletes train. They want the illusion. And we're feeding our youth into that myth."
>
> **Steve Courson**
> expert on sport doping, 2005

Anabolic steroids were fantastic for football, the bodybuilder told me. Within a year of multiple cycles, he said with certitude, I would gain 30 to 40 pounds of muscle, add at least 100 pounds to my bench press, and only get faster afoot.

Sounded great to me, very tempting, in the summer of 1982 at Southeast Missouri State University. I was 22, immature, and determined to live out a long-held dream: Play college football and *star* — be known for blasting rival guys on the field. I wanted to be a football hero, a big, bad man on campus, a self-image I'd coveted since grade school. Granted, at 22, I was lacking two full years for a bachelor's degree. Even so, I saw no rush to graduate, especially after this revelation would play right into my long-held fantasy. I would kick ass in college football, really revel in my manhood, and win an athletic scholarship.

I also anticipated the related awards of college football I'd heard so much about since boyhood, part of the game's built-in recruiting pitch for males: off-field pleasures. I wanted football to afford me an upgrade in local social status, to provide me access to both "football parties" and the Greek system, a most-happening scene featuring more chicks, alcohol, marijuana, and amphetamines than I could encounter as a non-player.

I craved it all — physical superiority on the football field, finances to pay for school, more parties and women. What more could a guy ask for amid the rocking early '80s at Cape Girardeau, a fun old river town of French-Spanish heritage on the Mississippi. I knew it could be mine through steroids, a bona fide shortcut. A magic potion really did exist.

A side of me wished it weren't true, and I did hesitate, as I had for years on the question of the use of steroids for performance enhancement. But greed won out, pulling me towards juicin' for football success. I knew I had to compete with guys who were already using to get there. I also knew that I was cheating the game, "plain and simple," as my Ozarks grandma would say.

Moreover, the scant literature I found on anabolic-androgenic steroids warned that the drugs could be dangerous. Much of the rhetoric was "scare tactics" that bodybuilders and football players told me to ignore, comical stuff overblown to "reefer madness" proportion, and most doctors stood by the fact that no clinical study had been performed on long-term risks for athletes who had juiced.

But health concerns, *fears*, seemed common sense to me, which is primarily why I had avoided steroids for years. I obsessed now, truly pondering using and the physical changes that would follow, perhaps mental changes as well. I already liked the size of my body, with no desire to get much bigger, and injecting steroids meant tissue-building hormones set loose in my bloodstream, cruising and attaching to tissue everywhere, including heart muscle and prostate gland. I couldn't believe that wouldn't mean serious consequences, at some point. And steroids definitely entailed short-term effects such as acne, hair loss, and shrunken testicles.

Ah, what the hell, I figured. *What's the big deal about a prescription drug? I've done worse.* I went for instant gratification, the American choice, juicin' on 'roids in my quest for football stardom, the classic male glory.

I. An Independent Scientist Emerges

When I first used anabolic steroids for small-college football, I felt sinister because of a certain naiveté, believing I was manipulating the sport through an unfair advantage, or "cheating" other players in particular.

Perhaps I did deny someone a spot on special teams, a non-steroid guy who could have made the game roster anyway. But I began to look at "cheating" in football differently; I began regarding muscle drugs as a necessity to compete.

For a coveted starting position, and the scholarship money attached, dopers had swept through college football top-to-bottom by the early 1980s. From the major programs into the lower levels of college football, juicers guarded the gate to starting status and potential stardom, for which any competitor aspired. And it was a myth that a guy had to think of lofty pro football goals before considering steroids; those players constituted a minute portion of the doping population. A guy only had to play competitive football, college or high school, to face the question of whether to juice.

By the 1984 season, I was finished as a player, having devastated my right knee with injuries requiring three surgeries. I worked as a student coach in the SEMO State program. By this time, steroid use was an inside joke for big-time college ball, but juiced competitors had become evident on every team in NCAA D-II, including ours, as well as in smaller federations such as the junior colleges and the National Association of Intercollegiate Athletics. I understood few Americans had a clue about anabolic or tissue-building substances in football [soon to change with unprecedented media exposure], and coaches and athletes were basically powerless to fight the problem short of complete solidarity in a walkout, which obviously wouldn't happen.

Ultimately, I found that when I tried to discuss football doping with people outside the game, the average fan either didn't accept the notion of widespread use or didn't want to hear about it. This realization was difficult for me. Typically, the topic was a one-way, dead discussion, and if someone would go as far as to affix blame for football doping, including the historic entrenchment of dangerous amphetamines, he or she blamed the players solely, absolving the football institution of any responsibility. The rationale carried that if I, for example, had been stupid enough to employ "speeders" and steroids for football, I was wholly responsible. Likewise, I was solely to blame for my physical disablement: a destroyed knee that encompassed foot paralysis. If I complained in the least to anyone besides my parents, I always heard the catch-all retort, "*You knew* what you were getting into." America was bound and determined to protect its holy blood sport, especially on issues of drugs and physical brutality.

In my worst moments, the football doping apathy made America seem crazed — in ludicrous denial. I knew, regardless of my character faults, I never would've touched steroids had I not played college football, and there had to be untold thousands of guys like me. So, as a fledgling writer, I filed the few articles gathered, with vague ideas about doing a book someday, but I was sure no one really gave a damn.

I was mistaken. Unbeknownst to me at the time, a young epidemiologist was on the research trail of doping in sport. Dr. Charles E. "Chuck" Yesalis, University of Iowa, was trying to sort out the myriad of mysteries. He had begun laying out sound information.

A fitness buff and former athlete who loved sports, Yesalis completed his bachelor's and master's degrees at the University of Michigan during the 1970s, followed by his doctoral degree for epidemical research at the Johns Hopkins University School of Hygiene and Public Health. In Iowa City, Yesalis joined the university's Department of Preventive Medicine and Environmental Health, with an interest in the medical issues of sport. An initial focus was the use of amphetamines for competition, but Yesalis encountered athletes more concerned, or curious, about anabolic steroids for performance enhancement. Prompted by their questions, Yesalis checked medical literature and found little was known about steroids, amazing him. No clinical data existed, for example, on the prevalence of illicit steroid use in any facet of culture, including sport.

Yesalis was profoundly intrigued. Decades later, he recalled: "As epidemiologists, what do we do? We count things. We look at numerators and denominators, incident rates, prevalence rates. And a concept that's really big in epidemiology is populations at risk. So who's the population at risk of using steroids? Who uses steroids?"

"There were these testimonials then, and rumors, and anecdotes and so on, but very little resembling what I considered to be solid science as to who's using. And before you decide to investigate health effects, both physical and psychological, or determining if it's worth doing that, you've got to know the magnitude of the problem relative to the population at risk."

Having arrived at his research calling by 1980, Yesalis took the lead for establishing scientific data on anabolic or tissue-building substances in sport and society. He developed worldwide reputation as a foremost expert in the field.

I first contacted Yesalis in January 2001, having relied on his research and expertise for years: the data, drug histories, published commentaries and news quotes. Yesalis was at Pennsylvania State University, 15 years a professor in Health Policy and Administration Exercise and Sport Science. I was a journalism teacher and graduate student at Central Missouri State University, completing a study in press coverage of muscle doping in football for my master's thesis. I had thousands of hours of study in the issue, specializing in football as a journalist and an academic, and I had amassed a personal library of news articles, books, documents, and more artifacts. I had used steroids as a college football player and discussed the drugs with hundreds like me, over the span of three decades — users in the pros, colleges, and preps. Additionally, I knew hundreds of juicers elsewhere in sport and culture. At the outset of the new millennium, I was among only a handful of American writers and scholars working sport doping, but I knew the time for the issue's public exposure was impending.

But I was humbled in meeting Yesalis, who had co-authored groundbreaking research on teen use of steroids, had written scores of journal articles and co-authored or edited books, including the imperative issue *Anabolic Steroids in Sport and Exercise* and *The Steroids Game*, and had interviewed a thousand steroid users, from seventh graders to elite athletes and men in their 60s. He had consulted for the White House, the Drug Enforcement Agency and a host of sports bodies such as the NCAA, the NFL, and the International Olympic Committee.

Yesalis really appealed to me as an honest scientist, independent and informed on performance-enhancing drugs, with big-picture perspective rooted, not coincidentally, in his thousands of hours of experience in gyms and weightrooms, exerting and challenging his natural limits of strength and size. A long-time lifter and strength coach, Yesalis clearly understood the limits of training and nutrition, and his news quotes always rang with insiders like me.

Among other so-called experts in sports doping, Yesalis was the iconoclast, virtually alone with feet firm in reality and no influence or outside agenda. The large majority of recognized doping experts — scientists, doctors, psychologists — were beholden to a business agenda, particularly in the selling of faulty urinalysis detection or dubious anti-steroid education to organizations, government, and the public. Most spoke in muted tones about everything, from pervasiveness of drugs to ineptitude of urine testing, but not Yesalis.

Drawing no favor or capital, Yesalis owed no one, resulting in free outspokenness and intellect, often searing and nailing anti-doping programs in the process — a godsend for me. Yesalis was neither patient nor tolerant of sport doping, with no use in his arguments for undue tactfulness and diplomacy. He could be merciless in the criticism of deserving athletes, coaches, organizers, drug testers, doctors, politicians, fans, and parents. Yesalis made no apology for truth, hard as it may be, because bluntness in important matters constituted family honor. Indeed, the scientist dedicated one book in part to "My father, Charles Yesalis, a great athlete, a warrior, and a patriot. He taught me to speak the truth regardless of the consequences."

It was heartening to know a recognized expert who shared my perspective of rampant anabolics in sport, especially football, and that society really did not care. Yesalis believed football's smoking-gun evidence was obvious in every televised game, as I did, with behemoths parading en masse for roaring spectators.

Twenty-five years previous, the NFL didn't have one 300-pound player, despite steroids' establishment in the game. The 300-pounders numbered 15 in 1987, when league officials acknowledged widespread use and began urinalysis testing. But by 2000, the NFL had 300 players weighing 300 or more, several approaching 400. "Now, anybody weighing less than 300 is going to have a tough time," said scouting combine director Duke Babb.

In the collegiate ranks, 300-pound linemen were standard at major universities and competitive junior colleges, and becoming so in NCAA Division II. The star linemen at high schools were enormous, as were standouts at other positions, particularly those gearing for college ball.

Urinalysis testing had failed in preventing anabolic substances, and any talk of eradication was falsehood. Yet football organizations claimed virtual eradication, both the NFL and NCAA, while typical high-school officials had never seen a problem.

Yesalis scoffed. "Nothing adds up," he said. "It's no secret athletes can get by drug testing. Football players are getting bigger, and there's no reasonable explanation other than drugs to explain this substantial increase in muscle mass."

The scientist heard so-called explanations of player sizes sans anabolics, including the contemporary claim of a Zen-like practice in strength training and nutrition. The routine involved always unspecified training techniques, power foods, and more that were lost on experienced weightlifters like Yesalis. In addition, no one openly marketed this allegedly wholesome approach to gaining mass, strength, and speed, although surely worth a fortune. Other excuses for football's ever-increasing sizes involved creatine or amino acids, "genetic wonder" specimens appearing in waves, along with "fat" athletes, and even an ungodly advance in human evolution since television.

"Smoke screens," Yesalis retorted, saying none could be a legitimate factor. He pointed to recent studies on anabolic steroids for performance enhancement, unnatural gains, as the only reliable compass. He proposed the example of a college recruit arriving on campus as a freshman. Presumably, the prospect was already trained in weightlifting and had his associated gains in mass, typically no more than 10 percent of optimum body weight. "After you've strength-trained for four or five years, you've already made your big gains [for life]. You're past your growth spurt," Yesalis said.

"So when I see a kid come to a big-time college program, and you hear, in a year, that's he's gained 20 to 30 pounds of lean mass. Well, that's just not possible. That's just absurd." Yesalis recalled the late Lyle Alzado, who observed that so-called natural monsters multiplying in the NFL were merely frauds on drugs. Yesalis said, "I would alter [Alzado's] statement to say that there certainly are not enough 'freaks of nature' to fill our Division I [football] rosters, baseball rosters, pro basketball and hockey rosters, and on and on."

If most Americans chose to believe fantasy, *aspiring athletes*, meanwhile, knew exactly what was up, once familiar with weightlifting and food consumption for gaining mass. Young athletes clearly understood their physical limitations at that point, knowing only synthetic substances could take them beyond.

Football fans could think and would do as they desired, Yesalis said, but that absolved no one of culpability for hazards befalling young athletes. Football culture was to blame, every principle party: the athletes, teen to adult, the organizers, including coaches, trainers and medical support, the capitalizing news media, and the consumer base — fans from small towns to stadium clubs.

"I can make a strong argument that as long as the drug use is not shoved right in the fans' faces, they really don't care," Yesalis said. "I think their primary goal is to be entertained. In fact, arguably, if they really saw the *consequences* of a drug-free sport, there wouldn't be anywhere near the big guys or gals, in some sports, doing bigger-than-life feats. Perhaps [fans] would even clamor for having the drugs back. [In football] just go back to the early 1990s or latter '80s; just look at the number of 300-pounders, then versus now."

Modeling effect ebbed and flowed throughout America's games, perpetually spurring athletes to observe, exchange, replicate. Athletes copied technique and style for running, jumping, handling a ball, hitting one, kicking — and using substances to enhance performance.

Celebrity users were only the surface of behavioral impact for rampant doping. Yesalis contended the athlete who used anabolics, any age of any arena, middle school and up, influenced others. With the Internet, pubescent youths understood big gains in sport were chemical-based, and when one joined in, accepting and employing muscle dope, he or she modeled for the next round of candidates.

"Clearly, there's a cascading effect," Yesalis said. "The sixth-grader knows what it takes to make the junior-high team. The junior-varsity player knows what it takes to make the varsity. The varsity player knows what it takes to make all-state and vie for a college scholarship. The freshman in college football knows what it takes to make the starting lineup sooner rather than later. The starter on the college team knows what it takes to possibly go on to a pro career. So the problem cascades down from one level to another."

"Look, all this is driven — besides our desire to look good and be winners — because these drugs *work*, and many work very well. … Anabolic steroids, in my strong professional opinion, will take athletes to heights they never would have attained naturally. The window of athletic opportunity is very small. You don't have five years to grow enough to get a college scholarship. If you're not big enough your junior year in high school to play Division I or Division II college ball, there aren't going to be any miracles out there, to make gains naturally."

After random urinalysis for steroids was instituted by college and pro football in 1990, the public rhetoric became very predictable, echoed by athletes, coaches, organizers, media, and fans in concert: Any users were an isolated minority bent on cheating, likely to be caught, because testing was always "state of the art." The storyline went that only a few steroid incorrigibles existed, hurting only themselves, but affecting none of the multitude of players following the rules.

But in reality the year-round dragnet was loose, and gaping loopholes existed in testing, including undetectable substances in low-dose testosterone, designer steroids, synthetic human growth hormone, insulin, and more. In 2001, the claim of scant use of powerful drugs in bloody football, for its spoils, was ludicrous, according to Yesalis.

"When you're talking about athletics, you either have to argue that [use] is either zero or a very small percent, or argue that it's a very great percent. ... And with the amount of money involved, if one person figures it out, you damn well have to think that *everybody's* going to figure it out."

An exact percentage of steroid use in football has never been known, yet for 20 years politicians and media always wanted an exact figure before making a judgment. Long-term health risks likely wouldn't be confirmed either, although questionable presumptions abounded in public — and Yesalis resigned that sports organizations didn't want to know. Not a single clinical trial had been conducted on steroid risks to athletes, largely for lack of cooperation that Yesalis experienced firsthand, through his repeated proposals for scientific analysis.

"That's one of the problems that people don't realize," he said. "We have yet to do an epidemiologic study of the long-term health effects of anabolic steroids. That study has not been done. I've proposed it on three occasions [to sports organizations], and I quit after being turned down three times. I think it can be done..."

"Why hasn't it?"

Yesalis paused then continued in a cryptic, sarcastic voice. "Maybe my science wasn't good enough. Interestingly, some of the same people that have turned me down for that, they ask me to give talks on a regular basis. But I gave up [proposing study] in the early to mid-'90s. After the third [rejection], I was done."

II. Praising Football, Chastising Baseball

A stark double standard was manifest in the new millennium: American outrage over baseball doping, in direct contrast to apathy for the very problem in football, assuredly more pronounced.

The phenomenon reared in stunning fashion, August 2005, around two star athletes. Baltimore Orioles' slugger Rafael Palmeiro, who tested positive for steroids, and Ravens' defensive back Deion Sanders, who acknowledged using the drugs to reporters. While negative reaction buried Palmeiro, particularly since he waved a finger in denial at Congressional hearings the previous spring, the nation ignored Sanders, an all-time great of football. Palmeiro likely would not see Baseball Hall of Fame induction at Cooperstown, but Sanders could keep yapping all the way to Canton and the shrine for pro football.

A most curious dichotomy, groundwork for the cultural hypocrisy, was laid decades before, when football responded to the growing crisis of muscle doping, even if superficially, but baseball plunged carelessly forward, doing nothing.

Steroid exposés exploded on the NCAA and NFL in the 1980s. Headlines fueled by open comments from players, coaches, doctors, police, other witnesses, and football officials perpetuated the myth that led to perfectly preserving booming business. Effectively establishing steroid policy from within accomplished this purpose, but it did nothing to educate and prevent usage. The football public-relations strategy for steroid scandal, modeled on the Olympic approach, called first for formulation of steroid rules and penalties, then deployment of urinalysis testing for anabolic steroids. Never mind that the detection technology and methodology were ineffective and muscle doping went on unchecked. Football's so-called random urinalysis was regaled by clueless media, ultimately proving to be golden for public image.

Critical for maintaining the American sports-media complex of big-business synergy, the blame for drugs in football stayed focused solely on players. The real issue was money, billions of dollars in U.S. sports content, exported as leading world entertainment.

Major League Baseball, meanwhile, was entering the wilds of unrestrained juicing on a wave of talented hitters and pitchers destined to obliterate power records as their bodies transformed. Several young stars charged ahead with the drugs, notably slugger Jose Canseco at Oakland, as steroids and HGH reshaped big-league culture, literally and figuratively, from player physique and performance to ballpark dimension and fan expectation.

The 1990s saw football largely escape public scrutiny for steroids and HGH, but baseball increasingly gained attention for large athletes and garish statistics. The 1998 home-run race between Mark McGwire and Sammy Sosa was watershed. Both shattered the longstanding season record of 61 by Roger Maris, with McGwire finishing at 70 and Sosa 66. Each had gained massive muscle since entering the big leagues. In addition, McGwire acknowledged using androstenedione, scientifically classified as an anabolic steroid but sold over-the-counter as a dietary supplement. McGwire and Sosa both denied muscle doping, and America went along for the happy ride.

However, suspicion heightened around Barry Bonds, the next rebuilt bulk blasting homers, and after his 73 homers in 2001, muscle doping in baseball was surfacing as it had in football. But because no policy existed between management and players to quell damning information, baseball began to suffer.

In May 2002, first-person witnesses stepped into the public eye with significant allegations. Declining star Jose Canseco, McGwire's old "Bash Brothers" teammate at Oakland, and former players Ken Caminiti and Chad Curtis told media that baseball was out of control with muscle doping.

"It's completely restructured the game as we know it," Canseco said. "That's why guys are hitting 50 or 60 or 75 home runs." Canseco would not confirm whether he used steroids, but promised writers to tell everything in a book he was planning — including about more star players, fostering speculation he had the goods on McGwire.

Caminiti, meanwhile, confirmed he used steroids in 1996, his National League MVP season for San Diego, and response from within the game was heavy. He quickly pulled back on his assertions to *Sports Illustrated* that half the major leagues was juicing. "When I said 'half,' I lied," Caminiti recanted. "I can honestly say that."

Major controversy ignited, nevertheless. "Much as we wanted to enjoy the power surge, there always was a certain suspicion to it," wrote Jay Mariotti, *Chicago Sun-Times*. "Now, the taint is exploding into scandal..."

Baseball was called upon to establish steroid testing, by players, fans, politicians, and media, with no one minding the technology's faults. Most sportswriters viewed testing as the complete solution, and others thought it better than nothing.

In Pittsburgh, however, radio host Mark Madden labeled testing worthless for prevention but effective as a feel-good measure for writers and fans. Madden felt no empathy for doping athletes anyway. "Baseball should do what football does: Institute testing for the sake of public relations," he wrote for the *Post-Gazette*. Continuing,

> The testing would be a sham, just like the NFL's testing. NFL players know how to beat a steroid test. Just use Human Growth Hormone, which is undetectable. Or take water-based testosterone, which quickly clears the system.
>
> But testing gives NFL fans a chance to believe their game is on the level. It gives pro football credibility. That would work in baseball, too.
>
> There is no way to truly solve baseball's steroid problem.
>
> In fact, I don't even consider it a problem. I don't care about the long-term health risks. I don't know these guys. I don't care if they live or die. Using steroids is their choice, and if they choose yes, and it provides me a more exciting athletic spectacle, great.

Baseball commissioner Bud Selig instituted steroid testing at long last, on the outcry over Caminiti and Canseco. And as soon as urinalysis began, revealing 5 to 7 percent of players tested positive, Selig proclaimed his program was ridding baseball of doping, mimicking rhetoric of late NFL commissioner Pete Rozelle, two decades before. Players union official Gene Orza parroted Selig.

Response was loud from critics, writers and doping experts ripping the shabbiness of baseball testing and the shallowness of claims by Selig and Orza. Fans were largely disinterested, leaving the "issue" primarily between baseball and naysayers in media.

"The public is not going to be pressing very hard for change because it wants to see impressive and muscular athletes," said Dr. Harrison G. Pope, professor of psychiatry at Harvard Medical School. "We would not be very happy to see athletes reduced back to their normal size."

Yesalis expected nothing to change. "Too much money involved," he said. "Look, we love our entertainment, and the only thing that I think would be the exception to that, is if there were an *extraordinary*, huge number of deaths *clearly attributed* [to anabolics]. And I don't mean one or two. Look, Lyle Alzado's death — I don't know any of my colleagues who said his death is attributed to steroids. ... So, unless there was just an unbelievable amount of deaths — and I mean they [athletes] would have to be dropping like flies."

Besides, America had already approved carnage in football by watching, for example, almost a thousand young people die of collisions since 1931, according to the National Center for Catastrophic Sport Injury Research. In addition, more than 600 died of complications related to football, including heatstroke, brain aneurysm, and heart disease.

"If the public really didn't like it, if the public were grossly outraged about it —

meaning if people turned off their television sets — you can damn well be assured something would change," Yesalis said. "But, again, [sport organizers] realize their fan base doesn't care."

As football season approached, many writers were unconcerned too, trumpeting its arrival while trashing baseball as drug-sodden. Bob Glauber, *Newsday*, declared the NFL's "steroids problem was taken care of 13 years ago," while Ira Kaufman, *Tampa Tribune*, intoned, "Stow the steroid issue and try to forget about Bud Selig for awhile."

NFL Has 'Gold Standard' Testing

By winter 2003-04, the issue of muscle doping in American sport exceeded bumbling Bud Selig and baseball. The BALCO lab scandal, unfolding in San Francisco, was milestone criminal proceedings. The Bay Area Laboratory Co-Operative, a multi-million-dollar business founded and operated by self-taught chemist Victor Conte, had rolled with an undetectable designer steroid for athletes, "THG," the so-named tetrahydrogestrinone. Big-name athletes were implicated across several sports, including baseball, football, cycling, and track and field.

A federal grand jury convened to investigate, and superstar athletes were paraded in public, arriving and leaving a San Francisco courthouse where they testified in closed proceedings. Gold medalist Marion Jones headlined for track, with the best-known NFL players in Bill Romanowski and Dana Stubblefield.

But scandal blew up over baseball all-stars under subpoena, including Jason Giambi and Gary Sheffield and particularly Barry Bonds, notorious home-run king, the self-centered local hero increasingly known at-large as an anti-hero. Many Americans perceived Bonds as the epitome of jocks "cheating" baseball through muscle drugs, egomaniacal individuals out to destroy the sanctity of records and, therefore, the game.

Sport doping was front-and-center in America with BALCO and Bonds. President George W. Bush stamped the issue for national spotlight in his State of the Union Address, January 20. Kicking off his reelection year in TV primetime, Bush discussed the war in Iraq, homeland security, taxes, the economy, education and healthcare, and then spoke about steroids in professional sports, chastising all levels of culprits.

"To help children make the right choices, they need good examples," the president said. "Athletics play such an important role in our society, but, unfortunately, some in professional sports are not setting much of an example. The use of performance-enhancing drugs like steroids in baseball, football, and other sports is dangerous, and it sends the wrong message — that there are shortcuts to accomplishment, and that performance is more important than character."

"So tonight I call on team owners, union representatives, coaches, and players to take the lead, to send the right signal, to get tough and get rid of steroids now."

Skepticism met Bush immediately, beginning with political pundits alleging a steroids stunt for votes, grandstanding through a high-profile topic that rated highly irrelevant. Other critics remembered Bush as soft on performance-enhancing substances in the past, particularly his administration's embracement of the supplement industry.

An NFL figure acted insulted by the president's accusations. "I don't know who Bush is talking about," said Gene Upshaw, head of the players union, "but he's not talking about the NFL, because we've already dealt with steroids, performance-enhancing drugs and all that." Upshaw failed to note four Oakland Raiders recently tested positive for THG, including All-Pros Romanowski and Stubblefield.

But overall the response was positive to President Bush, his naiveté aside about the impossibility of eradicating steroids. He picked a winner in steroids for the election year, a topic worth political capital with seemingly low risk for repercussion, and his White House would remain in the doping issue for the second term he would win.

"The president's remarks were a reminder of how fame, fortune and ESPN have carved out an unusual flow chart of influence in this culture," observed Mike Lopresti, Gannett News Service.

More politicians followed the news of baseball doping and Bonds, and as pitchers and catchers reported to spring training, the slugger's personal trainer Greg Anderson was among four people indicted by the BALCO grand jury, along with Conte. A report had Anderson admitting to investigators he gave steroids to unnamed players.

Bonds continued to deny using, saying MLB "can test me every day," but the dam broke March 2, when the *San Francisco Chronicle* reported Anderson allegedly provided steroids and HGH to Bonds, Giambi, Sheffield, and other athletes.

"The Giants' clubhouse is the epicenter of what has become baseball's worst nightmare," reported Wright Thompson, *Kansas City Star*. "There is a growing suspicion that a number of sluggers are using illegal performance-enhancing drugs. The foundation of the game — the significance of its most important records — is being shaken."

Selig placed a gag order on baseball, instructing all personnel to cease discussing steroids and related matters, namely BALCO, but the move only compounded bad press. "Don't talk about it and maybe the problem will go away," began a wire report. "That appears to be the stance Major League Baseball is taking on steroids."

The NFL was looking good by comparison, with commissioner Paul Tagliabue feeling compelled to promote the league for fair, clean play, a positive example for America's youth. In a posting for the NFL Web site, Tagliabue tossed bouquets to federal investigators for BALCO and to George W. Bush, making up for Upshaw's previous disrespect of the president. Tagliabue recycled time-honored league rhetoric on muscle doping, dating back to Rozelle, by claiming eradication was possible through "a comprehensive program of steroid testing, discipline, and education."

The critic Yesalis, meanwhile, was not buying the talk. "Let's state the obvious: If drug testing worked, we would not be reading about doping scandals on a weekly basis," Yesalis and colleague Dr. Michael Bahrke wrote in a commentary for *The New York Times*. "The major problem with drug testing is not that it marks innocent people as guilty (a false positive) but rather that it is unable to catch cheaters (a false negative)."

On March 10, both Yesalis and Tagliabue attended a hearing on Capitol Hill, before the Senate Commerce Committee chaired by John McCain.

The hearing's topic ostensibly was sport doping, but the committee's target was only baseball, and Selig suddenly seemed focused, offering lawmakers promises of improved drug policy. The most unpopular witness was Donald Fehr, representing the players union, who got fried by politicians.

Yesalis, however, was struck by something else at play, the sight of Tagliabue and Upshaw drawing praise from senators! NFL officials were being lauded for doping prevention: The league's "random" testing, shepherded by Tagliabue in concert with Upshaw since 1990, was being presented by politicians as worth emulating.

Doping critics did a slow burn, not the least of which was Yesalis, seated on the dais directly behind Tagliabue. Yesalis looked at the ceiling; he could not say anything in protocol of the setting. A veteran of congressional shows on doping, Yesalis knew what was going down, as did *Philadelphia Inquirer* columnist Bob Ford.

"By the end of the day's testimony, the senators had determined that Paul Tagliabue and Gene Upshaw, the NFL's commissioner and union chief, are great guys doing all they can to eliminate performance-enhancing drugs in sports. …," Ford would report. "The committee, chaired by Sen. John McCain of Arizona, did an extremely thorough job of oversimplifying the vastly complicated problem of drug use in sports."

At conclusion of the hearing, Yesalis rose from his seat, left quietly, and caught a commuter train back to Pennsylvania. On the drive home to State College, his cell phone rang. It was Dick Patrick, *USA Today*, seeking comment on the hearing. The scientist would not restrain himself now.

"The NFL came off as the gold standard [in prevention]," Yesalis told Patrick. "That was enough to make me gag."

Bob Ford called next, and Yesalis said, "It was clearly, 'Let's beat up on baseball.' Football got an undeserved group hug."

Yesalis was hearing himself repeat the same refrains on doping, decades running, and tiring of it. But he would not relent. "I've said for some time that I don't believe that, on a percentage basis, there are more baseball players using illegal drugs than players in the NFL and even the Olympics, there are so many [urinalysis] loopholes," he told Ford. "I've questioned all along the true sincerity of sports federations' desire to clean it up. Because cleaning it up would damage their business."

Politicians Target Baseball Players

As the 2000s brought unprecedented exposure of doping in American sport, football maintained its historical ability to deflect implication. The culture's gridiron religion was not interrupted, with fans generally accepting drugs as a prerequisite for the game, the players' resorting to massive amounts of painkillers, tissue-builders, and amphetamine-like boosters. Baseball fans mostly did not care, either, for they thrilled to individual performances chemically augmented, particularly the freakish numbers in homers. Governing all was cultural ethos, a society that embraced drugs or technology for every enhancement promoted, from physical and sexual performance to improving looks and preventing aging. Cops, doctors, and lawyers used steroids and growth hormone, as did politicians, entertainers, teachers. Humans juiced animals with powerful PEDs, injecting racehorses, fighting cocks, and dogs with steroids and other anabolic agents.

Yet baseball's doping was deemed an American travesty, primarily by sportswriters and politicians, and when BALCO revelations and a tell-all book exploded on two superstar sluggers during winter 2004-2005, the doping spotlight fixated on baseball and there it would remain. The president himself would face questions as a former MLB owner during the 1990s, as to whether he knew anything about muscle drugs' proliferation in the game.

The grand-jury testimony of Bonds had been a public matter for a year, since investigative sportswriter T.J. Quinn, *The New York Daily News*, reported overhearing portions from outside the courtroom. Now, the first weekend of December 2004, the Giants outfielder's testimony was fully exposed by *The San Francisco Chronicle's* Mark Fainaru-Wada and Lance Williams, investigative reporters who obtained the court-sealed transcripts from an unnamed source.

Bonds, the record holder for season homers and nearing Hank Aaron's career mark, testified he unknowingly used steroids. Bonds told the grand jury he thought substances provided by trainer Greg Anderson were flaxseed oil and rubbing balm. The revelations of Fainaru-Wada and Williams were historical in sport doping. They also publicized the testimony of Yankees sluggers Jeremy Giambi, who admitted using steroids and growth hormone, and Gary Sheffield, who said he unknowingly used "the clear" and "the cream," briefly.

The Bonds news blew worldwide, muting allegations against track icon Marion Jones by BALCO chemist Victor Conte, interviewed on ABC's *20/20.* Conte said he administered an undetectable drug protocol to Jones, among Olympic stars, including designer steroid "The Clear," or THG, and growth hormone. Conte blasted conventional anti-doping steroid testing, declaring that beating it amounted to "taking candy from a baby."

The planet's biggest headline for days was Bonds on steroids establishing sport doping as sexy modern expose, rendering mere Hollywood scandal passé in the cyber-enveloped landscape. Media editors and writers previously miscalculated sport doping, thinking consumers were lukewarm over stories of heroes drenched in PEDs, if not resistant to exposure. Now the fact was clear: While audiences apparently cared little about *reform* of drugs in sport, they devoured sensational disgrace of a personality by drugs. In addition, shrewd politicians recognized the issue's incredible public exposure potential, particularly when uncloaking superstar athletes.

Anti-Bonds rhetoric raged, but a few sportswriters warned against torching mere individuals for the cultural sin of performance-enhancing drugs in athletics, regardless of how famous the names. They argued a witch hunt or quickie "solution" would not invoke relief of the widespread problem, having already failed multiple times.

"[W]e all need to step back and give the 'steroid' controversy a little more thought," urged *Kansas City Star* columnist Jason Whitlock, a former college football player who knew steroid users. "Politicians are ready to pounce on the steroid media-feeding frenzy. ... Steroids form a complex problem for professional sports. You can't solve the problem with a simple-minded war."

"Bonds isn't the only cheater in baseball; he's just the latest to turn up in the dragnet through the steroids underworld...," observed Bernie Miklasz, *St. Louis Post-Dispatch*. "The genie is out of the steroids bottle, and there's no way to push Bonds and these other weird baseball scientists back inside. To single out Bonds is to deny the possibility that Mark McGwire dabbled in something more potent than andro, or that Sammy Sosa had some hidden kick in his bottle of vitamins."

The evidential net was entangling McGwire, threatening his run as an American hero. Millions still held to the idea of Big Mac as genuine in 1998, even overlooking his use of androstenedione, then a legal steroid available over-the-counter. But "andro" had since been classified a Schedule III controlled substance, defined by government as an anabolic-androgenic steroid, while baseball's festering scandal also chipped away at McGwire, with Caminiti and Bonds embroiled.

Then, early 2005, lingering Big Mac fantasy vaporized in a matter of weeks, against an onslaught of public disclosure about doping in the past.

In February, Jose Canseco's book *Juiced* rocked baseball and America, naming several big names as dopers or likely suspects, according to the author declaring himself as the supreme authority on the game's evolution into a muscle-doped environment. As baseball's self-anointed Godfather of Steroids from the 1980s to the 1990s, Canseco claimed to have personally injected drugs with several stars, including three favored for the Hall of Fame: Rafael Palmeiro, Ivan "Pudge" Rodriguez, and, of course, McGwire, his old Bash Brothers teammate in Oakland. Palmeiro and Gonzalez, still active in the majors, denied the allegations. Canseco even alleged President George W. Bush knew about steroids as part-owner of the Texas Rangers when All-Stars Canseco, Palmeiro, Rodriguez, and Juan Gonzalez allegedly juiced together on the team. A White House spokesman said Bush "was not aware of it at the time" and reiterated the president's anti-steroid stance.

But the book's weight fell on McGwire, retired and living in seclusion. His mega-legend, once built by capitalizing media, withered. The McGwire story surpassed the daily profile of Bonds and BALCO when New York reporter Michael O'Keeffe, *The Daily News*, broke Canseco's major allegations a week before the book's release. Media and consumers were tantalized that the mythic hitter might fully confess to juicing.

Politicians watched closely as the reclusive McGwire made two denials, particularly Rep. Henry Waxman, ranking minority member of the powerful House Committee on Government Reform. McGwire associates issued the second statement on February 13, Sunday, as Canseco aired his considerable claims on *60 Minutes* with Mike Wallace. McGwire, in the most publicized portion of his canned response, declared, "Once and for all, I did not use steroids or any other illegal substance. ... The relationship that these allegations portray couldn't be further from the truth."

But most Americans believed Canseco, one poll found, and McGwire neither sued nor emerged to answer questions from reporters.

Bonds, meanwhile, offered no confession whatsoever, only derisive denial, speaking to the media for the first time since his grand-jury testimony went public months before. "It's time to move on," Bonds said on February 22, in a contentious scene at Giants spring training in Scottsdale, as reported by Henry Schulman for *The San Francisco Chronicle*:

> He called reporters "liars" and likened their steroid stories to "Sanford and Son" reruns. He excoriated Jose Canseco's tell-all book as "fiction." He praised Major League Baseball and the players union for their new drug-testing agreement, but at the same time said he can't understand how steroids would help someone hit a baseball.
>
> In his first news conference since The Chronicle reported in December that he told a federal grand jury that he used clear and cream substances, similar to those at the heart of the BALCO doping case, Giants star Barry Bonds came out slugging at his critics Tuesday...

Two days later, Waxman acted in Washington, forwarding a letter to Rep. Tom Davis, Republican chairman of the Government Reform Committee, to propose a review of MLB doping by the large congressional body. "Jose Canseco's allegations about steroid use by Mark McGwire and other baseball players have received enormous media attention," Waxman wrote. "Many of the individuals have denied the accusations. Mr. Canseco insists his information is accurate."

Waxman chastised Selig for announcing MLB would not investigate the Canseco allegations. "There is a simple way to find the truth in this matter," Waxman, highly optimistic, wrote to Davis. "Our Committee should hold a hearing with Mr. Canseco, Mr. McGwire, and others and have them testify under oath. This would be an opportunity to find out what really happened and to get to the bottom of this growing scandal."

Waxman's idea was simplistic, uninformed, and unoriginal, decades behind anabolic steroids' entry into American sport and the beginning of a congressional inquiry. Waxman believed, or postured, that the Reform Committee could help baseball "halt the use of steroids and other drugs once and for all." The mission, Waxman asserted, was to deal with a heath problem that threatened "millions of youth who emulate athletes." He noted the committee's work on the stimulant ephedrine, following the 2003 death of Orioles pitcher Steve Bechler. "Given our committee's broad oversight powers, we can play an important role in restoring baseball's luster," Waxman concluded, "and keeping sports at all levels clean of these dangerous drugs."

The sensational baseball hearing was set for March 17 on Capitol Hill, although players and management did not share Waxman's rosy outlook and tried to avoid appearing, unsuccessfully, widening a rift between baseball and the committee. Baseball figures obviously did not want to reveal secrets, angering congressional leaders, but in fact the event's premise was faulty, naïve — or outright political grandstanding.

Politicians would not learn the big picture of baseball doping and, most importantly, had no hope for immediate prevention; none existed.

But the spotlight was not trained on government foolishness, but on the lineup of players subpoenaed to appear and testify: Sosa, Palmeiro, Canseco, Curt Schilling, and McGwire, marquee catch. America once speculated whether McGwire would catch Maris, but a new anticipation stirred millions: Would he confess to steroids?

Excitement mounted on new revelations by *The New York Daily News*, which bombed the Big Mac myth — and MLB credibility — in days leading to the hearing. "FBI informants say McGwire was juiced," the paper reported. The historical *News* sport investigations team hit the jackpot through their FBI contacts who gave McGwire's name, from an early 1990s steroid investigation, that netted a record 70 trafficking convictions, though hardly publicized. The newspaper's damning report, by O'Keeffe, Christian Red, and Quinn, detailed a hardcore steroid protocol sources said McGwire employed in the 1990s: "1/2 cc of testosterone cypionate every three days; one cc of testosterone enanthate per week; Equipoise and Winstrol V, 1/4 cc every three days, injected into the buttocks, one in one cheek, one in the other." McGwire's public support crumbled, and the hearing before Congress would finish it. The story of Big Mac would never sound the same.

Jocks Put Up a Wall

On St. Patrick's Day morning, sports-talk radio railed against athletes, but callers to C-SPAN TV's pre-hearing coverage took a different slant, nailing politicians. The sterile channel displayed scenes from the hearing room on Capitol Hill, in Rayburn House Office Building, where Government Reform Committee members gathered with media and spectators, and a succession of callers denounced lawmakers taking part.

A caller from Auburn, New York, ridiculed the grandstanding, incredulous that baseball players were scrutinized for doping. "NFL and NBA players abuse steroids a lot more than baseball players," he alleged. "They're the ones that should be brought in [to testify]."

"This is absolutely ridiculous, the whole thing," a man said contemptuously from Princeton, New Jersey, ticking off issues ignored by politicians. "They should all be voted out of office — Democrats, Republicans, all of them... Makes me sick."

And a caller from Tom's River, New Jersey: "This is very ludicrous... a dog-and-pony show," said the man. "They better find something that they can accomplish that will help the people of the United States."

Congress did achieve a television audience with the baseball hearing, millions of viewers tuning in for continuous coverage on ESPN2 and ESPNEWS. Committee chairman Rep. Tom Davis felt the TV cameras, slicking his hair as he sat at the center of the long desk up front. He called the baseball hearing to order at 9 a.m., and it would not adjourn for 11 hours; steroids in baseball would stand as the oversight committee's longest session for the entire 109th Congress.

Viewer patience was tested early, without players as initial witnesses. Davis, Waxman, and other politicians droned on in opening statements, maximizing face time and providing only common knowledge and false assumptions about doping. None mentioned the reality that no immediate prevention existed and never had, with anti-doping in sport an abject failure. Television share was strained on the first "panel" for testimony, consisting of one man, Sen. Jim Bunning, Kentucky, a 74-year-old Hall of Fame pitcher and congressional member. A conservative lawmaker who retired from MLB in 1971, Bunning said he never saw anabolic steroids in baseball and made no mention of amphetamines, the performance enhancer of choice in his era. No one asked.

The second panel produced dramatic sound bites in testimonies of parents whose sons committed suicide after they used anabolic steroids for sports. Some psychologists claimed steroids could cause suicide, and although unsubstantiated by clinical science, the theory was bandied about as fact in the hearing. The parents — Don Hooton and Rob and Denise Garibaldi appearing in person, and Efrain and Brenda Marrero present but communicating via statement — blamed steroids for psychological changes in their sons leading to the tragedies, and they laid heavy responsibility on stars of Major League Baseball, models for using steroids, they said, especially Bonds, McGwire, and Canseco. [Bonds was not subpoenaed for the hearing because of the ongoing BALCO investigation, according to the committee.]

Committee members heaped sympathy on the parents while projecting scorn for crass athletes, and viewers expected an afternoon barbeque of players to come, save for Schilling, whom Davis described as "an outspoken opponent of steroids," along with Frank Thomas, set to speak by satellite hookup.

After lunch, the featured suspects finally appeared from a side waiting room, within a solemn line of dark suits, mostly lawyers. Off camera, ESPN2 host Bob Ley commented on the procession: "And here they come — the players arriving with [legal] counsel, certainly." Schilling was the first player in line followed by Palmeiro, Sosa, and McGwire. Canseco was last, having been sequestered from the other players, who detested him and his book.

The still-hulking Canseco, dressed in V-cut suit and rumpled necktie, opened witness statements by reading nervously, eyes down. Canseco noted his published allegations and bemoaned his lack of immunity for testifying. He said he might plead the Fifth Amendment for some questions, being on criminal probation in Florida.

Following Canseco, the politicians hit headlong into jock denial, the sport's code of silence. Sosa embodied the dumb act during questioning, replying to Waxman: "I can tell you, Mr. [Minority] Chairman, I don't have too much to tell you."

Perhaps Sosa suddenly was incapable of speaking English, after yakking and grinning for years as Chicago Cubs icon, for he brought along an "interpreter" while attorney Jim Sharp read his statement. Now traded to Baltimore, the former camera-mugging slugger denied performance-enhancing drugs about himself, claiming no knowledge of use by anyone. Sosa offered his services in anti-steroid programs for kids, a modern refrain of jocks under doping scrutiny, and he expressed sympathy for families like the Hootens, Garibaldis, and Marreros.

Then McGwire's turn — he stood to raise his right hand, shockingly absent the former bravado and body posture of a world superstar, having lost the freakish muscle, swagger and *respect* as history's most feted baseball slugger. The shrunken McGwire donned a green tie for the Irish holiday, but exuded zero charm and seemingly expected none, looking wimpy, beaten, scared, "a sodden hunk of aged and post-verbal sadness," George Vecsey would recount in *The New York Times*.

McGwire quietly mouthed "I do" to the oath administered by Davis, sat down, put on eyeglasses, and easily surpassed Canseco for loss of composure in reading his statement. Saluting parents of children who were "victims of steroid use," McGwire paused to choke back tears, sigh and pull a small water bottle to his lips. He drank, put the bottle back down, and stammered, "My heart goes out to them." Excruciating to watch, old Big Mac under fire made for riveting television, framed in doping allegations swirling about him.

McGwire, 41 and four years retired from baseball, praised the committee for the hearing. "There has been a problem with steroids in baseball, like any sport where there is pressure to perform at the highest level," he said, "and there has been no testing to control performance-enhancing drugs if problems develop." Every aspiring player had to "understand that performance-enhancing drugs of any kind can be dangerous," McGwire stated. "I will use whatever influence and popularity that I have to discourage young athletes from taking any drug that is not recommended by a doctor."

But McGwire would not name names "implicating my friends and teammates" nor discuss his own history regarding PEDs. He paused, adjusted eyeglasses, drank water. "I do not sit in judgment of other players," he said, and would not "dignify Mr. Canseco's book." Specifically, McGwire said he and confidants would not become political pawns or criminal targets by his account. "Asking me or any other player to answer questions about who took steroids in front of television cameras will not solve the problem. If a player answers no, he simply will not be believed. If he answers yes, he risks public scorn and endless government investigations."

"My lawyers have advised me that I cannot answer these questions without jeopardizing my friends, my family, and myself. I intend to follow their advice." And so Big Mac had come to neither confirm nor deny steroid use, and politicians would not wrest an answer from him, though several would try in open questioning.

Theatrics continued in the player statements. Palmeiro was next, seated to McGwire's left, with his infamous positive steroid test only months away, and he would boldly rebuke Canseco and deny muscle doping. Eyes defiant, Palmeiro stood up, raised his hand for the oath from Davis, barely nodded, then plopped back down in his chair and began his defense, or offense, with attitude.

Palmeiro glared directly at Davis, committee chairman, pointing a finger, "Let me start by telling you this," he said," I have never used steroids, period. I do not know how to say it any more clearly than that. Never!" Darkly handsome, Palmeiro wore stylish blue pinstripes, white shirt, and speckled-blue necktie. "The reference to me in Mr. Canseco's book is absolutely false," Palmeiro hissed, impressively indignant. "I am against the use of steroids. I don't think athletes should use steroids, and I don't think our kids should use them."

Like Sosa, Palmeiro recounted his impoverished boyhood, noting his family fled Castro's Cuba to seek the American dream, and he was grateful for realizing that dream. Softening in tone, his gaze earnest, Palmeiro now addressed Davis respectfully — "Mr. Chairman" — and pledged to join an anti-steroid task force established by the committee, in a mission to save children. "I, for one, am ready to heed the call," Palmeiro said convincingly.

"Thank you very much, Mr. Palmeiro," Davis replied.

The committee remained hitless for any fresh confession of steroid use, and Davis hoped Schilling would open up the discussion. But this was not the same vocal Schilling, once alleging a serious problem in baseball for steroids and growth hormone. After taking his oath, Schilling voiced nary a negative about baseball; instead, he praised management and the union.

The Red Sox star fizzled as a witness, looking rather ordinary under the glare of doping allegations, at odds with his John Wayne image as a jock. Reading his statement rapidly, the World Series hero recited simple information: his team's White House visit, his admiration for President Bush and Vice President Cheney, his family's military history, his charity work, his self-made greatness, his concern for kids, his presumptions of steroid evil, and, of course, his 180-degree flop to praise baseball. Schilling, rather than criticize baseball, claimed "serious, positive, forward-thinking steps" were underway to eradicate doping. Schilling played shell games with testing data on baseball, suggesting invalidly that results could accurately measure use in the majors. Schilling purported around 2 percent of big leaguers used or wanted to, basically equal the rate of teen girls in surveys.

Davis turned to the final witness, "Big Hurt" Frank Thomas, the veteran White Sox slugger who avoided direct questioning by speaking from off site. The hulking Thomas, whom Davis introduced as "another outspoken opponent" of steroids, only joined Schilling in knowing nothing. Mustering the briefest of opening statements, Thomas warned kids about dangers and supported new MLB policy as "a very good first step in eliminating steroid use." He denied using steroids, "ever."

During the lengthy hearing recess, ESPN2 replayed McGwire's "emotional" opening statement in full, aired soundbites of others, and offered commentary by Ley, Buster Olney, and legal analyst Roger Cossack. The analysis anticipated witness remarks to come as if the second half of the Super Bowl was at hand.

Sponsor commercials showcased rippling models, suspects for steroids and growth hormone, and network promos featured jocks likely juiced. Network tags reminded viewers that congressional testimony of Canseco and McGwire was coming up. Then, back at the hearing, witness questioning commenced.

Rep. Waxman, the California liberal, called out Schilling, the conservative Easterner and aspiring politician, for waffling on steroid awareness in baseball — for contradicting his 2002 statements to *Sports Illustrated*, including, "You sit there and look at some of these players and you know what is going on" and "I know of guys who are mixing steroids with human growth hormone."

"Did players know?" Waxman demanded from Schilling. "You have spoken out about this. Did you know that other players were using steroids?"

Schilling replied in doublespeak, rebuking himself: "I think there was suspicion. I don't think any of us knew, contrary to the claim of former players [Canseco]. I think while I agree it's a problem, I think the issue was grossly overstated by some people, including myself."

Waxman: "Grossly overstated? Why do you say that?"

Schilling: "I think at the time it was a very hot situation, and we were all being asked to comment on it. ... But given a chance to reflect, when I look back on what I said, I'm not sure I could have been any more grossly wrong."

Politicians, effectively stonewalled, had only Canseco as an open witness, but he was scorned throughout the room, suffering credibility problems of his own. Doubt had been cast on his book allegations, particularly through believable denials of Palmeiro and Sosa, both persistent in claims they knew nothing. In addition, Canseco turned completely on his own book passages and began touting steroids and other PEDs as beneficial, especially for pro athletes. The pro-drug stance outraged politicians and the parents, inspiring easy verbal barbs at Canseco from players like Schilling, and so the author backpedaled, claiming steroids were bad and must be kept from kids.

But if Canseco gave McGwire an opening to outright deny the published drug allegations, the latter did not bite. McGwire refused to answer questions about steroids, including androstenedione, his former supplement, and confounded politicians by not invoking the Fifth Amendment. McGwire repeated versions of his statement, "I'm not here to talk about the past," a flimsy stance that would finalize his image reversal from cultural god to disgraced cheater. The jock's denial was characterized as "theatre of the absurd" by Rep. Tom Lantos, from McGwire's home-state of California. Lantos said "we *must* look at the past."

The final witness panel was anticlimactic, of no entertainment value, even boorish, with politicians verbally slapping Selig and Fehr but predictably avoiding a real discussion of measures to fight doping, or even if it were possible. Politicians made were predictable calls for tougher testing, stronger penalties, and responsibility to children. A few like Waxman blustered about government-imposed "Olympic testing." But, in the end, everyone went home the same as before save for McGwire, who absorbed most criticism in the hearing aftermath.

The fall of Big Mac became world headlines, again, but the media astute saw nothing constructive to report on the so-called fight against doping. Commentators gave thumbs-down on the hearing coast to coast, with Whitlock chortling disgust from Kansas City. The truly outspoken *Star* columnist ripped Congress' TV event as ridiculous drama providing no clear directives for children and parents.

"In their zeal to bludgeon baseball, talk tough in front of potential voters and promote a zero-tolerance policy for baseball drug testing, the politicians were seemingly unaware of how self-serving and simple-minded they looked," wrote Whitlock, seeing the only valid result as "McGwire, the one-time, single-season home-run king credited with bringing the game back, was flogged and disgraced."

Certainly, McGwire-bashing flourished across America, dominating media content and personal conversation. "Avoiding the Past, a Role Model Is History," headlined *The New York Times*, over Vecsey's column.

Politicians, baseball writers, and fans reared viciously on their defrocked hero, claiming a naiveté about McGwire's doping before he evaded steroid questions under oath. The rationale was faulty, given the athlete's androstenedione use and recent allegations by Canseco and FBI sources. Most new McGwire haters could not admit their old denial as fans, when they did not want to know.

America had Mark McGwire in its clutches, a powerful single sacrifice for everyone's problem, sport doping, historical and entrenched. Big Mac was burning, more superstars were following, and drugs for performance only proliferating.

Modern Scandal Confronts Football

Former NFL lineman Steve Courson had to laugh: Even he, a longtime expert on performance-enhancing substances in football and culture, had never imagined baseball would be labeled America's drug cesspool of sport. "With the elephant standing right next door — the NFL — how can you not see it there?" Courson said in March 2005. "I mean, if you can see it plainly in Major League Baseball..."

Somehow, the dots remained unconnected on a picture of football doping that was obvious. Many hundreds of news items involving football and muscle drugs had occurred since the 1980s, when Courson helped ignite history's biggest press coverage by detailing his steroid use and the widespread abuse in pro and college football, including his Super Bowl teams with the Pittsburgh Steelers. Now, the 2000s, football players, coaches, and doctors still were exposed as perpetrators, but officials for the pros, colleges and high schools continued to explain away steroids and the like as "isolated" in use.

Football officials continued to claim steroid use was limited to scattered individuals determined to cheat. Regarding growth hormone, they dismissed the logical presumption the substance was widely used, even though undetectable. They said the game's perpetually increasing sizes and athleticism were not drug-related, just the result of unspecified "advances" in training and nutrition. As usual, football officials proclaimed testing was effective and widespread muscle doping was in the past.

Bottom line, football officials still maintained the organizations held no real culpability for muscle doping and, as usual, football America went right along.

Meanwhile, Major League Baseball got pummeled publicly, with Selig the whipping boy for all U.S. sports executives. Selig's own advisors surely understood conventional anti-doping, from testing to penalties, was a futile preventative for any organization, but he seemed willing nonetheless. Therefore, every sport's poorly kept secret was intact: Nothing of impact could be done about muscle substances. And obviously most people did not care, noted Courson.

"BALCO has really exposed the frailty of drug testing," Courson said. "So the public knows, if you've got any brains whatsoever — you know when Bud Selig says 'We're going to clean the game up of steroids' — that's an out-and-out lie."

Courson saw the current steroids inquisition as "public theatre," and he agreed that Selig was the fall guy among sports executives. But he also surmised baseball was "being punished for not running as good a cover-up" as football. "Football was smart, 1989, when they went to random testing," he said, recounting milestone hyperbole. "OK, if it was disingenuous or not, it was still 'random testing' with 'state-of-the-art' technology. And it was before passage of the 1990 Steroid Trafficking Act."

"Baseball's emergence in the drug problem occurred primarily in the '90s, after the changing of law. And the fact that they *weren't serious* about their drug testing put them in harm's way. That's the big issue now. Where you say Selig is taking a hit for everybody, well, he made himself available for that hit."

However, the NFL faced its own modern scandal, brewing in the Carolinas, which threatened the league image on doping. *The State* newspaper reported that a West Columbia physician was under DEA investigation for illicitly prescribing steroids and growth hormone to as many as nine Panthers players, current and former, including some of the 2004 Super Bowl team. Agents found testosterone, HGH, and other evidence linking football players to Dr. James Shortt during a raid on his pharmacy. Short was being investigated for an alternative medical practice that allegedly led to the death of a female patient.

No names were yet available, but a lengthy prescription list of Shortt's patients had been forwarded to CBS reporters for *60 Minutes*, by a malpractice lawyer who described the doctor's business as "BALCO east." The attorney, Richard Gergel, said "professional football players knew this is where you get your steroids, and this is where you get your needles and syringes." Gergel alleged "widespread" dispensing of PEDs to professional athletes.

The NFL promoted its anti-doping policies as solid, but the scientist in charge of league urinalysis said otherwise. "People in the public assume all our testing is airtight and perfect, but that's not the truth at all," Dr. Don Catlin, director of the UCLA Olympic Analytical Laboratory, told reporter Charles Chandler, *Charlotte Observer*, adding, "There are loopholes. ... Anyone can get past a test. It all has to do with the timing and the kinetics."

Catlin, a premier engineer of testing technology, said anti-doping by organizations including the Olympics was limited and overwhelmed by substances and methods designed to evade detection. "The whole theme of drugs in sport is one that is worldwide in nature and scope," he said. "It spares no one — no country, no sport. ... There are very powerful forces at work out there. This is a huge problem." Growth hormone, designer steroids, and insulin were PEDs invisible to conventional technology, as was low-dose testosterone typically not subject to a special scan of carbon isotope ratio.

"It's not the fault of any team or any league or any lab. It's just the scientific means aren't there yet. ... When will we be there? That's a tough question," Catlin said, calling for new funding in research and development.

Money for advanced testing was not addressed by NFL commissioner Paul

Tagliabue, who responded from league meetings in Hawaii. "I think we have a very strong program and very pervasive testing and very severe penalties and a minimum number of violations," he said. "But is it perfect? No." Despite his affirmation, Tagliabue was altering his stance of a decade, dropping former rhetoric declaring or implying NFL testing as perfect.

The turn in the commissioner's perspective, in concert with Washington politicians' sudden grumbling about NFL testing, constituted a significant change for critics like Courson and his colleague Dr. Charles E. Yesalis, of Penn State.

Football was "going to get exposed big-time by *60 Minutes*," Courson said. "Baseball has raised the public's awareness to how the institution of sport lies about this problem. It's the age we live in, and [institutional denial] involved the little nuances where the public wasn't educated about steroids. Now the public has become educated through what's gone on in baseball with McGwire and Bonds."

Yesalis said, "There's no doubt in my mind the spotlight is going to shift from baseball to the NFL. ... I've been saying for four or five years that, as an overall percentage, there are a lot more drug users in the NFL than in Major League Baseball."

Media scrutiny of football doping was intensifying on events following baseball's hearing in Washington. Besides the Carolina situation, Saints' coach Jim Haslett said he used steroids about 1979, coming into the NFL, and Pittsburgh radio host Mark Madden pounced on Haslett's fresh claim about juicing on Steelers title teams. Steelers' owner Art Rooney II angrily denounced Haslett, as he had done Courson in the past for steroid allegations about the team. But Madden did not cower to the Steelers' brass and fans, telling his audience: "You want to asterisk Bonds' home-run records? You've got to asterisk the Steelers' four Super Bowl championships. ... I don't know if Rooney is lying. But I do think he's got it wrong." Madden noted the obvious, stating, "Given that size and strength are the most necessary elements for success in the NFL, does anyone really believe that steroid use isn't rampant in pro football today?"

Ron Cook, the *Post-Gazette*, criticized Rooney and others in the franchise and the NFL, calling the community "hypocritical as heck" about Bonds and furthering his argument by vindicating Courson, the Steelers pariah damned for telling the truth on muscle doping. "Rooney's contention that the Steelers didn't have a steroids problem because [coach] Chuck Noll preached against their usage is almost laughable if you believe Courson's book," Cook wrote, noting the Hall of Fame coach surely knew of steroid use. "If that's true, that doesn't make Noll a bad guy," Cook stated, echoing Courson. "It just makes him the same as any other coach who isn't against an edge that might help his team win a championship."

A few days later, March 30, CBS aired the *60 Minutes Wednesday* report on Dr. Shortt's dispensing of muscle drugs to NFL players. The story by Anderson Cooper named three Panthers' players for receiving banned steroids within days of Super Bowl 2004: offensive linemen Todd Steussie and Jeff Mitchell, and punter Todd Sauerbrun. A former employee of Shortt, Mignon Simpson, told Cooper she shipped HGH to unnamed players, with as many as six purchasing the undetectable drug from Shortt.

The Carolina scandal rose from warm to hot under national TV focus, as doctors and critics hammered the holes in NFL testing, especially for failing to detect stanozolol, the steroid bought by Sauerbrun. League officials declined to be interviewed, issuing a statement that read in part: "Is this a widespread problem? We doubt it." But league credibility took a hit. Tagliabue and the NFL had enjoyed 15 years of influential support for his random testing by media and lawmakers, but not anymore.

"The NFL is no longer flying under the steroids radar or in a position to brag about its program," Gary Myers opined for the *New York Daily News*. "The gold medal, for now, has dropped to bronze while the NFL and the DEA figure out what's going on down in Carolina."

Predictably, Congress called a hearing on steroids in pro football, by the House Committee on Government Reform, the same body that went after baseball, but with less vigor for attacking the NFL.

Politicians Love Football

By middle age, I was certain America wanted its football but nothing to do with fighting drugs in its football. I was 45, a writer and researcher on anabolic or tissue-building substances in football since my own steroids experience in college. I was practically resigned to trusting that nothing would be done. April 2005 reinforced my cynicism, when politicians made folly of "examining" steroids in the NFL.

The hearing's debacle was evident before it started, when the politician's witness list conveniently omitted Yesalis, America's foremost independent expert on sport doping. I was angry but not surprised, because Yesalis as a witness would have defied both Congress and the NFL, stressing the overriding fact that effective steroid prevention was likely never to happen. Yesalis would have strongly rebuked both politicians and NFL officials in their claims about fighting doping. Politicians contended that a "solution" was possible through "Olympic-standard testing," whatever that meant, while NFL yaks asserted they had already cleaned up muscle drugs through random testing.

Yesalis had rejected the tired propaganda of doping for years and as recently as a poorly publicized Washington hearing the month before. Appearing as a congressional witness for the fourth time in 17 years, Yesalis noted politicians first reviewed PEDs in 1973, "when Olympic athletes and professional athletes openly testified about the steroid and amphetamine use of that era." Drug detection had failed abysmally, Yesalis observed, while sport, lawmakers, and fans acted oblivious. "The most rigorous drug-testing systems have loopholes through which I could drive every M1 Abrams tank we own and not scrape the body armor," he said.

Consequently, Yesalis wasn't invited to the NFL hearing, and another absurd absence was that of Dr. Don Catlin, the testing guru in charge of league urinalysis results at the UCLA lab. Catlin, increasingly outspoken about the worthlessness of conventional anti-doping, had recently criticized NFL loopholes during a newspaper interview. Catlin wasn't invited to the hearing.

Without those earnest scientists, I knew the stage was set for grandstanding by politicians and their supposed adversary, the powerful NFL, the most influential pro sport around Washington. Additional signs included no NFL coaches as witnesses — just two coaches from *high schools* — and not one contemporary player. Bill Romanowski wasn't even summoned, the former NFL bad guy and confirmed steroid user whose autobiography was nearing release. Without popular jocks to squirm on camera, the football hearing on April 27 was relegated to delayed airing on C-SPAN.

Courson agreed to testify, but he wondered why Government Reform Committee leaders called him, since he'd retired from pro football 20 years ago. A committee member, Rep. Stephen F. Lynch, also questioned the lack of a single modern player, calling it a "glaring" deficiency. "I think this defect… will lead the public to come to question the commitment, thoroughness and fairness of this committee and this [steroids review] in general," said Lynch, the atypical politician for his proper study on the issue of football doping. His committee colleagues were largely ignorant, so the hearing was easy for pro football.

Following the model of the 1989 hearings, NFL officials skated by the issue. Led by Tagliabue and Upshaw, league and union brass denied a widespread steroid problem and proffered smoky excuses for worthless testing, the increasing sizes of players, and the Carolina scandal, simply overlooking the evidence of pervasiveness. Cheery politicians went along, mentioning federal intervention but not threatening it. Of course, Tagliabue and Upshaw declined that option politely but firmly.

Politicians heaped praise on the NFL figures, supposedly for tough anti-doping policies and their cooperation, in contrast to MLB officials. "I want to thank all of you for your testimony and your patience," said Davis, committee chairman.

Waxman, ranking minority member, said, "I want to commend… you for not just being here, but for the proactive way you have tried to deal with the steroid problem."

Rep. Christopher Shays praised Taglibue and Upshaw, gushing, "I kind of love you guys, and yet I shouldn't…"

After the hearing, only scattered sportswriters criticized the fan fest of politicians with the NFL.

San Francisco Chronicle columnist Gwen Knapp wrote that Upshaw and Taglibue "waltzed through drug hearings in front of the same committee that only six weeks ago left Major League Baseball face down in its own drool."

Skip Bayless, ESPN commentator, derided the hearing as "five hours and 56 minutes of funny-sad." He wrote: "What a waste of time. You've seen first-week NFL preseason games that were more meaningful. … Mostly, Tagliabue was a Park Avenue attorney talking circles around a gaggle — or giggle — of fawning fans masquerading as politicians. … This was a hearing without seeing."

Courson agreed the event was farcical after returning home from Washington. He had delivered a riveting opening statement lauded by journalists including Knapp, but only one politician was present to hear him, and the hearing's substance went downhill from there. Courson had predicted the event's flow ahead of time, saying, "The NFL gets its hand slapped a little bit, nothing like baseball went through, and life will go on."

The league was too powerful as usual, Courson said, in money and influence over lawmakers and sportswriters, to get called out for drugs. "We don't know, lobbying-wise, what's going down behind the scenes," he said. "And the media are only going to dog [the NFL] to a certain extent."

Cultural mythology insulated football from criticism. A groundless game view shaped by fans and disseminated by media had developed. Regardless of evidence of doping, the public classified it as a personal issue, starting and ending among individual athletes, with absolutely no systemic culpability for football.

Yesalis didn't watch the NFL hearing, having personally experienced such exhibition. "Everybody goes away, you know. The politicians do what they do, they move on to another sexy topic, another photo op." But Yesalis did see a "progress that can't be taken away," despite no immediate answer to drugs in any sport. "I think there are far more journalists that know what time of day it is," he said. "I think the majority of the population knows what's going on now. That's what's really been damaging and damning to the Olympics but especially the NFL and MLB: The *people* aren't as dumb as they were. Whether people give a damn about it, that's another issue."

III. Football Denial Survives a Fighter

Just before 11 o'clock a.m. on a gray Tuesday morning in southern Pennsylvania, November 2005, a white limousine bus approached Gettysburg. The travelers were middle-aged men and ex-football players, Steelers of yore, late for the funeral of former teammate Steve Courson. Now, one of the Men of Steel called ahead to the church, St. James Lutheran, where about 150 mourners waited. People had been gathering in town since Monday. Like a tardy schoolboy, he apologized on the phone, saying his group was prevented a timely departure from Pittsburgh, a four-hour journey. Some of them had risen before dawn but to no avail, he said, and he requested delaying the funeral until their arrival. Church officials relented and the holdup was announced, to the chagrin of many in the pews. A "busload of Steelers" was promised, exciting no one.

Entering old Gettysburg, the great battlefield spread about local hills, the ex-Steelers knew what, or who, awaited them: a potentially adverse situation with people unimpressed by football mythology. This would be no autograph session with loyal fans, no adoring fans celebrating the Super Bowl glory years. Instead, the funeral congregation was family and close friends of Steve Courson, people who understood the issue of muscle drugs in football, and who personally knew the deceased in his 20-year fight to shed light on its consequences. The Steelers' franchise and alumni players were not highly regarded by most people waiting at the church.

For ex-Steelers on the bus, steroid use on their historic teams was no secret today. Rather, it framed context for this funeral experience. Worse, a determined reporter waited at the church, Jeff Barker, *Baltimore Sun*, who sought to confirm Courson's allegations of steroid abuse among Steelers in the 1970s and '80s. Barker had already phoned a couple of the guys, inquiring whether they ever used steroids.

In 1985, Courson, as an All-Pro NFL lineman, publicly disclosed his anabolic-steroid use and football's widespread problem. He then waged an intellectual battle his remaining two decades. He became a lay expert on muscle doping and the blatant abuse of anabolic steroids, synthetic growth hormone, and other tissue-building substances in American football — high school, college, and the NFL. Along the way, he overcame alcoholism, obesity, and heart disease, coached football, counseled thousands of young people, wrote a book, and twice testified before Congress. But he paid to tell the truth and attack the machine, getting blackballed from pro football, losing more career opportunities, and dying in financial debt.

Courson, 50, had followed a simple code of right and wrong, believing honesty could make an impact in the superficial lives of a self-indulged people. Other old Steelers fashioned themselves warriors of conquest, victors upholding team and fans' honor, but Courson always disagreed. A few months before his death in a tree-cutting accident, Courson discussed a warrior's mission in a letter to a former teammate, a rider on the limousine bus. *Warriors throughout history, starting with even tribal cultures, protected the weak*, Courson wrote in an attempt to clarify for this football player. *Gladiators fight for spoils, ego, and survival.*

Courson did not mail the letter, perhaps because the former teammate and others would not budge off their code of silence on drugs. Old teammates never backed him in public but just continued in their livelihoods as businessmen, teachers, coaches, broadcasters, Christian speakers, and combinations thereof while watching him suffer alone on his path. They practiced and upheld football's denial of muscle doping, as practically everyone in the game had done for 40-some years.

Officials of the Steelers and NFL ignored Courson's funeral, and the "busload" of ex-teammates attending were conveniently late, thus avoiding any interaction with the waiting congregation beforehand — except for Jeff Barker, the reporter who greeted them outside the old church as the charter pulled up at 11:10 a.m. About 10 men exited down onto the sidewalk, several hobbling on arthritic legs. Most brushed past Barker, with a few pausing to deny knowing anything about steroids on the Steelers, and certainly nothing like Courson alleged. Had they discussed steroids on the trip? No, they told Barker, just "Steve stories" since leaving Pittsburgh. Then they entered the church clustered together like fraternity boys.

Silence and glares met them in the sanctuary, a reception hardly befitting Steelers' status in Pennsylvania, even if the men were shriveled and normal-looking, contrasting their former hulking physiques in black and gold. None fit the gridiron images in films, posters, photos anymore, but so what? To this day they saw those images pasted throughout Steelers Nation, hard copies and in cyber, testifying to their legends for real fans to worship.

Maybe they were the antithesis of true warriors, but they were *football heroes*, Super Steelers, and they would unite for that against anybody, including mourners of Courson. Their greatest nemesis was silent now, anyway, sealed in that coffin up front. And they *were* the only franchise representatives making an appearance, along with a couple other ex-players who came independently. Besides, the old Steelers accomplished plenty for fans and had even *helped Courson*, when he was down-and-out and ill from heart disease. It all justified their silence about performance-enhancing drugs in football and especially where the team was concerned. They were "protecting the game," as one scolded Courson in the past.

But their rationale had been groundless to him and was now for vast majority at the funeral, with their dead teammate's words standing in defiance. *It's not personal anymore because I am no longer the scapegoat*, Courson had written in the un-mailed letter, still incomplete and buried in a PC file. *The sad thing is if all athletes spoke out together, none of us would be [solely blamed]. ... Everyone has to do what is right for [his family], but a media and public once educated are also accountable for what they know. This is not just going to disappear. All I can do is relate what I know to help you understand it deeper. Sometimes the seemingly "safe" route in time becomes perilous.*

The old Steelers took a pew reserved for them in a forward row, and the service began, officiated by the Rev. Lois K. Van Orden, a Courson family friend. Rev. Van Orden endorsed Courson's example, comparing him to Job and the Apostle Paul. "Nothing could separate Steve from his confidence that something good comes to those who try," she said.

Steve's brother, Bruce Courson spoke. Both had been adopted as infants by their parents, Iber, deceased, and Elizabeth Courso, a retired nurse. Steve had been proud of his family. The 1973 Gettysburg High graduate regularly noted his mother's scientific rationale, and the military service of his father and brother, veterans of World War II and Vietnam. "Steve changed professional sports," Bruce said. "He changed me. I think he changed a lot of us for the better." Bruce saw several "heroic plays" by his brother, especially Steve's singlehandedly rocking the mighty football institution. "Certainly, the team owners weren't happy. A lot of the professional athletes probably still are not happy."

Down in front, the old Steelers sat quietly, seemingly oblivious to the glances their way.

I always thought that being recognized publicly for being truthful, in an effort to address this issue, was in essence part of regaining my honor as a human being, Courson had written. *It never really had anything to do with money. ... Sometimes, knowing too much about something is a difficult burden, but it is better than existing in a void absent of personal honor, serving a myth, even a popular one. Myth and fantasy I was forced to [discard] in 1985, when I was interviewed by* Sports Illustrated *about steroid use [in football]. I had a choice, tell the truth or lie. ... It's not complicated: Either you behave like a standup person or you don't.*

The short service concluding, the congregation joined in The Lord's Prayer. Then Rev. Van Orden said, "Let us commend Stephen to the mercy of God, our maker and redeemer. Into your hands, O merciful Savior, we commend your servant, Stephen. Acknowledge, we humbly beseech you, a sheep of your own fold, a lamb of your own flock, a sinner of your own redeeming. Receive him into the arms of your mercy, into the blessed rest of everlasting peace, and into the glorious company of the saints in light."

"Amen," the mourners answered.

The body would be cremated — there was no money for burial — and pallbearers escorted the coffin outside to a hearse. Most everyone stayed for refreshments and fellowship in the dining room downstairs. And still the old Steelers stuck together, moving by cluster to a table against a wall. Hardly anyone approached them.

A microphone was ready for comments about Steve, and his girlfriend went first, Denise Masciola. More testimonials followed, until expectancy in the room turned to the table of old Steelers that included self-avowed Christians.

The former teammates must have felt the burning eyes, for they got up, *all* at once, and approached the microphone in a cluster. Silence hung heavy and one of them stepped forward, resorting to standard football tales to break the pall. But this was not a VFW gathering, and recounting wild times of the distant past with Steve, or "funny stories" about living loose as young players, fell flat in the church. The audience was generally unresponsive, neither amused nor stirred.

A second former Steeler took the more appropriate tact of discussing Steve's religious faith. He said Steve "made mistakes" in life but, by returning to the path of Jesus, had found redemption. The teammate said nothing about steroids, football brutality or more problems his fallen friend had taken so seriously. The teammate did not address "mistakes" made by himself or anyone else in his group.

The fellowship session concluded and everyone departed. The old Men of Steel found haven in their bus for the return to Pittsburgh, leaving behind the silent inquisitors, having admitted nothing.

"I wish they could do that now to let [Steve] go peacefully," Masciola told Barker. "But I knew he would take it to the grave with him."

The former Steelers disgusted Charles Yesalis, Penn State, a close friend and collaborator of Courson. "They know how Steve felt, they know how he lived, and even at his funeral they dishonored him, by actively maintaining their fabricated existence," Yesalis said later. "They couldn't even hint at truth. They didn't have to go up to that microphone and give us a personal confession, but they couldn't even break ranks or acknowledge reality in a general way, at Steve's funeral."

"So they didn't attend this funeral to honor Steve. They attended it to maintain the façade. They honored Steve in no way, shape or form."

Courson, in his letter to the teammate, had written:

I think more and more players from our era are going to come out and speak their piece, especially those with weight-related ailments. I'm sure there are many NFL players from our time that feel exploited, abandoned by their union. They have some reservations about the NFL myth. It is almost unbelievable that an industry that exploited our health so dramatically in front of the public does not provide us lifetime health-care insurance. Webbie's demise [former Steelers lineman Mike Webster, Hall of Famer, died in 2002] and the similarities we shared in disability fights still don't sit well with me. ...

I believe the magnitude of doping in elite football will be eventually exposed. In many ways it already has been. Recent events in baseball will eventually take their toll on the “elephant in the room.” If the NFL is hit with another major doping scandal it may unravel, [although officials] probably have enough power, wealth and influence to weather the storm. But eventually there will be sacrifices because of the charade. I think certain ex-players in the sports media may be at risk. In a wholesale meltdown they would be the first to be cannibalized. …

Football with drugs or without drugs is society’s drug. I’ve said often in seminars that drug use in sport is a symptom of greater problems. I believe the system is broken and can’t be fixed. I also believe that the greater implosion is coming. It is just a matter of when, not if.

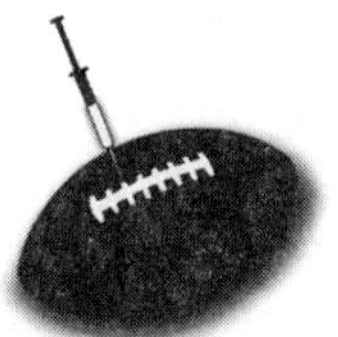

REFERENCES

A Service. (2005, November 15). A service of Christian Thanksgiving for the life of **Stephen P. Courson.** Gettysburg, PA: St. James Lutheran Church.

Alzado, L. (1991, July 8). 'I'm sick and I'm scared.' *Sports Illustrated*, p. 20.

Bahrke, M.S., & Yesalis, C.E. (Eds.). (2002). *Performance-enhancing substances in sport and exercise*. Champaign, IL: Human Kinetics.

BALCO Chief. (2004, December 3). BALCO chief on sports doping scandal. *ABC News* [Online].

Bamberger, M., & Yaeger, D. (1997, April 14). Over the edge. *Sports Illustrated*, p. 62.

Barker, J. (2005, November 16). Taking it to his grave. *Baltimore Sun*, p. 1C.

Baseballs Lively. (2000, June 21). Baseballs aren't juiced, just lively. *Kansas City Star*, p. D5.

Bavley, A., & Rock, S. (1998, August 29). McGwire's pills. *Kansas City Star*, p. A1.

Bayless, S. (1990). *God's coach*. New York, NY: Simon and Schuster.

Bayless, S. (2001, October 3). Survival of the fittest drives HR totals ever higher. *Knight Ridder/Tribune News Service* [Online].

Bayless, S. (2005, April 29). The NFL's comedy of errors. *ESPN.com* [Online].

Bhasin, S.; Storer, T.W.; Berman, N.; Callegari, C.; Clevenger, B.; Phillips, J.; Bunnell, T.J.; Tricker, R. ; Shirazi, A.; & Casaburi, R. (1996). The effects of supraphysiological doses of testosterone on muscle size and strength in normal men. *New England Journal of Medicine*, p. 1.

Boswell, T. (2005, February 8). Canseco is easy to read, hard to believe. *Washington Post* (reprinted in *St. Louis Post-Dispatch*) [Online].

Bosworth, B., & Reilly, R. (1989). *The Boz*. New York, NY: Charter Books.

Bouchette, E. (2005, March 24). Haslett admits to using steroids. *Pittsburgh Post-Gazette* [Online].

Bradley, J. (2000, April 3). Gen XXL. *ESPN The Magazine*, p. 84.

Canseco, J. (2005). *Juiced*. New York, NY: HarperCollins Publishers, Inc.

Canseco Reports. (2005, February 25). Canseco reports e-mail death threat. *Kansas City Star*, p. D2.

Carlton, J.G. (1998, August 30). In professional athletics, looking for an edge is part of the game. *St. Louis Post-Dispatch*, p. B1.

Chaikin, T., & Telander, R. (1988, October 24). The nightmare of steroids. *Sports Illustrated*, p. 82.

Chandler, C. (2005, March 22). Cheating players may slip through drug tests' big gaps. *Charlotte Observer*, p. 1A.

Chandler, C. (2005, March 23). Panthers link to steroids is traced to leak in court. *Charlotte Observer*, p. 1A.

Chaney, M. (1998, October 2). Big Mac steps up to the plate; steroids awareness steps back. *Kansas City Star*, p. C7.

Chaney, M. (2001, January 27). Despite drug testing, players get heftier. *Kansas City Star*, p. B9.

Committee on Energy and Commerce. (2005, March 10). *Steroids in Sports: Cheating the System and Gambling Your Health* (Serial No. 109-65). Washington, D.C.: U.S. Government Printing Office.

Committee on Government Reform, U.S. House of Representatives. (2005, March 17). *Restoring faith in America's pastime: Evaluating Major League Baseball's efforts to eradicate steroid* (Serial No. 109-8). Washington, D.C.: U.S. Government Printing Office.

Committee on Government Reform, U.S. House of Representatives. (2005, April 27). *Steroid Use in Sports, Part II: Examining the National Football League's Policy on Anabolic Steroids and Related Substances* (Serial No. 109-21). Washington, D.C.: U.S. Government Printing Office.

Cook, R. (2005, March 27). '70s Steelers are guilty like Bonds. *Pittsburgh Post-Gazette* [Online].

Cooper, A. (2005, March 30). Steroids and the NFL. *60 Minutes Wednesday* [Online].

Courson, S. (2005, March 7). Interview with author, Farmington, PA.

Courson, S. (2005, March 27). Telephone interview with author.

Courson, S. (2005, April 3). Telephone interview with author.

Courson, S. (2005, May 1). Telephone interview with author.

Courson, S. (2005, July 20). Letter to former Steelers teammate, non-delivered.

Courson, S., & L.R. Schreiber. (1991). *False glory*. Stamford, CT: Longmeadow Press.

Dahlberg, T. (2004, April 27). Steroids, terrorism concern Americans. *The Associated Press* [Wire].

Dutton, B. (2003, November 14). Baseball to penalize players for steroids. *Kansas City Star*, p. D6.

Dvorchak, R. (2005, October 5). Good uses for steroids overshadowed by bad. *Pittsburgh Post-Gazette* [Online].

Elias, P. (2003, November 25). Validity of MLB testing called into question. *The Associated Press* [Wire].

Emmons, M., & Almond, E. (2003, December 2). Pushing the steroid issue. *San Jose Mercury News* [Online].

Etc. (2003, July 22). Etc. *Kansas City Star*, p. C2.

Fainaru-Wada, M., & Williams, L. (2004, March 2). Slugger's trainer said to have given substances to several athletes. *San Francisco Chronicle*, p. A1.

Fainaru-Wada, M, & Williams, L. (2004, December 2). Giambi admitted taking steroids. *San Francisco Chronicle*, p. A1.

Finder, C. (2005, November 16). Courson's legacy is change. *Post-Gazette* [Online].

Ford, B. (2004, March 12). Senators make Fehr steroid whipping boy. *Philadelphia Inquirer* [Online].

Gag Order. (2004, March 4). Commissioner issues gag order on that baseball 'S' word. *Kansas City Star*, p. D2.

Glauber, B. (2002, July 22). Questions abound as NFL training camps begin. *St. Louis Post-Dispatch* [Online].

Gloster, R. (2004, January 21). Bush makes anti-drug appeal to athletes, pro leagues. *The Associated Press* [Wire].

Gloster, R. (2004, February 17). Trainer admitted giving steroids to baseball players. *The Associated Press* [Wire].

Goetinck, S., & Beil, L. (1998, August 31). Surge in sales of steroid-like supplement boosted by celebrity. *Kansas City Star*, p. D3.

Gonzalez Says. (2005, February 24). Gonzalez works out, says Canseco lied. *Kansas City Star*, p. D3.

Goodall, F. (2002, May 17). Canseco: Many players take steroids. *The Associated Press* [Online].

Goold, D. (2005, February 8). Canseco book draws fire. *St. Louis Post-Dispatch* [Online].

Goold, D., & Hummel, R. (2005, February 13). McGwire denies using steroids. *St. Louis Post-Dispatch* [Online].

Huizenga, R. (1994). *"You're okay, it's just a bruise"*. New York, NY: St. Martin's Press.

Kaufman, I. (2002, July 14). Now's time to welcome rite of summer: Football. *Tampa Tribune* [Online].

Keteyian, A. (1989). *Big Red confidential*. Chicago, IL: Contemporary Books, Inc.

Knapp, G. (2005, April 28). NFL drug success is relative. *San Francisco Chronicle* [Online].

LeBlanc, C., & Newton, D. (2005, March 13). Probe targets Shortt, Panthers. *State*, p. A1.

Litke, J. (2004, March 18). The calvary isn't on the way. *The Associated Press* [Wire].

Lopresti, M. (2004, January 25). State of the steroids. *Kansas City Star*, p. C12.

Lyons, R.D. (1984, June 14). Athletes warned on hormone. *New York Times*, p. D23.

Madden, M. (2002, June 1). What's wrong with steroids? *Pittsburgh Post-Gazette*, p. C3.

Madden, M. (2005, March 25). Were the Super Steelers 'Roided Up? *WEAE Radio* [Online].

Magee, J. (1999, October 31). The 300-pound lineman, once a rarity, is now the norm in the NFL. *Copley News Service* [Online].

Mandell, A.J. (1976). *The nightmare season*. New York, NY: Random House, Inc.

Mariotti, J. (2002, May 30). Truth starting to hit home. *Chicago Sun-Times* [Online].

Masciola, D. (2005, November 29). Telephone interview with author.

McCain, J. (2004, April 8). Postal correspondence to author.

Meehan, M. (2005, April 27). NFL is a model for cracking down on steroids. *The Hill* [Online].

Meggyesy, D. (1970). *Out of their league*. Berkeley, CA: Ramparts Press, Inc.

Miklasz, B. (1996, December 2). Telephone interview with author.

Morrissey, R. (1995, January 10). Drug suspicions still dog football. *Rocky Mountain News*, p. 17B.

Mueller, F.O., & Diehl, J.L. (2004). *Annual survey of football injury research.* Chapel Hill, NC: National Center for Catastrophic Sport Injury Research [Online].

MVP Used. (2002, May 29). '96 MVP says he used steroids. *Kansas City Star*, p. D5.

Myers, G. (2005, March 30). NFL not flying below radar screen anymore. *New York Daily News* [Online].

Nadel, J. (1993, August 26). Howie Long says steroid use down, growth hormone use up in NFL. *The Associated Press* [Online].

O'Keeffe, M. (2005, February 7). Canseco: I injected McGwire. *New York Daily News* [Online].

Oriard, M. (1993). *Reading football.* Chapel Hill, NC: The University of North Carolina Press.

Patrick, D. (2004, March 11). Expert: Let anti-doping groups do testing of pros. *USA Today* [Online].

Quinn, T.J. (2007, July 21). Jury's in on Bonds. *New York Daily News* [Online].

Reents, S. (2002). Determining the efficacy of performance-enhancing substances. (In Bahrke, M.S., & Yesalis, C.E., *Performance-enhancing substances in sport and exercise*). Champaign, IL: Human Kinetics.

Reilly, R. (1998, September 7). The good father. *Sports Illustrated*, p. 32.

'Roid Rage. (2002, May 31). 'Roid rage has Caminiti backing off. *Kansas City Star*, p. D2.

Rosenthal, K. (1998). Steroids: Baseball's darkest secret. *MSNBC* [Online].

Schulman, H. (2005, February 23). Bonds brushes off steroid questions, praises baseball's new drug rules. *San Francisco Chronicle* [Online].

Sheridan, P. (2003, November 16). Steroid stupor. *Kansas City Star*, p. C12.

Sidoti, L. (2004, December 13). Steroid issue puts McCain in the limelight. *The Associated Press* [Online].

Speech Text. (2004, January 21). The text of President Bush's speech. *Kansas City Star*, p. A1.

Steroids Hearing. (2005, March 17). ESPN2, ESPNEWS television.

Telander, R. (1989). *The hundred yard lie.* New York, NY: Simon and Schuster.

Thompson, W. (2004, March 3). Illegal steroids rattle baseball. *Kansas City Star*, p. A1.

Woolsey, G. (2001, November 13). Baseball ignores all the stuff about McGwire. *Toronto Star*, p. E6.

Vecsey, G. (2005, March 18). Avoiding the past, a role model is history. *New York Times* [Online].

Verducci, T. (1998, March 23). Man on a mission. *Sports Illustrated*, p. 76.

Verducci, T. (2001, October 8). Pushing 70. *Sports Illustrated*, p. 38.

Verducci, T. (2002, May 28). Caminiti comes clean. *Sports Illustrated* [Online].

Voepel, M. (2002, June 1). Recent steroids exposé is only latest in long line of incidents. *Kansas City Star*, p. D2.

Voy, R. (1991). *Drugs, sports, and politics*. Champaign, IL: Leisure Press.

Williams, L., & Fainaru-Wada, M. (2004, December 3). Sheffield's side. *San Francisco Chronicle*, p. A19.

Williams, L., & Fainaru-Wada, M. (2004, December 3). What Bonds told BALCO grand jury. *San Francisco Chronicle*, p. A1.

Wilstein, S. (1998, August 30). 'Andro' use OK in baseball, not Olympics. *Sedalia Democrat*, p. 6D.

Wilstein, S. (2004, January 22). Bush uses bully pulpit against steroids. *The Associated Press* [Wire].

Yaeger, D., & Looney, D. (1993). *Tarnished dome*. New York, NY: Simon & Schuster.

Yesalis, C.E. (2000). *Anabolic steroids in sport and exercise* (2nd edition). Champaign, IL: Human Kinetics.

Yesalis, C.E. (2001, January 17). Telephone interview with author.

Yesalis, C.E. (2004, January 22). Telephone interview with author.

Yesalis, C.E. (2005, January 22). Telephone interview with author.

Yesalis, C.E. (2005, February 7). Telephone interview with author.

Yesalis, C.E. (2005, May 3). Telephone interview with author.

Yesalis, C.E. (2005, November 23). Telephone interview with author.

Yesalis, C.E., & Bahrke, M.S. (2004, March 7). Where there is a will to gain an edge, athletes find a way. *New York Times* [Online].

Yesalis, C.E., & Cowart, V.S. (1998). *The steroids game*. Champaign, IL: Human Kinetics.

You Believe? (2005, February 14). Do you believe former baseball slugger Jose Canseco's allegations about widespread steroid use by top players? *Fort Lauderdale Sun-Sentinel* [Online].

Chapter 2 [Chemical History Anabolic steroids in football, 1950s-1979]

"I couldn't understand why [rookies] felt making the pros was so tough, until the veterans arrived. ... Two huge guys were standing in the locker room doorway. ... Their arms looked as big around as my thighs. I was reluctant to ask them to move aside."

David Meggyesy
former NFL linebacker, 1970

Contrary to a common assumption, athletes alone did not bring anabolic steroids into sport. Rather, the early predominant pushers were doctors, coaches and trainers, and especially in American football, a pioneer colony of a muscle-doping culture. During the 1960s, football officials and associates apparently instigated and nurtured the spread of anabolic steroids through every level of the game, professional, collegiate, and high school, and by decade's end, stories were surfacing in print.

A 1969 investigative series was landmark, by writer Bill Gilbert for *Sports Illustrated*, on the burgeoning use of performance-enhancing drugs across sports. Among revelations by Gilbert, he noted anabolic steroids entered pro football by 1963, when players for the San Diego Chargers began receiving Dianabol pills from team officials. The Chargers also gave Dianabol to at least one prospect in the college ranks, while another college player told Gilbert the majority of big-time linemen were juicing by 1968. The writer also learned of steroid programs in high-school football, part of product testing by pharmaceutical companies and physicians who provided the drugs to teens.

A steroids case in college football surfaced through David Meggyesy, disillusioned NFL linebacker turned author of *Out of Their League*, his acclaimed autobiography of football counterculture in 1970. Meggyesy had left pro football with no direct exposure to the use of anabolic steroids, later recalling that he neither witnessed nor heard of the practice. But while writing the book he learned about muscle doping through track-and-field athletes in California, and he met a college football player with sobering information.

Meggyesy was a guest lecturer for a class at UC Berkeley, a course on sport culture taught by critic Jack Scott, where one day the discussion turned to drugs in football. Jim Calkins, a Cal co-captain and tight end, said coaches and a team physician were providing him with anabolic steroids for gaining size and strength.

The author was alarmed but not surprised. In his football autobiography, Meggyesy asserted drugs like steroids were staple in a sport beset with risks for players. He blasted pro football, an easy mark, but Meggyesy also ridiculed the public's naive notions of college football. "Young men are having their bodies destroyed, not developed," wrote Meggyesy, a former player at Syracuse University, where he alleged football corruption extended across the campus in pursuit of national championships.

Meggyesy saw performance-enhancing drugs as another axle for football's evolving gladiatorial function. The NFL and ABC-TV were debuting *Monday Night Football*, leading millions to adopt another cherished rite constructed around a television circus, but Meggyesy was dismissing gridiron indulgence as damaging for society. Drugs, he observed, were shaping modern football's mediated illusion that smacked of comic-book characters, gargantuan heroes and villains performing superhuman feats in bloody clashes for victory. "The violent and brutal player that television viewers marvel over on Saturdays and Sundays is often a synthetic product," Meggyesy proclaimed, unchallenged by credible rebuttal.

I. Dawn of Muscle Doping: Testosterone Synthesis

Anabolic or tissue-building substances in sport began with the male hormone, testosterone. Victorian scientists recognized testosterone's potential to physically rejuvenate the human body, and by the 20th century a crude extract was harvested via methods such as crushing bull testes. Research progressed. In 1935, Dr. Charles D. Kochakian isolated testosterone in an experiment at the University of Rochester, confirming its chemical structure and anabolic or tissue-building nature.

American doctors sold this latest miracle drug for injection during World War II. Testosterone was considered beneficial as a treatment for medical conditions such as premature growth in infants, anemia, and male impotence. Women received it for menopause, premenstrual syndrome, and enhancement of sexual desire. Elsewhere, rumors surrounded the Nazi regime, with unsubstantiated reports that doctors performed research on prisoners, including extraction techniques. Adolf Hitler reportedly took testosterone for what ailed him physically and mentally.

Speculation focused on the effects of testosterone for athletic performance, and a researcher found an "athlete" to work with—a broken-down trotter horse, 18 years old, named Holloway. Benefiting from testosterone implants, Holloway resumed training and competing, winning or placing in several races, along with setting a speed record at age 19. In the 1945 book *The Male Hormone*, author Paul de Kruif discussed testosterone for improving human athletic performance. De Kruif, a former medical student turned writer who used the substance himself, wrote: "We know how both the St. Louis Cardinals and the St. Louis Browns have won championships, super-charged by vitamins [amphetamines]. It would be interesting to watch the productive power of an industry or a professional group that would try a systematic supercharge with testosterone—of course under a [doctor's] supervision."

American bodybuilders in California were injecting testosterone as the war era concluded, according to hearsay accounts, and competitive weightlifters likely were too. Evidence of anabolic augmentation in sport became more tangible during the 1950s, with documentation that athletes used testosterone for becoming bigger and stronger.

Russian athletes were competing in international sports for the first time, producing astonishing results in weightlifting. The U.S.S.R. lifters quickly dominated, scoring a convincing victory at the 1954 world championships in Vienna, and their American counterparts, deposed as champions, suspected testosterone as the opposition's edge. An American team physician, Dr. John B. Ziegler, later said Russian athletes were using catheters to urinate in Vienna, inserting the metal devices themselves. Their condition was enlargement of the prostate gland, so swollen it blocked off the urinary tract, and Ziegler said a Russian team doctor confirmed synthetic testosterone as the culprit. Ziegler said the U.S.S.R. program administered injections to athletes for performance enhancement.

Inspired rather than infuriated, Ziegler returned to America and contacted parties for discussing testosterone's applications in athletics. Ciba Pharmaceutical Company reportedly agreed to supply the drug. Ziegler tried injections on himself and U.S. weightlifters, conducting the trials in York, Pennsylvania, home of the Olympic program directed and funded by Bob Hoffman, a private businessman and leader of resistance training or "free weights," barbell workouts for strength. Hoffman's enterprises included York Barbell and supplement sales—his Hi-Proteen powder mix was widely popular—along with magazine publishing of titles like *Strength and Health*. Most of America's elite weightlifters held jobs under Hoffman in York, where they trained, and Ziegler injected several with testosterone. Initial strength results were unsatisfactory, and those coupled with strong androgenic or "male-producing" side effects caused Ziegler to abandon testosterone.

Pharmacologists continued work in America for developing synthetic forms of the male hormone with no harmful side effects. A goal was to create strictly anabolic steroids, envisioned to enhance body and performance without testosterone's androgenic or "male-producing" element, side effects such as acne, baldness, testicular shrinkage, and prostate ailments. Ciba technicians made a breakthrough, at least for mass marketing of anabolic steroids, by developing methandrostenolone, marketed under trade name Dianabol.

Released in 1958 for prescription treatment of medical conditions, "D-bol" pills exploded in off-label use as the classic muscle drug, even though production had failed to separate the androgenic effects from the desired anabolic mechanism. Dianabol was an anabolic-androgenic steroid, retaining adverse effects associated with testosterone injections, but bodybuilders and athletes flocked, nonetheless. Dianabol's big sell was its pill form, the first anabolic steroid for oral consumption, timing perfectly with consumer belief and appetite for pills to fix anything.

During this period, Ziegler renewed ties with both Ciba and the musclemen at York Barbell. "Clearly the pharmaceutical age of sport was on the horizon," wrote John D. Fair, weightlifting historian, in his book *Muscletown USA: Bob Hoffman and the Manly Culture of York Barbell*. Later, many accounts would cite Ziegler as the creator of Dianabol. "What was Ziegler's role in it? I would answer his role was simply as an experimenter with [Dianabol], with the athletes," said Fair, who worked with papers of both Ziegler and Hoffman. Apparently, Ziegler obtained Dianabol from a Ciba plant in New Jersey and gave the new pill to weightlifters at York, who displayed strength gains.

Soon the town in southeast Pennsylvania was attracting steroid-seeking athletes from across the country and abroad. Medical prescriptions for Dianabol were readily available around York, many signed by Dr. Ziegler, and some U.S. lifters were "juiced" for the 1960 Olympic Games in Rome, with Hoffman's approval. "It grew from a few people and spread into other sports," recalled Bill March, a former U.S. lifter at York and Mr. Universe winner in 1965. "Everybody used it to some extent. All the guys on the [national] team took Dianabol. It helped all of them. Anybody connected with the Barbell knew what was going on."

Drug companies began manufacturing new anabolic-androgenic steroids, and there was no turning back for the sports world. Available and usable, 'roids were the rage among elite strength athletes, who gobbled and shot-up whatever they could get, from D-Bol and Deca-Durabolin to Anavar and Winstrol V. And the drugs worked, making users bigger and stronger. Young athletes ignored warnings of danger, for they were *winning*.

Ziegler realized athletes were prone to abuse steroids, including lifters under his supervision in York. Ziegler would prescribe 5 milligrams of Dianabol one to three times daily, but athletes took as much as 10 to 20 times that amount, enraging him. The doctor started to backtrack on steroids, feeling less and less secure about the drug-sport phenomenon he helped spawn. The development of a certifiably safe anabolic steroid had not panned out. All creations that followed Dianabol turned out to be anabolic-androgenic, including nandrolone decanoate, trade name Deca-Durabolin. Ziegler had long heard of hazards associated with male-producing hormones, but his awareness heightened in the early 1960s, particularly about potential dangers to the liver and heart. He began publicly denouncing steroids through York's muscle publications, but Hoffman's weightlifters only increased their use in private.

Ziegler could do nothing to stop steroids' spread through the sports of America and abroad, sealing his infamy for doping history. He left York in 1967, disgusted with steroid-abusing weightlifters and other jocks. "I lost interest in fooling with IQs of that caliber," he said afterward. "Now it's about as widespread among these idiots as marijuana." Years later, the doctor expressed remorse. "I wish to God now I'd never done it," Ziegler said in 1983, a few years before he died. "I'd like to go back and take that whole chapter out of my life. Steroids were such a big secret at first, and that added to the hunger the lifters and football players had to get hold of them. I honestly believe that if I'd told people back then that rat manure would make them strong, they'd have eaten rat manure."

II. Modern Football Mandate: 'Bigger, Stronger'

Dianabol pills were coming available in 1958, but Ron Mix, a USC football player in his junior season, had not yet heard of anabolic steroids for gaining size and strength. Mix was just learning to lift weights, one of the few football players doing so in America.

Weightlifting had taken root on many college campuses, but typically only as far as curriculum classes in physical education, along with clubs or teams organizing for competitions in intramural or national competitions. The large majority of athletic coaches still condemned weightlifting for sport training, believing an invalid "muscle-bound" theory, or "that resistance training would somehow bind the muscles of anyone who trained with weights," wrote Dr. Terry Todd, historian on the muscle culture, for his journal article "The Expansion of Resistance Training in U.S. Higher Education Through the Mid-1960s." An exception in coaching was Knute Rockne at Notre Dame, pre-World War II, who sent some football players to lift under Father B.H.B Lange, the strongman priest who founded a gym on campus, equipping it with barbells and apparatus. Todd's comprehensive research determined that weightlifting helped mold an All-American as early as 1951, Piggy Barnes, who sneaked away from LSU football coaches for strength training under revolutionary trainer Alvin Roy in Baton Rouge.

Mix was a breakaway football player for the latter 1950s, thinking past conventional dogma to lift weights on his own. His motive was a personal challenge, being moved from end to the interior line by USC coaches. "After my sophomore year at USC, I was switched to tackle," Mix later recalled. "At the time I was 6-foot-4, 205 pounds. I thought to myself, 'I gotta gain weight,' and one of the ways I thought it could be done was by lifting weights."

The payoff in strength exceeded his expectations. "I didn't gain as much weight as I would have liked. I gained 10 pounds," Mix later recalled. "But I was so much stronger than anybody else, it was unreal." Mix emerged immediately as a tackle for the Trojans, a lineman to reckon with around the Pacific Coast Conference. He was big, athletic, and would grow larger and faster, a harbinger of football's move to fields full of mobile giants.

Mix had to leave campus for a weight room, finding none at the University of Southern California, despite SoCal's regional boom as the cradle of *physical culture* in America, a flourishing population of competitive lifters and bodybuilders. "But they weren't playing football," Mix said. So he joined local musclemen at a gym in Inglewood. "I really [lifted] religiously," Mix recalled, "every other day, the entire offseason of football."

Building on his football success as a junior, Mix continued weightlifing for his senior season, bulking up 10 more pounds to 225. A pair of USC teammates of Mix pounded iron with the same dedication, twin brothers Marlin and Mike McKeever, and in 1959 the three strongmen led the Trojans to an 8-2 record. All three made the All-American team. Mix said, "This is going to sound so immodest, but facts were facts: We were so much better than the people we played against, it was almost unfair."

The psyche thrived on superior strength of the body. "It was really helpful," Mix recalled, chuckling. "The truth is in those days, it was unusual to have a 250-pound lineman in college football. Most linemen weighed between 200 and 225, and I could press 300 above my head at this time. So the guy you're playing against, if you wanted to, you could lift him up and do reps. That gives you a lot of confidence."

Pro football courted Mix, his gridiron future bright and driven by weightlifting. At large, the iron game was staking a foothold in football, especially at colleges, to become a monumental imprint. College football players were frequenting weight rooms and gyms nationwide, according to Todd, with team strength programs underway at LSU, Maryland, Stanford, and Wake Forest. Soon, Texas would lead in the wave of athletic training facilities, establishing a massive weightlifting complex in Austin to primarily serve the football program of the Longhorn's coach Darrell Royal.

But elements came attached to weightlifting, including potential hazards. "So you move into weightlifting and then naturally you're exposed to other things," observed Mix, an attorney after football who represented former athletes in compensation claims for disability. "You start taking vitamins and start taking protein supplements, to gain weight. You become part of a culture, of not only lifting weights but taking things nutritionally that are supposed to help you get stronger and get bigger. So it's not that much of a leap to the steroids."

Anabolic Steroids, Doctors' Rx for Football

Bobby Waters, young quarterback in the NFL, held high hopes entering training camp for the San Francisco 49ers in 1962. The 24-year-old was vying to start in coach Red Hickey's "shotgun" formation, banking on his athleticism in the run-and-gun offense to win the job. John Brodie and Billy Kilmer also contended for quarterback, but both lacked Waters' ability to run with the football.

In a vicious flipside, however, the lanky Waters worried for his safety, as did any guy behind the center in pro football. Big, fast man-bulls chased down quarterbacks and pounded them, and while Waters' talent for running the ball served his aspirations, it increased his vulnerability to brutal hits. Taking off up field in the NFL, Waters met waves of *huge* tacklers, seemingly multiplying around the league. A tough, native Georgian, Waters was a lithe figure with speed, but he was too skinny, down toward 180 pounds on his 6-2 frame. He had endured broken bones since boyhood, among other injuries playing quarterback, but he was getting blasted by the athletic maniacs of pro football, flying at him from every direction, every play. Then the team doctor told Waters about pills that could "help you gain weight." Dr. Lloyd Millburn, 49ers physician and surgeon, offered a sample pack of Dianabol, the anabolic steroid, in low-milligram tablets.

Pills for withstanding the NFL gauntlet? Anabolic steroids were completely new for Waters and athletics in general. "No one had heard of them really," he later recounted, "or knew what they'd do." Waters accepted the Dianabol, consumed it, and experienced the physical gains. For the next two years, until 1964, Waters obtained steroid pills from Dr. Millburn, intermittently and mostly in sample packs, to maintain his bodyweight at 200 to 210. He knew of more steroid users on the 49ers, and practically all players received prescription medication from staff, including amphetamines, painkillers, and cortisone injections.

"You have to view this within the context of the time," said doping historian Charles E. Yesalis, discussing Waters and other early steroid users of football, in contrast to modern athletes labeled cheaters by popular press and opinion. "[Steroids] were considered not-at-all controversial drugs in the '60s. They were viewed more as super vitamins. It was an era when we were naïve, or overly optimistic, about drugs as safe. ... Viewed in context, anabolic steroids were very benign. It wasn't controversial, it wasn't considered illegal. ... That was the start of this significant trend in our being a drug-taking society for legitimate purposes, for human capacities: to help you concentrate, to help you sleep, or help you get awake, or make you look better. Again, to not view performance-enhancing drug use by athletes within that greater context is a grave mistake, because as a society we use and have accepted a lot of things."

Doctors brought anabolic steroids into football at every level, supplying players in high school as well as the pros. Dianabol reportedly hit prep football in 1959, soon after the drug's release by Ciba, according to a Texas physician who told Yesalis he provided the pills for a school team. Gilbert of *SI* reported a "clandestine" experiment of Dianabol's administering to prep players in the early 1960s, overseen by the team doctor in tandem with a pharmaceutical company; the program was shut down based on complaints to a state interscholastic commission. At Bloomington, California, in 1965, Dr. H. Kay Dooley organized a study involving three commercial brands of anabolic steroids for prep football players. "Dooley believes the drugs did increase muscle size and improve performance," Gilbert wrote, "and he says there were no undesirable side effects."

Dooley, who advised amateur and pro athletes, was a leading advocate of pharmaceuticals for performance in sport. "I don't pretend to be a researcher or a scientist," Dooley said in 1969. "I'm a practicing physician who is interested in athletes. A lot of physicians are stuffed shirts when it comes to sports. Athletes do want to perform better, that is what it is all about. If I know of something which may improve performance, a training or rehabilitation technique, a drug that is legal and which I don't believe involves any serious health risk, I see no reason not to make it available to an athlete."

College Players Adopt the Iron Game, Find Dianabol

A football sensation—and enduring legend—broke out for the Oklahoma Sooners on September 22, 1962, in their season opener at home against powerful Syracuse. Joe Don Looney, OU transfer running back, began the afternoon as an unknown, but he would end it as a celebrity.

Buried in the depth chart, Looney stewed on the sidelines. The irreverent, troubled young man had been on campus a month but was already in the coach's doghouse, informed he would not play in the game. But when Oklahoma trailed 3-0 in the fourth quarter, mustering no offense against the rugged Syracuse defense, Looney confronted stone-faced coach Bud Wilkinson along the bench. "Put me in, Coach, and I'll win the game," Looney declared.

The coach complied, impressed and desperate, and Looney quickly broke loose on a pitchout, banging through tacklers and sprinting 62 yards to score with two minutes on the clock. Oklahoma won, 7-3, and Looney was the story of college football, headlining sports news by suppertime in America. Wilkinson had a new starting running back, and Looney finished the season a football hero, an All-American.

J.Brent Clark attended the fabled OU-Syracuse game as a teen, and 31 years later he wrote the lauded biography *3rd Down and Forever: Joe Don Looney & the Rise & Fall of an American Hero*, after the provocative figure died of a motorcycle crash in 1988. "Joe Don was very fast for a big man, and we've got to keep in mind this was the early '60s," said Clark, a Norman attorney and OU alumnus. "Looney was an early day power-speed back. He had it all."

Looney possessed the genetics and motivation to become hulking. The son of former football star Don Looney, Joe Don was a chiseled 6-2, 210, with a speed of about 9.7 seconds in 100 yards. And while he could be indifferent about football, Looney loved strength training, according to Clark. "Joe Don got into weightlifting a long time before it was a prescribed regimen for any colleges," Clark said. "He had an ability to totally throw himself into any endeavor, and this was true throughout his life, even much later when he got into mysticism, Indian spiritualism. He would throw himself *totally* into it. And he did that with his weightlifting."

Looney was obsessed with getting bigger, stronger at OU, where he hopelessly sought to win paternal affection from the stoic Wilkinson. "He always looked to Wilkinson as a father figure, and Wilkinson was having none of that," Clark said. "Wilkinson was a patrician, a remote personality, and he was not close to his players. Certainly not to an enigmatic, emotional person like Joe Don. They conflicted, on the practice field and [elsewhere]." In addition, Clark noted, Looney was media literate, a voracious reader of newspapers, magazines, and books, fully comprehending his pop-culture status built on football publicity. "Again, Joe Don was figuring: If being 6-2, 210, and being able to beat Syracuse in the last offensive drive of the game, if that got some publicity, just imagine if I weighed 225 or 230 and was still just as fast. What would that do?"

"What drives young [football players] to take steroids, it's the positive reinforcement that they receive from women, from fans, from coaches," Clark observed. "It's their performance, you know."

And Looney already grasped the blossoming science of athletic performance, strength training and more bona fide techniques, still rejected by the vast majority of coaches, trainers, and physicians. Looney practically founded weightlifting for gridiron performance at Oklahoma, scrounging around on his own in 1962. "The fact that Looney, when he was at OU, he had to *find* some weights somewhere?" posed Clark, historian of Oklahoma athletics. "And he had to find a place, some dark corner of a storage area, just to work out? To me, that's amazing stuff."

Not surprisingly, iron-pumping Joe Don Looney was an early football convert to steroid use. "Whatever the latest technique was, he was into it," Clark said. "Looney was an explorer, he was a seeker." In research, Clark discovered Looney was among a small group of football players from multiple schools who gathered at Baton Rouge in the summer of 1963 to train under strength coach Alvin Roy—and consume Dianabol.

Muscle pills were circulating college campuses and host communities, if not always reaching football players. Weightlifters at Texas-Austin had obtained D-bol via Olympic athletes in York, Pennsylvania, according to Dr. Terry Todd, a 1960s power-lifter for the Longhorns who used the anabolic steroid. Todd, a UT professor and a leading authority on physical culture, said there were no juicers in Longhorns football during the school year 1962-63. "In fact, I don't think I had personal knowledge of any college football players using [anabolic steroids]...," Todd wrote in 2008. "We had a number of lifters and bodybuilders in our area who began using in the early '60s, and it seems likely that I'd have known about UT [football] players using such substances. You have to remember that many, if not most, of the college programs in the late '50s [to] early '60s didn't even do heavy lifting—which meant they weren't nearly as likely to be around the serious gyms."

Alvin Roy, meanwhile, boasted a serious gym of national reputation in Baton Rouge, a weightlifting hotbed garnering attention in the news media and in muscle publications such as *Strength and Health*, produced by Hoffman's York Barbell. Roy, a former U.S. competitive weightlifing assistant coach, remained a close associate of the York gang, including Hoffman, Dr. Ziegler, and Olympic lifters. Roy was a rising name in football for his position of "strength coach" at LSU, where his training program keyed big winning by the Tigers. Roy had founded football's first weightlifting program at Istrouma High in Baton Rouge, which produced LSU star Billy Cannon and more college players.

Roy stirred heated national debate for football, leading the movement of weightlifting for training. He espoused strength and size as wholly beneficial for football, not counterproductive, and his protégé, Cannon, stood in evidence, the Heisman Trophy-winning running back. A large, muscular athlete with a reported 9.4 time in the 100, Cannon was a legend in two sports for LSU. Cannon led the Tigers to the 1958 national championship in football, claimed the Heisman the following year, and pulled off an extraordinary feat of track and field, winning Southeastern Conference titles in the 100-meter dash, the 200-meter, and the shot put.

Cannon was Looney's model for both football and weightlifting, due to their common position on the field, running back. Each was manic for building strength and physique, and Roy represented Looney's ticket to superhuman status, available for training in his wondrous old gym down in Baton Rouge. From Norman, the Sooners' All-American followed both figures closely during the school year of 1962-63, reading everything he could find on Cannon and Roy in newspapers, magazines, and books. Looney cornered mutual acquaintances of the famed athlete and coach for eyewitness perspective on the entire scene of weightlifting in southern Louisiana, increasingly known for producing explosive, exciting athletes.

Looney saw enlightenment in the bayou region, opposite his own situation in Norman, where he constantly clashed with his head coach. Bud Wilkinson at OU led the passé, doomed anti-weights dogma of football, which surely Looney detested. Wilkinson wanted "lean and mean football players" with "pony backs" running the football, Clark noted, so Looney felt a coaching bias as a large ball-carrier, however fast he moved, not to mention being Wilkinson's first recruit from a junior college.

"Wilkinson in particular, who's a Hall of Fame coach… did not want kids lifting weights," Clark said. "And the Billy Cannon thing, in the minds of youngsters like Joe Don, changed all of that. Cannon was their proof that being strong did not necessarily affect your quickness and your speed… The Cannon Heisman Trophy, I think, is critical, the Alvin Roy gym is critical, as proof positive in itself that weightlifting could yield great rewards. "So, of course, Joe Don was down in Baton Rouge in summer of '63."

No OU teammates accompanied Looney to Louisiana, but he did bring along Gatlin Mitchell, his wild buddy for lifting and partying in hometown Forth Worth. Both were affluent Texas boys indulging themselves on a summer excursion to get bigger, stronger, and faster, all expenses paid by their parents. Mitchell even received Dianabol for the trip from his father, a physician, Clark found, although Looney's source for steroids would remain unknown.

Looney and Mitchell lifted weights under Roy's tutelage for more than a month, concentrating on major-muscle groups with the bench press, dumbbell press, power clean, dead lift, and squat. They also consumed steroid pills while working at the Baton Rouge gym. "Joe Don finally told me he was going to quit taking Dianabol," Mitchell later recounted for Clark, "because he was concerned that the drug might make his testicles shrink up." Looney was buff enough, anyway, a rippling 230 pounds, having added 20 in lean mass while increasing strength and speed.

Roy's summer session concluded for college players in Baton Rouge and everyone scattered, the athletes bound for campus towns and preseason, two-a-day practices in football. Roy packed up weights, apparatuses and everyday items in a truck then headed west for California, off to debut as a strength coach in pro football—and the steroid guru for an entire team.

Unfortunately for Looney, his dream for football greatness and Wilkinson's respect went awry in 1963 completely. He and Wilkinson engaged in an ongoing battle that the coach ended unceremoniously by dismissing Looney from the team following Oklahoma's loss at rival Texas, a month into the season.

The coach's stunning decision was likely unrelated to anabolic steroids, Clark concluded, and users remained on the OU roster. Charley Mayhue, a defensive back and quarterback, had done a short cycle during the summer at home in Ada, Oklahoma, a football-crazed town where he obtained Dianabol through workouts with college and prep players at the high school. "Nobody expressed any health concerns in those days," Mayhue later told Clark. Sooners' running back Lance Rentzel also embraced steroids, in the summer of 1964, employing Looney's prescribed regimen of weightlifting, running, and juicing. "When I arrived for preseason training, I weighed 215 pounds, far more than I'd ever been, and I hadn't lost a step," Rentzel wrote in his 1972 autobiography, *When All the Laughter Died in Sorrow*.

College players juiced at many schools in the 1960s, including Los Angeles State, California, and Colorado State. Gilbert reported Utah State player Ken Ferguson said in 1968 that a large majority of big-school linemen used steroids, and everyone who was headed into pro football. Arkansas defensive tackle Terry Don Phillips later recalled "very minimal" usage at the time.

Athletes at small schools were not immune, such as freshman Lyle Alzado of Yankton College in South Dakota, who was not performing well enough to make the team. Weighing only 195 pounds, the impoverished kid from Brooklyn, New York, needed a football scholarship to stay in school. Alzado committed to loading on Dianabol and working harder at weights than anyone he knew, and football opponents ceased pushing him around. By his sophomore year Alzado weighed 245, followed by 280 as a junior, when he moved from offensive back to the defensive line. Alzado had "blossomed" into a small-college star and pro prospect, big, strong, athletic, and the Denver Broncos drafted him in 1971. Alzado would abuse muscle dope the rest of his life.

Coaches' Dianabol Program Juices The Chargers

July 1963, Southern California, and the sun shone hot and dry on the hills around Boulevard, a dusty little town along Highway 8 east of San Diego. The area was an hour's drive out of the city, far enough into rural country, Chargers' head coach Sid Gillman figured, to get his young football team isolated and focused on training camp. The year before, the Chargers trained at the University of San Diego, amid plenty of distractions, and they went on to lose 10 of 14 games. Gillman planned on winning this season, so he made arrangements to hold training camp at "Rough Acres Ranch," a forsaken spot near Boulevard.

Likewise, in the pursuit of winning, Gillman hired pro football's first strength coach, Alvin Roy, to help the San Diego players become bigger and stronger.

The camp conditions were primitive at Rough Acres, a failed dude ranch, even for the chintzy American Football League. San Diego sports writer Jerry Magee would later remember the place as "inhumane." No grass grew from the ground of dry sand and rocks, so the "practice field" clearing was covered in sawdust and mulch. Old ranch buildings served as housing, and, since neither air conditioning nor women existed at Rough Acres, players and coaches moved about in various stages of disrobement, glistening in sweat. Buzzards swirled overhead, bugs infested the grounds, and snakes slithered about and through the buildings, scaring the macho men. When the Chargers' No.1 draft pick arrived at Rough Acres, All-American lineman Walt Sweeney from Syracuse wanted to go back home.

A most curious sight was Coach Roy, with his muscleman gait. Standing 5'6", Roy's physical stature was short, but at age 43 he teemed in blocky muscle, and though a personable fellow, he sought to project a hard-assed image. Roy set up weightlifting equipment outside, under the burning sun, and strutted around in tight T-shirts that broadcast his expertise, markers from Olympic events or world meets in locales like Russia, where he recently spent time learning about training methods. Gillman had considered team strength training for years, observing the success of players who pumped iron, such as Billy Cannon and Ron Mix, the Chargers' All-AFL offensive tackle. Then Gillman heard Roy speak about weightlifting and hired him for training camp.

Roy's zeal for pumping iron was new for the vast majority of Chargers; most had never picked up a barbell, and only a small group led by Mix lifted on a regular basis. But Roy also brought something foreign to every player: Dianabol.

When Roy joined the Chargers, Mix, a law student, was team captain and de facto representative. Later, Mix and other Chargers players would publicly discuss Roy's introducing anabolic steroids at Rough Acres Ranch, recalling a meeting where Gillman presented Roy to the team. Roy held up a bottle of Dianabol for the players, telling them that "Russkie" lifters won gold by taking it. He opened the bottle and held up a tiny but potent D-bol sample, proclaiming it as "the secret" for muscle building. Roy said the pink pills could assimilate protein, which the players understood built muscle. "He didn't say they were steroids," Mix said in 2008, "and if Alvin had said 'steroids,' we wouldn't have known, anyway. ... We hadn't heard of steroids, and something that just helps you assimilate protein sounded great to us."

After Roy's talk, Chargers players found D-bol waiting for them at every meal in the cafeteria, where brown plastic bowls full of the pills lined tables. The Chargers also started lifting weights as a team, adding another mandatory session to a day in training camp, besides the two practices in pads and strategy meetings. "We were told to take a pill after every meal, and we did," Mix said. "And they actually worked, in the sense that we were working very hard but still seemed to have more energy. Normally in training camp, I'd feel my strength going down, but it actually increased."

Every day for five weeks at Rough Acres, Mix and his teammates did as instructed, eating anabolic-androgenic steroid pills with food. "Everybody take your pink pills," Gillman would remind them in the dining hall. Everyone went along on the new strength fad, even sportswriter Magee, who lifted weights and asked the head coach about Dianabol. "Gillman cautioned me not to take the pills," Magee later wrote.

Then tight end Dave Kocourek showed some Dianabol to a neighbor physician, who strongly advised against use of the prescription drug by athletes. Kocourek took the doctor's message and literature to Mix, who was startled to learn of potential hazards. "That was the first time I understood it to be harmful and illegal," Mix said.

"So I showed it to Coach Gillman, and he said, 'You know what? Everybody's got an opinion. Our doctors say it's fine.' I said, 'Well, Coach, I gotta call a team meeting, let the guys make their own decision.' He said, 'That's fine.' So I called a meeting, told the guys about it, and the vast majority stopped taking it. I never took it again."

The team no longer made Dianabol mandatory for players, but kept the drug available for those who wanted it. Mix played at San Diego until 1969; team officials, he said, supplied anabolic steroids to willing players the entire time. Officials even provided D-bol to a college player, Howard Kindig, whom the Chargers later drafted and signed. "It's seductive; the stuff works," Mix said

Several factors converged for winning by the Chargers in 1963, as they blossomed from former AFL losers to league champions. The team matured with quality young players and the brilliant coach, Gillman, along with strength training under the visionary Roy. But while observers might deduce team muscle doping was also critical, Mix rebuked the presumption, contending that anabolic steroids provided no lengthy benefit. After Mix's team meeting about health risks, no player "confided in me that he continued to take the pills," he stated. "The reason I believe taking the pills did not have a beneficial impact in our championship season is because the benefits would have eroded within a few weeks of our stopping the ingestion. In subsequent years, I was aware of some players taking the pills but, again, it was very few."

Young Stud Juices Up, Makes Lombardi's Packers

Bill Curry Jr. yearned to play professional football in 1965, probably deserved to, but understood he was too small at 212 pounds, especially to play center, his best position in college for Georgia Tech. Curry was an elite athlete among Baby Boomers, the namesake son of William Curry Sr., champion weightlifter of the South. Bill Jr. was a complete player in his beloved football, skilled in running, catching, blocking, and tackling, but he had to get bigger and stronger, quickly, to succeed in his NFL tryout—for the Green Bay Packers of Vince Lombardi, no less.

Suddenly, his father's words made sense, the constant encouragement to lift weights for football, and Curry hit the iron to tutor under a gym owner and family friend. But the gym owner espoused something relatively new, "help" for gaining power and bulk: Dianabol. Young Curry readily accepted the pills, unaware his father knew of anabolic steroids and opposed them.

Curry gained 25 pounds of muscle in two months, and his father was impressed, saying, "You look great." Then Curry got out the Dianabol jar. His father grabbed it, walked to a toilet and poured in the pills. Senior told his son about world-class weightlifters he knew who were ailing or dead from abusing steroids. "I'm saving your life," Curry recalled his father saying, during a 2008 interview. "This was 1965, early spring, so he probably did save my life."

Curry made the Packers and played for other teams in a lengthy NFL career that led into coaching and broadcasting. He said he quit Dianabol following his dad's lecture and never employed steroids again; nor did he meet other users in Green Bay or elsewhere in pro football. "Nobody knew much about it," he said. "I never saw anybody doing it while I was playing. I don't remember anybody that had the [appearance]."

But anabolic steroids had disseminated through pro football, passing from one team to another among carrier athletes, coaches, trainers, and physicians, who exchanged the drugs and information. By 1969 the journalist Gilbert reported confirming users on teams at Cleveland, Atlanta, and Kansas City, while insiders told him steroids had hit every franchise in both the AFL and NFL.

Fred Dryer, defensive end for the Los Angeles Rams, used anabolic steroids in 1969, he later said. "It's a matter of choice and opinion; it's not a morality issue," Dryer told ESPN in 1990, as a television star after football. "It's one of just common sense to me. ... You can't do [steroids or any drug] for a long period of time and gamble on the accumulative effect, 5, 10, 20 years down the road. I just don't think it's a natural addition to the daily diet, just to eat a bunch of steroids."

III. Smash Hit: Juiced-Up Football on Television

No mere coincidence, televised football and anabolic steroids went mainstream America together in 1958, as Ciba's release of Dianabol pills jibed perfectly with pro football's arrival on network television, the Colts-Giants classic in New York for the NFL championship live on NBC.

A half-century later, into the new millennium, American football reigned in world entertainment, golden content on TV, video, cyber. The spectacle of gladiatorial athleticism was fed almost daily, summer into winter, big game after big game, starring pro and college players of cartoonish physiques. It was a speeding battle among giants and available by the minute on weekends, from stadium sites everywhere, fast-cut visuals packaged smoothly and bloodily for mass consumption.

And yet many media clung to a false ideal, repeating for decades, in response to football's chronic muscle doping, that America would reject the game if not cleansed of drugs. On the contrary, retorted experts, football *could not gratify* its vast consumer base without chemically enhanced players. "The notion that drugs have *not* played a major role in producing these legions of bigger-than-life athletes is, again, very naïve," Yesalis said in 2008. If muscle doping were removed from football, a purely hypothetical proposition, "the show, the spectacle, in my view, would take a huge hit," he said. "How financially stable would the NFL be if the players started looking like they did in the '50s? Same with baseball, same with basketball, same with track. You can never put the genie back in the bottle. ... The public's appetite for bigger-than-life people doing bigger-than-life things is almost insatiable."

"The notion that the public would be satisfied with never seeing any records broken again—or with seeing normal-looking individuals competing again—is wrong." Yesalis understood the business stance of football, the denial of doping for marketing and liability, because fans did not care and demanded supped-up performance. "If you took the sensationalism out of sport by getting rid of the drugs, I think a big chunk of fans would find other entertainment for spending their money. And when you talk of huge businesses, multi-billion-dollar entertainment, for them that's unacceptable."

Television, Steroids Make Over Football's Show in The 1970s

In prime time on a Monday evening, autumn 1973, households and taverns across America anticipated the start of *Monday Night Football*, the hip ritual of gathering to watch the game on TV. The NFL had eclipsed baseball as the culture's No.1 spectator sport, and its television programming was growing, enriching the one-time garage league and partner networks. Glitter events like the Super Bowl and *Monday Night Football* fed this TV beast.

At the top of the hour—9 o'clock Eastern, 8 o'clock Central and 6 Pacific—the calm of network ID segued into ABC's rousing intro for *MNF*, giving viewers their first adrenaline hit. With a mod music bed of keyboard, horns and guitars, the screen flashed a lighted stadium and moved into the ABC control trailer, where directors in headsets, facing a wall of monitors, made their rocket countdown to show time:

"Fifteen seconds to air."

"Stand by all cameras. Stand by videotape. Stand by slow-mo."

Announcer Howard Cosell flashed on camera, intense, cocky, nodding to viewers.

"Stand by to roll videotape in 5…"

Announcer Frank Gifford signaled ready, youthfully handsome, and the third booth man waved hello, "Dandy" Don Meredith, grinning in lapelled jacket and big bowtie.

"And roll tape: 4, 3, 2, 1…" — trombones, trumpets rose higher — "Take tape!"

Da-da, da-da, da-dun-da!

A crowd's roar opened football highlights in groovy graphics, screens of color melding over gridiron action like Joe Namath on his familiar drop-back to pass. Player movements pulsed on notes of keyboard and horns.

The 45-second intro hit crescendo gave way to a live shot of Cosell, Gifford, and Meredith from a raucous stadium, in matching yellow ABC Sports blazers and clutching big microphones, talking over the din of fans in the background.

For millions of Americans, Monday night had been made over. *MNF* "was a smash hit," said Art Modell, the Cleveland Browns' owner. "It was historic. The atmosphere, the venue was unreal. It had a Super Bowl atmosphere. It was something new — Monday night used to be *I Love Lucy*. Then we came on the scene and captured the country."

Roone Arledge, president of ABC Sports, transformed coverage of athletic action with *MNF*, instituting viewer pleasures like slow-motion instant replay, close-ups from hand-held cameras, and microphones for the game and the crowd. And he put brash New Yorker Cosell in the booth, along with dashing former players Gifford and Meredith.

American football and television had realized their mutually lucrative relationship as a business empire. Gate attendance for both the pro and college games was increasing, but football had struck its cash cow on television, and vice versa. The NFL and NCAA were giddy over dollars every time they renegotiated TV rights to their games, while the networks enjoyed lucrative ad sales rated on a huge market share delivered by football.

Pro football's juggernaut through TV began inauspiciously in 1939, when NBC broadcast games locally, picked up by a thousand sets scattered around Manhattan. The DuMont Network aired NFL title games beginning in 1951, and NBC paid $100,000 for telecasting the NFL Championship in 1955, when the country had 32 million sets. A year later, CBS began its long association with the NFL, televising regular-season games in select markets, and the weekly product caught on. The birth of a national mania for the NFL, according to many observers, was NBC's telecast of the 1958 championship game between the Giants and Colts, their fabled sudden-death title game at Yankee Stadium on Sunday evening, December 28. Baltimore running back Alan Ameche hit the end zone in overtime to win for the Colts, and a national audience was indoctrinated with pro football.

Television money exploded around the NFL and AFL in the 1960s. The two leagues merged in 1970, when commissioner Pete Rozelle's dream of *MNF* debuted on ABC, and the new NFL reaped riches for 26 franchises. "By 1972, pro football had boomed, becoming the most popular sports programming on TV," Gene Klein, billionaire Chargers owner, wrote in his autobiography. "That year Rozelle, Modell, and I negotiated a four-year deal with CBS and NBC for $2.1 million a year per club. Four years later we were able to double that to $5.2 million a year per club. In 1980, we signed the historic $2.1 billion contract, which escalated to $16.2 million a year per club."

The steroid issue escalated along with the profits in the 1970s, a decade that opened on a civil court case that embarrassed the NFL. Former lineman Houston Ridge sued the Chargers franchise for $1.25 million, alleging his career was ended prematurely because of its wrongful administering of drugs to him, ranging from painkillers to anabolic steroids. Team officials countered that the suit had no merit, but they settled with Ridge for $295,000. The NFL was developing a reputation for doping, and Rozelle, a sun-tanned former PR writer for the Rams in Los Angeles, countered the negative publicity by unveiling his plan for drug prevention. The policy language banned black-market amphetamines, although not *prescription* speed, and no mention was made of anabolic steroids. Rozelle's plan was hailed in public, but it proved to be cosmetic and incapable of stopping systemic drug use. Team doctors and trainers continued prescribing or administering drugs, including anabolic steroids, cortisone steroids, amphetamines, and pain-killing barbiturates.

Football's drug problem did not resolve itself. Muscle doping was accelerating because of several factors: increased availability of anabolic steroids, many potent types, sought by a new generation of iron-pumping players who thrived on the drugs; the general establishment of weight rooms and strength training in football; and the success of juicer performers at Olympiads in Rome and Munich, models for athletes in every sport.

"The question of whether it was going on [in the NFL]? Uh, yeah. How many people were doing it? Quite a few," said Bruce Laird, Colts and Chargers safety from 1972-82, during a 2008 interview for this book and the author's historical article published by the *New York Daily News*. Anabolic steroids "were very, very plentiful in our day," Laird said, adding he was not a user.

Former Cardinals linebacker David Meggyesy retired in 1969 but stayed close to the league in work for the union. "I never saw [anabolic steroids] or heard about it on the Cardinals," he said. "We were doing other drugs, mostly speed, various painkillers, that sort of thing. ... Then, of course, in the early '70s I think it changed very quickly because the track guys were getting into it, doing steroids. And then it really came into the line positions of the NFL."

Pittsburgh offensive lineman Jim Clack discussed his steroid use in 1973, during an interview with author Roy Blunt, Jr., for his book on the Steelers, *About Three Bricks Shy of a Load*. In high school Clack was a tall, skinny kid until taking up football and excelling. After college ball at Wake Forest, Clack signed as a free agent with

Pittsburgh in 1971, under head coach Chuck Noll, and likely would not have made the team without steroids. "Noll called me up and said 'How much do you weigh? I said, '228.' At the time I weighed 214. He said, 'That's great. I'd like you to report at 235. Seven pounds shouldn't be too much to gain.'" Clack told Blunt he used steroids, ate food and frequented the weight room. "I'd lift two and a half hours a night. Three and a half. Jon Kolb and I — we'd work so hard we'd have each other crying. That's no lie. When I showed up Art [Rooney] Jr., who'd scouted me, didn't even recognize me. I'm up to 248 now." Clack said his wife made him stop juicing. "She says [steroids] don't do any good, but they do," he told Blunt.

Clack was the first of several Steelers to be revealed for steroid use, spanning three decades, but team officials, led by Noll, would repeatedly deny any knowledge. Mike Webster, Steelers center bound for the Hall of Fame, juiced "for a very short time" in the 1970s, according to correspondence between doctors. Running back Rocky Bleier used Dianabol while lifting to add size and speed, for fear of losing his job in pro football. "I did not abuse it. I got the ability I wanted for a short period and got off it," Bleier said a decade later, to Ed Bouchette of the *Pittsburgh Post-Gazette*. Bleier told Bouchette he obtained Dianabol by prescription from his personal physician and used it in the preseason for about six years with the Steelers. "My feeling is this, under a doctor's control, taken the way it should be taken, there are no side effects," Bleier said. "You have a right to do what you feel is best to get the most out of your abilities. I was staying at 200 pounds. There's a mental something that coaches have. They look at you, if you're 5-10, 200 pounds and run a 4.8 [40 yards], you're too small to play, you'll take a beating. But if you're 5-10, 200 and run a *4.5* or are 5-10, *220* and run a 4.8, then you can play. There's a perceived difference [by coaches]."

Rivals of the Steelers employed steroids for performance in the 1970s, players at Dallas, Houston, Los Angeles, Denver, Cleveland, and New York, but there was no investigation of league-wide abuse and culpable parties. Congress broached the issue of PEDs in football a couple times but made no demand for reform. Media generally did not care, or were blissfully ignorant. Sportswriter Doug Krikorian later wrote: "When I covered the Los Angeles Rams throughout the 1970s, it wasn't exactly a secret that many players in the NFL used steroids, including I'd say some of those on the Rams." Fans were oblivious or acted so. For football-loving America, safety issues or questions remained no real concern, as always.

College football was also awash in TV money—and anabolics. Gridiron revenue poured into big-time athletic departments of the NCAA, and many football teams chased more money through winning. Some schools, at least, distributed steroids to athletes.

At the University of Utah, the athletic department administered anabolic steroids to football players. Later, Utes coaches and department officials said few athletes were involved, with school mission being to "protect" them from juicing gridiron opponents "unnaturally big." Utah personnel interviewed football players, identifying those who desired to use steroids, then contacted the parents. Players and parents signed waivers prepared by university lawyers, and the athletes used steroids under a doctor's supervision.

At the University of South Carolina, summer camp 1973, a 230-pound freshman arrived from Gettysburg, Pennsylvania. The kid was a bona fide freak of nature, large and ripped, low body fat, athletic. Seventeen-year-old Steve Courson struck a gorilla posture at 6-foot-1, long-armed and muscular with a big head. The lineman-linebacker could dunk a basketball and run a 40 in 4.7. He was an extraordinarily natural weightlifter, largely self-taught, able to bench-press 400 pounds. Yet Courson would need more to stand out at this level.

Paul Dietzel, Gamecocks head coach, had led national champion LSU during the time of Billy Cannon, with Alvin Roy as his strength coach. At South Carolina Dietzel was expected to replicate his LSU success. "The whole environment was a distant cry from the high spirits and high jinks of high school football," Courson recalled in his 1991 autobiography, *False Glory*. "Bigger people, bigger pressure, bigger business. And let me tell you: This was *serious* business." The teen went right into game action on Saturdays, serving as backup defensive tackle. Courson was tough but recognized his limitations against larger players, particularly when that translated into physical defeats, even beatings. He was thrashed against Houston, for example, overmatched in facing star offensive guard Everett Little, 6-5, 285.

Courson enjoyed a successful freshman season, but understood his growth spurt was over through nature and augment weightlifting. His power was already peaking for life. "By the time I got to SC, strength-wise I'd pretty much hit the wall," Courson said years afterward. "I could've gotten bigger over time when I was in college, but I probably only would've gained 10 more pounds. And it would've taken a long time to do it." The youth had known about anabolic steroids since the age of 12, when he met a hulking, user football player from Texas. So in summer 1974, working out in Columbia before his sophomore season, he seriously considered the drugs for the first time.

A Gamecocks assistant coach suggested Dianabol, pointing to blue pills in plain sight at the team weight room, filling a bowl. But first Courson visited a team physician, inquiring about steroids. The doctor said nothing, basically, as he took the 18-year-old's blood pressure and handed him a prescription for Dianabol: 30 pills in 5-milligram dosages. Courson went to a pharmacy, where once again no one asked questions, and the university was billed for the drugs.

Eating one 5-mg pill of D-bol per day, along with fanatical training and eating, Courson gained 30 pounds of lean mass in a month. His speed improved to 4.5 and his bench-press went up 50 pounds, reaching 450. Steve Courson became one of those big, bad dudes, then went out and dominated opponents. Within two years, he was captain of the Gamecocks. By 1977 he was a member of the Super Bowl Champion Pittsburgh Steelers, living the NFL dream on his home turf of Pennsylvania.

Muscle doping was evident to Courson throughout pro football, especially among linemen, and he continued juicing. "Absolutely," he recalled in 2005. "You saw people with strength parameters [of steroids], more of them that made you contemplate their training regimen. ... To me, it wasn't intimidating or anything, because I was at their strength levels when I walked into the league." Many players would have weighed closer to 200 pounds without drugs, instead of 275 and up. "I knew a bunch of lesser-known linemen who fit that mold, from my era. ... The ones that were natural, if they were, I would say they were the extreme exception to the rule. I'm not saying that there weren't any, but I'd have to see it to believe it."

Around the league, sentiment labeled the Steelers as the Steroid Team, but Courson dismissed that criticism as simplistic and hypocritical. What the Steelers did do, he said, was set a model standard for dedication in the weight room. Pittsburgh linemen lifted year-round. Strength training "was already entrenched in football and steroids had been used for a decade," Courson said. "But the way we trained validated everything with the success we had. People always copy something successful. We probably were not doing anything different in training than what Alvin Roy was teaching back in the early days. We just had a bigger, more committed group. We were definitely into the power movements." Courson said anabolic steroids were widespread among Steelers linemen, like any team. "There were probably a few guys in the league playing on natural ability, and technique," he said. "On my team, the only guy that I knew... was Gerry Mullins, and I took his job, OK?"

Historian Terry Todd quoted an anonymous steroid user in pro football of the 1970s, for an article published by *Sports Illustrated*. "I doubt if the NFL will ever try to stop it," the player said. "The rule against it is just ignored now. But I've always told the doctors I was on testosterone, and nobody paid any attention." Anabolics were "great for football," the player said. "I lost my family, but I think I'm a better player now. Isn't that a hell of a tradeoff? But the use of steroids has grown steadily since I've been playing. I hear more and more about them."

Alvin Roy was an influence through the 1970s, having long ago left the Chargers to build upon his reputation of helping make title teams. Talk of steroids followed him always.

In San Diego, Roy's strength training was hailed as a key in the Chargers' winning the 1963 AFL title, but Sid Gillman paid him mostly for training camps. After Kansas City lost the first Super Bowl, Roy made his pitch to Chiefs coach Hank Stram, expressing certainty he could provide the edge for a championship. Stram hired Roy as a full-time strength coach, and the Chiefs immediately organized pro football's first "minicamp." In spring 1967, Kansas City players reported to learn how to lift weights under Roy's instruction. The following season, team officials "asked" the players to live year-round in Kansas City, so they could train year-round with Roy. The Chiefs returned to the Super Bowl in 1970 and manhandled a supposedly physical Vikings team, winning by two touchdowns.

Roy's job prospects were hot. His next employer was the Dallas Cowboys, and they won the Super Bowl in 1972. Within a few years a majority of Cowboys linemen used anabolic steroids, according to tackle Pat Donovan. Roy died of a heart attack in 1979, age 58, while strength coach for the Oakland Raiders.

IV. IN RETROSPECT: CONFESSIONS, CONCERNS, EVASIONS

Users of anabolic steroids in football often defied stereotypes, from the very beginning. Skill players, ball-carriers, for example, were prominent among earliest known cases, including star running backs Joe Don Looney and Lance Rentzel of the Oklahoma Sooners. They were preceded by a steroid user in professional football, 49ers quarterback Bobby Waters, who accepted Dianabol from a team physician in summer 1962 to gain bulk for withstanding the relentless tacklers of the NFL.

Waters hardly fit the image of a football juicer, particularly in the perception of future generations. No lineman or linebacker, Waters played quarterback, the game's dignified position of higher intellect. He was no psycho behemoth but a slender, nice guy; a Southern gentleman who respectfully met a young woman's parents over dinner in Lafayette, California, before taking her out on a date—and then later marrying Sheri Gidley. Waters fashioned no grand scheme about anabolic steroids, no plans for super feats on the field and a rich payoff. Instead, Bobby Waters represented the common man's quarterback, a hard worker from small-town Georgia by way of Presbyterian College in South Carolina, trying to carve out his niche in pro football. And steroid use did not guarantee longevity for Waters, not in the NFL, where he lasted five injury-marred seasons, mostly as a substitute. His pro career ended with a shattered right arm in 1964, requiring surgical insertion of a metal plate and screw. He gave up playing and entered college coaching.

Eventually, in an act genuinely rare for football, Waters publicly discussed his steroid use, even while waiting until stricken by the fatal illness amyotrophic lateral sclerosis, or "Lou Gehrig's disease." In the 1980s Waters became part of an extraordinary ALS cluster, three victims from one football team of the past, the 1964 San Francisco 49ers. After Waters watched two former 49ers mates succumb to ALS, Matt Hazeltine and Gary Lewis, he waged war against the dreaded disease.

Waters strove foremost to raise awareness of ALS, a creeping paralysis that cut off motor function in incremental muscle groups, while the brain remained fully cognizant. But he also chased a cure for saving himself, a virtually impossible dream. "The only other choice I have is to lie down and wait for death, and I'm not ready for that," Waters told *People* magazine in 1987. "My goal is to get well." The former quarterback, tough as an Appalachian pine knot, continued working as the head football coach at Western Carolina University. The school's most successful football coach in history, Waters believed the job kept him alive.

Waters was diagnosed with ALS following three years of symptoms. He lost use of his arms as the disease advanced, taking him down slowly. By early 1987 he was still moving upright on sound legs, but his quest for information, to locate a common denominator among the ex-49ers with ALS, had taken the urgency of a man on short time. Hazeltine and Smith were gone and media were listening to Waters, picking up this sensational story of three men once together on a football roster of 48, whose shared disease averaged 1 or 2 cases per 100,000 Americans.

No cause was known for ALS, but a popular theory focused on environmental exposure to toxins. During media interviews, Waters said possibilities for the 49ers cluster included a fertilizer on practice fields and toxic batches of dimethyl sulfoxide, DSMO, the topical ointment to numb pain. He also pointed to the team's mass dispensing of pills and other treatment to players during the 1960s, including cortisone injections, painkillers and anabolic steroids. Waters revealed his use of Dianabol to reporters such as Bill Brubaker, *Washington Post*, saying he knew more juicers on the 49ers but offering no names. "I doubt that Bob was the only player using anabolic steroids," his widow, Sheri Waters, said later, "but I truly don't know who else. There was some talk, but not much."

In 1987 Bob Waters and the 49ers skirmished over team records, but an accord was reached and the parties worked together to raise ALS awareness as well as research funds. "He didn't really feel like the 49ers had anything to do with his disease," Sheri Waters recalled in 2008. "He wanted to have [experts] research the coincidence between him and two teammates. ... The 49ers office originally sort of stonewalled Bob's questions, because they thought he was trying to build a lawsuit. But I think once they realized that was not the case, they were pretty straightforward with it."

A research team examined the 49ers cluster, led by Dr. Stanley H. Appel, an ALS expert who treated Waters and chaired the neurology department at Baylor College of Medicine, Houston. "I was denied almost all medical records by the 49ers medical staff," he later stated. "However, we could not attribute the ALS to any of the substances we did investigate such as DMSO and 'Milorganite' [fertilizer]." Appel confirmed Dianabol was dismissed as a possible agent, writing that "no form of steroids, including anabolic steroids, has been documented to cause or to aggravate ALS."

Sheri Waters volunteered alongside her husband for the drive against Lou Gehrig's disease. "We were really working hard to find a needle in a haystack," she said. "I think what we did accomplish was, we drew a lot of attention to that particular disease, and the Muscular Dystrophy Association started giving a larger percent of its money into [ALS] research. Research doctors started pooling the information for sharing advances."

Confined to a wheelchair at the end, paralyzed and disfigured, Bob Waters continued appearances and interviews, generating publicity for the cause. He died in 1989, distinguished for his football career and courageous fight against ALS. "Bob really put himself out there and gave up his vanity to get people interested," Sheri said admiringly. "I think he'll always have the legend of that football coach, or player, who died of Lou Gehrig's disease and did what he could to try to figure it out. So I'm very proud of that." Sheri Waters said her late husband harbored no grudge against football, and neither of them believed steroids contributed to his ALS.

Concern lingered, however, for other football players and families of the era, people wondering about harm for users of anabolic steroids in the 1960s and '70s. Former college and pro player Greg Harris wondered about the effects on him; he gained 60 pounds on steroids at the University of Montana, where he played from 1971-75, and 30 more in the NFL. "Now I'm full of tumors, but they are all benign," Harris told *The Kalispell Daily Inter Lake* in 2008, adding "one friend died in Missoula."

Secrecy shrouded the issue, and no scientific evidence existed in doping's aftermath, but controversy and lawsuits flared around the health problems of NFL retirees, including former steroid users who suspected or blamed the drugs. The famous example was Lyle Alzado, who expressed certainty his extended abuse of muscle drugs caused fatal brain cancer in the early 1990s. From college ranks, former Towson State linebacker Joe Vitt believed his juicing on steroids at Towson State in the mid-1970s contributed to his two bouts with testicular cancer by age 34. Vitt, an NFL strength coach, would not disclose further details to media. "It's a personal thing," Vitt said. "I'm not trying to scare anybody, but I want my players to know that it can happen."

A cancer case with a stronger connection fell under the national radar, evidence and medical opinion supporting a link to anabolic steroids. Jim White had been a strapping offensive lineman in college and pro football, reaching 6-4, 275 pounds, but by age 31 he was dying of rare hepatocellular carcinoma, an aggressive liver cancer. Doctors treating White in Denver in 1981 targeted three likely causes, according to an account 14 years later by writer Rick Morrissey, the *Rocky Mountain News*. In questioning White, doctors ruled out two possibilities, alcoholism and hepatitis.

But when they asked White about the third suspected cause, anabolic steroids, the quiet man confirmed he used the hormones for at least eight years, beginning in college at Colorado State and continuing through his pro career that ended with the Broncos in 1976. "If you want to be a lineman, you've got to be big," White said in the hospital. Previously, a causal relationship was made between oral anabolic steroids and hepatocellular carcinoma, in a case review of afflicted patients who had consumed the drugs for aplastic anemia. Typically, the cancer might strike 1 among 100,000 people.

White's death did not make big news, but when Morrissey revisited the matter a decade afterward, interviewing doctors, family, and friends of the deceased athlete, they believed collectively that steroids were the culprit.

"Jim White either had liver cancer due to steroids or liver cancer due to bad luck," said Dr. Alan Rosenberger, who treated White as a resident physician. "It's tough to say he had bad luck." Rosenberger had heard the response about no scientific proof. "The answer is, 'They're right, we don't have any proof,'" he told Morrissey, continuing, "We don't even have the kind of proof you'd like to have with a cigarette, where you've got 400,000 cases a year. This is one case and one guy who might have had bad luck. And Lyle Alzado might have been one case of one guy who had bad luck. But it seems the linemen in the NFL who used steroids have more bad luck as they get older than other people."

White's family members never heard about steroids from him, but a doctor contacted them several years after his death, and they began to recall possible signs. White had told his sister, Marva White-Neal, that pharmaceuticals were necessary to play pro ball. Anabolic steroids seemed logical to her, in retrospect.

White's mother, Connie, had always admired her son's motivation for football; now she thought it was likely based in his steroid use. "Football was the greatest thing in his life," she said. "From grammar school up, that's all he went out for. He just loved it. It wouldn't surprise me [that he took steroids] because that's what he wanted, to play football. I guess someone told him that they would make him stronger, if he would take it."

Elsewhere, long-term health was a public issue for some former Chargers who played under 1960s coach Sid Gillman. Retirees Ron Mix and Walt Sweeney made headlines for substantial allegations against Gillman's regime in San Diego, particularly about the dispensing of drugs like anabolic steroids, speed, pain-killing shots and pills. Mix, a member of the Pro Football Hall of Fame, penned a widely read account for *Sports Illustrated* in 1987, offering new details on the Dianabol program of Gillman and Roy exposed by Gilbert two decades previous. Anabolic steroids were "agents of future death," Mix wrote.

Sweeney, mired in chemical dependency and hobbled with a bum knee at middle age, filed a 1995 claim in federal court for full disability benefits from the players union. Sweeney had been an All-Pro lineman for the Chargers in the 1960s and '70s, relying on the team's drug distribution to start 140 straight games. In his disability claim, Sweeney alleged a lifetime drug addiction was fostered by the San Diego staff—Gillman, assistant coaches such as Roy, trainers, and team doctors—to keep him on the field through injury and illness. A former No.1 draft pick, Sweeney said he began abusing steroids and amphetamines like Dexedrine upon his arrival at Rough Acres training camp. Soon he moved into regular use of painkillers, including highly addictive Seconal, which, he alleged, a team doctor provided him non-stop for five years by repeatedly filing the same fraudulent prescription.

Lawyers for the union's $400 million pension and disability fund acknowledged Sweeney was chemically dependent, but they contended not until 1990 and thereby not because of football, since he worked jobs such as a drug counselor after the game. Lawyers also argued the union fund had no connection to team drug dispensing and should not be subject to Sweeney's problems.

Sweeney won round one in San Diego, with federal judge Rudi Brewster awarding him $500,000 in disability payments retroactive to 1976, along with $4,000 per month for the rest of his life. In his decision, Brewster wrote that NFL teams faced "incredible pressure to win," creating heightened risk for players like Sweeney "who may be unusually susceptible to chemical dependency." This danger is "knowingly assumed by the NFL teams," the judge determined. But union fund lawyers appealed the ruling, and Sweeney's case dragged on until 1998, when he lost in federal appeals court in San Francisco. The court did allow the continuance of the player's original $1,800 per month in disability from the union, for his wrecked knee, but any chemical dependency was classified as non-football related.

Gillman himself largely avoided comment on doping allegations surrounding his San Diego teams of the past, but in 1991 the Hall of Fame coach, age 79, addressed the subject with reporter Mike Fish, *Atlanta Journal and Constitution*. By then several former players had alleged Gillman oversaw drug use on the team, and former owner Gene Klein had stated he fired the coach over amphetamines. In contrast, Gillman told Fish he was unaware of anabolic steroids among his players. "They used every vitamin in the book," Gillman said. "Beyond that and salt pills, I don't know."

Pete Rozelle briefly discussed the Sweeney case with Joe Burris of the *Boston Globe* in 1995. The retired NFL commissioner had discussed doping for decades, mostly in private meetings and closed hearings, learning about anabolic steroids, amphetamines, and various painkillers. In public he had seen court cases, testified before Congress, and participated in 1980s media coverage documenting widespread drug abuse in his league—at one point, Rozelle even acknowledged "widespread misuse" of steroids. Yet Rozelle told Burris he did not know the scope of drug use in Sweeney's era, and he blamed the union for obscuring information.

"I know we took action anytime in any case we would find," Rozelle said. "We felt we had created deterrence with the actions we took." Rozelle died the next year at 70, hailed worldwide for his genius in marketing football through modern media.

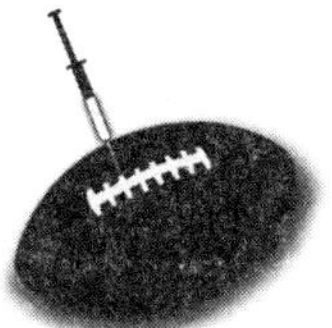

REFERENCES

49er Case. (1987, February 2). The 49er case. *Sports Illustrated* [Online].

Allen, K. (1989, August 29). W. Carolina coach follows a tough act. *USA Today*, p. 1C.

Alzado, L. (1991, July 3). Interview with Roy Firestone on 'Up Close.' *ESPN-TV*.

Alzado, Broncos. (1972). *Topps football card No. 106*. Brooklyn, NY: Topps Chewing Gum.

Alzado, L., & Edwards, W. (1991, July 29). Fourth down and long. *People*, p. 52

Alzado Funeral. (1992, May 15). With Alzado funeral. *The Associated Press* [Online].

Alzado, L., & Smith, S. (1991, July 8). 'I'm sick and I'm scared. *Sports Illustrated*, p. 20.

Appel, S.H. (2008, June 8). E-mail correspondence to author.

Arledge, R. (1973). Monday Night Football. *ABC-TV*.

Armstrong, J. (1999, November 28). Roy and weights turned LSU's Cannon into a Renaissance man. *Denver Post*, p. C12.

Bahrke, M.S., & Yesalis, C.E. (2002). *Performance-enhancing substances in sport and exercise*. Champaign, IL: Human Kinetics.

Barnhart, A. (2002, November 9). Last week's 'MNF' party needed more Cosell. *Kansas City Star*, p. E1.

Barnhart, A. (2002, December 6). Innovator who altered TV's presentation of sports dies. *Kansas City Star*, p. D1.

Black, B. (1989, June 22). Utah athletic director thrilled Gadd acquitted of charges. *The Associated Press* [Online].

Blount, R., Jr. (1974). *About three bricks shy of a load*. Pittsburgh, PA: University of Pittsburgh Press.

Bouchette, E. (1985, May 15). I used steroids, Bleier says. *Pittsburgh Post-Gazette*, p. 21.

Brubaker, B. (1987, February 1). Players close eyes to steroids' risks. *Washington Post*, p. C1.

Burris, J. (1995, October 3). Lost in the shuffle. *Boston Globe*, p. 43.

Chaney, M. (2008, June 16). Dianabol, the first widely used steroid, turns 50 this year. *New York Daily News* [Online].

Clark, J.B. (1993). *3rd down & forever: Joe Don Looney & the rise & fall of an American hero*. New York, NY: St. Martin's Press.

Clark, J.B. (2008, June 9). Telephone interview with author.

Clark, J.B. (2008, August 5). Telephone interview with author.

Coming Clean. (1986, November 5). Coming clean about steroids. *New York Times*, p. D24.

Courson, S. (1991). *False glory*. Stamford, CT: Longmeadow Press.

Courson, S. (2005, March 27). Telephone interview with author.

Courson, S. (2005, May 23). Telephone interview with author.

Courson, S. (2005, June 22). Telephone interview with author.

Covarrubias, A. (1995, July 7). Sweeney's drug disability claim before federal judge. *The Associated Press* [Online].

Curry, B. (2008, June 7). Telephone interview with author.

de Kruif, M. (1945). *The Male Hormone*. New York, NY: Harcourt, Brace and Company.

Dvorchak, R. (2005, October 2). Steroids in sports: Experiment turns epidemic. *Pittsburgh Post-Gazette* [Online].

Fair, J.D. (1999). *Muscletown USA*. University Park, PA: The Pennsylvania State University Press.

Fair, J.D. (2008, June 2). Telephone interview with author.

Farmer, S. (2003, December 26). Ravens owner Modell helped shape NFL. *St. Louis Post-Dispatch*, p. D7.

Fimrite, R. (1987, August 24). The battle of his life. *Sports Illustrated* [Online].

Fish, M. (1991, September 29). Rooskies' big secret: Red pills. *Atlanta Journal and Constitution*, p. F3.

Fitzpatrick, F. (2002, November 4). How the steroid game got out of the bottle. *Ottawa Citizen*, p. A9.

Gaudelli, F., & Esocoff, D. (2003, January 15). History of ABC's Monday Night Football. *ABC Sports Online*.

Gilbert, B. (1969, June 23). Drugs in sport, Part 1: Problems in a turned-on world, *Sports Illustrated*, p. 64.

Gilbert, B. (1969, June 30). Drugs in sport, Part 2: Something extra on the ball. *Sports Illustrated*, p. 30.

Gilbert, B. (1969, July 7). Drugs in sport, Part 3: High time to make some rules. *Sports Illustrated*, p. 30.

George, T. (1993, June 27). Strength and conditioning coaches: The force is with them. *New York Times*, p. 8—2.

Grogan, D.W., Faber, N., Leviton, J., & Powell, L. (1987, February 9). An incurable killer strikes three ex-49ers, and an anguished victim doubts it's a coincidence. *People*, p. 94.

Hazeltine Dies. (1987, January 17). Matt Hazeltine, 53, is dead: Former linebacker for 49ers. *New York Times*, p. 1—15.

Hennell, C. (2008, February 7). It's official: Harris inks with Griz football. *Kalispell Daily Inter Lake* [Online].

Johnson, W.O. (1985, May 13). Steroids: A problem of huge dimensions. *Sports Illustrated*, p. 38.

Kerkhoff, B. (1999, November 28). Sports in the '90s: Remote controlled. *Kansas City Star*, p. C9.

Klecko, J., & Fields, J. (1989. *Nose to nose*. New York, NY: William Morrow and Company, Inc.

Klein, G., & Fisher, D. (1987). *First down and a billion*. New York, NY: William Morrow and Company, Inc.

Kochakian, C.D., & Yesalis, C.E. (2000). Anabolic-androgenic steroids. In Yesalis,

C.E. (Ed.), *Anabolic steroids in sport and exercise* (2nd edition). Champaign, IL: Human Kinetics.
Kreisler, F. (1973, September 8). 'Beware of mossback tactics,' Hunt cautions NFL. *The Sporting News*, p. 56.
Krikorian, D. (2007, March 5). Make me the boss and I'd correct Arte. *Long Beach Press-Telegram* [Online].
Krueger, C. (2008, June 11). Telephone interview with author.
Laird, B. (2008, June 5). Telephone interview with author.
Lederman, D. (1989, June 28). Steroid program for athletes confirmed by U. of Utah. *Chronicle of Higher Education*, p. A26.
Lineman Loses. (1998, August 8). Lineman loses drug claim. *The Tampa Tribune*, p. 7.
Lipsyte, R. (2007, February 2). Telephone interview with author.
Magee, J. (1999, October 31). The 300-pound lineman, once a rarity, is now the norm in the NFL. *Copley News Service* [Online].
Magee, J. (2001, January 29). Svare wants to lay '73 scandal to rest; ex-Chargers coach says Rozelle later gave back his fine. *San Diego Union-Tribune*, p. D1.
Magee, J. (2001, August 12). Surviving the furnace that was rough acres. *San Diego Union-Tribune*, p. C7.
Magee, J. (2002, June 3). Baseball could learn from football's steroid policies. In *Pro Football Weekly* [Online].
Magee, J. (2002, December 22). 'Junction Boys' no match for '63 Bolts. *San Diego Union-Tribune*, p. C10.
Magee, J. (2007, December 16). Steroids: Cold War era Commie training tip. *San Diego Union-Tribune* [Online].
Mandell, A.J. (1976). *The nightmare season*. New York, NY: Random House.
Marks, S.M. (1993, May 24). Medical correspondence to Charles Cobb.
McDonough, W. (1999, September 10). He gave NFL a lift. *Boston Globe*, p. D10.
Meggyesy, D. (1970). *Out of their league*. Berkeley, CA: Ramparts Press, Inc.
Meggyesy, D. (2008, June 7). Telephone interview with author.
Mix, R. (1963, September 16). I swore I would quit football. *Sports Illustrated* [Online].
Mix, R. (1987, October 19). So little gain for the pain. *Sports Illustrated*, p. 54.
Mix, R. (2008, June 10). Telephone interview with author.
Mix, R. (2008, August 26). E-mail correspondence to author.
Mix, R. (2008, September 28). Sports letters: Ron Mix's viewpoint. *San Diego Union-Tribune* [Online].
Moldea, D. (1989). *Interference*. New York, NY: William Morrow and Company, Inc.
Morris, G. (2008, June 13). Weightlifting leads Hatch to La. Hall of Fame. *Baton Rouge Advocate* [Online].
Morrissey, R. (1995, January 10). Ex-NFL player paid for steroid use with his life. *Rocky Mountain News* [Online].
NFL Chronology. (2001, May 23). History 101: Chronology of how the modern-day

NFL came to pass. *CNNSI.com* [Online].

Parrish, B. (1971). *They call it a game.* New York, NY: The Dial Press.

Phillips, T.D. (2006, May 16). ARNS interview with Terry Don Phillips. *Arkansas Razorback Sports Network* [Online].

Possible Link. (1987, February 6). Possible link between fertilizer, disease needs investigation, expert says. *The Associated Press* [Online].

Rentzel, L. (1972). *When all the laughter died in sorrow.* New York, NY: Saturday Review Press.

Rozelle Dies. (1996, December 12). Rozelle dies of cancer. *Kansas City Star*, p. D1.

Thomas, R.M. (1987, January 19). An awful mystery. *New York Times*, p. C2.

Todd, T. (1983, October 1). The steroid predicament. *Sports Illustrated*, p. 64.

Todd, T. (1988). Watershed days in weight training: Billy Cannon and Istrouma High. *North American Society for Sport History*, p. 34.

Todd, T. (1992, January). Al Roy: Mythbreaker. *Iron Game History*, p. 12.

Todd, T. (1993, January). The history of strength training for athletes at the University of Texas. *Iron Game History*, p. 6.

Todd, T. (1994, August). The expansion of resistance training in U.S. higher education through the mid-1960s. *Iron Game History*, p. 11.

Todd, T. (2008, June 2). E-mail correspondence with author.

Trussell, R. (2004, January 10). Factory-fresh footballs. *Kansas City Star*, p. F1.

Utterback, B. (1987, September 2). Battle against steroids picks up steam. *Pittsburgh Press*, p. B1.

Wade, N. (1972, June 30). Anabolic steroids: Doctors denounce them, but athletes aren't listening. *Science*, p. 1399.

Waters, S. (2008, June 5). Telephone interview with author.

Waters, S. (2008, June 9). E-mail correspondence to author.

Weisman, L. (1989, June 2). 1,600 pay respect at Waters' funeral. *USA Today*, p. 9C.

Weisman, L. (1990, June 27). 49ers going strong on banquet circuit. *USA Today*, p. 2C.

Willing. R. (1997, January 21). Football led to addiction, suit says. *USA Today*, p. 3A.

Wilstein, S. (1987, January 15). Former teammates' deaths lead Waters to make plea. *The Associated* Press [Online].

Yesalis, C.E. (Ed.). (2000). *Anabolic steroids in sport and exercise* (2nd edition). Champaign, IL: Human Kinetics.

Yesalis, C.E. (2008, June 3). Telephone interview with author.

Chapter 3 [The Spectacle

Social factors sustaining doping in football]

"Football has been so enshrined as a spectator sport, both in college and professionally, that it would be impossible for revisionists to alter it without protests of an almost revolutionary character."

James A. Michener
book author, 1976

On occasion when I was a football player, the game's brutality startled me, jerked me awake from the fantasy. During a game in high school, I witnessed a crushing hit on a kid running the football, an opponent. My teammates drilled him high and low, and the cluster of them went down with his blood-curdling screams. He lay shuddering, holding a leg perfectly still for a compound fracture near the foot. Two white bone shards protruded from his sock slit in ribbons, bloody prongs of fibula and tibia, lower-leg bones, snapped off near their union at the ankle and jabbed through skin.

I was shocked, nauseated instantly.

Then I heard *cheering* from the stands. Some fans applauded our first-degree assault on a 17-year-old, and my concern began to subside. The moaning kid was carted away to an ambulance, out of sight, and a referee blew his whistle. Play resumed immediately. "Huddle up!" yelled our defensive captain. The shared football fantasy rolled on, for it was strong, resilient enough to easily obscure the life-altering injury for one teen in this game. More seriously injured kids could follow too, and the game would continue until no precious time was left on the clock.

My concern was gone, and a couple series later I sacked the quarterback, ramming into his head as he stumbled, trying to flee another pass rusher. Adrenal sensations shot up my spine and through my head — my first "head rush" on a football field — intense feelings of pleasure, as though floating. My high was narcotic-free, "a natural," a feeling of reigning over my immediate world, that football field. I *knew* I couldn't be stopped. I was tingling, hardly able to wait for the next snap of the football. The experience was *power*. Never before had I felt like this, doing anything, anywhere.

The quarterback got up slowly, and my teammates slapped me joyfully. We were awash in victory frenzy, so sweet. The opposing players were mostly older and bigger. They were supposed to beat us, to deny us our crack at the conference championship, but we were flat kicking their asses. We were pounding them. And, for the first time, I heard fans cheering for me, *real fans*, other than my mom or some goofy girl. Fans adored my play. I wanted more of this entire scene, the physical, mental, and emotional, much more.

Six years later, I was a guided missile in college football, highly aggressive and zeroing in on everyone with my facemask. I meant to knock people unconscious including myself, if necessary to finish a kill. Seeking and destroying opponents was very gratifying for me, exhilarating, as a young man insecure about buckling down to live real manhood, to be truly responsible and productive in my life.

But I couldn't shake troubling doubt over football, particularly when a severe knee injury ended my 1982 season abruptly, right before the homecoming game. Then I had nine days in a hospital to think about my football reality. I understood the fans for craving some ass-kicking out there. We players wanted that. But I also had to wonder, question, whether I was crazy along with society over this fucking game. I was flat on my back in a hospital bed, my right leg encased in blood-soaked plaster, a cast I would wear for 23 weeks. Just days ago I was The Big Man On Campus and on the brink of becoming a Football Hero. Now I was headed home to my parents, for a long while, and my mother would have to bathe me again.

That hospital bed reduced me to sniffling in regret, overcome with self-pity. A sad pastime was watching bloody fluid drip from out the cast, through long tubes sewed-up in my surgical wound — a week after surgery, that tubing was embedded in mending tissue, but apologetic nurses had to yank it out. I sat up yelping, an energy reflex to searing pain.

The nurses also stuck me with needles, constantly. But,what the hell. By then I could recall using needles to inject myself with anabolic steroids.

Jesus, why *did* I play football?

I. Base Appeal of Football: Violence

Dr. Michael Oriard, an academic critiquing football as spectacle in America, stirred controversy in 1983, writing a guest commentary for the *New York Times*. Oriard contended that violence and casualties were football's base attraction, for fans and players alike. Americans wanted brutality packaged sanitarily before their very eyes. Football was mere violence but sanctioned, seemingly benign, revered and consumed by the culture as a civilized pastime. "Injuries are not aberrations in football, or even a regrettable byproduct," Oriard wrote. "They are essential to the game." Oriard did not need his Ph.D. to make the connection; as a former NFL and Notre Dame lineman, he had long understood the culture's obsession with spectacular, bloody football. In boyhood Oriard experienced "intense pleasure" from the game's physical contact, smashing other kids.

Former football players speaking out like Oriard had faced society's reaction, which was typically unfavorable. Americans, they found, really did not want to hear about any problem of consequence in the game. Fans discussed and argued the trivial constantly, such as a referee's call, a coach's ability to win, a player's contract holdout, but their desire and energy vaporized for addressing big-picture troubles. Most Americans avoided making a public issue about any problem of football, so Oriard drew criticism for his *Times* viewpoint. Football organizers and fans wanted to dismiss him as a malcontent, just another former player harboring a grudge. At least one person reacted by writing a letter to the newspaper.

David Jenkins, self-described as "a British import" and obviously still learning about American football, believed that a player always controlled his own health. Jenkins, ignorant of coaches' control, saw a player as "a fool to himself" for risking injury, "especially when 30 of his colleagues on the sidelines can replace him." Jenkins' remedy was to abolish the helmet, "the main injury-causing weapon." This fan saw Oriard as causing more harm than good for football. "Injuries are not 'essential to the game,' and are not in any other game either," Jenkins opined. "Such a disturbing attitude as Mr. Oriard's can only encourage reckless and brutal behavior on the field."

Oriard responded to Jenkins: "Rather than simply condemn or defend sports like football, I wanted primarily to point out a cultural dilemma: We can't have sports whose appeal depends in part on their participants' physical courage without accepting the consequences — frequent injuries." Reform to eliminate injuries, Oriard noted, was out of the question for football. That "would require rule changes that remove physical risk altogether," he observed. "I cannot imagine that happening without a profound change in the entire culture. Rule makers are very conscious of what fans want."

Jenkins' fantasy of American football aside, the oblivious Brit wanted the same as every fan and player. Physical risk, in fact, was football's initial allure for the boy Mike Oriard.

Growing up a Baby Boomer in the Northwest, Oriard discovered the game in typical fashion for the young male. Football was a social force around his native Spokane, for all ages, and the game and its scenes made profound impressions on the boy. A gifted youth, Mike excelled intellectually as well as physically. He competed hard in school, amassing straight A's, and his motivation for football was likewise powerful. "From the very beginning, football was more than a game," Oriard recalled in his 1982 autobiography, *End of Autumn*. "Softball and tag and red rover and kickball were games. Football was something more."

The game was no make-believe for a youth who attempted it. Football posed physical confrontations at high speed, blocking, tackling, and running with the ball, and Mike discovered the consequences were real and immediate. Exhilaration and pain came often in the same instant, such as when scoring a touchdown while getting hammered by tacklers. Football confronted young Mike in his perception of masculinity, and he strove to meet the challenge, to prove his manhood. He succeeded, at least in becoming respected, even feared, on a football field.

Mike first played "sandlot" football in his neighborhood, open games among boys in vacant lots and yards. Tall for a 7-year-old, Mike faced older boys in sandlot, and while he took some lumps, he won enough collisions to become smitten with the thrills. Football affirmed Mike's self-worth differently than other games, through legitimate drama. "Scoring a touchdown was a real event that required no pretending to be meaningful," Oriard wrote. The game "grabbed my imagination and deepest longings in ways baseball never did. Football players seemed to me braver, more heroic, than other athletes."

Football inspired Mike Oriard the child, and he would go on to pursue dreams with vigor, including playing the sport at its highest levels.

Oriard Reconstructs Football Phenomenon of America

Dr. Michael Oriard, professor of English at Oregon State University, released his *Reading Football: How The Popular Press Created an American Spectacle* in 1993. A qualitative study, the book clearly identified football's cultural power. The lifeblood of this sport, Oriard discovered, lay in its grand storylines produced by mass media, typically more myth than hard fact, and consumed by Americans for more than a century. Oriard achieved the book's scholarship through Herculean reading and analysis of old football stories and illustrations by the thousands, dating to the founding of the sport at elite college campuses following the Civil War.

Imperative to football's establishment in America during the latter 1800s, Oriard found, was its ability to serve as a "major cultural text," or a perpetual drama of recurring media themes that overall served as feel-good mythology for the country. The print stories had to be compiled and delivered in tasty versions of the reality on the field, a game of violent moments, often thrilling, broken repeatedly by boring stretches. Football, therefore, became the great American spectacle, thanks especially to the Golden Press. The newspapers and magazines capitalized on special content possibilities offered by the sport, producing the stories to spawn enduring football fantasy. "That the popular press was primary, the game itself secondary, in football's extraordinarily rapid emergence as a popular spectacle and cultural force is one of the inescapable conclusions of my inquiry," Oriard summarized. For marketable content, "the games themselves are authentic in ways that no commodity can be," he observed, adding, "Those who describe professional football players as "entertainers" — a familiar claim — ignore the fact that their injuries are real, their careers short, their livelihoods at stake when they play. ... Fans know the difference between football games and movies."

Football fans did anticipate the violence but wanted positive meanings attached to the bloody acts, and football writers obliged the masses willingly, loving the game as fans themselves. They sought to rationalize carnage too, and developed popular themes to serve the purpose. In media stories, football really was not violent in the depraved sense; rather, it was Necessary Roughness for a boy or young man, a strenuous physical activity that built character, even if it tore apart his body. A coach was not a tyrant, not a sadist; rather, he represented Coaching Genius, a moral leader who taught and motivated young men to perform and achieve as a team — a widely popular storyline for industrializing America. In addition, a football player was not a thug; he was Gladiator Hero, exhibiting positive qualities every young male should emulate. Fans, moreover, needed to feel good in their role, so the media portrayed football as Social Event for Americans, a must-see, wholesome, patriotic happening — not a public bloodletting.

The game was not always spectacle, having begun humbly, to be merely played, not watched or marketed. American football's original architects were well-heeled college males, students in the Northeast who borrowed elements from rugby and soccer — the latter being known abroad as "foot-ball" — to develop a fast and rough game for themselves. Quickly, however, the stimulating scenes of American football attracted spectators.

College football's inaugural game, recognized as such, was in 1869 between Rutgers and Princeton. The Rutgers club issued the challenge, and Princeton "foot-ballers" accepted, making the bumpy carriage ride of several hours to Camden. Host Rutgers used its own version of football rules to win by a score of 6-4, but the next week Princeton was game host, employing its rules in defeating Rutgers, 8-0. Each team put 25 men on the field for these games, which drew several hundred spectators.

Club teams soon formed at other regional colleges, including Harvard, Yale, Columbia, Wesleyan, Tufts, and Pennsylvania. While football's gate potential was apparent locally, no historical evidence suggests anyone thought the market would expand from the region, or even beyond the affluent class of people who played and watched. Not one national media entity existed; the "mass media" was still formulating in daily newspapers and periodical magazines to become known as the Golden Press. America was largely unaware of *foot-ball*, outside elitist circles of the Northeast.

Early football resembled soccer, without much ramming contact, but that was unappealing for most players and fans. Harvard's rugby-style rules were the rage, featuring blocking, tackling, and daring ball-carriers. Thus, the sport's first major debate was over violence, or what type of game should be officially sanctioned for a planned federation of football schools. Violent collisions carried easily, with the Harvard community leading popular support, and the American Intercollegiate Football Association, established in 1876, adopted rules of the British Rugby Union.

Also for the emerging spectacle, the convergence of the mass media was at hand. American football would go nationwide, riding on more refinement of rules influenced by an explosion of press coverage.

A limit of 11 players per side was mandated in 1880, and two years later rule makers determined that only one team could have ball possession at any given time, a measure that eliminated rugby's "scrum" while producing football's "line of scrimmage." In addition, a first down was awarded when a team advanced the ball five yards on three consecutive plays [a rule later amended to 10 yards on four plays]. The playing field was revised, patterned after English soccer, to new dimensions of 140 yards long by 70 yards wide and a goal placed at each end — a crossbar 10 feet above the ground linking two upright posts. [By 1912, the field's measurements were finalized at 100 yards in length by a little over 50 wide, with 10-yard end zones for receiving passes to score.]

College football spread west in the late Victorian Age and in step with print media's growth into mass industry, as documented a century later by Oriard and sport communication analyst Robert McChesney, whose fundamental conclusion that, "media made sport," was indisputable in the case of football. Newspapers and magazines sprang up in every city and many thousands of small towns, and writers happily disseminated the gridiron legend already blossoming into a cultural mythology.

Golden Press media framed football stories to uplift the game rather than dwell on negatives. From the beginning, the sport's vitality radiated through writers and illustrators who glamorized it in the form of tale and exaggerated imagery. Communities and schools started teams and leagues everywhere, the most rural of places, inspired by *mediated* football rhetoric of heroism, manhood, education, and nationalism.

In turn, football helped transform media. Team games were the rage in 19th-century America, a society sensing loss of a "rugged individualism." With outdoor frontiers disappearing in the advance of urbanization and industrialism, Americans felt cloistered, channeled in their being, and a burgeoning sector turned to sport games for recreation.

The New York newspaper publisher Joseph Pulitzer identified the trend and took action in 1883, organizing media's first sports department, complete with "sporting editor," for his newly purchased *World* daily. Pulitzer shrewdly made other innovations in entertainment content, including placing comics and women's features in their own sections. His sports pages drew droves of readers — and advertisers — and college football became the lynchpin content for the entire newspaper. *World* circulation numbers rose astronomically under Pulitzer, from 15,000 to 150,000 in two years. In 1892, the publication reported two million readers, an unprecedented audience for a single entity.

Pulitzer rode on football to establish the Sunday newspaper, another idea of his to become an industry staple. The colleges played football on Saturday, and game stories and illustrations anchored Pulitzer's fat Sunday World. On autumn Sundays, editions showcased football on the front page. Other days of the week, readers demanded and received coverage on football's "Big Four" of the time, Harvard, Yale, Princeton, and Penn.

Sportswriters anointed football to be a national treasure, and they produced volumes of grandiose but basic storylines to construct the football legend. They painted football as an epic occurrence, even if on a regular cycle, and thusly the culture perceived it. The writers' standard themes of football were framed in morality, and a favorite of theirs was portraying the game as an education for players, an applied science. The storyline's key elements included Coaching Genius, the common belief that only a mature, forceful, intelligent man could lead a group of spirited boys to victory on a football field. Writers wrapped the sport in nationalism, labeling it a supreme demonstration of patriotic spirit by coaches, players, and fans. The very best of college players competed for "All-America Team" honors, anointing them national heroes.

Football as civilized warfare was a sensational narrative, with the coach as calculating field general and his players as brave foot soldiers. Indeed, the Golden Press touted football as a young male's proper substitute for war, also romanticized as a requisite for manhood. Sportswriters and illustrators loved to cast mere football games as historic clashes of armies. "YALE AGAIN OUTPLAYS HER ANCIENT FOE," screamed a *Herald* headline, hyping two football teams barely 20 years old at the time. A sub-head declared this Yale-Princeton game was the "Hardest and Most Scientific Football Battle on Record." In the newspaper's main story, the writer compared Yale players with historic warriors at Waterloo. The writer even portrayed extraordinary powers surrounding Yale's 6-0 victory, for sex and healing:

> There came a brief moment of miracles. Men who had never wept before burst into an exaltation of tears. Pretty girls who never behaved so surprisingly before threw themselves into their escorts'

> arms. And behold! The crippled substitutes of the Yale team who had been about on crutches threw them away and leaped into the air with joy.

The thematic catalogue of football fantasy offered many possibilities. Sportswriters molded the game as a symbol of progressive America, the Social Event worthy of altering a religious holiday. College football's Thanksgiving Day game moved to New York City in 1880, for determining the championship in America's print-media capital. The "Turkey Day Game" in New York became a national tradition by the 1890s, attracting 50,000 spectators at the gate and millions more through newspapers. A *Herald* writer touted the event as a new religion, surmising it "would have been quite an impossible feature of the Thanksgiving Day of the past." The writer continued:

> The town went football mad, and yesterday it exhibited its crazed mentality on Manhattan Field.
>
> In these times Thanksgiving Day is no longer a solemn festival to God for mercies given. It is a holiday granted by the state and the nation to see a game of football.
>
> No longer is the day one of thanksgiving to the Giver of all good. The kicker is now king and the people bow down to him. The gory-nosed tackler, hero of a hundred scrimmages and half as many wrecked wedges, is the idol of the hour.
>
> With swollen face and bleeding head, daubed from crown to sole with the mud of Manhattan Field, he stands triumphant amid the shouts of thousands.
>
> What matters that the purpose of the day is perverted, that church is foregone, that family reunion is neglected, that dinner is delayed if not forgot? Has not Princeton played a mighty game with Yale and has not Princeton won?
>
> This is the modern Thanksgiving Day.

Beyond many Americans' newfound necessity for football on a holiday, the sport also kept them in touch with the Romans, thanks to mythmaking by the Golden Press. Writers and illustrators could not resist making comparisons between football and Old Rome, and readers loved the tales, given the frequency. A *World* report on a game between rivals Harvard and Yale evoked imagery of "volcanic apocalypse," Oriard mused, and in faulty grammar:

> An Aetna of humanity, bellowing with the combined thunder of a dozen tornadoes. A huge quadrangular crater filled to the brim with the hoarse tumult of human passions and blazing with blue and crimson fires. In this crater great black drifts, that heaved and swayed and rolled like earthquake-shaken hills, and under all the deep diapason of voices, the thousand inarticulate cries of grief and joy and quick, sharp shrieks of rage. A battery of 40,000 feverish

> eyes focused with the intensity of burning glasses on a bare plot of withered turf, where twenty-two gladiators were fighting the fag end of a royal battle.

Oriard noted, "This is Harvard-Yale, not the last days of Pompeii. ... Football's simple narrative structure was now supporting cultural narratives of hyperbolic extravagance, college football players transformed into Roman gladiators."

Football players saw their heroic manhood documented before society, and enthused to read females were unflinchingly aroused. Sexual meanings, particularly regarding the prowess of players, ran throughout writings that set female figures as pleasurable adornments within football's world, and this attracted male spectators, storylines depicting pretty women flocking to games. In a *Herald* story on the 1892 Harvard-Yale contest at Hampden Park in Springfield, the writer raved about females in attendance, touting football as nothing less than their aphrodisiac: "Everywhere among the tiers of seats, where the cheers were loudest, were grouped most divine specimens of the American 'best girl,' no longer demure and retiring, but roused to a high state of tension by the unwonted scenes of excitement about her."

Newspapers and magazines gushed with sexism in football content, including the placing of females as sexually subservient to football players. A favorite theme was beautiful young women tending to wounded football heroes in erotic scenario. *Life* magazine sold the sexy motif in an 1897 illustration of two gorgeous coeds doting over a bandaged, limping, handsome football player, as they led him into a bed chamber with a crackling fireplace. Male readers could fantasize about Saturday evenings on campus post-game, being Football Hero enjoying his spoils. The caption for the alluring sketch advertised: "Some advantages of a college education."

Football Fends Off Abolishment at Century's Turn

Despite merriment, masculinity, sex, and more appeals of an American spectacle, football was in serious trouble by the turn of the 20th century. Critics were numerous by then, many were prestigious people, and their most common solution was simply to banish the sport.

Opposition haunted colleges already accustomed to marketing the sport for substantial revenues. Period critics howled about abuses, especially the casualty rates among student players. Fatalities alone were rampant, with 20 or more players dying of collisions in some seasons. Horrified teachers protested, and a Harvard committee issued a condemning report.

Other football problems plagued campuses. Impropriety or lawlessness was an element from the beginning, with athletes and coaches committing acts that would ring timely a century later. The advertised concept of amateurism in big-time football, for example, was as much a charade in 1900 as in 2000. Victorian Era teams paid players, including non-student mercenaries available to the highest bidder. Athletes and coaches, driven to win by whatever means necessary, cheated game rules and plotted to hurt opposing players. Any lessons of discipline, citizenry, were apparently lost on many football players, those engaging in assaults, drunkenness, gambling, and abuse of women. Football abolitionist Shailer Mathews, a professor at the University of Chicago Divinity School, said "there arises a general protest against this boy-killing, man-mutilating, money-making, education-prostituting, gladiatorial sport."

Some journalists of the Golden Press were not enthralled by football. They thought the game pathetic and rejected any notion it was educational or beneficial. In New York, E.L. Godkin wrote, "What we need in our youths is the capacity for high resolve, and noble aims, and the firm courage which does not need to be stimulated by bets or gate money." Other media rode the fence. *Outlook* magazine, apparently relying on positive football content to boost circulation, publicly condoned the field violence as "manly" but condemned urban hooliganism led by college students, "disgraceful exhibitions" attached to the sport that beset New York City streets each Thanksgiving.

Injury rates topped all controversy about football, prompting newspapers to concoct publicity stunts. For a Yale-Princeton game, Pulitzer's *World* hired two ambulances toting stretchers and a military surgeon. The 1897 football season was marred by excessive football fatalities, and newspapers ran lists of game casualties under headlines like "Maimed and Injured" and "The Injured Players — None of Them Will Die."

Football supporters were undeterred, meanwhile, and dug in for the fight. They believed the game's benefits for society far outweighed negatives. Supporters labeled football danger as a sound maturation process. "To bear pain without flinching, and to laugh at the wounds and the scars of a hotly-contested game, is very good discipline, and tends to develop manliness of character," opined *Frank Leslie's Illustrated Weekly*.

By 1901, football supporters boasted political clout in President Theodore Roosevelt, a fiery, hugely popular big stick for their side. Although T.R. did want to alleviate injuries — "I wish we could learn... to make the game of football a rather less homicidal pastime" — there was no mistaking that this president loved football. A Harvard graduate famed internationally as America's icon for rugged individualism, Teddy Roosevelt lauded football as a laboratory for boys in need of the strenuous life perceived to be vanishing.

Roosevelt was angered by much of the criticism targeting at football, and he blasted injured players who complained. "I have a hearty contempt for [a male] if he counts a broken arm or collarbone as a serious consequence when balanced against the chance of showing that he possesses hardihood, physical prowess, and courage," he said.

Another powerful voice echoed T.R., Oliver Wendall Holmes, U.S. Supreme Court justice, who likewise saw football as bloodshed with merit. "Out of heroism grows faith in the worth of heroism," Holmes said. "Therefore I rejoice at every dangerous sport which I see pursued."

Many collegiate leaders backed the game, including MIT president Francis A. Walker, who said it developed "something akin to patriotism and public spirit" in a young man. Illinois professor Edwin G. Dexter theorized that a football player might hear the "Call of the Wild... echoing down from a thousand generations."

Fortunately for football, public opinion largely favored the sport rather than opposed it, and the game overcame a tempestuous incubation period. On order of President Roosevelt, colleges established the Intercollegiate Athletic Association in 1906, forerunner of the NCAA, with a stated mission to make football safer. "The outcry against football brutality was great, but concern over the possibility of an emasculated American manhood greater," Oriard observed. "Football was saved not by eliminating all violence but by compromising on an acceptable degree of physical danger."

Americans were satisfied with "reform" and loved their football spectacle.

"Basically, the coaches and [athletic officials] had pulled a slick one on the public and universities," wrote critic Rick Telander, for his 1989 book *The Hundred Yard Lie*. "By making rule changes that made the game safer (though certainly not safe), they had also effectively killed protests about the game's ethics and its place on campus. Indeed, by the 1920s the complaints about college football became little more than a nuisance, part of the background din..."

Football had survived to become a major cultural institution by the end of World War I, assured of glorious coverage in the popular press. The game's enormous audience was testament, filling towering stadiums and consuming media content. Settling into the social fabric, football was celebrated with games, homecomings, parades, and more pageantry. College and prep teams stood anointed as fine symbols for schools and communities. [Professional leagues were operating, like the newly organized National Football League, but the pro game was decades away from popularity with the press and public.]

Football, once the private domain of rough college boys, had matured into a social mandate for America, a cherished autumn ritual.

A Boy's Socialization For Football

I read Michael Oriard's cultural criticism on football in my latter 30s, and his work was a roadmap to the cultural influences that drew me into the game as a child. Like Oriard, I perceived football players as heroic, brave as soon as I saw players trotting onto a field. I was 4 and swept up in the excitement of high-school games in Potosi, Missouri, a town of a few thousand in the hilly lead-mining country south of St. Louis.

The year was 1964. In pro football, players were fed hard drugs on a daily basis, while colleges and high schools were experiencing their deadliest decade in the game on record, with deaths of contact injuries to exceed 200. But for me, the boy, little else could match a football game on Friday night for the Potosi High Trojans. Play on the field was spectacular and the grandstand scenes stirring, with shapely female cheerleaders leading fans in rooting for the Trojans.

The teen players seemed enormous and gloriously armored, faceless behind the cage masks, their helmets shimmering under pole lights. In my mind, these valiant guys battled for Potosi's honor against an enemy wearing different colors, and the concept both thrilled and frightened me. I knew I wanted to play football in high school, but primarily to wear the uniform and trot out to applause. The constant collisions were very intimidating for this preschooler; later, I would realize my natural talent for hitting and tackling, along with a tolerance for pain.

My immediate family had no football history or tradition. My father played basketball and baseball in college, and my older brothers were still too young for football. But, no matter, the sport gripped me, particularly the appearance of its players, and I enjoyed access to every game. My father, Louis W. Chaney, was principal of the high school, attending all sporting events at home, and I usually went along. Even when Potosi lost in football, about 90 percent of games during the mid-1960s, I loved the show.

My father was not the type for pushing any of his four sons into a sport, particularly football, which he knew little of and cared less about. And while Dad never played football, he was quite masculine. Dad commanded respect for excelling as a school administrator, and people remembered him as an outstanding athlete. I, however, lacked confidence in someday reaching my own manhood. At a very young age, I came to believe if I could prove myself on the football field, then I would achieve masculinity — a notion reinforced to me by a variety of influences, including adults, children, and media. Indeed, someday Oriard would determine manliness to be the theme most affixed to football, by any source.

Football certainly represented manhood in Charleston, Missouri, a Southern town where my family moved as I entered first grade. Located in the northernmost flatlands of the Mississippi River Delta, Charleston was a cotton town, complete with a club of millionaire landowners and hordes of impoverished families. The poor folks relied on either low-paying farm jobs, which were diminishing locally in favor of mechanization on increasingly large operations, or collecting welfare. The town's population of around 5,000 was split about 60-40 between whites and blacks, and racial tension was constant, given the local history. The familial background of most folks in the community, black and white, included Alabama or Mississippi and the defunct landowner-sharecropper system. Stark differences between races began from there, with anger or hate always percolating.

Whites lived east of the railroad tracks, the clean portion of town that encompassed retail businesses, city government, churches, schools, parks, and safe neighborhoods. Blacks crowded together on the west side, along dirty, rough streets lined with tilting sharecropper shacks — basically gray wooden boxes — once hauled into town from the old plantations. That side of the tracks was "Nigger Town," I was told by other white boys, grade-schoolers with me, and I repeated the phrase in my own ignorance, until learning better.

Dad was hired as assistant superintendent for the school district. He was part of a new administration charged with completing the desegregation of local schools, 12 years after the Supreme Court ruling in *Brown versus Topeka*. As Dad began his new job in August 1966, Charleston High opened with blacks in the student body for only the second year.

The town's desegregation trial posed many problems, but not so much on the football team, where young blacks and whites immediately felt camaraderie. Together they endured the game's grinding demands such as two-a-day practices in summer. Most of the team's seniors were African-American, and the Blue Jays of Charleston High had an exciting season, drawing fans of both races in winning six games.

Football, demonstrating its social dexterity in Charleston, was one of the few elements bringing races together with at least some feeling of accord and mutual interest. The game's unifying dynamic also worked at the grade-school level. I attended Mark Twain Elementary, a neighborhood school where I interacted with black children for the first time, and through tackle football at recess, I made a fine friend in Bobby Joe Clark, whose African-American family included outstanding scholars and athletes. The Clark Brothers were a local force, hugely popular kids, models for schoolwork, competition, personality, and citizenship. And they were bad-asses if the situation required, always ready to put down bullies. I rode a school bus with the Clarks, Bobby Joe and his big brothers, and they "took up" for me in conflicts with other kids, black and white. I was tight with the Clarks, forever.

Blue Jays football took hold of me in the 1967 season, firing my emotion and ambition. I was a second-grader attending every game on Friday nights, home and away, and the images and sounds stayed with me for days. I'd lay awake in bed, or daydream at church, replaying the previous game. There were long runs by senior quarterback Charlie Babb, my idol on the team; ecstatic fans, celebrating every good play by Charleston; and gorgeous, bouncing cheerleaders, following their gladiator heroes on the field. A Blue Jays victory was a stupendous conquest for me, especially their win over mighty Poplar Bluff, 7-6, snapping a 21-game win streak for that team, considered the best in Missouri.

With every win for the Jays, football enthusiasm revved up in the school and community, fostering loyalty. To rally pep, cheerleaders led night-time bonfires at the practice field and victory parades through town. Football coverage increased in the weekly newspaper, and merchants posted signs proclaiming their support.

I fawned over the star Charlie Babb, as did several sandlot buddies, and he did not disappoint any of us. Several kids and I reported our every "Charlie" sighting in town, and the teen was a positive role model who imprinted my life, at least. Friendly, polite, and a top student — while also a great competitor in three sports — Charlie always greeted me warmly, whether cruising by in his jacked-up Camaro or arriving at church with his family on Sunday. Sometimes he'd ask me about my own football or baseball exploits, and I'd feel important. Charlie was a big friend to me, always leaving me happy and motivated.

Charlie was named an all-state honoree in football at Charleston and headed to Memphis State, where he starred at safety. This guy's body was built the old-fashioned way, through genetics, good diet, and hard work. He was rock solid and muscular, rippling but taut, not hulking. Whenever Charlie came home from college, where he lifted weights, I thought he had to be the most muscular guy on the planet.

Charlie's girlfriend and future wife was Leslie Ashby, a teen goddess in my eyes. Leslie recognized my adoration for Charlie and treated me kindly, sweetly, always personable and charming. Leslie was athletic, charismatic, and *very pretty*. I swooned, dreaming of someday meeting a girl like her.

My own football potential, meanwhile, was showing as a grade-schooler. I was quick with good hands, and I excelled in running and catching the football during sandlot games. I could kick and throw the ball, so I signed up for "Punt, Pass and Kick," a new competition for boys sponsored by the Ford Motor Company. Trophies were offered to top finishers in each age group, a big deal, and I was runner-up among 8-year-olds. The trophies were presented a few days later at the local Ford dealership, and we recipients lined up for a picture to appear in the week's newspaper. I took that little silver trophy home and admired it so, the shiny metal, the little football man resembling an Oscar in an old helmet, standing at attention with a determined look, clutching a football at one side. I looked at that trophy every time it came into view, over and over.

Among football skills, I was finding the physical side of self, first as a ball-carrier learning to move around and break through pursuit. Escaping or blasting tacklers was my indoctrination of football toughness, and I loved the challenge. I also recognized intimidation in the boys trying to stop me, a respect I relished. I played football every day, from the summer start of school until the winter snowfall.

Blocking and tackling did not begin as specialties of mine, but I steadily grew aware of my body as a weapon against male peers. Neither tall nor big for my age, I was solidly built with strong legs and hips, a thick chest, and a large, hard head. Grasping the physics of leverage, I gauged on the run where to best ram an opponent for toppling him, usually striking his chest area.

Physical prowess in football was profound for me because I got pushed around off the field. Outside sandlot football I scared virtually no one, boy or girl, what with my medium build, easy-going nature, and thick eyeglasses. "Mister Magoo" was a nickname from other kids. My parents were not exactly peace-niks, but they were pacifists who forbade street fighting by their sons. They regularly told us, "Walk away from trouble," which wasn't difficult for me because I also abhorred street fighting. The prospect of punching another boy with my fist seemed chaotic, and when I did attempt the act on occasion, I would only stop and flee in order to avoid further conflict. I learned to make hard hits on the football field, where my violence was both sanctioned and celebrated, by young and old. Mom and Dad had little understanding of football, but they did accept the societal belief that the pastime was constructive for youths.

Frustrated by my ineptitude for fighting, I pulverized boys in sandlot football for gratification and masculine redemption, especially boys who picked on me elsewhere. In those cases my motive was revenge, and that emotion would last through college, where I likewise sought paybacks on the field for avoiding conflicts off it. A college teammate who angered me in everyday life — "talking shit" to me at a party, or "messing" with my girlfriend — became a priority target the next time we were in pads together. I made sure I blasted that guy at practice, often switching places in contact drills so I could line up against him.

Beyond football's direct socialization for me in boyhood — high-school games, sandlot play, people's talk — powerful indirect influences promoting the game reached me through media, print and broadcast.

Televised football was my passion, despite our black-and-white TV subject to grainy reception in southeast Missouri. We could pick up only three stations, but each carried a major network, and that was enough for a football fan. The "Ice Bowl" title game between Green Bay and Dallas was perhaps the first TV game I watched, and by the 1970 season I was a 10-year-old perusing the week's listings ahead of time, so not to miss a football telecast. I usually caught parts of the feature college game on Saturday, while on Sunday the NFL was my true religion, not church. I watched the afternoon pro game from start to finish, rooting hard when it involved either of my favorite teams, the old St. Louis Cardinals or the Kansas City Chiefs. *Monday Night Football* quickly became a weekly goal, persuading my parents to allow me to watch at least the first half before bedtime.

I tuned in to highlight shows such as *This Week in Pro Football*, with peak action of multiple games condensed into an intense stream. I savored productions by NFL Films, featuring crisp editing by Steve Sabol and voice-overs by John Facenda, legendary narrator. Facenda's dramatic employ of words helped transform NFL action into important conflict. His articulation was deep and rhythmic, theatrical, and set in writing by Sabol to play perfectly over beating music and snap edits, making pro players figures of heroism for the audience. They ran and collided on film, looking dirty, bloody, magnificent; a camera shot would roll in ultra-slow motion, bodies flying about with cymbals clashing, and Facenda's voice would flex in time.

NFL Films cast quarterbacks such as Johnny Unitas and Bart Starr as field generals indifferent to danger, heroes displaying "the courage to take punishment," Facenda declared. The line of scrimmage was a "no man's land" and "the lair of the linemen." Linebackers were "search-and-destroy men." Facenda was grand for a show's climax, speaking in one episode over a heartwarming montage of scenes from sunny stadiums on Sundays, camera shots of boys, fathers, granddads, and NFL players. "The game is a time warp..." Facenda intoned, "where the young dream of growing up, and the old remember youth... And for a few hours on Sunday, neither fantasy nor reminiscence seems foolish."

Transfixed by the images and sound, I envisioned myself the doer of gridiron deeds. Watching at home, I hopped and yipped about our living room, juggling a football and diving over furniture. Psyched to play, I phoned kids to organize a sandlot game — and looked forward to physically pounding them.

For newspaper reading, I found a morning treat waiting daily in the sports section. We received the *St. Louis Globe-Democrat*, where I searched football stories and stats on the Cardinals, Chiefs, and the Missouri Tigers of coach Dan Devine, my favorite college team. I heard Tigers' games on radio, since TV broadcasts of Mizzou sports were few in our area. Sometimes Dad subscribed to sports magazines, mainly for us boys, and I clipped and taped on walls the vivid photos of football players, gladiators fighting it out for supreme glory — of exactly what, I couldn't comprehend. I just understood football heroism rated big in America.

Books were another favored medium of mine, since before kindergarten. I read and reread my complete collection of football books targeted for young boys, produced by Random House in partnership with the NFL, called "The Punt Pass and Kick Library." My favorite titles were: *Star Quarterbacks of The NFL*, *Star Pass Receivers of The NFL*, *Star Running Backs of The NFL*, *Great Moments in Pro Football*, *Great Upsets of The NFL*, *Great Linebackers of The NFL*, and *Super Bowl!*

For my ongoing game indoctrination, the classic fantasy themes of football resonated throughout these books, including Necessary Roughness, Gladiator Hero, Coaching Genius, Social Event, and Sexual Conquest.

The manhood stuff was most important for me. I read of injured guys, men unable to sleep the night before the big game because of throbbing pain, only to miraculously be ready to go by kick-off — and chomping at the bit, no less. I savored a storyline on quarterback Joe Kapp, an NFL favorite of mine who led the Minnesota Vikings to their first Super Bowl. Author John Devaney captured much of what I yearned for, a dreamy football lifestyle, in his portrayal of "colorful" Joe Kapp:

> A tough-talking guy who liked fast cars and all the luxury things in life, Joe had come out of the University of California to play football in Canada. There he won a championship and picked up the nickname Injun Joe. He looked like a battle-scarred Indian.
>
> His chin was crisscrossed with the scars of dozens of battles, on and off the football field. He came to the Vikings from Canada in 1967. He gave the team a relaxed, happy attitude that it had lacked. Once he and middle linebacker Lonnie Warwick were arguing.
>
> "I'm right," Warwick yelled.
>
> "I'm right," Kapp yelled.
>
> "Let's go outside and settle this."
>
> They went outside the hotel room. Warwick looped a right-hand punch that dropped Joe Kapp to the floor. Injun Joe got up slowly, rubbing his bruised chin.
>
> "You're the toughest man I've ever met," he said to Warwick.
>
> "Let me buy you dinner."
>
> And Joe threw an arm over the startled Warwick's shoulder and took him out to dinner, the fight forgotten.

Man, I wanted to be Joe Kapp! At least that version of him, Star Quarterback, Speed Racer, Street Fighter, Cool Dude, and even Indian Warrior — which conjured Cowboys and Indians, another distorted fantasy of this Baby Boomer. Kapp seemed to be one guy having it all. How could life be more exciting than his?

I had no clue about reading football as a cultural text, but as a boy I felt the effects. I dreamt of someday living the storyline of Football Hero, and in 1971 a TV surprise heightened my passion. Charlie Babb came back into my focus, this time through television, which really left an impression. One night I flipped through our total four stations to find a collegiate all-stars broadcast from the South, the annual

Blue-Gray Game. And there was Charlie! Now he was an All-American safety for Memphis State, making plays and having his name announced, as usual. A few months later, I was thrilled to read that Charlie was chosen by Miami during the NFL draft; hopefully he would make my new favorite pro team, the Dolphins, who had just lost the Super Bowl to Dallas.

Charlie made the Miami squad, becoming the sport's first "nickel back" under defensive guru Bill Arnsparger, an assistant to head coach Don Shula. The Dolphins achieved their perfect 17-0 season, thanks in part to a big play by Charlie in the playoffs.

In round one of the postseason, the Cleveland Browns tested the Dolphins in Miami. Early in the game, Browns All-Pro punter Don Cockroft took a snap and stepped forward to kick — then I saw jersey number 49, Charlie Babb, streak in for the Dolphins. "AND IT'S BLOCKED!" screamed a TV announcer, with the Orange Bowl crowd exploding. Charlie picked up the loose ball and strode into the end zone. "TOUCHDOWN! CHARLIE BABB!" Watching TV, my younger brother and I alerted family members in time for slow-motion replays of Charlie's glory. "Look at him!" I said. "Boy, he's happy." I had taped the play on audiocassette, wrapping the microphone cord around the TV dial, and I would listen repeatedly in years ahead.

I wanted to be a football player. To be merely a spectator seemed no worthwhile prospect to this American boy.

II. Playing Football: Passion, Disillusionment

For young Mike Oriard, football was a personal quest he could not find in other ventures, including academics. "I read Latin and Greek and Shakespeare, discovered the fundamentals of chemistry and physics, studied history and religion," he recalled. "But through football I discovered myself. And proved that in a public arena." Playing the high-school game during the 1960s in Spokane, Mike transcended his normal identity as a shy, awkward adolescent.

One afternoon in varsity practice as a second-teamer, Mike repeatedly defeated a starting player, an older boy who was popular in school. A coach harshly scolded the starter, questioning his manhood, while praising Mike, who happily accepted affirmation of his masculinity. Although intelligent, Mike suspended his sensitivities for football; by knocking around the upperclassman, he felt "no compassion, only exultation," he recalled. And vanquishing this particular teammate was antidote for some very personal, larger struggles. "In the [school] hallways I could not show my resentment and envy of the fact that he seemed self-assured while I was insecure, that he was 'cool' while I was not," Oriard wrote. "On the football field, I could express those resentments without even admitting I was doing so."

Mike became a standout defensive end for Gonzaga Prep, and after graduating high school in 1966, he followed his dream to play football for Notre Dame University. A 6-5, 200-pound freshman, Mike was versed in the football legends of Notre Dame, and he loved the famed symbols like Touchdown Jesus, the oval brick stadium, Knute

Rockne, and The Gipper.

But as a walk-on player in South Bend, a non-recruit with no scholarship, Mike's reality was to struggle to prove himself and get playing time. In practice he took his lumps on the "meat squad," the non-roster players lined up as cannon fodder against the starters, but he returned punishment and steadily acclimated himself to big-time college football material. Off the field, he lifted weights feverishly in Notre Dame's antiquated training facility, slowly adding pounds to his lean frame. After two seasons as a practice player, Mike made the team under Fighting Irish head coach Ara Parseghian.

In the fifth week of his junior season, 1968, Mike Oriard was named starting offensive center for Notre Dame, and the significance was not lost on him. He was truly part of gridiron legend now, down to the act of donning the fabled uniform:

> As I put on the various knee pads, thigh pads, and hip pads, then slipped the shiny gold pants over my blue nylon knee-high socks, I took on proportions and brilliance that made me feel larger than life. When I looked in the mirror, I was someone who impressed even me.

Mike pulled on shoulder pads and his dark-blue Irish home jersey, number 54, and listened to Coach Parseghian's pregame talk and a prayer by a university priest. He put on the renowned golden helmet of Notre Dame, then charged out of the locker room with teammates. Mike basked in cheers from 59,000 in the famed oval stadium, living his cherished goal, experiencing the ultimate in American spectacle. He wrote:

> Playing football at Notre Dame was a private experience, but it also forced me to see beyond the narrow boundries of my own world. ... The pageantry, the crowds, the chanting and cheering and booing and singing reminded me that playing football at Notre Dame was not only my private communion with the past but also a public celebration in the present that engaged thousands, even millions, of people.

As a senior for the Irish, Mike was offensive co-captain and, with help from the university's promotional machine, named a *Sporting News* second-team All-American. Pro scouts took notice, and he was selected in the 1970 NFL draft as a fifth-round pick of the Kansas City Chiefs, who had recently won Super Bowl IV. His remaining naiveté about football was set to expire.

Oriard's Ambivalence: Burned by Football Business

In 20th century America, a boy could embrace football as a sacred passage, a virtuous adventure in life growth. A boy could see football as his chance to become a man, even a hero, believing the cultural chant of role models, mentors, authority figures, societal leaders, media. His overall experience may well have been positive in the sport, particularly if his career ended in high school. Football's common mystique remained intact for many former high-school players, often the sincerest compatriots of this game.

But a male who grew to play football in college or beyond might have seen the glorious wrappings unravel, fall away. He may have become one of football's disillusioned, or one like Dr. Michael Oriard, English professor. "I consider myself a beneficiary of my football career, but am aware that too many others have not been," Oriard wrote in correspondence, 2008. "I can only be ambivalent, not entirely cynical or outraged about football." Oriard did walk away from pro football in one piece, without a debilitating injury, but departed with some innocence lost. The NFL was little of the football he beheld as a boy, pining for older guys to let him play, or the gridiron romance he embraced at 17, of grand personal conquests while wearing the hallowed uniform of Notre Dame.

Experiences and abilities guided an individual's destiny, and Michael Oriard found his as football critic, even if he preferred the moniker "cultural historian" of the game. Indeed, Oriard became a *critical* football critic, given his important work regarding the game's pervasive impacting of society, and the player's disillusionment, Oriard's, was the essential here.

Oriard was among several authors on football who played the game during the Vietnam era. His own autobiography of disillusionment, *End of Autumn*, was not an expose in the class of Meggyesy's *Out of Their League*. It was not psychoanalysis of self and football culture, such as Gary Shaw's *Meat on The Hoof*, and it lacked the investigative analysis, judgment, of Telander's *Hundred Yard Lie*. Oriard's book illustrated his own inner makeover by the game, from his holding passionate faith to finding disenchantment.

The football dream was not damaged for Oriard at Notre Dame, where he lived a fantasy of many players and fans. Oriard's success story at Notre Dame, his rise from obscure walk-on to co-captain, was the stuff of a *Rudy* movie never made. Oriard's story was better, in fact. He was a gifted, disciplined student who was able to treat football as a part-time activity, and the time and place helped, the latter 1960s at Notre Dame University, where a football player could be late for practice because of academic work. Oriard graduated with high regard for his professors and sport coaches, especially Parseghian, and he still believed the college football experience could be valuable for young athletes.

The NFL, however, changed Oriard, teaching him, he recalled, "that professional football as a *business* was a very different game from the one I was used to." Oriard was reluctant to accept reality. "I did not relinquish my emotional commitment to the game easily," he wrote.

Oriard was a gung-ho rookie in entering training camp with the Chiefs in 1970, but in the next five years acquired a veteran's seasoned cynicism, including the necessity to watch out only for himself. As a taxi-squad player who worked into roster positions of backup center and special teams, Oriard experienced the rip-off shenanigans of coaches like Hank Stram, one of football's most image-conscious, and the authoritarian rule of powerful ownership in the game, in this case Chiefs' owner Lamar Hunt, the calculating Texas billionaire-in-making regarded as a folk hero around Kansas City. [Notably, Oriard said exposure to drugs was not a factor for him in pro football. While use of anabolic steroids was alleged of Chiefs' players around 1970, with Alvin Roy as strength coach, Oriard recalled in 2002 he did not use the drugs as a player and that neither Roy nor anyone else mentioned the topic to him. Oriard stated in his 1982 book he never saw Chiefs' players use pills of any type, including steroids or amphetamines.]

In pro football, Oriard felt the pain and sorrow of fellow players and families in their misfortune, over injury or outright loss of employment, but could really do nothing except await his same fate. It came in the 1974 preseason. Stram released him following a contentious NFL labor strike, when Oriard led players demanding job conditions standard for other workers across America. Oriard played that year in Canada, for the Hamilton Tiger-Cats, then retired after 18 seasons in organized football. Oriard was ready to move on in life anyway, with a healthy perspective and fine prospects.

Oriard's dedication to scholarship was paying off. Since joining the Chiefs, he had utilized off-seasons to continue his graduate studies in English, and he was nearing completion of a doctoral degree in American literature at Stanford University. He was teaching and writing critical analysis, looking forward to university rank and salary as a professor. Oriard left pro football as an exception among retirees, completely focused on his future. "When football is exchanged for a new career, the athlete must adjust," he wrote. "*All* football players must make these adjustments. All must give up the familiar rhythms, the physical intensity, and the basic simplicity of their football world."

Leaving the game could be particularly troubling for football's most talented players, an exit typically premature because of injury. "Theirs is a physical rather than an intellectual genius, but genius nonetheless," Oriard stated, "and to have to give it up so early can be difficult." Oriard noted peril for the player was to believe he was truly indestructible, ignoring the certainty he was not:

> Detachment is key — being able to see your own football career from outside, rather than being totally caught up in it. Football can be a seductive siren, whispering in players' ears the words that will drag them to their doom.
>
> "You're special," it breathes. "You're a hero; the world admires you and wants to take care of you. Don't worry about anything; sign autographs and let people buy you drinks. You can play forever."
>
> The athlete cannot afford to believe such lies for very long.

Oriard, writing as a professor in 1982, understood the white-hot fire that was the American football spectacle for the athlete. Oriard had relinquished his central role willingly, but, he admitted, there remained scattered moments of longing to be a player again, battered and bruised but feeling *alive*. Former players of any level could identify. "I sometimes regret the loss of the physical pleasures of my football-playing days. ... I will never again be as strong, as fast, as able to endure prolonged physical strain as I was when I played football. I have lost a physical mastery that I can never regain."

American football remained important to Oriard as research, providing him a rich, charged field of communication content representing ideology of not just a game, but of a super-civilization. Playing football was relatively fleeting, but *reading football*, analyzing the game's texts and power for culture, Oriard could do that for life.

Oriard remained concerned about football fantasy, such as the claim of benefits for young athletes. Decades after playing at Notre Dame, he could no longer see evidence that his positive college experience could be replicated, particularly at the major levels due to the interests of enormous money. Writing for the *New York Times* in 2001, Oriard expressed "grave doubts" about the game's effects on players in major colleges, those so-called student-athletes generating billions in revenue for the NCAA, member universities, and associate multi-media conglomerates. Oriard questioned the colleges' year-round training for football, their lengthy game schedules in autumn and winter, and their unrelenting emphasis on winning.

And he worried about the multitude of giant young bodies "manufactured to meet the specs for today's football."

Courson: Teen Gladiator, College Football

On a weekend visit to his girlfriend's in Pittsburgh, 49-year-old Steve Courson met friends of her teen daughter, including a male he figured to be 17 or 18. Courson was nationally known as an expert on anabolic steroids, with a very public stance against teen use of the drugs. Most adults would be intimidated to approach Courson, the former Steeler and steroid user, for initiating shop talk on how to use muscle dope, yet this kid went right to the point. "He was talking about how he had Winstrol at home, and he wasn't even an athlete," Courson said afterward. "He was asking me about it. I said, 'Well, you don't want to be taking that.' Courson, in his experience, may not have been surprised by the teen, but he was disappointed. The kid "was real nonchalant about it," Courson said. "He says, 'Yeah, I want to cycle, I want to get tight abs, da-da-da.' I was like, 'Oh, great.'"

Courson did not condemn the teen; he empathized. Three decades before, Courson was a youth heading into anabolic steroids for meeting a goal, though his competitive environment differed. This contemporary teen was seeking looks for enhanced attraction in a culture intoxicated by image. Courson had wanted size and power enough for supremacy in football, and he succeeded before it almost consumed him.

In boyhood, Courson envisioned someday dwelling in a warrior's world, either the military or big-time football. He was the second adopted son of Iber and Elizabeth Courson, native Pennsylvanians and Lutherans. Iber was a World War II veteran who had played college football, and Steve's older brother, Bruce, was a Vietnam veteran.

Military and football "were the two things that were in my mind," Courson said in 2005. "Both of them have a kind of rigid discipline to them. So that kind of fit into my scheme of looking at the world." Young Steve was an A-grade student, Boy Scout, and avid reader, particularly of books on military history, but he realized he would not fight in Vietnam, where he believed the U.S. government, uncommitted to winning war, was exploiting brave troops. By the time Steve's family moved from Massachusetts to Gettysburg, he was in high school and focused on playing major-college football.

The sport, in turn, was literally set up to capture boy athletes like Steve. "The game is a symbol of our industrial-military complex: That's *huge* in the spectacle," he said. "Football was one of the last vestiges, as I saw everything growing up, where something was presented as an honorable combat. That drew me toward it, the fact it was socially acceptable, where Vietnam was not."

Pennsylvania was a storied hotbed of football, with schoolboy legends like Ditka, Namath, and Blanda, and Steve enjoyed the local gridiron tales, particularly while emerging as a star himself at Gettysburg High. Furthering his socialization for football, Steve devoured sports pages and pro football on television. "I watched [the NFL] on TV, grew up with it, loved it, you know," Courson recalled. "My football heroes were guys like Butkus, and the Fearsome Foursome, and the Purple People Eaters. I grew up watching a very unique era of professional football, where money hadn't taken it over yet. It was about the game."

Steve embraced weightlifting during high school, believing the activity was imperative to athletic success. The year was 1969, and pumping iron made Steve an oddity, but he was ahead of the curve for prep football, correctly identifying that the training lifestyle, getting bigger and stronger, would line his path ahead in the sport. "I was a nut because I worked out with weights," Courson said. "I understood at a very young age the benefits, you know. I had that part figured out. I hadn't even considered the steroid aspect of it."

Steve strength-trained mostly alone and without drugs, virtually self-taught, but he was genetically blessed, extraordinarily, and bull-minded. He progressed to bench-pressing 400 pounds at the age of 17, when he graduated high school in Gettysburg, forever establishing himself among America's strongest teens sans chemical aid. At 6-foot-1, he weighed 230 solid pounds and could run fast and leap high. He was one of Pennsylvania's top college prospects.

The University of South Carolina recruited Courson diligently, competing against schools like Kansas State, Penn State, and Colorado, and he visited South Carolina on a weekend in late November, leaving cold weather behind in Gettysburg. On a sunny Saturday in Columbia, Courson watched the Gamecocks knock off a ranked team, Florida State, winning on a field goal. He had never seen such football excitement and was highly impressed with the Gamecocks' facilities, first-class for training and games. "I was witnessing, you know, the whole flavor of college football: The South, plus the weather, plus the facilities. And it was a pretty intoxicating," Courson said. "I wanted a part of it."

Courson signed with South Carolina, and in August 1973 he reported for summer camp on the campus in Columbia. Previously, as a pampered recruit, Courson had felt the fantasy of Gamescocks football and the affectionate solicitation of coaches; now, as a freshman grunt under *control* of those coaches, he was confronted by challenges most males of any age would not endure.

Gamecocks practice opened in the repressive Carolina heat and humidity, and Courson encountered the program's pack of screaming assistant coaches, swarming to berate players tired or hurting. These men ensured that two-a-day football practices in the South could still be defined as sadistic. Actually, it was three-a-day practices for the Gamecocks. Each morning and afternoon, a contact session in full pads lasted at least two hours on AstroTurf, which could fire up to 120 degrees Fahrenheit under scorching sunshine. The coaching staff reserved a practice in shorts and T-shirts for the cool of evening, adhering to the old idea that full pads in direct sun made players tougher. The players were supposed to appreciate the "light practice" at night and they did, regardless of how much the coaches yelled, cursed, and made them run.

On one hot morning Courson keeled over, dropping to the ground. The freshman defensive lineman was carried off, and medical personnel hospitalized him for heat prostration. The coaches decided Courson needed no lengthy care, however, and summoned him to practice the next morning, in full pads. They worked him like a mule and made snide cracks about his collapse. He considered quitting but would not. "To be honest, I liked playing football," he said. "Despite all the bullshit, I liked the game, you know. There's something about it. Personally, it was the camaraderie and the challenge. ... You pour yourself totally into that game, it's real hard to step back."

The coaches recognized young Courson's determination and talent, and when the Gamecocks opened their season at home, he played much of the game as a backup defensive tackle. "I got thrust into it at age 17, right away, so that was a huge smack in the face," he said. "It's an electric feeling when you've never played a game on AstroTurf before, and your first experience in a college football game is in front of 56,000 people, under the lights, playing a school like Georgia Tech."

Courson had reached big-time college football, and at times it seemed much as he had expected, glory and fun in the grand spectacle. The player could not avoid elements of the game's dark underside, however, beginning with crazed, demon-eyed fans packing the enormous stadiums. In high school he had felt warmth from the stands, a steady support through victory or defeat imparted by family, friends, and community. In the arena of major-college football, players amounted to gladiators for fans who paid high prices to enter. From the perspective of these consumers, no real persons existed out on that field, just beings for staging combat entertainment — beings to be booed, cursed, cheered at whim. Courson grasped he was faceless for fans, soulless, just another fighting machine covered in armor; that was how they wanted him. "The fans in college... It was the Roman Coliseum," he surmised. "It was heavy-duty, win-at-all-costs atmosphere. The difference between that and the pro level? Put it this way: There was a huge difference between high school and what I experienced out there in South Carolina. But there was a very small difference, as far as intensity of the fans, from college to pros. It was very similar. The difference was marginal."

Fans in the stands may have bellowed blood lust for football, but they risked nothing. From their safe perch above the fury on field, spectators got to vicariously experience the violence, celebrate it then go home unscathed.

Down at the spectacle's underbelly, meanwhile, young players lay in the wake of every game, beaten and injured. Wallowing down there, players pondered how to end their misery, and the surest thing they knew of was anabolic steroids, which were reaching every team in big-time football. Indeed, everyone playing at this level was encountering drug-aided behemoths, if not joining the growing crowd. "I was so beaten up after some of those games," Courson remembered. "I knew I had to do something."

Courson was not concerned with merely surviving in college ball. He also would not accept being merely good in the game. Rather, he was determined to be one of the best. South Carolina teammates told him to use anabolic steroids, drugs available through the football program, and the final urging came from a young coach. "I think the big thing, what really gets obscured in all this, is athletes respond to their environment," Courson said. "And, if you look at my drug use throughout my career, I responded to my environment and my challenges. I was just thrust into an environment where I was up against bigger, older guys, as a kid. I knew I had to get bigger to do what I needed to do, and that led me to it." The team physician wrote a prescription for Courson, and he did the only steroid cycle of his college career. Courson consumed one 5-mg Dianbol tablet every day for a month, along with training manically and gorging on food, and grew from 230 pounds to 260 while increasing strength and speed.

The impressed coaches moved Courson to the offensive line, where he blossomed at guard. Facing Clemson the final game of his sophomore season, Courson, just turned 19, played like he envisioned he would on drugs — dominantly.

Webster: The Winning Game Consumes 'Iron Mike'

Mike Webster became iconic for Pittsburgh's legendary Men of Steel, instantly recognizable No.52 in black and gold, baring his big biceps in cold and snow, the offensive center for Steelers' teams that claimed four Super Bowl championships in the 1970s. After retiring, Webster was elected to the Pro Football Hall of Fame, but he did not live long enough in age to reach his jersey number.

Webster died in 2002, reportedly of a heart attack, and once again doping allegations swirled around Super Steelers of old, but the volume was louder in public this time, more persistent. In the past Pittsburgh media gave benefit of doubt to the Steelers franchise over steroids, often generously. Courson had been mostly ignored during the 1980s and '90s, his allegations and general insight, or, when acknowledged, he was typically disparaged by local scribes and broadcasters.

"Webbie" was different, a Steeler beloved, and the decade was different. What was known or presumed now, about both the individual and drugs in sport as a whole, rendered illogical the former good faith. Pittsburgh media took up the issue in force following Webster's death, for several years, into events like BALCO, steroids in baseball, congressional hearings, and the Carolina Panthers. Some local columnists and commentators blasted the Steelers and football, and predictable denials by old players and team officials did not quell the uprising. "The irony is that most of the intelligent public, when it comes to Steeler linemen, has figured this out," Courson observed. "The guys are caught in the public-relations lie, very sad but also very shallow. ... They don't have to proclaim their use from the rooftops, but in our circles let's be real."

Webster's personal problems post-football were documented. He suffered dementia, depression, hearing loss, and other ailments doctors linked to concussions, or "frontal lobe syndrome." Trapped in a wrecked body, gripped by chemical addiction developed as a player, Webster's life was constant physical pain shrouded in mental anguish. The Pittsburgh community was shaken by Webster's arrest for forging pain-killer prescriptions, and to learn he sometimes lived out of his pickup. Reporters found him sleeping in stretches at the Amtrak station downtown. At death, Webster was deeply in debt, facing lawsuits, and divorced from his wife, basically homeless. Rumors he had abused steroids had circulated the town for years.

"Mike Webster was too young to die," declared John Steigerwald, *Tribune-Review* columnist. "Did football kill him? Did he ask his body to take too much punishment for too long? Would he have died of a heart attack at 50 if he had been a football coach instead of a football player? ... And the big question, the one that nobody seems to want to answer, did he shorten his life by using steroids?" Steigerwald beseeched Steelers officials and former teammates of Webster — 20 to 30 still resided in the area — to step up and attest he did not use steroids. Apparently, none would. "Their silence is deafening," Steigerwald wrote.

Confirmation of Webster's steroid use surfaced in late 2004, through court documents that stated he told doctors he "experimented" with the drugs as a player. The deceased NFL legend's family was suing the players union in a disability claim making national news. Courson, for his part, had not divulged the names of Webster and other users among former teammates, but publicity of the court case led him to open up some about his late friend.

"Now it's out there that he used steroids," Courson said at his remote cabin south of Pittsburgh, where Webster bunked occasionally. "The bottom line with Mike Webster is, it's a real shame. Here's a guy that gave 17 years to the league, and you know the reason why he's no longer with us: the fact that the win-at-all-costs mentality in football, as much as anything, killed that man. The combination of the head, the medication, everything that went on: I mean, he's the prime example. We still don't want to be honest about the reality of what goes on out there. ... It's got to be embarrassing for the organization. It has to. That was so unnecessary."

Courson — widower, former NFL lineman, former steroids user, former cardiac patient, book author, doping expert, and, incredibly, a stud physical specimen nearing age 50 — was no sentimentalist, but the misfortune of Webster, his great teammate, was emotionally difficult. Among endearing qualities, Webster was honest, humble, intelligent, strong, caring, loyal — personifying the definition of honor for Courson. "Webbie" covered Courson's back against malevolent coaches and writers. He consoled Courson when the latter was released from the NFL and later diagnosed with cardiomyopathy. When Courson was overtaken with serious illness, Webster organized a benefit roast to defray medical bills. In turn, Courson was among former Steelers who helped care for Webster, caught in his own demise. Ufortunately, the man known as Iron Mike was beyond the saving graces of anyone, and he succumbed.

In the Webster estate's claim against the $1 billion NFLPA retirement and disability plan, family members, primarily Mike's four grown children, sought $1.14 million compensation for the 5½ years following his retirement in March 1991, a period not covered in previous payments by the fund. The plan's board members had determined a start date of September 1, 1996, for Webster's compensation, but friends, associates, and doctors argued Webster was incapacitated at the time he retired, after playing his final two seasons in Kansas City.

"He couldn't sell; he couldn't talk," Steve Truchan, who worked with Webster in a laser-painting business during the summer of 1991, told Chuck Finder of *The Post-Gazette*. A physician who treated Webster in 1996, Dr. Chuck Kelley, concluded the football player's mental faculties began degrading as early as 1989, predating retirement. "He had frontal-lobe syndrome," Kelley said. "It was injured from repeated blows to the forehead... where all your executive function comes from. The chronic symptoms begin to accumulate." Estate lawyers told Finder that a neurologist certified by the NFL disability and retirement board, Dr. Edward Westbrook, assessed Webster as disabled in 1991.

Some people viewed the case "as a transparent, after-the-fact money grab," reported Greg Garber, *EPSN.com*, who compiled an in-depth series on Webster post-football, but estate administrator Sunny Jani dismissed such criticism. "The kids deserve it because of what their dad went through," Jani said. "They basically sacrificed their father to this game."

The writers of football spectacle could glean no glory theme here, but Webster's former wife saw plenty of analogy to Old Rome, grounded in the harsh reality she knew of American blood sport, NFL style. "Mike's story needs to be told," Pam Webster said from Wisconsin, where she lived with their children. "I don't want this man to die in vain. They're gladiators. When the game is over, these guys have to go home. And when it's over, a lot of them don't have a home to go to."

A federal judge in Maryland ruled in favor of the estate in April 2005, awarding $1.18 million in retroactive benefits. Lawyers for the disability plan contested, but the ruling was upheld in December 2006 by three judges of the U.S. Court of Appeals for the Fourth Circuit. Estimates for the final award approached $2 million, including interest, legal fees, and court costs.

The case set a precedent for work-related compensation of brain trauma in professional football, according to some participants. "I'm very excited," said Bob Fitzsimmons, the estate co-counsel who worked with Webster before his death, "not only for the Webster family but all the NFL players that in particular had head injuries — for them, it gives them some hope."

III. Modern Media Maintain Football Fantasy

The autumn NFL season brought soothing relief for Americans frightened by the world at large, sports columnist Michelle Kaufman purported in 1990. Constructing a narrative for *The Detroit Free Press*, Kaufman lamented bad happenings in the world, including illicit drug abuse and violence affecting kids. For those social ills, Kaufman asserted, "a Sunday afternoon football game can offer tremendous therapy."

Typical of most Americans, Kaufman viewed the game of football as not only innocuous, but goodness to behold. Kaufman saw no drug abuse — not even in pro football — no violence, nothing wrong with chemically bloated men beating each other before 75,000 screaming fans and a much larger TV audience, including children. This was the spell of football spectacle, reality distorted in front of the entire nation, aided and abetted by everyone who chose to ignore the warts. Blind loyalists constituted the American majority, and Kaufman was counted in the ranking, her writing under the illusion.

Evidence suggested an armor of rhetoric immunity enveloped football, shielding it from damaging criticism, spoken or written, and communication studies had a name and model for the force. Narrative researcher Dr. Ernest G. Bormann outlined the concept of "rhetorical vision," which he defined as "a unified putting-together of the various scripts that gives the participants a broader view of things." Therefore, the central theme in the communication of football in America — *football word*, the avalanche of exaggeratedly positive messages from print media, cyber, television, radio, film, software, licensed products, personal conversations — portrayed and protected the game as a symbol of success.

The rhetorical vision of football carried the sport onward as an impenetrable ship, repelling all torpedoes. Glory themes served as feel-good scripts for media, fans, athletes, and organizers, allowing the unified mass to rationalize or ignore the negatives, dismissing factors such as deaths as incidental aside to football's vital function in society. Oriard observed, "Boys today learn what football means from television, magazines, newspapers, and books; they learn from parents and peers, coaches and teachers, relatives and friends and strangers, all of whom in turn have learned from a similar range of possible sources." Oriard believed the general communication of football spoke to a meta-narrative preferred by society, a cultural mythology of glorious storylines that any reformers would be hard-pressed to change.

Applying a singular football theme in Bormann theory, a singular gridiron theme like a classic identified by Oriard, could function as a category of "rhetorical fantasy" for loyalists seeking to maintain their grand vision of football. Media or fans could rationalize the gore, for example, by viewing it as Necessary Roughness. Bormann, as part of his "symbolic convergence" theory, stated a rhetorical fantasy "refers to the creative and imaginative interpretations of events that fulfills a group psychological or rhetorical need." Football writers and fans shared many rhetorical fantasies that fit their perspective of purity about the game.

Regarding doping, a rhetorical fantasy nurtured by organizers was to blame only players for muscle drugs. The illusion, widely accepted on face value, followed that cheating players were an isolated minority treading upon a vast majority of "clean" athletes who would not dare. In this version the system held no responsibility, the problem was easily dismissed as personal in nature, and everyone could continue enjoying football with a clear conscience.

Not surprisingly, the players' use of hard drugs and their suffering injuries at astounding rates continued into the new millennium. Although essentially underground, those problems remained potentially damaging for the spectacle if allowed to escalate into money issues. America's rhetorical vision of football held firm against criticism, however, sustaining the sport, noted a relative few writers, as it had for generations.

Injuries were no image problem for football, had not been since the game's establishment as spectacle in the 19th century. Casualty rates of the 1970s, for instance, confounded author James A. Michener, who speculated what would happen if physics classes taught in schools were to annually kill 28 students and injure 86 percent nationally. "I think it obvious that physics would be eliminated as a subject, and within a very short time, for such a cost would be deemed excessive," Michener surmised for his *Sports in America*. "But there is no cry to end football, nor will there be, because every society decides what it is willing to pay for its entertainment."

Americans chose to be oblivious about muscle doping in their football. "I don't know that society wants the story out," said Bernie Miklasz, veteran NFL writer in St. Louis. "And that doesn't excuse reporters, but do people want these stories told? In the years I've been in it and with what I've seen, I don't think, generally speaking, the American public wants to hear it. *This is our legal drug*. People don't want to be bummed out by sports. They want sports to make them feel better." Miklasz worked across multiple media, *The Post-Dispatch*, radio and television, and in 1996 was an exception among writers in speaking openly about media coverage of anabolic substances in American football.

During the 1990s news media did not work much on doping in football, other than compiling simple stories that parroted officials and players claiming random testing had eliminated steroids. Sportswriters overlooked provocative developments the entire decade. Pro and college players were arrested with quantitities of steroids, human growth hormone, and paraphernalia, and well-founded books were released, detailing the systematic drug use. A milestone scientific finding, coupled with data of players' weights, demonstrated the ever-increasing sizes of players in the NFL and NCAA were surely unlikely without muscle doping. Urinalysis testing for anabolics was exposed as woefully inadequate for preventing such cheating, and lawsuits by retired players over doping rattled NFL management and the players union. A cover-up surfaced, wherein NFL management and union agreed to keep secret failed drug tests for at least 16 players. The Internet proved to be a ready source for obtaining anabolics, going along with established venues like black-market street dealers and crooked physicians. The unregulated supplements industry created legal sales of some anabolic steroids and other enhancers, right over the counter.

Yet football writers hardly budged on the issue of doping, even when prompted by an NFL star in Kansas City. Derrick Thomas, the Chiefs' All-Pro linebacker, told *Sport* magazine that steroids were foremost among problems for the league. Kansas City media ignored completely this statement by Thomas, while otherwise producing massive coverage on the Chiefs, especially Thomas, and football in general. National media did not sniff.

Football media were too cozy with the sport. Big money was at stake, after all, for every party invested in football spectacle, with media reaping profits second only to the sport's organizers. "There's a real synergy," Miklasz said. "There's an event, and people write about it. Then there's another event coming up, and people hype it. And it's just a cycle that goes on and on." Researchers in economics and communication identified this business synergy, the high-revenue exchange between major sport and attendant media, as the foundation of what they labeled the *sport-media complex*, a business hegemony that industry critics decried for insurmountable conflicting interests, profits versus journalism.

"I mean, the hands are locked," Miklasz said. "There's no question about it. There's a partnership, whether people want to acknowledge it or not. And obviously it's a business partnership where TV and radio are concerned. They pay for the right to broadcast, televise these games. There's an actual business relationship, where it's in TV's best interest to make [football] players god-like, because they also stand to gain from it financially.

"I think there's a lot more independence in newspapers because there really isn't a direct business relationship. However, I think sports writing's always been about myth-making. You go back to... Red Smith, he referred to it as 'godding-up' the ballplayers. There's still a lot of that, although I do think that print journalism, more than any other [media], has a more discerning eye about the issues and will actually investigate things, and occasionally will actually *de-mythologize* athletes and these games. [*The Post-Dispatch* purchased a small ownership in the Cardinals baseball franchise after this interview.]

Miklasz continued, "Still... this is true of every paper: If your baseball team is in the pennant race, or gets to the playoffs or the World Series, you sell more newspapers. So you directly benefit from the success of your team. And so, when the team's doing well and you're selling more papers, the editors are saying, 'We want more stories, we want more photos, we want more space. Let's get out this special section. Let's jump aboard this train.' It's like no money is changing hands per se, but there's a flow chart. When a team's doing well, the newspaper sells more papers, they get to print special editions. writers write more. Everyone's excited. More money comes through the till at the newspaper. Advertisers take out ads in special sections, like when the Cardinals go to the playoffs or World Series. Everybody in the business does it; we hype the special event that's coming up. When the Rams came into St. Louis [in 1995 and won early], we sold a lot more papers on Monday, the day after a Rams game. And we adjusted our section accordingly, to sort of capitalize on that."

Televised American football featuring the NFL and the NCAA major schools generated enormous capital by the 1990s, for organizers and host networks alike. The Super Bowl alone garnered almost half of American viewers as the most-watched show in history, and upwards of a billion people tuned in worldwide. Miklasz said muscle doping was a definite no-no for TV networks paying billions for football rights. "This product's got to fly or they're going to take a bath on it, and I'm not passing judgment on these people. ...," Miklasz said. "To achieve these means, are you going to hire some investigative reporter to go to the locker room and break stories about players bulking up on steroids and cheating, and state they're all going to die or be deformed in several years? Or do you want to roll out 50,000 features a year on John Madden's bus, and his cooking turkey?

"I mean, what are you going to do if you're a businessman? You're going to go with the Madden cruiser and turkey recipes. You're not going to worry about steroids. Sports are our drug. You *want* the audience to feel good. You don't want them to be bummed out about what you're uncovering, right?"

This sentiment of sports fans, to be entertained by games rather than outraged, ran deeper than adult consumers. Children were at the center of everyone's concern, and the sport-media complex particularly understood the magic of games would be gone without its ability to enrapture children. Sport content had to appeal to kids versus appalling them, and so editors would steer away from themes like athletes as drug-abusing cheats. Sports writer and pundit Leonard Koppett addressed content and kids in his 1981 book, *Sports Illusion, Sports Reality*. "Carried to a logical conclusion... stripping sports of their romantic and idealistic elements and making them less appealing to children would be a form of fairly quick suicide for the mass-entertainment sports establishment," Koppett wrote. "The industry's sense of self-preservation is rather strong, and so is that of its numerous allies, so the resistance to muckraking [journalism] is both powerful and effective."

Business entities vested in football, including many media, typically were obstacles for journalists seeking to expose systematic abuses of the game, but so were fans in multitude. The power of football spectacle confronted Dr. Charles E. Yesalis, Penn State epidemiologist, as a critic of doping, but he also felt the affront as a college professor. He saw faculty pressured to be lax or fraudulent in grading football players, and he knew of football-friendly networks on campuses, professors, and even departments identified by coaches and players as showing favoritism. Yesalis also served on a committee with Linda Bensel-Meyer, English professor at the University of Tennessee, who in 1999 suffered publicly and privately for exposing academic improprieties involving 37 football players, including all 22 starters on a Vols team. The FBI reported Bensel-Meyer's house was broken into and her phone bugged, and she and her children were threatened. She was trashed daily by Tennessee sports media, radio, Internet, and newspapers. "This thing has consumed my life," she said. "I can't go to the grocery store without getting harrassed. It's devastated my marriage. My husband couldn't understand why I wasn't protecting myself."

Yesalis, in every region of the country he visited, encountered fans of big-time college football. The adult fans were of every ethnicity, every socio-economic class, every profession. Yesalis imagined the vast majority to be reasonable people concerned about ethics in their jobs, but, in their alternative persona as football fans, these people could insult him. The teacher and scientist resented football fans who approved, tacitly or directly, the game's ethical violations in academics and doping, thusly pushing professionals like himself to forego integrity.

"Their morals really are not affected like the morals of faculty," Yesalis said, "because they're wanting *us* to be pimps, so they can enjoy their entertainment. They're asking us to pass these people along, to pretend that they're true student-athletes. They really don't care, as long as there aren't huge scandals that can't be swept under the rug. It doesn't bother them that faculty are agreeing willingly to go along with the system, or pressure, or whatever. Because they value the entertainment more than the other. And it's not their integrity actually besmirched. It's *mine*."

The view fans held for football aligned with that of writers, a dynamic of no coincidence. The public's values for football, framed in themes that never threatened the institution itself, were manifest in media stories because fans demanded it. Among daily calls or e-mails to a newspaper, for example, complaints and requests over football content could exceed all inquiry, topping those regarding crime, education, government, or religion.

Miklasz said fans of major-college teams were particularly vigilant, if not belligerent, in their see-no-evil attitude, and writing was impacted. "The pull is to put on a happy face and sort of go along with the crowd," Miklasz said, "and you make your readers happier that way." The topic of doping on college football teams was not entirely avoided by sports writers. National publicity had generated around steroid scandals at Vanderbilt, South Carolina, and Notre Dame, but little was made of significant allegations involving dozens of other programs, including Southern California, Texas, Oklahoma, and Michigan State.

At any level in football, the journalist's task was daunting for investigating the use of anabolic substances. Scant hard evidence existed for such stories, if any, and officials released little information willingly. In a college town where a probe targeted a revered team, the reporter could expect stiff resistance led by powerful alumni and other boosters. "It creates mostly grief when you stick your nose in and get a little dirty by going after a story that might not be so pretty to readers, and especially fans of a particular institution or team," Miklasz said. "I don't know that as a business it pays off to pursue these stories."

Certainly not, said New York author Robert Lipsyte, a former sportswriter who compiled *SportsWorld*, unprecedented criticism of sport media and business released in 1975. Decades later, Lipsyte said sportswriters, broadcasters, and editors still did not qualify for journalism, highly overrated in itself as a public trust. "I hate to piss on sports press, specifically," Lipsyte said in 2007, "because I've seen how city hall press, and White House press, foreign press, all operate. And they will very often pull their punches because they want future access, or in the case of Judy Miller, some kind of combination of careerism and ideology. It leads you into incredibly unethical behavior. But I think that… you have to almost immediately discount television, most of television, because they're *co-owners*. They're absolutely financially in bed with the sport-industrial complex."

Print media could be just as bad, warned Lipsyte, a former *Times* sports columnist, especially beat reporters too comfortable with the athletes and officials they cover daily. "I was never really a beat reporter, but I shoulda been smarter in the '60's, when I was going into pro-football locker rooms and figuring, 'Oh, well, the guys have pimples on their shoulders because the shoulder pads are chafing them.' Yeah, right. But I didn't know better [about steroids], and I didn't keep going in. And of course now we have the example in another sport, of all these baseball writers, ya know, writing their mea culpas: 'Yeah, I shoulda known. Yeah, I shoulda been on it.' Bullshit. I mean, it's kind of a combination of denial, not wanting to believe what you're seeing, being a fan at heart. Ya know, like all the guys now who are viciously attacking Mark McGwire, who were jerking off over him in 1998, the Summer of Swat."

The selective moralizing by sport media, their pretense as a public watchdog applied inconsistently to individuals only, was their historic fatal flaw, Lipsyte charged, and completely revealing of a business agenda to please the general American consumer. The topic of performance-enhancing drugs was a prime example. "On the one hand, you have the media, which take such moralistic postures on [doping]," Lipsyte said. "On the other hand, you have athletes, who, in my experience, have never seen drug use as an ethical issue."

Lipsyte understood anabolic steroids on a personal level, as a testicular cancer survivor who had injected testosterone for 35 years. "So in some ways — and now I lose my media card — in some ways, it's a good thing. Certainly, we're talking about a medicine here, ya know? So the point is that I don't think the media was either aware of this or wanted to be aware, of any of this. And they are still locked in to some sort of 19th century idea of a level playing field. Well, that's kind of bullshit. What's a level playing field? And how can there be a level playing field? ... The media has kind of locked into these outworn concepts."

Sport in America was long distorted into a dangerous, economic power that exploited children, Lipsyte charged. "Certainly we indoctrinate kids, and condition kids, with the values and definitions of sport, which then go from field house to White House," he said. "I write young-adult novels, that's always been the other strand of my career, and I have a new book out called *Raiders Night*. It's a young-adult novel about football which has been banned in a lot of places, not so much for the fucking and the drugs and all that stuff, but for the *dark look* at high-school sports, which is becoming a real revenue center for a lot of districts around the country."

Media accepted crass commercialization in Hollywood, including abuse of child actors, but that was unacceptable for prep athletics, at least according to sportswriters, lawmakers, and special interests. "For some reason, there's the idea that some sort of magic in club sports helps condition the kids," Lipsyte observed. "Nobody is saying that the way Jack Nicholson fucks around is damaging the moral fiber of America. But they *are* saying, ya know, that steroids will wreck us."

Football Culture Blames The Individual, But Courson Perseveres

During the 1990s, media analysts criticized sportswriters for their shoddy coverage of anabolic substances in American athletics, especially football. A fault, critics said, was media's penchant to blame only individuals for the problem, completely absolving systems such as the NFL and the NCAA, powerful private enterprises of football spectacle subsidized by taxpayers.

In a graduate thesis study of print coverage on muscle doping in football from 1983 through 1999, by this book's author, the primary finding was that sportswriters generally viewed the problem as organizers portrayed it: individual in nature, involving isolated players who cheated, with the institution having no culpability whatsoever.

"That was the strategy of journalism and sport in what I think was a willing collaboration," Yesalis said. "In the large majority of sports journalism on this issue, the focus is on the so-called few bad apples among athletes."

As football's rampant abuse of anabolics escalated unchecked, any insider talking openly on the subject invited trouble, particularly the relative few players who did so in the public eye. These athletes had to expect hits in press stories; after all, it was their own choosing to use anabolic steroids to enhance performance. Users who were willing to come forward were also prone to malicious attacks by writers — ignorant, unethical, or both — who compiled narratives that blatantly protected the football organizations.

No one individual player absorbed more blame, for systemic muscle doping in American football, than did Steve Courson. He was the first active NFL player to break the league's rigid code of silence on steroids, fully disclosing in 1985 his long-time use as a lineman for the Steelers and Buccaneers. For an historic first-person account in *SI*, Courson, a 6-1, 285-pound offensive guard at Tampa, told writer Jill Lieber, "A lot of guys won't talk about their steroid use. They won't even tell their wives. I'm talking about it because I don't want to be hypocritical, because I believe in telling the truth." Courson spent a dozen hours with Lieber, speaking on-record about the widespread use of steroids in the NFL, especially among linemen, although he discussed only himself. Courson also contemplated the possibility of suffering adverse health effects in the future. "But you do what you have to do, otherwise you don't have your job," he said.

Twenty years later, Courson was a corporate fitness trainer and foremost lay expert on doping in sport and society, busy granting interviews, researching, writing, and speaking. He had been through a lot, however, since Lieber's story, and his trials began with the premature end to his NFL career, specifically an apparent blacklisting by the league. He suffered a life-threatening heart ailment and lost a 1990s disability claim against the NFL and union, becoming an unpopular figure with the press, amid a decade of zenith popularity for the league. Courson was always subject to misinterpretation — or misrepresentation — for his progressive, well-researched writings and statements on performance-enhancing substances in culture, not merely sport. Many writers, ill-informed or outright sycophantic to football, automatically ignored Courson's testimony and other evidence and narrowed blame strictly upon his shoulders.

From the late 1980s through the 1990s, Courson was made an example by the forces of football spectacle, the organizers, coaches, players, sycophant media, and fans in contempt of the message he brought out. Courson told America its beloved sport of football was rife with muscle doping, and the messenger got pummeled, particularly in Pittsburgh. "When it came to the Super Steelers, they were treated with an almost manaical reverence, and still are," said Yesalis, a close friend of Courson. "And Steve was just pilloried." Courson made anti-steroid presentations and outlined the fallacy of NFL drug testing, and fans confronted him, including children. Refusing to accept his evidence, Courson's detractors offered none to refute him. They just did not want to hear the truth.

In media study, the case of Courson was textbook for the theoretical spiral of silence, wherein one who openly addresses a taboo topic is met with negative fallout. Within a spiral of silence surrounding football, a forbidden subject such as anabolic doping is broached at peril for the messenger. Courson broke the football code and took the wrath; he messed with The Spectacle.

"Right, I understand that," Courson said in 2005. "But why did I mess with The Spectacle? I think my reasons were very sound. ... I look at what I did while I was still playing, and it had negative repercussions. And people say that. But there are times in your life where you've got to speak your piece. That's the thing right now, is finally I feel like I'm experiencing vindication. Because it's not a money issue with me. It's an issue of honor. And I feel like the system dishonored me for being truthful."

Football did not break the righteous Courson, and no one was taking cheap shots anymore. A peaceful, articulate man, Courson talked at his log-cabin home in mountainous southwestern Pennsylvania. This was no luxurious lodge, and Courson possessed modest means. He had what he needed. An avid outdoorsman, the woods were at his door, and always nearby were Courson's companion black Labradors, Rufus and Rachel, both as big and friendly as he. Stacked and stowed around the little house were his research items on doping, a PC with Internet, news and journal articles, books, photographs and more. There was no visible evidence anywhere of Courson's glory in football, other than two gold Super Bowls rings on his fingers.

Once reviled by the press, Courson was respected by sportswriters, locally and nationally, and he appreciated his due respect, even when it buried him during hot news cycles for doping stories, such as baseball. His phone rang constantly then, from media and others seeking insight. "It's a huge difference," he said, smiling. "I'm no longer on the defensive. I don't have to be."

Courson saw tremors shaking football's foundation again because BALCO showed the public that current urinalysis was inept to stop cheating through designer steroids, low-dose testosterone, and HGH. It showed that athletes were involved from several sports, including the NFL, and Courson was not surprised. If anything, he expected more bad news to surface from American football, because of its long-time reliance on muscle dope and other substances for performance by athletes.

"What I've been trying to get across in this seemingly endless education process of the public, the main emphasis — and the purpose of my book, *False Glory* — was to show that it was equally institutionalized as much as it was individualized," Courson said. "And that had a personal note to it, because I was tired of being labeled as some kind of jerk when I knew I was telling the absolute truth. The system is not blameless here. Nobody wanted to deal with it, although they're being forced to now. BALCO is helping that. But my mission now is not so much to hammer that drumbeat, as it is to make sure people understand that I was right in that assumption *but incomplete* in that assumption. Because [anabolics use] is more *societal* than it is institutional. And that's the real issue."

Concern for users of any type prompted Courson, but the thought of children at risk motivated him most. That really drove him to go on-record with *SI* as a younger man, and, in middle age at 49 with no children, Courson's will for the cause was stronger than ever, and for good reason. Time was running out for any effort against abuse of anabolic substances, not only in games, but throughout the culture. The substances were pervasive and gene doping was ahead, a new form of muscle enhancement that experts predicted could be employed by the 2008 Olympics. In addition, studies were showing that people's pursuit of improved looks had overtaken athletic performance as the top reason for using steroids and other PED's in the United States.

Back in the 1960s, American athletes in track and field and football knew anabolics answered their need for physical power. By 2005, a society obsessed with "look-ism" wanted the drugs for altering physical image. Children, young adults, the middle-aged and older were consuming massive inventories of anabolic substances — legal and illegal steroids, growth hormone, and more — in their quest to look better, feel better.

Researchers believed at least one million school-age children in America had cycled on anabolic steroids, including upwards of 100,000 eighth-graders, or about 2.5 percent nationally. In a shift of dominant trend, the mechanism in most cases was teen vanity, not a desire for improving athletic performance. Children understood anabolics were available and recognized juicer models in person and indirectly. Media content was chock full of chemically augmented people, or imagery, from sports to music, movies, television shows, and advertisements. Children knew what they were seeing, hearing, and reading; one study found 50 percent believed their athletic heroes were on steroids, as part of the fake sheen covering icons throughout culture.

Courson saw danger in adolescent awareness, the potential for use, of course, but also the cultural hypocrisy teaching deception, denial for responding to a complex issue. "What is the greatest dishonor? The fact that athletes used drugs, or the fact that athletes use drugs and we pretend they don't?" he said.

Courson did detect a reckoning for football spectacle, despite protective forces in society. "Here's what the NFL's facing right now... " he said. "It is an organization which holds cities hostage for franchises. They basically have priced the average fan out of the stadium. They are making obscene amounts of money — owners, players, and announcers — at a time when people are struggling financially. The game's violence is at an all-time high. At the same time, the size and speed have gotten insane, into an unbelievable realm for what I call athletic parameters, because of [muscle doping]. They basically have drug testing as a public-relations shield, and most people know that, OK?

"Then, baseball entering at this time, the hearings before Congress, has raised the public's awareness to how the institution of sport lies about this problem, to see how embarrassed the baseball players and the owners were in Congress. It was a total sham. They had no credibility whatsoever. It's the age we live in. And [the evasion] formerly involved the little nuances where the public wasn't educated about steroids. Now the public has learned much about steroids through what's gone on in baseball with McGwire and Bonds.

"Plainly, on the radio, I've heard repeatedly that we can't test for growth hormone and designer steroids. I mean, I wrote about that how long ago? Chuck [Yesalis] has been saying it for how long? And now you're hearing it commonly said, consistently. ... Then, here's the other thing about all of this: One side of the coin you have a million teenagers using steroids. And the other side, performance-wise, we have genetic engineering. It ain't a pretty picture."

Courson's honesty, his accurately portraying the picture of football doping over the previous decades, had cost him. He likely lost NFL career time, a season or two minimally, and personal bridges were burned, snuffing out opportunities and damaging friendships. Courson maintained decent relations with former teammates in western Pennsylvania, all things considered, but he was the odd man out among Super Steelers. "I understand why, and I don't put them down for that," he said.

Even though Courson had named no one for steroids, a certain uneasiness loomed over encounters with former teammates, such as at the 2004 Dapper Dan sports banquet in Pittsburgh. "What I read in some of them, especially some of ex-teammates who are more active in their community and churches — and they were [steroid] users — they're really uncomfortable around me, because they know what I know," Courson said. "And it's like, I'm not going to say anything, but I know I make them uneasy in their walk because they're not admitting the truth. And they're unable to."

The Super Steelers still included Courson in their event plans. Mel Blount, a Hall of Fame defensive back who led charity drives around Pittsburgh, invited Courson to his upcoming celebrity roast, but Courson would not attend because of the tension his presence created. "I'm not going to do that to them," he said. "They chose to live the myth, you know. I can't help it."

In late March 2005, former NFL player Jim Haslett ruffled the Super Steelers by alleging, inaccurately, that they pioneered steroid use in the league during the 1970s. Haslett, head coach of the New Orleans Saints and a Pittsburgh native, discussed his own use of steroids around 1980 as a Buffalo linebacker. Haslett estimated 50 percent of NFL players in the 1980s used steroids, including all linemen. "It started, really, in Pittsburgh," Haslett told Ed Bouchette of *The Post-Gazette*. "They got an advantage on a lot of football teams. They were so much stronger [in the] late'70s, early '80s... Steve [Courson], Jon [Kolb] and all those guys. They're the ones who kind of started it."

Courson laughed heartily, reading he was a godfather of steroid use in the NFL; Haslett's revised history completely omitted the 1960s and true pioneers such as strength coach Alvin Roy and the Chargers. "OK, Haslett was misguided in a couple of his points, but he was just trying to speak his mind on what the truth is," Courson said, his phone ringing non-stop. "I admire Jim's honesty and laud his courage. ... "It's been an interesting week around here, kind of crazy. Haslett's remarks lit the fire a little bit."

The fireworks featured Steelers owner Dan Rooney's taking shots at Haslett —

who apologized to the franchise — and his defending former head coach Chuck Noll regarding steroids. "Chuck Noll was totally against it," Rooney contended. "He looked into it, examined it, talked to people. Haslett, maybe it affected his mind."

Rooney's damage control had little of the intended effect around Pittsburgh, where some media members, prompted by Haslett, once again hammered the Super Steelers and their fans. Courson's book was standing tall now, detailing how most of his old crew of Steelers O-linemen pounded iron and abused 'roids, amphetamines, painkillers, and alcohol. *False Glory* shone in contemporary light at Pittsburgh, where historic alteration was underway for the fantasy themes of football. Now doping was forever part of the Steelers stories too, joining the established narratives promoting virtue, teamwork, and greatness.

Post-Gazette columnist Ron Cook ripped local football fandom and the entire NFL spectacle. The Super Steelers "were our heroes," he wrote. "They were our heroes. They won four Super Bowls. They made us proud. It wasn't the steroids. It was all talent and hard work. That's our story and we're sticking to it." Cook challenged believers to pick up Courson's book published in 1991. "It was a fascinating read then and is even more fascinating now. Courson, who played for the Steelers from 1977-83, detailed his and his teammates' steroids use.

"If you're looking for another Jose Canseco tell-all book, you're going to be disappointed. Courson did not name names. He didn't out teammates the way Canseco did to McGwire. The purpose of his book wasn't so much to make money as it was to shine a light on a longstanding NFL problem and maybe, in the process, educate a few young athletes about steroids. He had made national headlines six years earlier by admitting his steroid use in *Sports Illustrated*."

Courson was amazed by Cook's commentary, seeing his words of 14 years ago resonate "like a delayed-action fuse," he said. "I mean, Cook's commentary basically outed the Steeler organization. Nothing can get at the legend more than that, and the writer put his own ass out there, too."

A few days later, juicy details of the Panthers' steroid scandal were broadcast on *60 Minutes Wednesday*, and the NFL had joined baseball within the nation's contemporary focus on sport doping. Congress requested drug-testing records from the NFL, NCAA, NBA, and other federations in preparation for a capitol hearing.

Football's hard-core sycophant media were ready, and they emerged again in defiant defense of the game. For a commentary on *ESPN.com*, senior NFL writer Len Pasquarelli criticized Congress for worrying about football and steroids, contending lawmakers should be concerned with other national issues. He opined that the NFL and commissioner Paul Tagliabue "long ago took care of business in regards to steroids." Pasquarelli was smug in taking the NFL merely at its word on the issue. "[T]o suggest that the NFL has a serious steroid problem, because of the allegations that originated in Columbia, S.C., involving some Carolina Panthers players, is perhaps even more despicable than the contentions of the '70s that the entire league was juicing up," he wrote.

Pittsburgh's education in Steelers and steroids notwithstanding, the football spectacle held firm across America. Devout fans, including writers like Pasquarelli, were determined to maintain the mythology of goodness, but football players and more impressionable youths knew better, Courson argued, constituting a definite national issue. "The myth, it's wonderful for the storyline and the entertainment," he said, "but those who are training, or who aspire to be part of this, they know the reality. Because it's been around too long."

For delusional adults, Courson posed some points: "Do we really care that our mercenary millionaire athletes are doing this to entertain us? No. Do we care about the fact that some of our school kids are emulating that? Yep, we should. And that's where we're at. One million-plus kids are doing steroids, and, bio-technically, we're on the doorstep of genetic engineering. If we can't wake up now, we can't wake up."

IV. Game Plays On, Until No Time Left on The Clock

In just four months, six former NFL players died in their 40s of natural causes, from Christmas 2004 through mid-April 2005: Reggie White, Charles Martin, Reggie Roby, Todd Bell, David Little, and Sam Mills. Ailments included heart disease and cancer. Steve Courson had his suspicions, considering the dead as a group, particularly because all had played as large specimens for their frames. The giantism of modern football concerned him foremost, body frames with excessive mass ranging to 150 percent above recommended weight on the body mass index scale.

Regardless how added weight was acquired, and whether it be fat or muscle, Courson was sure health consequences and even death were becoming manifest in some players, retired and active. "What I fear about the NFL, the bodies are just going to implode," he said. "Especially now that we're on the doorstep of genetic engineering. We're walking into a very scary bio-technical world." The modern game's terrible contact injuries had to be expected, Courson said. "The size and speed denominators are just getting nuts. Modern training combined with the advances in pharmacology, you're creating missiles and weapons of a different dimension."

Courson predicted a collision death for contemporary pro football, and exactly one week later it happened, claiming a 26-year-old player in the Arena Football League.

Sunday afternoon, April 10, 2005, the Los Angeles Avengers hosted the New York Dragons before 11,000 spectators in the Staples Center. During a first-quarter kickoff, Avengers lineman and team leader Al Lucas, 6-foot-1, 300 pounds, was struck in the head while making a tackle. Lucas lay motionless with a severed spinal cord as trainers and medical personnel tended to him. Worried teammates looked on, some kneeling in prayer. After 10 minutes on the carpet, Lucas, a husband and father, was immobilized and removed from the field.

Football reality thusly witnessed, play resumed immediately, the shared fantasy rolling on in the arena. A referee blew his whistle, two teams huddled up, and fans awaited the next snap. The Spectacle was so strong.

Around halftime of the game in progress, Lucas was pronounced dead at a hospital in Los Angeles. Later, the Avengers won, 66-35, and Lucas' teammates were finally informed of his passing, "creating a tearful scene in the corridors outside the locker room, with players and employees leaving the arena dazed by the news," reported Chris Foster for the *Los Angeles Times*.

"I just wish this was a bad dream," said Avengers receiver Tony Locke. "I want it to be over."

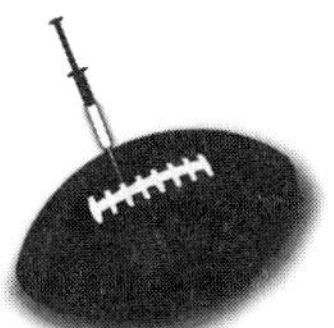

REFERENCES

Anderson, S. (2004, November 7). '79 Steelers found a home right here. *Pittsburgh Post-Gazette* [Online].

Anderson, S. (2004, November 8). '79 Steelers like current team. *Pittsburgh Post-Gazette* [Online].

Arena Death. (2005, April 11). Football player dies during Arena game. *Kansas City Star*, p. C2.

Berger, K. (2005, April 1). Congress to probe NFL testing. *Newsday* [Online].

Bernstein, V. (2005, March 30). NFL is seeking tougher steroid rules. *New York Times* [Online].

Bormann, E.G. (1985). Symbolic convergence theory. *Journal of Communication, 35* (4), p. 128.

Bouchette, E. (2005, March 24). Haslett admits to using steroids. *Pittsburgh Post-Gazette* [Online].

CHS Yearbook. (1967). *Blue Jay*. Charleston, MO: Charleston High School.

CHS Yearbook. (1968). *Blue Jay*. Charleston, MO: Charleston High School.

Chaney, M. (2001). *Sports writers, American football, and anti-sociological bias toward anabolic drug use in the sport*. Warrensburg, MO: Central Missouri State University.

Chaney, M. (2004, November 7). Corporate welfare for stadiums burdens Missouri. *Sedalia Democrat*, p. 16.

Christopher, H. Jr. (2004, January 25). Sports station guru reveals play book. *Kansas City Star*, p. E2.

Christopher, H. Jr. (2004, February 6). Mad counter wants to dim Plaza lights numbers. *Kansas City Star*, p. E3.

Coach Firings. (2004, December 22). UNK study finds increase in high school coach firings. *The Associated Press* [Wire].

Cook. R. (2005, March 27). '70s Steelers are guilty like Bonds. *Pittsburgh Post-Gazette* [Online].

Cooper, A. (2005, March 30). Steroids and the NFL. *CBS 60 Minutes Wednesday* [broadcast].

Courson, S. (1988, November 14). Steroids. *Sports Illustrated* [Online].

Courson, S. (1991). *False Glory*. Stamford, CT: Longmeadow Press.

Courson, S. (2005, March 7). Interview with author. Farmington, PA.

Courson, S. (2005, March 16). Telephone interview with author.

Courson, S. (2005, March 20). Telephone interview with author.

Courson, S. (2005, March 27). Telephone interview with author.

Courson, S. (2005, April 3). Telephone interview with author.

Courson, S. (2005, May 12). E-mail correspondence to author.

Courson, S. (2005, June 5). E-mail correspondence to author.

Courson, S. (2005, June 22). Telephone interview with author.

Devaney, J. (1971). *Super Bowl!* New York: Random House.

Dunn, M. (1989, July 10). Athletes' drug use could tax short organ supply. *The Associated*

Press [Online].

Fabregas, L. (2002, September 28). Webster's death fueling steroids speculation. *Pittsburgh Tribune-Review* [Online].

Finder, C. (2004, November 7). Former Steeler Courson at heart of big turnaround. *Pittsburgh Post-Gazette* [Online].

Finder, C. (2005, March 13). Webster's estate will tackle disability rulings. *Pittsburgh Post-Gazette* [Online].

Finder, C. (2005, March 14). Attorney is a staunch defender of the Plan. *Pittsburgh Post-Gazette* [Online].

Finder, C. (2004, March 14). Steve Courson — Witness without a hearing. *Pittsburgh Post-Gazette* [Online].

Finder, C. (2005, March 16). Steve Courson — Steroids and society. *Pittsburgh Post-Gazette* [Online].

Finder, C. (2005, March 20). The surveys say steroids affect kids more and more. *Pittsburgh Post-Gazette* [Online].

Finder, C. (2005, April 27). Webster estate beats NFL in benefits case, but appeal seems likely. *Pittsburgh Post-Gazette* [Online].

Finder, C. (2006, December 14). Appeals panel gives Websters win in disability case. *Pittsburgh Post-Gazette* [Online].

Flaccus, G. (2005, April 12). Avengers teammates remember Al Lucas. *The Associated Press* [Online].

Foster, C. (2005, April 11). Arena football player dies after injury. *Los Angeles Times* [Online].

Freeman, M. (1999, August 30). Tapes show that NFL looked the other way on drug tests. *New York Times* [Online].

Funk, K. (2000). Faculty group seeks reform for athletes. *Kansas City Star*, p. C1.

Garber, G. (2005, January 24). A tormented soul. *ESPN.com* [Online].

Garber, G. (2005, January 25). Blood and guts. *ESPN.com* [Online].

Garber, G. (2005, January 26). Man on the moon. *ESPN.com* [Online].

Garber, G. (2005, January 27). Wandering through the fog. *ESPN.com* [Online].

Garber, G. (2005, January 28). Sifting through the ashes. *ESPN.com* [Online].

Glauber, B. (2005, March 15). NFL to help DEA investigation of steroid doctor. *Newsday* [Online].

Goldberg, D. (2005, March 30). NFL wants upgraded steroid test standard. *The Associated Press* [Online].

Haslett Talks. (2005, March 24). Saints' Haslett says he tried steroids. *NFL.com* [Online].

Hilliard, D. (1994, February). Televised sports and the (anti) sociological imagination. *Journal of Sport & Social Issues* [Online].

Jenkins, D. (1983, December 11). Letter to editor. *New York Times*, p. 5 — 2.

Keteyian, A. (1998, August). Mass deception. *Sport* [Online].

Kaufman, M. (1990, September 14). Wisecracks aside, being a woman sportswriter is still a great job. *Detroit Free Press*, p. 11D.

Knapp, G. (1997, September 16). Football is a guilty pleasure. *San Francisco Examiner* [Online].

Koppett, L. (1981). *Sports illusion, sports reality.* Urbana and Chicago, IL: University of Illinois Press.

Lieber, J. (1985, May 13). Getting physical — And chemical. *Sports Illustrated*, p. 50.

Lipsyte, R. (1975). *SportsWorld.* New York, NY: Quadrangle Books.

Long Confesses. (1991, December 4). Long admits using steroids. *The Associated Press* [Online].

Luder, B. (2001, January 22). Not just fun & games. *Kansas City Star*, p. C1.

Madden, M. (2005, March 25). Were the Super Steelers 'roided up? *wtaeradio.com* [Online].

McChesney, R.W. (1989). Media made sport. In Wenner, L.A. (Ed.), *Media, sports, & society* (p. 49). Newbury Park, CA: Sage Publications.

Michener, J. (1976). *Sports in America.* New York: Random House.

Miklasz, B. (1996, December 2). Telephone interview with author.

Mueller, F.O., & Diehl, J.L. (2004). *Annual survey of football injury research.* Chapel Hill, NC: National Center for Catastrophic Sport Injury Research. [Online].

Murray, K. (2005, March 30). Steroid heat now turns to NFL. *Baltimore Sun* [Online].

Myers, G. (2005, March 30). NFL not flying below steroid radar screen anymore. *New York Daily News* [Online].

NFL Survey. (1999, February). National Football League players survey. *Sport* [Online].

Noelle-Neuman, E. (1995). Public opinion and rationality. In Glasser, T.L., & Salmon, C.T. (Eds.), *Public opinion and the communication of consent* (p. 33). New York, NY: Guilford Press.

Oriard, M. (1982). *End of Autumn.* Garden City, NY: Doubleday & Company, Inc.

Oriard, M. (1983, November 20). Why football injuries remain a part of the game. *New York Times* [Online].

Oriard, M. (1983, December 11). Response to letter to editor. *New York Times* [Online].

Oriard, M. (1993). *Reading Football.* Chapel Hill, NC: The University of North Carolina Press.

Oriard, M. (2001). Football glory and education are a team no more. *New York Times*, p. 8 — 11.

Oriard, M. (2008, September 2). E-mail correspondence to author.

Pasquarelli, L. (2005, April 1). Tagliabue, NFL won't be fazed. *ESPN.com* [Online].

Passon, J. (2006, February 4). Super Bowl memorable moments. *Kansas City Star*, p. D4.

Rock, S. (1997, October 8). NCAA doesn't require medical supervision. *Kansas City Star*, p. A1.

Rogers, T. (1985, May 17). Altered state. New York Times, p. A22.

Ross, B. Jr. (2004, December 18). 'Holy huddle' helps football fans keep the faith. *The Associated Press* [Wire].

Sabol, S. (1994). *The legendary voice of John Facenda.* NFL Films.

Shapiro, L., & Maske, M. (2005, March 31). NFL looks to shore up drug policy.

Washington Post, p. D3.
Shaw, G. (1972). *Meat on the hoof.* New York: St. Martin's Press.
Steigerwald, J. (2002, September 28). Silence surrounding Webster deafening. *Pittsburgh Tribune-Review* [Online].
Steroids Prescribed. (2005, March 29). Steroids prescribed to NFL players. *CBSNEWS.com* [Online].
Tagliabue Talks. (2005, March 22). Tagliabue: Talks at 'dead end.' *The Associated Press* [Online].
Telander, R. (1989). *The hundred yard lie.* New York, NY: Simon and Schuster.
T.R. Speaks. (1997, October 8). Overheard. *Kansas City Star*, p. A8.
Weiner, E. (2005, April 1). Congress should leave NFL alone. *NBCSports.com* [Online].
Wenner, L.A. (Ed.) (1989). *Media, sports, & society.* Newbury Park, CA: Sage Publications.
Yesalis, C.E. (2005, January 22). Telephone interview with author.
Yesalis, C.E. (2005, March 23). Telephone interview with author.

Chapter 4 [The '80s
Muscle doping in football, 1980-86]

"If me and King Kong went into an alley, only one of us would come out, and it wouldn't be the f---ing monkey."

Lyle Alzado
NFL lineman, circa 1980s

Steve Courson strode into the Pittsburgh neighborhood drugstore, looking huge and menacing, in gym shorts and tank top. Other customers gawked at Courson's massiveness, the muscles bulging on muscles — *He's a Steeler*, they assured each other, noting the Super Bowl rings — but he paid them no mind. Though gentlemanly, respectful of people, Courson was in no mood for pleasantries or even eye contact; it was the NFL offseason, 1982, and he had come to the pharmacy to purchase anabolic steroids.

No steroid prescription was required, not for Steelers at this drugstore. Courson quietly scanned the inventory, reading labels on plastic bottles and boxes of vials, asking nothing of the compliant pharmacist hovering nearby. This football player needed no advice about juicin'. He knew exactly what he wanted, ordering plenty of steroids for himself, his O-line teammates, and his power-lifting friends.

Into the shopping bag went Dianabol, Anavar, and Anadrol in pill form, and for injectibles, Deca-Durabolin, Winstrol V, and the testosterone esters cypionate and propionate. Courson picked out other compounds, human chorionic gonadotropin to stimulate testosterone production, antiestrogens to counter side effects of cycling on anabolic androgens; he then finished with a box of hypodermic needle-syringes. Courson wrote a personal check for the total amount, grabbed up the bulging bag, and walked out.

For football fans around that pharmacy, the NFL's ever-growing problem with muscle doping in the 1980s was as apparent as Courson's physique. Fans, however, ignored what this scene really meant. They just admired a young athlete and his sport.

Decades later, a middle-aged Steve Courson shook his head at the thought. "Can you imagine the sight of me back in those days, about 285 all ripped-out, coming out of the pharmacy? I'd walk out with a shopping bag full [of steroids]," he said. "Nowadays, people would be like, 'What are you doing?' Back then, nobody had a clue."

At the time, Courson and other Steelers were immersed in off-season weightlifting and, like a multitude of NFL players representing every team, cycling on anabolic steroids. They were preparing for the coming season, but pros like Courson would also enter a made-for-TV event dominated by the Steelers, the strongest-man competition for NFL players.

Moreover, Courson was amid a chemical breakthrough, perfecting his acquired science of "stacking" steroids in combinations for maximum muscle-building. In eight years since college football, Courson had cycled a half-dozen times, never in-season nor more than once annually, and always at or near therapeutic dosage levels. "The first year I competed in the strongest-man competition [1981], I cycled on D-bol and Deca; it was really light," he recalled. "The following year, '82, was the first year I hiked it up pretty good."

Courson mixed testosterones with potent anabolics such as Winstrol and Anavar, concocting a special tissue-pumping synergy. Consuming pills and taking injections like never before, he experienced abdominal cramps and increased irritability, but the performance enhancement paid immediate dividends for his particular job: Courson added about 15 pounds in lean body mass and his strength shot up. When bench-pressing 405 pounds, Courson increased from 6 repetitions to an astounding 14. "That taught me. I learned something there," Courson said of the accelerated cycling. "That's when I definitely knew that no matter what I did training-wise, there was nothing that I could do to compare to this. I was totally sold. There was just no way to train to match that."

Players everywhere were figuring it out, including at colleges and high schools. Any period of "isolated" steroid use in higher competitive football was over, if that had ever held longer than briefly at any level. The chemical-arms race was on, thoroughly covering leagues from the colleges to the pros, and hitting hard at high schools. Many users had advanced beyond cowboy chemistry. In the NFL, steroid sophisticates like Courson were becoming common. "They were on many [teams]," he recalled. "At the time, the early '80s, I was savvy... I knew the game. I understood it. I read about it. I wouldn't just pop needles into my butt without thinking."

In his autobiography, Courson declared "unequivocally" that 75 percent of his offensive line mates in Pittsburgh used anabolic steroids at least once. Courson, a Steeler from 1977 to 1984, named no names, but media reports would confirm other period linemen in Pittsburgh, Jim Clack, Mike Webster, Rick Donalley, and Terry Long, while implicating Jon Kolb and Steve Furness.

Rival NFL players called Pittsburgh the "Steroid Team," but league-wide abuse rendered that charge hypocritical. Every season in Dallas, for example, the Cowboys' Super Bowl hopes relied not so much on the skills of Coach Tom Landry as on numerous drug-using players, from "yoking-up" linemen to "dabbler" backfield players. Landry's strength program had a confirmed steroid user as a coach, and at least one of his juicing players was bound for Canton, the Pro Football Hall of Fame. Decades later, media and politicians fretted, rather fashionably, over muscle doping's effects on records in *baseball* — after winning in pro football was affected through the TV age. "It was everywhere," Courson said in 2005. "Back then [the 1980s], it was so wide open. That's why for people to deny it was out there, you had to live in a bubble."

Offensive linemen were not the only culprits. Defensive stars of the period said to have used steroids in varying degrees included Bills linebacker Jim Haslett and Cowboys safety Charlie Waters, along with linemen Joe Klecko and Mark Gastineau of the Jets, Randy White and John Dutton of the Cowboys, Steve McMichael of the

Bears, and Lyle Alzado, who played for the Broncos, Browns, and Raiders.

Klecko discussed steroids for the 1989 book *Nose to Nose*, which he authored with former Jets teammate Joe Fields and sportswriter Greg Logan. Klecko estimated a large majority of offensive and defensive linemen used steroids, and he believed the training method "became commonplace in the NFL in the late seventies and increased during the next decade to the point where it became a major health issue," the book stated. Klecko added, "I can't prove it, but based on my experience, I'd say there were a high number of steroid users."

Many more NFL insiders of the time corroborated Courson and Klecko about steroid prevalence, collectively portraying that a significant amount of players used, if not a majority.

There existed no steroid policy. The league, franchises, union, and players had done nothing to curb anabolic steroids' spread in the game, since the drugs' arrival in the early 1960s. Management, in fact, had long publicly purported that performance-enhancing drugs were under control in the league, a problem of the past, and were not proven to work. "Amphetamine and steroid use in the NFL is said to be down dramatically from the early '70s. This was due in large part to game films, players seeing that they actually were being hindered rather than helped by drugs in games," *Washington Post* sports columnist Ken Denlinger reported inaccurately in July 1982, as monsters like Courson and Klecko headed to training camps.

In reality, NFL players relied heavily on performance enhancers, especially steroids, painkillers, "speed," and more so than ever before, whether or not writers and fans could believe it. "I don't regret anything I've done as far as pharmaceutical use is concerned," Courson told *Sports Illustrated* in 1985. "It's very easy for people on the outside to criticize. But it's different when it's your livelihood, when it's your job to keep a genetic mutation from getting into your backfield."

The jungle was only getting deeper, for survival of the fittest in football. The anabolic era was flying out of control, forever perhaps, and many players were preparing themselves, becoming equipped, to whip King Kong.

I. Steroid Issue Fires Up on NFL Advisor's Letter

In late August 1983, doping controversy struck at the Pan American Games in Caracas, Venezuela, where new urinalysis was unveiled for detecting testosterone levels. The upgraded steroid testing surprised athletes and coaches, and 15 competitors tested positive, mostly weightlifters. Even more athletes withdrew from the games before facing testing, led by a dozen Americans who checked out and returned home, inviting press attention.

In the United States, athletes were regulars in drug news, but for street narcotics, not performance enhancers. And while steroids and amphetamines were commonly accepted within American sports, news accounts reaching the public were scattered; fewer still, accurately depicted the reality of the big picture.

The Caracas scandal was met in America by anger. Stark facts were exposed about doping, tainting U.S. track and field, and speculation quickly moved to other sports. Football players were obvious suspects, and a big story broke in New York on the NFL.

The Times obtained an internal letter by the league's medical advisor, Dr. Walter F. Riker, Jr., who wrote that he believed use of anabolic steroids to be "extensive among football players at all levels." Reporter Michael Janofsky contacted active NFL players for a story. With no drug policy and sanctions in place, players were able to discuss doping freely, and several told Janofsky steroid use was a part of pro football, occurring mostly among offensive linemen, defensive linemen, and linebackers.

"Sure, it's being done," said Jeff Van Note, Falcons center and president of the NFL Players Association. "You would have to be naïve to believe they're not being used." Van Note said he did not view the matter as a problem, but "more a quiet thing." Tom Condon, Chiefs' offensive guard, said, "Usually the people who need to hold their weight, the people in the big-man positions, are the ones who would take it."

Two players requesting anonymity spoke with Janofsky. "I've used them under a doctor's care and made great gains," said a Raiders lineman. "I wouldn't consider it a dangerous drug. But I would consider it, in some ways, damaging if misused." A defensive player on the Chargers had recently changed positions, needing massive weight fast to keep his NFL job, and he reported adding 45 pounds using Dianabol. "Sometimes the game dictates drastic measures," he said. "It's sad, but you have to make a choice. If someone asked my opinion about using steroids... I wouldn't make any recommendation that somebody else take them."

The players generally viewed steroid usage as minimal in the NFL, Janofsky reported, and other than Riker's written observation, coaches and officials downplayed the notion that it was widespread. Jim Williams, strength coach for the Jets, said that he was unaware of any steroid use by his players, but those on the fringe were susceptible. "Most of the time I've seen steroids used on this team have been by rookies who didn't make the team," said Williams, presumably oblivious to veterans such as Klecko and Fields. Pete Rozelle, NFL commissioner, expressed concern about anabolic steroids, but he also noted "a firm policy" would have to be hammered out with the players' union. "We have to start out with education, tell the players the potential bad effects," Rozelle told Janofsky.

The NFL's monitoring system for steroids relied on reports by team physicians, who had produced little information. Rozelle ordered a fresh internal assessment, but before he could release the results, another story blew up in Dallas, where young sportswriter Skip Bayless had gathered extraordinary information about the Cowboys.

Steroids were important for many players on America's Team, Bayless revealed in a column for *The Morning News*. Bayless, a marathon runner and weightlifter, had struck up a friendship with the Cowboys' strength guru Robert "Dr. Bob" Ward, a former coach in collegiate track and field who held a doctorate degree. Ward, rippling at 225 pounds, told Bayless he used steroids and that about 25 percent of Dallas' players had cycled or were doing so. "Man was not created equal," Ward said, "so why shouldn't he use every form of technology to get better?" The strength coach would be reprimanded by his superiors for his interview with Bayless.

Bayless continued, quoting Dallas defensive lineman John Dutton, who cycled during preseason two-a-day practices. "I felt real strong," Dutton said. "I'd get a second wind in the afternoon practice. I was looser. Lifting was easier."

All-Pro and future Hall of Fame defensive tackle Randy White "was the most successful of several Cowboy steroid users in the late '70s and early '80s," Bayless would write in his book *God's Coach*. White had packed on heavy poundage beginning in his college days at Maryland, but claimed on-the-field pressure to use began for him in the NFL, pointing the blame at the usual suspects, the Pittsburgh O-linemen who fired at him in face-offs in the Super Bowl. "Man, I'd look across the line at those Steelers with their sleeves rolled up on those huge arms and, well, I had to do something," White said. "I figured they were using steroids, too."

Bayless checked with Landry, the famed Texas Methodist, one of America's most respected Christian speakers and a top draw on the Billy Graham circuit. Bayless called him Mount Landry, describing a man who consciously cultivated his public image. Landry devoted himself to Christian religion as much as to a Sunday game plan, the popular storyline went, but he was in a fix over Bayless' nailing down steroid use on his Cowboys. Bayless wrote, "Landry, who tightropes between his religious image and Super Bowl realities, takes a see-no-evil stance on steroids." Landry preferred not to address drug use of any sort on his team while, at the same time, he preached against narcotics, alcohol, premarital sex, and adultery in his Christian ministries. Landry did nothing about the same issues plaguing his football team, according to Bayless' research, and he opposed intervention at the league level: "We don't want to develop a police state," he had said, in discussing possible NFL urinalysis for drugs.

Facing Bayless, Landry said the Cowboys organization did not dispense steroids, so team officials had no knowledge — besides Ward, apparently — of any use by players. [In 2005, Charlie Waters, a Dallas safety during the 1970s and 1980s, said former team GM Tex Schramm told Cowboys players that he condoned their use of performance-enhancing drugs like steroids, but not street drugs.] Landry talked of opposing the use of anabolic steroids on the Cowboys, citing associated health hazards. However, he added, "The bad thing about sports is that people are afraid to get behind. If they hold, you gotta hold, too. That's not right, but that's the American way."

Bayless' scoop on juiced Cowboys went national, and Rozelle tried to counter the negative publicity from NFL headquarters in New York, announcing that a new league assessment had found that the "non-medical" use of steroids by players was not a problem. In a letter to NFL teams and players, Rozelle stated: "The League recognizes that in certain circumstances physicians may prescribe anabolic steroids for valid medical reasons." The commissioner had never said much about anabolic steroids in the league; media had rarely inquired, and he had fairly evaded any questions asked. Now, in staking a significant stance on the topic, Rozelle said anabolic steroids were OK when legally prescribed. "When it is under a doctor's care, steroids can help rehabilitate injuries," Rozelle told media. "We have never found a heavy order by the clubs for it, but that's not to say they couldn't have gotten [steroids] on their own."

Meanwhile, in California, newly hired Raiders internist Rob Huizenga was trying to sort out the team's messy distribution of prescription drugs. Oakland players were accustomed to powerful painkillers in unlimited quantity, for example, and they often found Huizenga unwilling to go along, he would later recall in his book *You're Okay, It's Just a Bruise*. The administering of pain-deadening cortisone also concerned Huizenga; the shots were routine for Raiders players, especially at the hands of Dr. Robert Rosenfeld, long-time team physician and confidant of owner Al Davis. Regarding amphetamines, Huzienga encountered heavy use among the Raiders, including alarming consumption by mammoth defensive lineman John Matuszak.

Abuse of anabolic steroids became apparent to Huzienga, of course, throughout the NFL, and he broached the topic upon meeting other team physicians at the 1984 league combine, his first. "I was struck by the fact that none of the doctors had looked into the effects of anabolic steroids, though they acknowledged their universal use in the league," Huzienga wrote.

The internist dealt with Alzado on the Raiders, a mercuric personality prone to keeping everyone on edge. That year at training camp in Santa Rosa, Huizenga happened onto a bag of used needles in the hallway outside Alzado's room. Huizenga, a former All-American wrestler in college, had already exchanged words with Alzado over steroids; now he confronted and berated the defensive tackle, who rationalized the doping. "Doc, I've been taking steroids since college," Alzado said. "I wish I didn't have to. But it's a decision I've made, something I've gotta do to stay competitive."

Steroid use in pro and college football could neither be stopped nor kept quiet. Players, coaches, and insiders were talking too much. Soon a major scandal emerged among universities in the Southeast, igniting unprecedented media scrutiny that would carry through the decade. Not until both the NCAA and NFL established random testing, however faulty, would the public be appeased and the allegations diminished in the press.

II. Juice in College Football Jars Teams, Officials

Performance-enhancing drug use was part of NCAA football by the end of the 1970s, at colleges large and small, occurring often at the behest of coaches, trainers, and other officials. America had just not heard much about it, not from bubblegum sport media, those writers and broadcasters who persisted in the telling, for example, of "what a great man and great role model Babe Ruth was," sneered Howard Cosell, the egotistical, iconoclastic journalist. In routinely ripping sport media, Cosell would reference *SportsWorld* analysis by cultural critic Robert Lipsyte, who the book of title about a dumb America hooked on fantasy spun by writers and illustrators, hyping trivial games and players. Cosell believed that media taught the culture "hogwash" about athletics. "It's ingrained in the American people that there exists a special world that is pure and a necessary Camelot in the daily travail of human life — SportsWorld. It's absurd," Cosell said.

Brent Musburger, CBS sports announcer, took offense to such criticism. He said sport media enjoy games while standing ready to tackle the tough issues. "It angers me, when there is a perception that those of us in sports can't do this or are not willing to do this," Musburger said, after covering the controversial 1983 Pan American Games in Caracas. Musburger's performance there was commendable, but in defending sport media as a whole, he got little support from a superior, Neal Pilson, president of CBS Sports.

Pilson spoke with unusual frankness about television's dealings with sports. Media critics screamed about conflict of interest with sport, and Pilson affirmed there existed an internal clashing of values, a network's business interests versus free-press duty. "When you are sponsoring sports events and generating profits, you can create conflicts and problems," Pilson told the *New York Times*. "In CBS Sports, we have major business relationships that are worth in the billions of dollars and are renewable. You cannot use people associated with CBS Sports to investigate the morals of people you do business with." At the time, CBS held broadcasting rights for the NFL, NCAA, NBA, the Olympics, U.S. track and field, and more.

Pilson's comments unnerved TV executives at every network, humoring Cosell, who said that the unwritten code was violated. "Neal Pilson was the honest one," Cosell would remark. "He said, 'We're partners with [sport organizations]. We do business with them.'"

Coverage on sport doping, however, had begun to change, progress, even if slowly. Prodding came in part from college athletes who brought their doping stories straight to the press, forcing the issue into the light.

One was Florida State basketball player James Bozeman, who quit the squad and told reporters how team officials had doped him to compete. "I've been injured and given drugs so I could play — Novocain and cortisone," said Bozeman, a senior sociology student; even Freon was used on him, in a failed attempt to freeze out the pain of a ravaged ankle. Other improprieties of collegiate sports, he said, included grades fixing and cash payments: "I've been given money. The important thing is that it doesn't happen again.... It's not just Florida State. It's everywhere." Bozeman spoke at a New York press conference, accompanied by sport's activist Dr. Cary Goodman, who implored of President Reagan and federal agencies to probe "rampant drug abuse in sports."

NCAA Steroid Scandal: Vanderbilt, Clemson, Coaches and Pharmacist

On October 19, 1984, Clemson University track athlete Augustinius Jaspers was found dead in his dormitory room. No sign of foul play, the death would be classified of congenital heart disease, but investigators recovered capsules of the prescription drug phenylbutazone, or "bute," a powerful anti-inflammatory popular for treating athletic injuries. An autopsy detected traces of phenylbutazone in Jaspers' bloodstream, and South Carolina authorities were intrigued because the distance runner had no prescription. A probe quickly expanded to anabolic steroids, with investigators moving beyond the state border, into Tennessee, tracking a prescription-drug pipeline from

Clemson back to Nashville and the athletic department at Vanderbilt University.

Two Clemson coaches resigned quietly in December, a graduate assistant joining them in the exit, and a month later the full story broke in Nashville, where lawmen told reporters about interstate distribution of anabolic steroids to college athletes, including a large number of football players.

"We know generally about four different kinds of drugs were diverted to South Carolina from Vanderbilt," said Arzo Carson, director of the Tennessee Bureau of Investigation. "We are looking at any and all drugs that may have been used without lawful prescription. ... That would cover steroids."

Vanderbilt announced that athletics strength coach E.J. "Doc" Kreis had requested a leave of absence. Kreis, 32, was a former linebacker at Clemson, where he was a close friend of Sam Colson, 34, who had recently resigned as Clemson strength coach, joined by track coach Stanley Narewski, 35.

Law authorities said they were focusing on "one person" at Vanderbilt, and suspicion surrounded Kreis, who declined to meet with media. A Kreis co-hort, local pharmacist Melvin "Woody" Wilson, confirmed to reporters that he was the original source of the drugs. Wilson said he delivered anabolic steroids to the Vanderbilt campus in his van, either meeting football players directly or going for drop-offs at the McGugin Center, which housed athletic offices. "I'd have to say it wasn't a secret," Wilson said. "The kids knew of its availability in the weight room, and also they knew it wasn't coming from the [football] coaches. It was between Doc and me."

Addressing the drugs reaching Clemson, Carson of the TBI said, "It started in the weight room at Vanderbilt, where the drugs were dropped off and were delivered on out. Then, after two or three of those shipments, it became more direct between Wilson and Colson."

Vanderbilt officials initially expressed surprise over the case. "I have no reason to believe we have a staggering wholesale problem," said athletic director Roy Kramer. Head football coach George MacIntyre refuted Wilson's claim that about 50 of his players received anabolic steroids over two years — police would document 32 of those names — referring to the allegations as "ludicrous."

Kramer and MacIntyre would reverse within days, however, as information continued coming to light. Media reaped a bevy of provocative details. *United Press International* reported:

A former appellate judge and an ex-convict were among the colorful crowd which made use of the now-closed Vanderbilt University weight room, where drugs were sold. ... A frequent visitor to the weight room was M. Woody Wilson, a Franklin, Tenn., druggist who admitted selling anabolic steroids to Vanderbilt athletes. Wilson used the facility as part of his rehabilitation after shoulder surgery.

Wilson is the key figure in the TBI investigation to determine the source of illegally dispensed steroids...

Speaking with the media, Wilson portrayed his pride for Vanderbilt athletics — "My blood runs black and gold," the pharmacist declared — and discussed his friendship with Kreis, strength coach and popular local figure. "I have strong feelings for Doc," Wilson said. "As little as gets out will be in his best interest and mine."

Kramer, within a week of learning about the police probe, moved toward establishing what seemed a fix: steroid urinalysis for athletes at Vanderbilt. "This is a problem that has been around for a long time and that may have been enhanced in recent years," he said. "Maybe we are at the forefront of solving this problem." Kramer refused to disclose how many football players received anabolic steroids. "Numbers are secondary. I know who, what, when and how, but that's for me to know."

The athletic director said his internal investigation had been an eye-opener personally, discussing performance enhancement with young athletes and others. "I've learned a lot of things that affect the use of these steroids," Kramer said. "There is the pressure of growing up and getting a college scholarship, the desire to come back from an injury and the possibility that, as coaches, we have taken off-season programs and made them an end in themselves."

MacIntyre caught heat for initially denying that his football players used steroids, but steroid author Bob Goldman empathized. "Coaches are in a very difficult position," said Goldman, who wrote *Death In The Locker Room*. "They are told by the alumni that if they don't have a winning season, they're going to lose their job. And they're also told by parents that if they give drugs to their children they're going to get fired.

"On top of that, athletes come to them and want to take the drugs."

MacIntyre had led the Commodores program to winning, rare for football at Vanderbilt, a staid, privately endowed institution with a lengthy history for losing in football. MacIntyre was candid with *AP* reporter Skip Latt, regarding the rapidly accelerating parameters for size and strength — and the associate realities for football training. "These kids want to get bigger, stronger and quicker, and when we, as coaches, see them doing it, we congratulate them," MacIntyre said. "I mean, what are we supposed to say, 'Aw, now, you're getting too big. You'd better stop that.' Or... 'You better slow down.' That's ludicrous."

The steroid predicament left young assistant coaches especially vulnerable to trouble, much like lesser-ranking soldiers in a Mafia organization. Jack Harkness, former Clemson graduate-assistant strength coach under Colson, discussed his part in steroid distribution with a South Carolina newspaper. "I was told to make the drug available and that is what I did," Harkness told the *Greenville News*, speaking by telephone from abroad, at his native home near Toronto. Harkness, a former Canadian national champion in the discus throw, had competed in track and field for Clemson. There as a GA coach during 1984, Harkness recalled, he provided steroids to five Clemson football players, all linemen, on the orders of Colson. Harkness said Clemson athletes fully understood the drugs were available for them. "I think that was the whole key to it — it was there if they wanted it," he said.

The drugs had come from Nashville, where Colson's buddy Doc Kreis had a steady steroid connection in Woody Wilson, the Vanderbilt fan and druggist. The Greenville story with Harkness ran on Sunday, January 20; the same morning, the *New York Times* published a lengthy analysis on the Vanderbilt-Clemson scandal.

The next morning, Monday, Clemson athletic director Bill McClellan announced a new drug-testing plan for athletes, while head football coach Danny Ford reacted in strong denial of the Harkness allegations. "The *Greenville News'* story implies significant involvement of our football coaches with the distribution of steroids," Ford said. "That is totally false. ... I assure the parents of our current players and the parents of the players we are recruiting that we have never even suggested to our players that they should use steroids or any other drug to become bigger and better football players. Winning is certainly not that important."

Lawmen, meanwhile, were examining whether the prescription-drug network included athletes at more universities; they apparently had met a University of Tennessee football player, for example, who told them he used steroids to improve his performance. The TBI believed the sheer quantity of illegally dispensed drugs could not have been consumed by athletes merely at Vanderbilt and Clemson. There were as many as 100,000 pills and 1,600 viles originating from Wilson's shuttered pharmacy.

Steroid use in football was making regular headlines in Tennessee, and a pair of young professional players entered the discussion: Steve Bearden, a linebacker who had played for Vanderbilt, and Reggie White, former defensive end for the Tennessee Volunteers. Both men played for the Memphis Showboats of the United States Football League, an upstart pro circuit, and each had encountered steroids since college. "I knew of some players who used them when I was still playing at Tennessee," said White, who added he did not partake. "They were linemen, linebackers and running backs." At Vanderbilt, steroids "were readily available," Bearden said. "And I had been aware that players were using them." Bearden said he cycled for eight weeks in 1983, the summer before his senior season for the Commodores, but Doc Kreis did not provide the drugs. White and Bearden alleged steroids were employed on their USFL team, though Bearden said he was "certain that none of the Showboats coaches or trainers are aware of anybody using them."

At Clemson University, athletic officials had been cognizant. On March 11, 1985, former strength coach Sam Colson and former track coach Stan Narewski each pleaded guilty to 10 counts of possessing and distributing prescription drugs, including anabolic steroids. They were placed on probation, fined, and ordered to perform community service. Jack Harkness, the former graduate assistant to Colson, was charged but could not be extradited from Canada. In an aside to the plea hearing, Clemson football coach Danny Ford again denied his staff had anything to do with Harkness' delivery of steroids to five of their linemen.

At Vanderbilt University, officials allowed E.J. "Doc" Kreis to remain an employee until he faced criminal charges. Finally, the inevitable came down on April 19, when a grand jury's indictment charged Kreis with seven counts of illegal distribution of steroids.

Deposed druggist Melvin "Woody" Wilson was indicted on 90 counts, and a former pharmacy employee was named in five, though police described that person's role as minimal in the distribution. All charges were misdemeanors.

Early the next morning, Kreis resigned as strength coach of Vanderbilt athletics, without appearing before the media. Kreis did not "want any controversy about him to affect the university or the athletic department," said Roger May, his attorney. "Doc cares about Vanderbilt University."

Athletic director Kramer said: "I have accepted [Kreis'] resignation in the spirit that it was offered — in an attempt to do what is best for the future of our athletes and Vanderbilt athletics." Kramer stressed to reporters the department had begun testing for steroids, and he professed having "a very positive feeling about that testing."

Deplorable circumstances surrounding young athletes had led to the steroid investigation at Vanderbilt and Clemson, involving strength coaches, a pharmacist, and likely others never named in public. Tennessee prosecutor Thomas Shriver charged that steroids had fueled a Vanderbilt mission for winning at football, to "build players to compete successfully in the Southeastern Conference. ... Some of those guys would never have made it without steroids." Shriver said coaches and players had discussed "specific type, quantity and duration of the administration of drugs."

Serious allegations notwithstanding, the matter concluded benignly for punishments administered. The NCAA enforcement division was not interested, displaying its aversion to probing sport doping, so Vanderbilt and Clemson were not sanctioned. And the last two primary criminal defendants "got off relatively lightly," opined *Sports Illustrated*.

Strength coach Kreis and pharmacist Wilson each pleaded guilty to one count of misdemeanor steroid distribution, a shipment of Dianabol to Colson at Clemson. Kreis and Wilson were each sentenced to one year of unsupervised probation. In exchange for their pleas, Shriver dropped one conspiracy count against Kreis and 95 counts of possession and distribution against Wilson. Circuit judge Bobby Capers concluded Kreis' role in the entire matter amounted to "a favor to a friend." Kreis had plenty of friends around Nashville, with several prominent individuals testifying to his character before the judge.

Kreis then spoke to reporters for the first time in a year, apologizing to the university and anyone "touched by my mistake." He told the *Nashville Tennessean*: "I have failed 30 fine Vanderbilt athletes, and for that I am truly sorry. I did something that was against the law. The fact that all I thought I was doing was helping a friend doesn't matter."

In spring 1986, a few months after Kreis had pleaded guilty of steroid distribution, he was chosen to be part of a contingent of U.S. coaches representing the country on a trip to Russia. That summer he returned to NCAA athletics as volunteer strength coach at Middle Tennessee State University, where head football coach Boots Donnelly called Kreis' addition "the most positive thing to happen to this football program in a long, long time."

Kreis quickly moved into a full-time job at MTSU, and, in 1992, after winning multiple NCAA coaching awards, he ascended back into big-time sports, hired by the University of Colorado.

College Coaches Catch Heat, Deflect It Over Steroids

Anabolic steroids pervaded college football and everyone involved knew it, coaches especially, according to a pair of NFL linemen interviewed in the spring of

1985 by *Sports Illustrated.* "Vanderbilt is the straw [scandal] that broke the camel's back," observed the Bears' Steve McMichael, who said he used following his senior season for the Texas Longhorns. "There are [players at] a bunch of other schools who are doing steroids, too. The whole college deal has gotten out of hand." Pat Donovan, retired lineman of the Cowboys, charged that head coaches at colleges "know about it and encourage the abuse or they look the other way and don't counsel the kids."

Other witnesses discussed doping in college football with *SI.* Charles Radler, a convicted steroid dealer whose million-dollar operation had gone national through mail order, said he started hearing from college teams in 1983, as his business took off through word of mouth and exposure in national media. "That surprised me at first," Radler said in jail. "Now it would surprise me if there was a college football team out there that isn't using steroids."

The magazine quoted Richard Sandlin, a former user and consultant, who said NCAA athletes and coaches continued contacting him for how-to information on cycling. Sandlin named two dozen major schools associated with the callers: LSU, Alabama, Auburn, Texas, USC, Washington, Washington State, California, Arizona State, Nebraska, Arkansas, Oklahoma, Texas A&M, SMU, Pittsburgh, Virginia, Clemson, Tennessee, Kentucky, Louisville, Georgia, Vanderbilt, Florida, and Florida State

Steroid controversy erupted at Baylor, on the revelation that men's basketball coach Jim Haller had instructed a player to use steroids, and discussion moved to football teams in the Southwest Conference. Use probably existed at every school, concluded an informal survey of athletic officials by the *Waco Tribune-Herald.* "Most head football coaches said they believe at least some athletes on most SWC teams used steroids, but they carefully avoided any finger-pointing," reported *The Associated Press.*

Opinions varied among the football coaches. Steroids had been eliminated from the Houston team, according to coach Bill Yeoman, who credited in-house urinalysis and other monitoring. In Austin, Longhorns coach Fred Akers said he had no idea about the extent of use in the conference, while at A&M, coach Jackie Sherrill contended the whole issue amounted to nothing.

Other coaches differed. "I don't think you can sit back and say it's not happening to us," said Southern Methodist coach Bobby Collins. "It's probably more widespread than we would all think or like to think." Jim Wacker, TCU, said, "I'm sure if I said none of our players used steroids... it would be the most ridiculous statement I could make. No coach knows who has and who hasn't.

"Steroids are very prevalent."

Juicing at Nebraska: Popular Old Rumor Confirmed as Fact

In the fall of 1983, the story went, an assistant football coach at Clemson University approached the strength coach with a picture of Nebraska's offensive line, saying he wanted his linemen to be as big and strong. The strength coach, Sam Colson, took the directive as "tacit approval" for Clemson players to juice. Clemson football coaches denied the incident happened — a lawyer related the alleged conversation during Colson's court case — but only to defend one of their own, not the Nebraska Cornhuskers.

Indeed, rumor and innuendo had long swirled around the physical Cornhuskers. Nebraska players were huge, standing out even in a sport riddled with muscle doping, and savvy observers felt sure of what that was about. "The Cornhuskers," UCLA coach Terry Donahue said, "were not typical college football players." Donahue, Clemson staffers and other college coaches were not above reproach, but the court story about Nebraska linemen rang true throughout football.

Tom Osborne, Nebraska head football coach, and his trusted strength coach, Boyd Epley, had for years heard the steroid talk but did not respond publicly. They continued to focus on churning out mammoth young men from their program's training complex, thousands of square feet of weights, racks, and lifting platforms adorned in the Big Red color scheme. The NU weightlifting facility became legendary in the game, a shrine of iron dedication. What materialized was one of the most fearsome offensive rushing attacks ever known to the game. Nebraska football under Osborne epitomized the steam-rolling offensive line, enormous, fast specimens leading the running game downfield, grinding defenses underfoot. However, football's steroid issue finally caught up to Nebraska officials in the 1980s, Osborne foremost, when incidents started making headlines nationwide.

Osborne, a Ph.D in educational psychology, struck a dignified appearance with his reserved manner. A future Congressman from his native state, Osborne strove to project unquestioned authority in the fall of 1983, going public with his disdain for a planned NCAA study on steroid use by football players.

Steroid stories had soiled the Pan Am Games and the National Football League, and momentum was growing within NCAA ranks for action on the drugs in college sports, football specially. The Michigan State study, which would survey college players, was endorsed throughout the association by coaches, athletic directors, and academic officials.

Osborne declined, nevertheless, suggesting a knee-jerk response at the collegiate level, or anti-steroid hysteria. Holding lecture with media in his office in Lincoln, Nebraska, the community and state fondly referring to him as "Dr. Tom," Osborne outright dismissed the steroid controversy. "I think there's always a reaction, sometimes an overreaction, to publicity," he said. "So I'm not sure it's entirely appropriate. As far as I'm concerned right here at Nebraska, I would just as soon they would let us handle those things ourselves."

The well-built, professorial Osborne, a former NFL receiver who donned spectacles at his desk, personified the classic gridiron theme of Coaching Genius. The man acted and appeared capable of winning as the head of any program or organization, sport, academic, or governmental. Yet as far as handling steroids at Nebraska, Osborne and his staff would prove to be secretive, sloppy, and ineffective.

Nebraska players ranging from linemen to running backs used anabolic steroids. Ultimately, the school's three renowned All-American linemen of the 1980s would confirm their involvement: center Dave Rimington, 6-3, 288, a No. 1 draft pick for Cincinnati in 1983; offensive tackle Dean Steinkuhler, 6-3, 273, No. 1 pick for Houston in 1984; and defensive tackle Danny Noonan, 6-4, 280, No. 1 for Dallas in 1987.

Steinkuhler would tell *SI* that steroid use was significant on the Cornhuskers in 1983 and 1984, his junior and senior seasons. In a separate interview, Osborne would deny widespread use occurred, but he would affirm noticing "suspiciously substantial weight gains made by about a third of Nebraska players in 1984."

The program began selective urinalysis for steroids in the 1984 preseason, testing about one-fourth of the team, and coaches announced all players were clean. "We're very pleased," said NU head trainer George Sullivan. "People have been making claims on us, so we'd like to know. It makes us feel good to prove them wrong." A Cornhuskers' player backed up his coaches, fullback Tom Rathman, who said: "We don't have illegal recruiting and we don't have illegal drugs. We have as clean a program as anybody and this is one way to show it."

Before the football season ended, however, intense steroid scrutiny was brewing for the Huskers, following an arrest at the California border, a crossing station from Mexico. The suspect, Richard Anthony "Tony" Fitton, was not a drug smuggler commonly encountered by U.S. Customs, although western authorities knew patented anabolic steroids were staples on black markets, purchased for pennies over the counter in Mexico. An enormous cache was recovered from Fitton's rental car, hundreds of thousands of Dianabol pills, reportedly, along with additional brand names in muscle dope. Authorities classified Fitton as perhaps the world's biggest steroid dealer, with an illicit network across sports and bodybuilding in America and abroad.

Fitton's clientele included Nebraska football players, some who reportedly ordered steroids from him prior to an Orange Bowl game for the national championship. Fitton, a former track runner, was a globe-trotting, fast-living Briton in his mid-30s who sold cases of steroids from hotel rooms during weightlifting meets, customers lining out into hallways. Fitton was first arrested entering the U.S. in 1981, Atlanta International Airport, where more than 200,000 steroid pills were found in his luggage.

Fitton did not receive jail time in that case, but the political climate for steroids was changing by early 1985. American law enforcement clamped harder on steroid trafficking, and Fitton, in connection to the border-crossing arrest, faced prison after pleading guilty of two counts of distribution. Fitton fled before sentencing, jumping bail, and continued to sell steroids. His business ledger included at least one Nebraska football player and other college athletes. After six months on the lam, Fitton was back in custody and sentenced to 4 ½ years in prison, for unlawful flight, tax evasion, conspiracy to import steroids, and possession of forgery paraphernalia.

Behind bars in San Diego, Fitton granted an interview to writers from *Sports Illustrated*. "Fitton said he had sold or given counsel on the use of steroids to strength coaches or athletes at Baylor, South Carolina, Virginia, Temple and Nebraska, among other schools," the magazine reported. Fitton said Nebraska was no worse for steroids than other NCAA football programs. "Anabolics are going to be taken," he said. "It's a fact of life."

Fitton expressed affinity for Nebraska football players to whom he peddled steroids in 1983 and 1984. "I had contacts in the Lincoln gyms," he said. "I got people referred to me." Fitton was described as knowing "several" Nebraska players, whom he counseled on how to pass the program's urinalysis for steroids. Fitton said he express-shipped pills of methyl testosterone in time for the 1984 Orange Bowl, won by Miami over the Cornhuskers for the national crown.

The allegations of Fitton drew out Osborne for his first interview about steroids with a national media entity, *Sports Illustrated*, in December 1985, regarding specific allegations against his program. "If I had known that...," said Osborne, responding to Fitton's claim about rush-shipping testosterone for the Orange Bowl, "I would have busted [any players] on the spot."

Football was buzzing in the bowl season: Would Nebraska get nailed for muscle doping?

"The National Collegiate Athletic Association doesn't have specific rules governing the use of steroids, leaving that to the individual schools," reported *The Associated Press*. "But that could change." Association officials did not comment on Nebraska, but they pledged to address the general doping issue at the upcoming annual convention for NCAA delegates.

On December 17 in Lincoln, Osborne discussed steroids in a news conference as the weekly *SI* edition was hitting newsstands and mailboxes. "We have yet to find anyone who tested positively," he said. "I don't believe we have widespread usage of [steroids]. But any time you have 150 individuals [on a team], you might have a few." Osborne said he strongly opposed steroid use because of health hazards and fair competition. "[W]e feel it's essentially a form of dishonesty, where you're trying to obtain an edge over your opponents or fellow teammates through chemical means."

Osborne was concerned about public perception surrounding football doping, suggesting overplay as a news topic. "I'm afraid this kind of thing is going to lead people to believe that anybody who's big and strong or is a good football player must be on [steroids], and that really isn't the case." Osborne adhered to the stance of isolated use, saying Nebraska's testing over two years showed no evidence to the contrary. "We will certainly not try to whitewash anything," Osborne promised. "Anybody that's proven, or in any way we know, we will deal with it."

Soon after Osborne's high-profile vow, in spring 1986, he and his staff certainly dealt with a steroid matter involving star players — they tried to keep it quiet. Lincoln police, searching for missing jewelry on the Nebraska campus, entered the dormitory room of football defensive linemen Neil Smith and Lawrence Pete, reportedly finding stolen items and "several plastic bottles containing pills," later determined to be steroids. No drug charges were filed, misdemeanor theft charges against Smith and Pete would be dismissed, and no press reports initially transpired. Television reporters for WOWT in Omaha found out anyway and broke the story in late August, as the Cornhuskers prepared for their nationally broadcast season opener against Florida State.

Osborne, forced to address media about Smith and Pete, said he had believed their excuse, that they only obtained the steroids for experimentation and had not consumed any pills. Osborne said one of the players could bench-press 495 pounds and wanted the D-bol pills for reaching 500. "Now you either believe him or you don't," Osborne said. "But everything I've ever dealt with him on, and some things have been unpleasant, he's told me the truth. So I tend to believe players unless I have evidence to the contrary." Osborne said Smith and Pete subsequently passed urinalysis for steroids and received counseling. He said their parents were notified and the players would face suspension for further impropriety. Concluding the press conference, Osborne said he hoped the players would be ready for Florida State; Smith had an elbow ailment while Pete was ill with a virus.

Nebraska could not get away from steroid speculation. Attention returned in October, on a comment by Oklahoma head coach Barry Switzer, Osborne's rival in the Big Eight Conference. Speaking about the UCLA Bruins, Switzer wisecracked, "They're not like Nebraska. They haven't discovered steroids yet." When the quote hit print in *SI*, Switzer called Osborne to apologize, but the new story had life.

Reporters sought out Osborne. "I don't like to see our whole program indicted by what some people may suspect, or rumors, or two or three guys who have gotten out of line," he said, still fielding questions about Smith and Pete. Steroid testing at Nebraska had produced one positive result, according to Osborne, from an unnamed player who was no longer with the team. "We tested all of our big people, anybody that was under any suspicion because we had heard rumors," he said, adding, "Now I'm not naïve enough to believe that in three years' period of time we've only had one player that's ever used steroids. I know that's not true." Osborne declared that he and strength coach Epley were "dead set against" the drugs: "Boyd has never been involved in any of that... He and his people have done everything they can to discourage it."

Osborne and Nebraska appeared under siege for a day or two, but the net effect of his defensive posturing was to discourage scrutiny from outside the program, if not steroid use on the inside. Once again, NCAA enforcement — and the football public — passed on headline allegations of steroids and the Cornhuskers.

III. Fast Forward: 'Isolated' Talk on Capitol Hill, Again

In April 2005, Congress began to investigate doping in the NFL. I found myself, once again, disturbed about the so-called hearing on anabolic steroids, growth hormone, and other performance-enhancers in the league. As always in this issue, most of the public talk was nothing more than word games, lies, or willful ignorance, very little substance. I felt let down, which of course, was my own fault by now.

I had expected nothing worthwhile from football officials before Congress, hauled in once again by a committee to "testify" about muscle doping in the sport. In addition, this time I had ample warning of the charade, 16 years following the first on Capitol Hill. Days before the event, I learned that Dr. Charles Yesalis, the foremost independent expert on anabolic substances in American football, was not asked to sit on the panel of scientists who would critique the NFL's drug policy before the U.S. House Committee on Government Reform.

The NFL had dodged a bullet in the omission of testimony on the part of Yesalis, the Penn State scientist who would have provided irrefutable testimony about loopholes in "state-of-the-art" steroids testing — and of how only anabolic drugs could generally produce the enormous sizes en masse of football players. The omission of Yesalis from the hearing reeked of information control, or power of The Spectacle, American football's amazing cloak against damaging facts and criticism.

Without Yesalis around to object, dogmatic football officials misled lawmakers and America. Football officials asserted, without rebuke, that the league's self-administered, random urinalysis for patented steroids was effective in preventing muscle doping, the ever-increasing sizes of players was no indication of a problem with anabolic substances, and user players still were isolated individuals, decades into the game's doping, acting without any systematic pressure.

These excuses were essentially the same as what Congress had heard from football officials in 1989, during the Senate hearings over doping events of that decade. Collegiate officials in 2005 implied that around 1 percent of NCAA football players used anabolic steroids, based on results from testing and surveys of athletes. NFL officials suggested the league rate was measurable by the ridiculously low amount of positive test results, about 0.0008 percent, during 15 years of random urinalysis.

I knew the rhetoric, had expected as much, but it was outlandish, the continuing claims of football witnesses before lawmakers. Even in my own experience as a member of a small college football team in 1982, I knew that about 10 percent of the players used steroids, including me, and that use continued to skyrocket in football and other sports thereafter.

Nonetheless, anabolic substances remained no concern for football in 2005, officials conveyed. Everything was under control, they said, despite several factors to the contrary. Patented steroids remained in use, recently purchased by Panthers players in quantity and repeatedly. Undetectable designer steroids were of unknown variety and count, circulating in elite sports through drug gurus and amateur chemists. Human growth hormone was available to athletes and citizens via both illicit and legal channels, and no reliable test existed. Players employed still more undetectable anabolic substances, including insulin.

Those elements were just waved off by NFL commissioner Paul Tagliabue and union director Gene Upshaw. As for the politicians assembled in committee, they fell in line with the NFL, happily it seemed. Virtually every elected government official, while addressing Taglibue and Upshaw, went out of his or her way to praise the league and its policy on doping.

The stance of the football officials where steroids were concerned had become an odd, illogical, and contradictory matter. Many officials and the media finally acknowledged rampant abuse during the 1980s but still avoided the obvious conclusion that random urinalysis had failed, miserably, given the fact that football players of 2005 were much larger and stronger than in 1985, no matter the level — professional, collegiate, or high school. In addition, it had become clear that substances were more available than ever, especially with universal use of the Internet.

At what point would the officials and media ask the obvious questions...What special ingredient of training had contemporary players discovered? What secret did they know that we had not, two decades before?

I had to laugh in disgust, watching the 2005 hearing on C-SPAN, as football-fawning politicians contemplated the question of doping's prevalence in the NFL. Historically, that had been a stupid question. Anabolic steroids were prevalent in football by the 1980s, in the pro ranks, in colleges, and in high schools. They were everywhere, particularly influencing the upper stage of one-on-one competition, where players battled to gain and hold starting positions. Moreover, many coaches were involved because steroids impacted their livelihoods; their win-loss records that determined employment and upward mobility.

I witnessed steroids' irreversible wave consume small-college football in the early 1980s, during my involvement as a player and student coach at Southeast Missouri State University, a member of NCAA Division II. [The school joined NCAA Division I in 1990.] Our team was just average for the steroid storm. A significant portion of starting linemen for any winning program in D-II had cycled at least once, and so had many linebackers, safeties, tight ends, and fullbacks. At Southeast Missouri in 1985, I conservatively estimate at least half the starting linemen and several skill players were users, on a losing team.

The most common adjectives for accurately describing steroid use in competitive D-II football were prevalent and widespread; no honest insider would have ever used "isolated" to describe the problem. Twenty years later, 2005, the use of the word "isolated" to describe use in pro football amounted to willful ignorance.

At the time, my friend Steve Courson again embarked on a major public educational tour on the issue of football doping. He spoke directly with players both powerful and common as well as to Paul Tagliabue and D.C. politicians, Steelers fans, and teenagers. He appeared on TV, talk radio, and was quoted throughout print media. Steve testified on Capitol Hill, once again. I was pleased to assist him, and he read early drafts of this book chapter, along with hundreds of 1980s texts I had forwarded, and information from mainstream media and other literature he'd never seen, including published denials by former juicing teammates. He made good use of my "rollin' blog" of e-mail forwards on contemporary events in the world of sport doping.

"The sports federations, they're saying the same thing," Steve said in June, over the telephone. "When you read through all this [past information], I think what reaches out and touches me, from being heavily involved in all of that, is basically it's the same rhetoric today. In other words, the old adage 'We've got it fixed *now*.' In the '80s, they were saying it then, ya know. Like, 'Yeah, it *was* bad in the '60s and '70s, but we've got it fixed *now*.'" Steve paused, laughed out loud. "Hello."

"Boy, we're hearing it now," I said. " 'It was rampant *then*, but not today.' "

"Yeah..." Steve said, sarcastic. "Ya know, I guess the big thing when you underline the facts here, when you really look at the training *facts*, and historical facts, and you combine them: The fact that resistance training hasn't changed any. The fact that diet hasn't appreciably changed any. People eat the same way, train the same way. And now the fact that we admit during the '80s [football doping] was rampant. Now, the parameters size-, strength- and speed-wise have taken *another leap*. And what other way do we have to explain this?"

"In other words, the evidence is obvious. But there are sycophants and the administrators of sport who still want to use the term 'isolated.' Where, what evidence do they have to support that? I'm talking from an evidence standpoint? *Especially* acknowledging the gigantic holes in drug testing."

For years, Steve and I on our converging paths, insider critics in football doping, encountered up-front demand for our evidentiary support in arguing that use was widespread and the responsibility multi-level, not merely of athletes. And we each appreciated the request and provided what we had to media, politicians, other power brokers, and fans.

The same authority was never asked of our opponents, those voices, especially from within football, continuing to claim muscle doping as static and isolated. Their rhetoric was privileged in the debate, unduly credited, always, while our arguments had to be upheld with supporting fact, expert opinion, and witness testimony.

"Right," Steve said, "because there's *denial.* Because [players] can pass the idiot's [urinalysis] test. I mean, looking at the quantity and quality of evidence that's out there today, when you put it together, how could any rational human being possibly believe that the use of these drugs, in any sport, is isolated?"

IV. NCAA Proclaims Reform, But Steroids Cast Doubt

In January 1985, "reform" was the buzzword for the NCAA national convention in Nashville, with delegates vowing to eliminate institutionalized vice in areas such as recruiting, grades, gambling, and street drugs. Performance-enhancing substances were a lesser concern for most officials. While testing for anabolic steroids was a discussion item on agenda, the 1,500 delegates representing 600 institutions were largely clueless about the drugs. They could have learned much that week in Nashville, where steroid scandal was unfolding at Vanderbilt University through the revelation of the drug pipeline that reached Clemson University. NCAA delegates ignored the code-red warning, the story playing out before them, and balked at implementing steroid policies and testing.

Some delegates said the steroid proposal confused them, while many thought street drugs should have been the priority for prevention by the NCAA — sport media were reporting plenty about jocks on cocaine and marijuana. The delegates were also concerned about potential legal action over positive steroid results, which would render offender athletes ineligible to compete for 90 days. Most significantly, delegates strongly opposed policy language that penalized coaches or other staff members for steroid use by their athletes. Speaking on the convention floor, Wilford Bailey, faculty representative for athletics at Auburn, said "there are obvious flaws in this legislation, so therefore I recommend it be sent back to committee."

Action against steroids was tabled until further notice by the NCAA, which was made up of a powerful bureaucracy of coaches, athletic directors, faculty representatives, and, entering the mix in 1985, college presidents from across America. On any given issue, NCAA delegates preferred to please every one of the 797 member institutions of various sizes, missions, and resources. The 70 or so major schools at the top wielded heavy influence upon the NCAA administration because of their football and men's basketball programs, the only two lucrative college games.

A monetary motivation fueled the drive to win by whatever means necessary, and higher education wallowed in hypocrisy over its relationship with sport as entertainment. Steroid abuse became manifest in the impetus for victory, by athletes who were not necessarily qualified students, particularly at major schools, while the NCAA cloaked the impropriety in marketing efforts focused on portraying amateurism and education.

Critics in 1985, as in other periods, easily established the NCAA model of amateurism to be a sham. "The smoke of recurring scandals in big-time college sports proves the existence of a corrupt system. ...," Ary J. Lamme III, a geographer and editor at the University of Florida, wrote for the *Christian Science Monitor*. "It is ironic that higher-education institutions dedicated to the search for truth close their eyes to the situation." Lamme called for universities "to sever the connection between athletic and academic programs."

No chance of that. The perspective of Lamme had been ignored in America for more than a century, particularly when the target was college football. The academic and athletic members of the NCAA continued forming committees, meeting, voting, and boasting about straightening out their monumental mess. They continued preserving the NCAA image.

The steroid saga did not coincide with upholding a good facade for collegiate athletics. The spring of 1985 brought more bad press for the NCAA over steroids, and university administrators felt the public consternation over stories of their doping athletes, especially football players. "Recent events indicate that steroid use on campuses is prevalent indeed," observed *Sports Illustrated*, "in spite of denials by many college coaches in football and other sports." Muscle-doping reports melded into the ongoing, voluminous coverage of NCAA problems in business and ethics, and the association's Presidents Commission responded to the PR fiasco by announcing an emergency national convening of delegates June 20 in New Orleans.

"I do not believe I can overstate the level of concern that presidents and chancellors feel regarding the integrity crisis in college athletics," said John Ryan, Indiana University president and chair of the commission. Arliss Roaden, president of Tennessee Tech University and NCAA vice president for Division I, said, "If you can't believe in the outcomes of games that have been played fairly and honestly, then what can you believe in?" Roaden said he and fellow presidents would "cleanse" themselves of "guilt" by passing needed legislation.

Few, however, considered anabolic steroids a priority for reform, despite sobering statements by John Toner, the University of Connecticut athletic director who headed the Special NCAA Committee for a National Drug Testing Policy. "We feel we have a serious problem with anabolic steroids...," Toner remarked during the convention's opening session. In an exceptional acknowledgment by an NCAA official, Toner pointed strongly to systematic or environmental pressures leading athletes to steroids. "We want to prevent non-users from feeling forced to use drugs just to remain competitive," he said. "I think it's safe to say that on the [proposed] list of banned drugs, some are in use in every athletic program." Toner's committee proposed a new NCAA drug policy that included steroid urinalysis and suspensions, to begin in the school year 1986-87, along with screening for street drugs.

Then news broke to affect the testing discussion from East Lansing, Michigan, where findings of research sponsored by the NCAA served to downplay organizational concern about college athletes and drugs — particularly anabolic steroids. Two researchers at Michigan State concluded estimates of steroid use were overblown, their findings suggesting individuals and society were at fault, not the NCAA system, for athletes' use of all drugs. The study's authors were William Anderson, an MSU professor of medical education, and Dr. Douglas McKeag, a physician who treated athletes at the university. Anderson remarked, "There are people going around saying that 70 to 80 percent of college football players use anabolic steroids. I've got a great deal of trouble with them going around touting those figures. It's flat out wrong." McKeag said, "I think by and large what we are saying is 'Yes, there is a problem, but it is not epidemic.'"

More than two thousand athletes at 11 universities answered the study's anonymous questionnaire, and 4 percent overall confirmed using anabolic steroids in the previous 12 months. From football, all divisions, 8.4 percent of players confirmed their use. Anderson said, "For drug use at the college level — I'm talking about the use of performance-enhancing drugs like amphetamines and steroids — we found from our data that use rates are much, much lower than touted in the press."

The same day the study story was released, NCAA delegates decided to again table the issue of doping. Toner's committee was told to further its work. The convention ended with new by-laws on the books, designed to prevent cheating by athletic programs, but none concerned performance-enhancing drugs like steroids or amphetamines.

Walter Byers, NCAA executive director, gushed with characteristic hyperbole, calling this convention "an historic moment in intercollegiate athletics." Rather audaciously, Byers claimed cheating of any sort was isolated, committed by only a "hardcore minority element." Byers, portraying the large majority of programs as rule-abiding, said, "There's a rejuvenation of the spirit and desire to conduct an honorable program. It gives support to the coaches who want to run an honorable program and don't want to be dragged down into... cheating to be competitive."

Critics remained skeptical about so-called reform, and steroids in football figured prominently in their objections. The Anderson-McKeag survey, for example, fell under doubt over its methodology. "Many athletes feel compelled to experiment with the anabolic-androgenic steroids whether or not they like the idea of their use. ...," wrote Dr. Donald L. Cooper, health services director and team physician at Oklahoma State. "An intuitive guess... tells me this figure [4 percent] seems much lower than it actually is."

NCAA Delegates Approve Steroid Testing For PR Coup

After a couple of years of debate, NCAA delegates finally approved testing for anabolic steroids in January 1986, and the positive reaction was immediate. While urinalysis was invalid for prevention, the NCAA leaped ahead in the image game of football doping. Officials basked in glowing publicity for unveiling the sport's first steroid testing at an organizational level. The *Christian Science Monitor* declared "the National Collegiate Athletic Association has issued a stern warning to competitors that drug use will not be tolerated." NCAA head Walter Byers gloated, saying, "Somebody had to step in and break the [steroid] chain in high school to get scholarships to college and in the college area to get a professional contract."

College football players, however, were hardly deterred from anabolic drugs. They understood there would be no testing until December, and only then for selected teams appearing in bowl games. Users of limited knowledge understood they could consume steroid pills until about two weeks before a test. Players in the NCAA still injected testosterone and even the detection risk Deca-Durabolin, which left trace evidence in a body system for six months or longer. Moreover, undetectable human growth hormone, though expensive, was already in use among major-college players.

Widespread abuse continued. The 1986 college football season opened to the cheers of crowds, TV viewers, and media as doping athletes thrived on teams such as Oklahoma, Notre Dame, South Carolina, and Duke, witnesses would later recount.

The NCAA began testing athletes for steroids in November, at the national championships for cross country, and football was targeted in early December. Testing personnel visited 20 schools randomly chosen from among the 36 bound for bowl games, and at each stop urinalysis was administered to the 22 players with most game minutes, along with 14 others on a random basis. Most schools received notice seven days before the tests, which would detect anabolic steroids, diuretics, amphetamines, and street drugs such as marijuana and cocaine. Each urine collection was divided in two, with one sample frozen so, in case of a positive result, it could be checked for confirmation. School officials were told the football collections would undergo laboratory analysis at UCLA and the University of Quebec in Canada, and they could expect complete results in the mail. A confirmed positive result would lead to a player's suspension for 90 days from NCAA football, or effectively through the bowl season.

About 720 football players were screened at major colleges, and NCAA testers also headed for playoff teams in the lower ranks, Divisions I-AA, II, and III. Each test cost around $250, including about $170 earmarked for laboratory analysis; officials conceded the process was an expensive, logistical challenge.

On December 5, two small-college players became the first football suspensions announced by the NCAA for positive results in steroid urinalysis. Both were starting linemen for defending D-II champion North Dakota State University: senior offensive tackle Tom Smith, 6-3, 265 pounds, and junior defensive tackle Flint Fleming, 6-4, 262. In a prepared statement, each player acknowledged using steroids the previous summer, and each reportedly had added 20 to 30 pounds. "They definitely made some gains as far as strength and weight," said Earle Solomonson, head coach of the undefeated Bison, "but we knew they had worked hard on the weights during the summer, so it was nothing... unusual." The coach laid blame squarely on the players. "We're constantly discouraging our young men from the use of any kind of drugs," Solomonson said. "They did it on their own. They feel terrible now."

Two suspensions were announced of Division III players, from Salisbury State and Concordia College, and in Division I-AA five players tested positive, all linemen, from Eastern Kentucky, Nevada-Reno, and Georgia Southern.

Major colleges began receiving testing results, and before the complete information was released, the biggest steroid story began breaking on Christmas morning in Norman, Oklahoma. As the Oklahoma Sooners boarded a plane bound for Miami and their Orange Bowl date with Arkansas, two-time All-American linebacker Brian "The Boz" Bosworth was not in sight, and an OU official confirmed he would not play in the game. The NCAA was in the process of suspending just 12 major-college players for positive steroid results, less than 2 percent of the number screened, but one of them was a big fish, Bosworth, the most publicized, notorious figure in all of football.

Suddenly, NCAA steroid urinalysis was a hit with the public. It had taken down The Boz, that arrogant publicity hound strutting around with muscles and a Mohawk. Americans were delighted at Bosworth's demise, even if generally enraptured with the antihero role played by the jock and perpetuated by sportswriters. Indeed, The Boz was at his peak for attention in this steroid tempest.

Media converged, clamoring for details. A few reporters practically clung to the Sooners' plane as it departed Norman, and a horde awaited Switzer and university officials in Miami. Bosworth himself was not yet available for comment; he had learned about the NCAA ruling the previous day and headed for his parents' home in Irving, Texas.

Switzer disembarked the plane in Miami and went straight into a press conference at the airport. The coach had concerns other than Bosworth because two more of his players had been suspended for steroids, both reserves: offensive guard Gary Bennett and defensive tackle David Shoemaker. The defending national-champion Sooners may have been ranked third in the latest AP poll, but they led the nation in positive results for steroids.

Reporters had no real interest in Bennett and Shoemaker; they just wanted to ask Switzer about The Boz. "Of course I warned him," said the coach, clarifying that he understood Bosworth and other Sooners to be steroid users. "I talked to him in January about the new rule. I knew they took steroids to be bigger and stronger." Switzer offered his distinction between performance-enhancing hormones and street drugs. "I certainly rather it be steroids than cocaine or marijuana," he said, adding he supported the new testing.

Sooners strength coach Pete Martinelli said the team had been warned about the steroid policy, but he blamed players for forging ahead with the drugs anyway. "They can't sink it into their heads," Martinelli said. "They all think they've got S's on their chest. They think 'This can't happen to me.'"

Oklahoma players expressed surprise at the news about Bosworth, the junior who had repeated that season as the Butkus Award winner, signifying the nation's premier collegiate linebacker. Rumor was already circulating that Bosworth, a superior student due in May to complete his undergraduate degree, would enter the NFL supplemental draft the following summer. "We're not going to blame him for [the suspension] or anything. ...," said Sooners fullback Lydell Carr. "I just feel sorry for him."

In Dallas, meanwhile, media reported Bosworth family members said the athlete took injections of an anabolic steroid eight months previous, Deca-Durabolin, from an unidentified physician.

The Boz Meets Media in Miami, Tells a Different Story

Brian Bosworth hit Miami a day after the Sooners, December 26, landing like a rock star at Miami International Airport, where the 21-year-old evaded reporters and led them on a chase to the Fontainebleau Hilton on Miami Beach. [Reporters were told Bosworth paid for the flight and lodging himself, following NCAA rules for an ineligible athlete, but

Bosworth later alleged Switzer paid for the plane ticket.] A press conference followed at the ritzy hotel, and The Boz strode in "wearing his blond hair in a punk style with red and black arches dyed above his ears," reported *The AP*. Dark sunglasses covered his eyes and three earrings draped his pierced left ear. The cocky jock surveyed some 50 reporters and a dozen cameras jammed into the conference room, then remarked, "I thought we'd have a bigger turnout."

Reading from a statement, Bosworth said he had used injectible nandrolone, Deca-Durabolin, under a doctor's care nine months before urinalysis, for six weeks from February to March, when he could not lift weights because of injuries. He said that he did not know at the time he would be tested for steroids in December, or that nandrolone traces could remain in the body for so long. He said OU had tested him for steroids in September, during the football season, and his results were negative.

Bosworth refuted a pair of assertions made by Switzer the day before: that he had used steroids to gain size and strength, or a competitive advantage, and that Sooners players had been properly apprised of the new NCAA doping policy. "This could hurt me a long time," Bosworth griped. "I'm plastered across the headlines from here to Russia."

Switzer, sitting next to Bosworth, did not say much — one photographer captured the coach grimacing, scratching his head as The Boz expounded. Switzer neither confirmed nor denied his players were fully apprised of NCAA testing, whatever that really meant. The coach was, however, going along now with Bosworth's key edit on their steroid story — that the linebacker used steroids for medical purposes, not performance enhancement. "We don't support any athletes taking any sort of drugs," Switzer said. "But [Bosworth] had a prescription to help him recover from an injury. He thinks that steroid helped." Switzer said Bosworth was under the care of a private physician with no connection to team personnel. [Other doctors, commenting for media, refuted the steroid prescription Bosworth described, saying there could be no legitimate medical reason for his using the drug as an injured athlete.]

Reporters asked Bosworth to name his physician, but he refused. Loathe to admit cheating, Bosworth stuck to his rationale that his "legal" use of the steroid was not for gaining competitive advantage. From January until March 1986, Bosworth contended, he took weekly nandrolone injections to maintain a size and strength and that was his "right." The Boz, who had acted as a spokesperson for anti-drug messages, said, "I'm not condoning the abuse of a drug. I'll continue to fight against abuse of drugs, recreational drugs that are destroying society. Steroids aren't destroying society."

Reporters were hardly impressed by the folks from Oklahoma, but media let Switzer off the hook, the coach with three national championships, by basically allowing him and other OU officials to walk away from the potential doping scandal in his program. As was typical for a steroid case in football, many key questions were left unanswered.

Several writers skewered Bosworth, sticking to form, by hating the player, not the game. Craig Neff of *SI* characterized the athlete as ignorant or uncaring about a publicized fad among boys in Miami, "to load up on anabolic steroids and transform themselves into thickly muscled Bosworthian hulks." Neff believed Bosworth should have utilized the press conference to raise awareness about steroid dangers, instead of choosing to give "a rambling self-defense."

A *New York Times* editorial slammed Bosworth, calling it "fitting" he received the lion's share of media focus on steroid suspensions. "He had gone out of his way to attract attention, sporting wild haircuts and depicting himself as a free-spirited maverick. ...," the newpaper opined. "Steroids gave Mr. Bosworth an advantage unavailable to his opponents who didn't have access to the drugs or feared their side effects. His exceptional strength and his success were, to some extent, the product of drugs, not hard training. That's not fair."

Bosworth sought to lay blame for his suspension on a czarist NCAA, but in Miami he did not allege systematic steroid abuse in big-time football. He hedged on disclosure, shielding Oklahoma and other programs, and avoided placing much blame on his coaches. He failed to cite the growing field of qualified critics who said evidence about elite football already added up to a competitive environment dominated by users, leading more and more players into doping.

Bosworth waited two years to make such charges, in his memoir *The Boz*, published after he entered the NFL. Bosworth then estimated the NCAA could catch 70 percent of football players using steroids, if so inclined, and he stated the drugs were as common as aspirin in Switzer's program. Writing in his book, long removed from that press conference in Miami, Bosworth ripped his old school. "The University of Oklahoma hung me out to dry. Left me alone on an island to fend for myself," he fumed. Bosworth discussed his and Switzer's public misrepresentations around the doping matter, their charades in Miami and afterward.

In writing and promoting the book, Bosworth stuck with his line about using steroids himself only for medical purposes, and he claimed that while the NCAA had a steroids epidemic, his current employer NFL had wiped out the drugs through urinalysis. Once again, virtually no one gave credence to The Boz regarding anabolic steroids in football. For decades to come, Brian Bosworth would remain the only college football star suspended for steroids by the NCAA.

Athletes, Coaches and Officials Comment in Testing Aftermath

Beyond The Boz, the Sooners, and their circus accompaniment in Miami, other player suspensions for steroids were mostly overlooked in the bowl season. Nine more athletes were ineligible for bowls because of positive results: offensive guard Jeff Bregel, a two-time All-American for USC; defensive end Roland Barbay, an honorable-mention All-America for LSU; offensive tackle John Zentner and defensive tackle Tony Leiker, both of Stanford; offensive tackle Jim Davie and defensive end Morgan Roane, Virginia Tech; defensive tackle Richard Bear, Arizona State; linebacker David Dudley, Arkansas; and offensive tackle Pat Johnson, Auburn.

Most of these players commented for stories that appeared under much smaller headlines, and they gave the range of explanations for using steroids, from the old medical excuse to insinuations or allegations of institutional encouragement. All guarded their comments to media, and several hedged on facts about their usage, even if making confessions of sort.

Barbay filed a court case against the NCAA, the first for a football player involving steroids, but it backfired. Seeking to overturn his suspension, Barbay initially employed the medical excuse, saying he had used physician-prescribed steroids for injury rehabilitation. A judge threw out the case, upholding the NCAA ruling, after the introduction of a sworn deposition wherein Barbay testified he had received the steroids from a body-builder and had injected himself. Like Bosworth, Barbay formerly made public-service messages for the NCAA denouncing drug use.

Probably the most open comments from a deposed player were by Johnson, a 6-foot-2, 265-pound sophomore trying to establish himself as a starter at Auburn. Johnson, laying low in Tampa following his suspension from the Citrus Bowl, told the *Huntsville Times*: "It was just a mistake I made like a lot of other people who have to sit out bowl games. I wouldn't do it again." Johnson said Auburn head coach Pat Dye informed him of the positive steroid test on Christmas Eve. "He said he was very sorry, but that he couldn't take me to Orlando under the rules. Coach Dye sounded very sincere that he felt bad for me. He just said he would see me when I got back to Auburn. ... I'm sure hoping Auburn won't hold this against me. It was a mistake, no doubt, but I certainly hope my career isn't over. I still feel like I can play at Auburn and contribute."

Johnson said he understood the risk of juicing while facing testing. "I knew there was a chance this could happen. I started using steroids [last] summer in workouts. I used them because I wanted to play so bad. When you take them you're able to work the muscle harder because it recovers quicker. You get stronger because you work the muscle harder than normal. I felt like I needed more strength to play. I tried to find out as much as I could about it, but evidently I didn't find out enough. ... I knew we would be in the bowls, but I thought there would be enough time to get it out of my system.

It stays around a lot longer than I thought. ... The way I look at it, I was trying to make myself better. I was trying to get better and make myself stronger."

In other voices, head coaches speaking with the media generally approved of the NCAA steroid testing, and they suggested or stated directly that players were wholly responsible for the drug use.

Steroids were "probably unnecessary if a kid has the patience to build up his strength," said Joe Paterno, Penn State coach. "It's when they're pressured to play quickly that there comes a problem."

"I don't have total agreement with the NCAA drug testing program," said Earle Bruce, Ohio State coach, "but I think it's a start and I believe in the rules." Bruce expressed sympathy for the players suspended and the teams affected, particularly Bosworth and Oklahoma. "I don't think a drug testing program is supposed to punish young men," he said. "I think it's to educate them and try to help them solve their problem. And, the next step is counseling if they have a problem. But, that's not easy to come by."

Bruce, however, saw steroid use by college football players as a problem of individual nature, not systematic. "I think every young man walks in his own shoes," he said. "He should be taught, he should be helped, but he makes certain decisions on his own. I don't think a coach or an administrator can be held responsible for the actions of a young man."

Jackie Sherrill, Texas A&M coach, believed anabolic steroids were quite manageable through testing. He was thrilled with the NCAA screening and expelling of Bosworth. "It's something that needed to be done, and I have to applaud them," Sherrill told reporters. "You could spend millions in advertisements and it wouldn't have the impact [Bosworth's punishment] will." None of Sherrill's players tested positive for the NCAA, and he boasted about A&M's in-house testing, over which he had presided as moonlighting athletic director for five years. Effective urinalysis "is the responsibility of the head coach and athletic director," Sherrill said. "We took a lot of steps to educate our players. And we spend $25,000 testing them. ... We started the testing program because I was more concerned with street drugs than steroids. Street drugs can kill you. You can get off steroids."

Among the NCAA hierarchy, officials were congratulating themselves. "We're convinced our new drug-testing program has already had a major impact," said Wilford Bailey, an Auburn faculty member making his speech as the incoming president of the NCAA. "We think the NCAA is unique in its position to make an impact on society in this area of great concern."

Byers was equally optimistic. Speaking in San Diego before delegates, the NCAA executive director said: "We believe we have the most comprehensive and effective testing program of any sports organization in the United States today. Its objectives are very clear — to ensure clean championship competition and protect the health and welfare of the student-athlete. ... We think that drug usage and efforts to combat drug usage in sports is one of the most significant issues of the day. We think it's not only important to the welfare of the student-athlete, but it's extremely important for the welfare of the country and young people to persuade those who have been swept up in the drug culture that that is the wrong way to go. ... [Urinalysis] is clearly interrupting the use of anabolic steroids. It's also treating the [street-drug] problem. My own hope is the NFL will step in and begin testing for anabolic steroids."

Critics would beg to differ about effectiveness of urinalysis for steroids, but the media were impressed by the collegiate initiative. "The heavy logging of college football players came courtesy of the NCAA, which last week proved its drug-testing program wasn't to be trifled with," Neff opined for *SI*.

Nevertheless, in the same magazine layout on bowl games, a sidebar story demonstrated that steroid controversy had not ended for college football, especially not Tom Osborne and Nebraska. In an interview with *SI* writer Armen Keteyian, NFL lineman Dean Steinkuhler discussed how steroid cycles and strength training in college at Nebraska helped him become an All-America.

Steinkuhler personified a specific star-out-of-nowhere tale which occurred often for the Cornhuskers, a storyline football fans everywhere had read or heard: Unknown Nebraska boy comes to Lincoln, yearning to be Football Hero for the mighty Huskers. Displaying an unbelievable work ethic in NU weightlifting, the boy emerges as a monstrous man laying waste to opponents and living his dream — and that of fans statewide. Amazing individual success at Nebraska often entailed steroids, Steinkuhler suggested. The drugs definitely made a difference in his becoming the second pick overall in the 1984 NFL draft, by the Houston Oilers. Steinkuhler signed a lucrative, guaranteed contract with Houston as a 6-3, 273-pound offensive tackle. A few years earlier he came to campus a 225-pound fullback, per the script for Super Cornhusker, after growing up in Burr, Nebraska.

Switched to the offensive line, Steinkuhler ate and lifted for three years, raising his weight to 260 pounds, he said, before hitting a strength plateau and turning to steroids. "I wanted to be the best I could be," he said. "I wanted to be better than anyone else. I thought I was a good enough athlete, but I needed something to get over the hump." Steinkuhler, using various steroids during his junior and senior years at Nebraska, found his best results with a six-week cycle stacking three types: Dianabol and Anavar, in pill form, and injectible testosterone. Steroids filled out Steinkuhler to 275, and his bench press increased from 300 to 350. "I never really gained that much strength," he said, "but it really gets you fired up about working out."

Firsthand, Steinkuhler said he knew minimally a half-dozen steroid users on the Cornhuskers of 1983. He knew of a few less in 1984, though he said steroid use "kinda took off" on the team. Steinkuhler believed Coach Osborne was aware of the steroid use but did not grasp the extent of it in the program. "The worst thing is what people will start to say about Nebraska," Steinkuhler lamented, anticipating his comments appearing in *SI*, the world's most popular sport publication. "But [steroid use is] everywhere. Things have happened, you know, that I'm not proud of. But I wanted to get this off my back."

Osborne, with the steroid issue back in his lap, denied Steinkuhler's accusations. "I'd like to make it very clear that I was not aware that Dean Steinkuhler or any other players were using steroids," Osborne said. "I was aware that there's always the possibility, but I did not know of any specific players."

Osborne said he became aware of talk about Cornhuskers and steroids as early as 1976, and in time he confronted a few players. "All we had to go on was rumors," he said. "I heard rumors about two or three players, and I took them aside, and in every case they denied it. There was nothing I could do.

V. Courson: A Trade, Illness, and Phone Call from SI

Steve Courson, in giving his all for seven years as an offensive guard for the Pittsburgh Steelers through two Super Bowl championships and one All-Pro season, had seen his accomplishments ultimately draw no acknowledgment from head coach Chuck Noll. Courson had learned not to expect a grunt in salute from Noll, another Coaching Genius by virtue of four NFL titles. The game was pro football, after all, strictly business, and most players agreed that Noll was a cold fish, if not an arrogant jerk. The more Noll could insulate himself from players, the better.

So Courson knew something bad was up when summoned to Noll's office at training camp in 1984. *Chuck must really be pissed*, Courson figured, considering his ongoing personal battle with the legendary coach, dating back to the previous season.

Noll and Courson had never gotten along. The coach was always prone to ridicule the player in down times, when Courson made mistakes or was too injured to perform. Noll oozed contempt in 1983, beginning with what would be Courson's last full season with the Steelers. In training camp, Noll exploded when Courson pulled a hamstring running a 40-yard dash "for time" by a stopwatch. "All you want to do is body-build and take steroids!" Noll said, berating the 285-pounder loudly — and hypocritically, given the obvious doping by many Steelers present. Courson said nothing this time, but he and Noll were on a collision course.

Courson opened the regular season with a solid performance through four games, but he injured his right knee in the fifth, hobbling him, and from there practiced and played through pain to finish the schedule. Trainers and coaches knew of Courson's gimpy knee but expressed little concern — Noll certainly did not — and a team physician determined no need for surgery. Courson himself was optimistic, anticipating that off-season recuperation and rehabilitation were the remedy required for his knee.

Courson carried out the plan in training for the 1984 season, but it was for naught. That summer at Steelers camp, he found out that the knee was broken down, demanding medical attention. Courson could not go full speed without jarring instability in the joint, radiating major discomfort. Staff personnel were indifferent. Courson was given anti-inflammatory pills and informed that he either practiced and played, right now, or lose his job.

Courson tried again, suiting up for the next workout, but it was fruitless and dangerous. The knee was coming apart, and he heeded its warning to stop before a blowout. Miserable, Courson limped off from a running drill, leaving the practice field in pain, then angrily crashing his helmet to pieces inside the locker room. Now Noll paid attention to Courson, but indignantly, chasing down the injured player to rant, rave, and dismiss any explanation. "There was not one iota of sympathy or concern on his part," Courson wrote in *False Glory*. "He wasn't even addressing me as a human being..."

Noll did not ease up, carrying his grudge into a team meeting and ripping Courson without provocation and in front of everyone. Fully within his power, Noll added a $100 fine for the injured player. Now Courson was enraged, insisting Noll discuss the matter with him, one-on-one, but their meeting brought no satisfaction. "I was so upset that my voice was cracking," Courson wrote. "I had gone to war for this man, and he was prepared to discard me like an old uniform. ... I knew that my days as a Steeler were numbered."

Seeking a different medical opinion, Courson visited a hospital where a doctor said the knee was damaged, requiring at least arthroscopic surgery for assessment. Back at camp the next morning, Courson informed his line coach of the second opinion, and the Steelers had a response. At lunchtime, Courson was in the weightroom when he heard from two people that Noll wanted to see him. He had always known his end with the Steelers was inevitable, but even now as he walked that plank, he found the experience of being discarded almost unbearable. In Noll's office, the coach looked up from his desk, "distant and forbidding as ever," Courson recalled, and wasted no time with human sensitivities.

"Steve, we just traded you to Tampa Bay for Ray Snell," he said, blankly. "Thanks for the seven years." Courson, limp, felt Noll shake his hand while ushering him back out the door. Someone directed him to a phone call from a Bucs official. After hanging up, he made his way through the hall outside the coaches' room. A meeting was in progress with Noll presiding, and Courson saw the assistants glance at him then turn away, saying nothing.

That hurt as much as anything. Just a few hours ago, Courson reported here for the workday as he had for years, while contributing to phenomenal success for the organization. Now, crippled and emotionally stunned, he was being shipped out to a new employer a thousand miles away, like some inanimate package. Moreover, for a final indignity, he was leaving to the silence of formerly trusted associates. "Some of these men were my friends," Courson wrote. "Yet not one of them had the brass to look me in the face and wish me well. Not one of them wanted to buck their head coach. Not one of them was willing to do the right thing."

At Tampa Bay, team officials opted immediately for surgery on Courson's injured knee. The "scope" operation was successful, removing chips of bone and cartilage, along with general tightening of the joint, and in one month Courson returned to football practice, enthused to play again. For the first time in his career, however, he cycled on steroids in season, to recover quickly from the injury. He was in the Bucs' starting lineup by the third game and went on to complete a solid season for Tampa Bay.

Courson moved to Colorado to work out during the offseason, highly motivated. He pounded iron twice a day, six days per week, with steroids his obvious foundation for inhuman training. Courson employed cycling science detailed by Dr. Fred Hatfield, a well-known author in the rising genre of how-to books for using anabolic substances, including human growth hormone. [Apparently, by the mid-1980s, many football players in the NFL and NCAA were consulting the written guidance of doping gurus like Hatfield and Dan Duchaine, co-author of *The Underground Steroid Handbook*; such information was a common tool of training in Olympic sports, power-lifting, and bodybuilding.]

Embracing a new year, Courson tried to forget the immediate past, particularly the trauma of being dropped by the Steelers, but 1985 would truly rattle the young man. Events would extinguish his career in pro football, threaten his life, and, ultimately, redirect his thought and purpose for living.

First, abuse of anabolic steroids would take Courson to the very edge. Increasing intake, he cycled twice in four months, for performance football and power-lifting, a new sport for him. Competing in the Colorada State Powerlifting Championships, Courson finished second in the 275-pound class, where his marks included 745 pounds in the dead lift. Then, for the first Bucs minicamp, Courson embarked on his largest cycle ever, four hefty injections per week: 4 cc of testosterone cypionate, 4 cc Winstrol V, 4 cc Deca-Durabolin, and 4 cc liquid Dianabol. "I knew it was a lot," he later wrote, "but it seemed worth the risk, and I had yet to experience any major negative side effects. My intention was to enter the '85 season at 285 pounds — able to bench press more than 600 pounds, squat about 850, and dead lift about 900."

Courson did not anticipate, however, his resting heart rate's rocketing to 160 beats per minute, compared to his normal of about 72. A physical exam at Bucs minicamp signaled the condition, and an alarmed cardiologist in Tampa grilled the 29-year-old athlete about substances he was consuming, especially alcohol or medication. Courson confessed to drinking beer excessively — and to currently cycling on a large amount of anabolic steroids.

"You've got to stop taking these drugs immediately," the doctor warned.

Courson was shocked into acknowledging his mortality, on the spot, along with the absurdity of his football existence. Driven back to Bucs headquarters, he sank in the seat. "I was confused and scared; my mind was racing," he recalled. "I wondered if all the drugs I had taken in order to compete were destroying my body. I always wondered if there would be any consequences."

Was there a direct causal link to steroids? Physicians and scientists had their suspicions but could not be certain. Medical literature about muscle doping by athletes was thin for case studies and non-existent for clinical data, and would remain so into the future. Courson definitely had blown up his body to grotesque dimensions, even if in the largely lean mass of a genetic specimen on chemicals. Clinical evidence was accumulating regarding the strain of an enlarged mass on body organs and systems, a cause of heart disease, among other potential ailments.

That was common sense to Courson, the health risks of becoming so big. Now, seemingly facing a consequence, Courson felt exploited by football, and he made a decision before the car ride ended. Upon reaching Bucs offices, he walked in and told head coach Leeman Bennett he was retiring from football, immediately.

The coach left open the door for Courson's return, and the young man's concern eased when medication returned his heart rate to normal range, allowing him to resume training. Courson began to favor staying in the NFL. Then a chance encounter shook him again, forcing him into deeper realizations about the widespread extent of steroid usage, not only in football but society at large, and what role he might have played in the cultural dilemma.

In the locker room of a local health club, Courson discovered a pair of teen football players injecting each other with testosterone. He did not know what to say and left the room, feeling terrible, wondering if he held responsibility. "Wasn't I supposed to be a role model?" he wrote in *False Glory*. "Didn't youngsters take their cues from professional athletes? If we were so blasé about taking these drugs — and let's face it, contrary to NFL pronouncements, kids do know that we're taking them — how could we expect them to do as we say, not as we do?"

Besides harm to youths, Courson was growing to detest the personal compromises made for football, particularly doping. Courson understood the teams and league unofficially approved of anabolic steroids. He had discussed the drugs with physicians for both the Bucs and Steelers, used them with numerous teammates and even opponents, discussed them with countless more players, down into small-college ranks. Courson felt caught up in a danger he courted, nonetheless; he loved the results of steroids, which enabled him to compete in a job environment saturated with the drugs, but he hated forsaking inner beliefs to do it. He believed most user players experienced the same inner conflict, including bitterness about management, and went on without protest. Not him. *I'm not a freakin' attack robot for these assholes*, he told himself.

From turmoil, Courson was formulating resolve. Conditions both external and internal were leading him to mobilize against anabolic steroids in sport and society, to personally raise cultural awareness. He was like dynamite set against football's wall of denial, given his quickly evolving attitude on the issue, his lifelong conviction about honor, and his regretful experience with the drugs.

Sports Illustrated writer Jill Lieber became the trigger mechanism when she dialed his phone number. Lieber explained that she and other *SI* writers were contacting players across the league for an investigative series on anabolic steroids in the NFL.

Twenty years later, Courson summarized his circumstances as a pro player at the time that Lieber called. "The game is full of compromises," he said. "We compromise ourselves when we go to training camp. We'd rather be at the beach. We compromise when we have some jerk-off coach run you down in front of your teammates, humiliate you, because it's all part of making the team better, and you hold yourself back. You compromise when they stick the pain-killing needle into your knee, when they need you to play. So the drugs are just another compromise. And, for me in 1985, I make all those compromises to play that game, then I'm starting to have some health problems, and I don't know what the score is. I'm sitting in this no-man's land, between Chuck Noll, blowing me out in front of my teammates, and a team in Tampa, saying they're going to do liver enzyme tests on me.

"And I'm caught between these extremes here, and... now I'm asked to tell the truth about [steroids]. I'll compromise to a point, but I'm not going to lie about it. I was willing to compromise to do what I did, use the anabolic drugs. I would do all of that for them, but not lie for them."

When Lieber called Courson, no NFL player had opened up about anabolic steroids for performance enhancement. No one had discussed the environment surrounding the drug within the NFL nor the full history of their own use, and certainly not on the record with the use of their name. Lieber asked Courson if he would.

"Yes," he said.

VI. Rozelle Oversees a PR Fiasco in Steroids

He surely was no genius about anabolic steroids, but who could be? Pete Rozelle, the 59-year-old NFL commissioner, must have felt humbled by the muscle hormones that swept his league irreversibly. Despite his expertise for spin, despite America's unabashed devotion to his football product, the old PR writer could not control this story, particularly against some determined sportswriters and publications.

As a young man Rozelle trained in a Hollywood seminary for the selling of NFL fantasy on America: Los Angeles, working for then-Rams hype-master Texas E. Shramm. Since 1960, Rozelle had steered the crafting of modern football mythology, The Spectacle on camera, by capitalizing on his close, powerful associates in television, greatest myth-making device in human history. The league had expanded from 12 franchises to 28 under Rozelle, becoming "the most powerful organization in the United States," said Howard Cosell. "They're on all three networks. Their control of the print medium is astounding." But Rozelle the image master was stymied trying to gloss-over muscle drugs in his NFL. He had dealt with anabolic steroids in public for years, but the story persisted. He could not stamp out evidence of institutional culpability, only hope it forever passed under surface. Rozelle was but a man who helped launch monster product in the modern NFL, with fields of drug-augmented players playing role of Superhero.

The issue went high profile in May 1985, when *Sports Illustrated* published an in-depth trilogy of articles on anabolic steroid use in American sports including the NFL, based in part on compelling information obtained from interviews with 25 active players such as Courson. The article succeeded in tainting the league along with its personnel from Rozelle on down to coaches and players.

The layout of the three stories in *SI*, by lead writer William Oscar Johnson with Lieber and Keteyian as contributors, surveyed the steroid problem throughout American sports. "It is a spreading wildfire that is touching athletes at every level of sport," the introduction began. "From NFL stars to iron pumpers in small-town gyms, from high school bench warmers to college All-Americas, thousands of American athletes, both male and female, are routinely ingesting or injecting anabolic steroids to increase their strength or improve their all-around sense of athletic and personal self-worth."

Football was the series' primary sport of discussion, the NFL, the USFL, and NCAA, and damaging testimony was quoted from players, a coach, a former steroid consultant, and a convicted dealer. They generally viewed use as widespread in professional and college football, with players in high school being affected.

"On some [NFL] teams, between 75 and 90 percent of all athletes use steroids," said Lyle Alzado of the Raiders, a 14-year defensive lineman. "Steroids create more raw power, speed, endurance. Some of the old-time players have gotten by without using them, but a player cannot compete today at a top-notch level of football without an aid of some sort."

"Steroids are very, very accepted in the NFL," said Pat Donovan, retired Cowboys lineman who played from 1973 through 1982. "In my last five or six years it ran as high as 60 to 70 percent on the Cowboys on the offensive and defensive lines."

Other player estimates ran lower. Fred Smerlas, Buffalo nose tackle, believed about 40 percent of NFL players had juiced.

Steroids apparently had permeated the new United States Football League. "You can find steroids in every pro locker room," said Kent Hull, center for the New Jersey Generals. "It is not a minute thing. It gets to a point where some guys, especially at the pro level, think they have to do it to make it."

Former power-lifter Richard Sandlin had first used steroids to become world ranked, then for income as a usage consultant. He told *SI* he had advised about 40 pro players in the NFL and USFL, along with college coaches and players. "They want to know what type of cycles to go on and how long to stay on the cycle. And they want to know basically what drugs to use, what drugs are harmful, what combinations are harmful, what combinations are best," Sandlin said, maintaining he ceased using and consulting.

Kim Wood, strength coach for the Cincinnati Bengals, pointed to the influence of head coaches in the NFL and NCAA. "They pressure the strength coaches and say, 'How can we get big and strong?'" Wood said. "Strength coaches justify giving steroids to their kids this way: 'It's my job to get them good stuff, not let them go to some scumbag on the streets.' They say, 'Steroids are the individual's decision,' but somehow the drug always seems to be there."

League officials, conversely, said they saw no real problem, basically sticking to their stock view that any "non-medical" users — athletes seeking increased size and strength — were isolated individuals. Johnson wrote:

> Rozelle says he doesn't think they're widely used. Gene Upshaw, the executive director of the NFL Players Association, who for 16 years was a star guard with the Raiders, also takes a see-no-evil approach and issues a string of denials. "I never knew any guys who took steroids."
>
> And: "There's no black market of steroids." Again: "I don't think steroids are a problem in the NFL."

One active player joined Rozelle and Upshaw in their stance, Chiefs offensive guard Tom Condon, the NFLPA president, who said, "Steroids might be a problem in colleges. They might be a problem in track and field. But they're a non-factor in professional football. I've never seen anybody take anything. I don't know about them."

But Courson, a friend of Condon, told *SI* everything he knew about anabolic steroids, including his current use and recent health scare. "I think everybody faces the question: Do I want to go on [steroids]? It happens to everybody at some point in their career. At every level," Courson said. "It's like you're cheating when you use drugs, but then again, everyone else is cheating, too. We'd all be better off if steroids weren't around — everybody would be better off." One story in the layout, "Getting Physical — And Chemical," focused entirely on Courson and was mostly a running narrative of direct quotes. "Steroids are a different realm of drug from speed or painkillers," he said. "They enhance your natural ability. They are a building block. They can take you somewhere. I can't condone steroid use, but I can morally accept it as an aid."

In the national debate on steroids in football, colleges had absorbed the brunt of bad publicity thus far, particularly Vanderbilt, Clemson, and Nebraska. But the *SI* stories hammered the NFL, rattling the league.

Upshaw, leader of the players union, responded by saying athletes were getting a disproportionate share of blame for steroids. He charged that management was just as guilty, suddenly displaying at least some knowledge of the problem. Not that the union boss was confirming widespread use; Upshaw claimed again that anabolic steroids were not a serious concern. "[A]t least not as big as *Sports Illustrated* made it out to be recently," Upshaw said, during a speech to youths at a football camp in Nashville. "The problem is steroids are a legally prescribed drug, which you have to separate from the others. Warnings are in every playbook not to use steroids. Enforcement goes back to the team level and, in some cases, teams are guilty of looking the other way. Unless you go through a black market, prescriptions are required for steroids. And players get prescriptions from somewhere."

Upshaw firmly opposed random urinalysis in the NFL, noting the current collective bargaining agreement called for a player to expect only one test annually, for street drugs, at training camp. "The owners have no right to spot checks," Upshaw said. "If there is reasonable cause, an athlete can be sent to an outside facility. We have one in every city."

Rozelle did agree with Upshaw on one point: Neither wanted the league to get involved with urinalysis for steroids. Within a year following the *SI* exposés, however, spring 1986 — after the NCAA had approved steroid testing for football players, winning loud approval — time was running out for the NFL to get moving on the issue. Media were criticizing Rozelle about steroids, but he stubbornly fixated on cocaine, marijuana, street narcotics — his platform for preventive action against chemical-substance abuse by players.

Along the way, some cursory attention was paid to amphetamines, but Rozelle persisted in largely ignoring steroids. He could afford to do so only a little longer.

Bad Press Punishes Rozelle, NFL For Lack of Steroid Policy

In late June 1986, Pete Rozelle apparently saw a PR opportunity, with no idea how badly it would backfire. Don Rogers, talented young safety for the Cleveland Browns, died of a cocaine overdose. Rogers' tragedy drew extensive publicity, occurring only a few days after NBA draft pick Len Bias died of a cocaine overdose.

Rozelle jumped to push his agenda on street drugs, announcing his "first" plan in pro sports for "mandatory random urinalysis." Rozelle's "comprehensive" drug policy included screening players for traces of narcotics such as marijuana, cocaine, heroin, LSD, and Quaaludes. Players now faced two unscheduled tests during the regular season, along with the scheduled test they already had at training camp per the collective bargaining agreement.

Rozelle unveiled his plan the Monday morning following the July 4th holiday weekend, and the story received front-page coverage by media returning to work and looking for a scoop. Rozelle denied he was exploiting the Rogers-Bias controversy, or the current media obsession over athletes' losing their lives or careers to street drugs, cocaine in particular. "Our concern," he said, "is the health and welfare of the players — those taking drugs and those injured by taking drugs." Rozelle said he had developed the new policy for a year, although union leader Upshaw was a dissenter regarding random testing.

Rozelle contended that an NFL player had a civic duty to avoid street drugs. "In the unique world of professional sports you give up some rights of privacy to participate," he said. "Whether or not they know it, these players are role models." Street narcotics posed a "serious potential economic problem" for owners, Rozelle said, threatening gate attendance and TV revenues, but he refused to "speculate" about the scope of use by players.

Upshaw, viewing random testing as an invasion of privacy, vowed to fight the plan that Rozelle promised to mandate under unilateral authority of the commissioner. Rozelle said league bylaws and the bargaining agreement obligated him "to protect the health and welfare of the players and preserve the integrity and public confidence in the NFL."

Battling anabolic steroids, meanwhile, was not a priority for any NFL official. Amphetamines would be screened under Rozelle's plan, but a positive result could only lead to education and counseling, not punishment. Anabolic steroids, absent from the testing list, would continue to be handled via the "reasonable cause" process, rarely employed, wherein a team physician would identify a steroid user through observation and recommend counseling. Steve Courson was the only NFL player known to be questioned in the process by league officials — but *after* he had spoken openly with *Sports Illustrated*. Previously, when Courson discussed steroids with team physicians in both Pittsburgh and Tampa Bay, no one mentioned "reasonable cause" or intervention. Rozelle's underlings said anabolic steroids would likely be added to testing the following year, 1987.

If the NFL expected public approval of Rozelle's new drug policy, they were disappointed. Positive feedback was almost non-existent while critics pounced from all over the country. Thomas Boswell of the *Washington Post* derided the initiative, calling it "a cure-all grandstand policy." Boswell wrote:

> No street corner in America has any greater need of a tough, caring, comprehensive drug program than the locker room of an NFL team. Players often seem chemically endangered from every direction. Yet, thanks to years of neglect, the problems have become diabolically hard to fix.
>
> Now, Rozelle feels the enormous pressure of public outrage. The NFL should have addressed the issue of amphetamines 20 years ago, of steroids 15 years ago, of painkillers 10 years ago and cocaine five years ago. But it didn't.

Rozelle and the NFL absorbed bad press from California, through politicians and a high-profile star of the Oakland Raiders, for failing to act constructively on anabolic steroids. The West Coast was overcome with illicit drug trafficking, with countless conduits in and out for smugglers, and the Mexican "pharmacies" across the border from California were legendary sources for steroids. After police in California busted large-scale steroid operations, allegedly involving sales to a football coach and players at Fullerton Junior College, legislators in Sacramento postured on the issue, drafting legislation and ripping the NFL's stance on tissue-building hormones.

Rozelle really felt the barbs from Oakland All-Pro defensive tackle Howie Long, a media favorite who complained bitterly about the league's ignoring steroids while testing for narcotics like cocaine. Speaking from the Raiders camp in Oxnard, Long pointed to a mission of damage control versus ensuring health and fair competition for players. He said fans saw a lie on the field in so many chemically augmented specimens. "Some of these guys are playing in a test tube. I want to know who the real guys are," Long charged in an *AP* interview. "I don't really think they [league officials] want to test for it. I think they're content with giving the fans a beefed-up product. They're concerned more about league image than anything. ... I'd say in the big positions, I'd say over 50 percent [of players use steroids]. It's just my guess. You know how many God-given 6-5, 270-pound guys there are who run a 4.7 [seconds in the 40-yard dash]? Not many. I can't push enough for the testing of steroids. The big guys are taking it. Some of those guys aren't really big guys. It's like going to a plastic surgeon. ... A lot of these guys just aren't the real deal. There are more than a few."

Long presumably was a genetic wonder, enormous, powerful, and fast, and the 26-year-old maintained he did not juice: "I don't need to take steroids. I roll out of bed at 275 pounds." Long said he recently began lifting weights for the first time, and karate also figured into his gaining about five pounds of muscle for the season. "I've gotten a lot bigger in the chest, arms, and shoulders," he said.

Following Long, another critic of Rozelle's drug policy, New York writer Sandy Padwe, made waves with his treatise "Drugs in Sports: Symptoms of a Deeper Malaise." Padwe, *SI* editor of investigative reporting, had his 2,500-word analysis published in *The Nation* magazine in September, opening month of the 1986 NFL regular season. Padwe was one of a few writers to criticize media and fans along with football organizers for the problem.

Padwe accused Rozelle of "pure hypocrisy" for his inactivity in policing performance enhancers. Padwe, a nemesis journalist for Rozelle in New York City, where they had faced off for years, alleged the commissioner only acted whenever forced, such as recently, in the wake of highly publicized deaths of athletes attributed to cocaine abuse.

Padwe recounted the historical time frame of doping exposed in the NFL, primarily the amphetamine scandals at San Diego and Washington in the early 1970s. Afterward, Padwe charged, Rozelle and other officials always referred to fines imposed as proof of their tough anti-doping efforts. "But the fines had little effect on the players, who understood that the league's drug policy was basically cosmetic, aimed at placating public opinion. Drug use hardly changed, according to [Pat] Toomay and several other players active at the time," Padwe wrote, continuing:

> As long as the drugs involved in sports were only amphetamines, steroids, painkillers and a little marijuana here and there, and as long as the books being written about the subject were by [NFL] dissidents such as [David] Meggyesy and [Peter] Gent — or, in baseball, Jim Bouton — the commissioners felt no discomfort.
>
> The same could be said of the directors of athletics at colleges and universities. Stories of cocaine abuse moved the stories to another level. They outraged the public, made TV advertisers nervous and caught the interest of the sporting press. To a lot of editors, coke was a hotter, trendier drug than amphetamines or anabolic steroids. The use of the latter was limited to enhancing one's performance, and in the anything-goes world of athletic competition no one cares about how players excel, as long as they excel.

The well-written commentary of Padwe, a foremost American journalist on sport doping, was timeless. His personal qualifications included extensive journalistic experience on PED use in elite sport, his perspective of sport media's ignoring problems, an understanding of fans' crass self-indulgence, and sharp analysis of flimsy fantasy that was the football spectacle.

Padwe, alarmed by talk of the so-called solution in urinalysis, warned of the faulty technology's use as a PR tool by football. Testing, he noted astutely, "is not the simple answer in sports," continuing:

> There are questions about the testing procedures themselves that have not been answered. The tests are hardly infallible. And, then, do you test for [street] drugs or performance-enhancing drugs too? Rozelle's plan does not call for steroid testing, which is laughable given the evidence available about steroid use throughout the league
>
> The N.F.L. says it is still working on the testing methodology.

Padwe was not the typical critic regarding the modeling effect of celebrity athletes. He saw no real responsibility for them to set positive examples for youths, particularly in their private lives, or to act like moral characters when a majority were not. Instead, Padwe identified the most destructive harm as fans' relentless idol worship — and consumer patronage — of players and games like football. Padwe wrote:

> The public must realize that athletes are not heroes. Simply putting on a uniform does not make them better people or give them a greater standard of behavior to uphold. Too many athletes are over-pampered individuals who have been told all their life that they are special because they can throw a ball or run swiftly. They are eased through colleges and universities when they should be learning to read and write.
>
> Not only do they accept it, they expect it. They are the recipients

> of money, clothes, cars, women and drugs from all manner of people, while teachers, coaches, administrators and even some parents look the other way. Many athletes fully understand sport's amorality and don't even try to distinguish right from wrong.
>
> If college and pro teams look away while the players pump themselves full of steroids, painkillers and amphetamines so they can play when they are hurt, why should athletes think there is anything wrong with doing coke with friends to relax? To be consistent, the press and the fans should be as concerned about athletes' use of painkillers or performance-enhancing drugs as they are about cocaine.
>
> Does the reason they aren't have anything to do with America's love affair with winning? Athletes are revered for scoring touchdowns, runs and baskets by a group of individuals to whom winning — or covering the point spread — has become an end in itself. Players get the message: Use whatever means it takes to get the score in your team's favor. Such an attitude skews values completely and bleeds all the beauty from our games.

Padwe concluded by accurately predicting no end in sight for sports' ills like doping — not until the entire culture, the real drug addict, accepted and dealt with its own malaise. Mere athletes and games, Padwe contended, would never achieve morality for everyone, and sports institutions could crumble under the expectation, if not a culture of costly indulgence. He wrote:

> For their part, the teams and schools expect the athletes to be paragons of virtue and role models. They make the players live this hypocrisy in order to receive financial benefits. As the system unravels — and it is unraveling faster than Roger Clemens can throw a baseball — the impulse will be to reach for a panacea like drug testing rather than to deal with much deeper, much more complex problems, which go to the core of sport in America. Instead of calling for testing, the people with the nooses should be checking the foundation. It's about to collapse.

Fortunately for Rozelle, the Padwe piece was published outside the mainstream press, but there was no hiding NFL irresponsibility while the steroid problem only festered, blowing up again in a series of events that produced negative headlines for months.

A steroid squabble among NFL players became news when Bill Fralic, offensive guard for Atlanta, confessed in a media interview to using the anabolics during college. The *Atlanta Journal* newspaper published Fralic's quotes on October 30, and the story went national. Fralic, a second-year player from Pitt, was already a vocal critic of steroids in the NFL, but previously he had not discussed his personal culpability in the problem. He decided to go public about his own use, he said, because of talk that he had been "caught" and was forced by NFL management to speak out in favor of steroid testing.

"I've heard that rumor, and I'm irritated by it," Fralic said. "It's just not true. Period. The reason why I speak out against this junk is for one reason and one reason only: It's wrong."

Fralic told reporters he used steroids for only one month in college, between his sophomore and junior years at the University of Pittsburgh, where he became an All-America. Fralic said the drugs helped his weight increase from 275 to 290, but he could not use them in "good conscience," especially for fear of adverse health effects. "I experimented with them because I thought I wanted to be bigger and stronger," Fralic said. "I got caught up in the mentality of football in the weight room. All my friends were taking them, or quite a few of them. They kept saying how great they were and I decided to see for myself." Fralic insisted he quickly ceased steroids. "I'm not on top of a ladder preaching," he said. "I'm not saying I'm a perfect human being. I'm not saying I'm not dumb enough to take steroids, because I was dumb enough, and I can see how somebody can fall into that trap. All I'm doing is voicing an opinion."

The Falcons star got some backup in Atlanta, where Georgia Tech head coach Bill Curry admitted he once used steroids, as an NFL rookie lacking size in 1965. "It was Dianabol," Curry recalled. "In two months, I gained more than 20 pounds. I looked great. My shoulders, legs and arms were all bulging."

Sports Illustrated came back firing at the NFL in early November, publishing football writer Paul Zimmerman's scathing "The Agony Must End," an analysis of the league's rising injury rates and contributing factors like anabolic steroids. An editor's lead-in to the story touted the perspective of Zimmerman, a former college football player and veteran pro football scribe, who investigated because "injuries in the NFL continue at an unacceptable rate." Zimmerman's article needed no introduction to the magazine's five million-plus readers, especially those of Football America. The cold facts and sensational details demanded attention and got it, and the unfavorable reaction would finally swing the NFL toward instituting steroid testing. While NFL injuries were Zimmerman's central focus, he labeled a fundamental cause to be anabolic-steroid abuse widespread in the league, and his inside sources like Howie Long agreed. "Today's [natural] 240-pounder is a pumped-up 280," Zimmerman wrote, continuing with sharp prediction: "In five years maybe he'll be 300, moving even faster, inflicting greater damage."

Dolphins trainer Bob Lundy observed that the formerly two types of NFL player had morphed into a Frankenstein combination. "It used to be that you either had a good athlete or a big guy," Lundy said. "Now you have to be both."

"Steroids are the worst problem in the NFL," said Colts linebacker Johnnie Cooks. "I just want to play football with the body the Lord gave me. Some of these guys we play are nothing but muscle. When you get hit by them, something has to go."

Long was fairly convinced the game's increasing sizes meant future health trouble for athletes. "You put 50 pounds of muscle on a player, and he goes from a baggage carrier in the jungle to Tarzan, and he says, 'Wow, this is great,'" he said. "But something has to give. ... It's tampering, voodoo. You're either going to pay now or pay later."

Many were paying an immediate price, as Zimmerman documented, with 183 starters sidelined in the season's first half. Former player and veteran Dolphins' coach Don

Shula believed brutality had ratcheted-up in the NFL. "Some of the collisions I've seen are really severe," Shula attested. "I've been happy for quite a while to be on the sidelines. I'm not anxious to put on a uniform again. It's a tough game for everyone. Real tough."

Steroids were the likely X factor in the trend, but, Zimmerman's story notwithstanding, most football insiders remained quiet about the topic, other than to complain in coded language or without directly mentioning the hormones. Even among admitted users, almost without exception their common story was about trying steroids only briefly, "experimenting," as they called it. Zimmerman hypothesized many players used steroids but did not admit it. "That's about right," Long said. "I don't know about the speed positions, but I've heard they've used there, too."

Wrapping the analysis, Zimmerman offered his solution directly for the football commissioner: "To Pete Rozelle — begin steroid testing right now. Get rid of the freak show in the NFL." The cultural impact of Zimmerman's piece, or the *SI* effect on contemporary issues in sport, was immediate.

Bad press buried the NFL, including a bomb launched in-house by the Patriots' general manager Patrick Sullivan, who accused league owners of ignoring steroids. Sullivan, of the Patriots' ownership family, minced no words during a speech at Merrimack College in Massachusetts. "There is no concerted look at the steroids issue," said Sullivan, whose franchise had been vilified for cocaine binging by players. "I personally consider it as big a problem as the cocaine-marijuana-alcohol abuse problem. The fact is that owners and coaches have chosen to take the problem and put it underneath the table. "They don't want to rock the boat and they don't want to disrupt their team, and they think they can continue to win."

The *New York Times* quoted an unidentified team executive about doping and injuries. "It's scary," the official said. "We've created a whole league of 275- and 280-pound players who used to be 245 to 250. What we're seeing are injuries caused by the inability of the bones and joints to support the size of muscles that are enlarged by steroid use."

An insurance company joined the fray, grabbing the attention of both the league and union, by dropping NFL players for permanent disability coverage. State Mutual Assurance Company of America officials, citing "a rash of career-ending injuries," said larger, heavier players and the spread of anabolic steroids were factors in their decision. "So many people have been injured with career-disabling injuries, that [we] ask, 'Does this still represent for us a reasonable business opportunity?' " said Steven Kurlansky, group coverage director of the company that underwrote permanent-disability for about 40 percent of the NFL players with such plans; Lloyd's of London underwrote the others. State Mutual was also reconsidering the permanent-disability policies it held with college players.

An industry official, Ted Dipple of American Sports Underwriters, said, "The odds are stacking up against the insurer; it's difficult to make a profit. To me, there are five basic reasons: [street] drugs; steroid abuse; artificial turf; players are more dispensable now that the USFL is out of business; and while the equipment is safer, it also gives the players more confidence [at contact] than ever before — they're braver."

Union officials regretted the insurance company's pullout, but executive director

Doug Allen said permanent disability should be the domain of franchises. "Our main approach to the problem, since we have no control over insurance companies, is to make sure the players are protected by the owners of the NFL," Allen said.

VII. Rozelle Follows Political Wind, Hypes Steroid Testing

The shadow of anabolic steroids stalked pro football, a constant source of media criticism, and NFL owners fretted for the public image of their mega product. Pete Rozelle finally acted. His office announced steroid testing on November 21, 1986, the same day an insurance company canceled its disability coverage in the league. The NFL urinalysis for anabolic steroids would begin in 1987. With a typical spin, a league spokesman said that the development had nothing to do with recent press coverage. "All we were waiting for was a new [steroid] testing methodology," said Joe Browne.

Sports Illustrated was highly skeptical. "The NFL has suddenly reversed its field on anabolic steroids," editors noted, attacking the "avowed reasons... rather suspect." *SI* rejected any possibility that the league could only now learn of widespread abuse and acquire urinalysis technology. "It appears that Rozelle, having sensed which way the winds are blowing, has put up a sail and gone with them."

In December, while the NCAA reaped glowing headlines for unprecedented steroid testing of football players that bagged The Boz, the NFL and Rozelle continued taking flak from multiple directions, including players who *supported* testing, interviewed by Paul Domowitch, the *Toronto Star.*

"Steroids are the biggest problem the league has right now," Bill Fralic said. "Bigger than cocaine, bigger than marijuana, bigger than amphetamines, bigger than booze, bigger than anything."

"It's always been a hush-hush issue that nobody's really wanted to talk about," said Michael Carter, 49ers' defensive lineman. "But something's got to be done."

Fralic was skeptical of Rozelle: "He told me he had just become aware of the problem recently. He said he was looking into it and would address it. But it seems to me it hasn't been addressed. It has been sidestepped. Because the public isn't as aware of [steroids] as the people on the inside are, I don't think the league has felt compelled to deal with it. ... Everything the league does is motivated by money. They're not concerned about our welfare."

John Spagnola, Eagles tight end and players representative, believed the NFL "tacitly endorses" steroid use. "The truth is," he said, "they like to see players bigger and stronger and faster."

Competitive pressure on the field was enough of a dictate. "It's not like [coaches and others are] forcing steroids down the players' throats," Fralic said. "It's the players who are taking them. On the other hand, the players are taking them because they feel they have to keep up with the Joneses. They feel they need them to survive."

"It's very prevalent, no question about it," Spagnola said. "I can't say how many guys are doing it and how many aren't. But chances are, if you're an offensive or defensive lineman and you're not doing it, you're not going to be around very long. This is a very competitive game. If you want to play, you look for any edge you can find. [Steroid use] has been going on and will continue to go on unless something's done about it."

The players echoed Steve Courson, retired because of apparent blacklisting after nine years in the NFL and four in the NCAA. The 31-year-old was moving forward, though, as an authority on sport doping. Courson knew much about performance enhancement through his own abuse of anabolic steroids and other chemicals, competing at football's highest levels, but now he researched the complicated big picture at work, all influences, from user player to consumer fan. Manually searching for documentation and other evidence, years before Internet access, Courson visited libraries and other research sources across the country. He constantly communicated with active players in private, names never to be revealed. Courson gathered literature pertinent to anabolic steroids and learned what he could about human growth hormone, recently introduced in a synthetic version and undetectable by testing technology. Courson had not used HGH, but players verified that it was being used in pro football.

Living in Jackson Hole, Wyoming, Courson was writing a book unprecedented for its strict focus on football doping and for the complete honesty of the author regarding his own experiences. And when new steroid testing by the NCAA and NFL became news, reporters tracked him down for comment. He saw no hope for controlling and stopping steroids in football. He well understood urinalysis technology had huge holes for evasion — in Olympic sports, steroid testing was proven a failure after a decade — and he understood that the entire culture's raw pursuit of winning drove the abuse.

"It's no longer a game, no longer fun," Courson said. "They've made the average athlete a killing machine. The drug use is a sad tribute to the intensity of the game. Society puts pressure on you to win. It's how competitive and rough the game has become. ... Athletes are going to do what they have to do to compete, and doctors are going to prescribe drugs to put you on the field to complete."

To solely blame players for steroids, the mindset of football officials and most coaches, was inaccurate and destructive, Courson contended. No rule in the NCAA, for example, specifically held a coach or institution accountable for the drugs; only an athlete could be penalized. The NFL, of course, would never label franchises as culpable. "The NCAA and the NFL ought to take a closer look at the game, instead of just pointing the finger [at players]," Courson said. "They should look at why guys are doing it. It's hypocritical. ...

"What these guys are doing is trying to compete at a higher level."

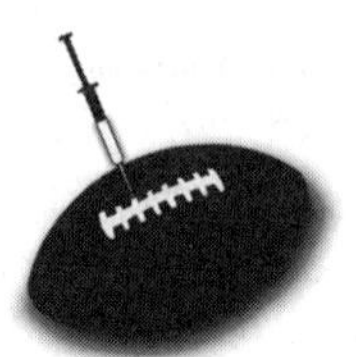

REFERENCES

1985 Survey. (1985, May 22). NCAA survey shows press reports exaggerated use. *United Press International* [Online].

Aldrich, M.W. (1985, May 16). Kreis pleads innocent of drug charges. *The Associated Press* [Online].

Alfano, P. (1983, August 30). CBS's Pan Am balancing act. *New York Times*, p. D20.

Alfano, P., & Janofsky, M. (1988, November 19). A guru who spreads the gospel of steroids. *New York Times*, p. 1 — 1.

Alzado, L. (1991, July 8). 'I'm sick and I'm scared.' *Sports Illustrated*, p. 20.

Anderson, D. (1986, November 30). X factor in N.F.L. violence. *New York Times*, p. 5 — 1.

Asher, M. (1985, January 14). NCAA to delay starting any drug-test program. *Washington Post*, p. D2.

Asher, M. (1985, June 21). Colleges push for reforms. *Washington Post*, p. E1.

Asher, M. (1985, June 22). NCAA passes most severe sanctions. *Washington Post*, p. D1.

Asher, M. (1986, January 12). Little opposition expected to NCAA drug proposal. *Washington Post*, p. G2.

Asher, M. (1986, January 14). NCAA approves testing for drugs. *Washington Post*, p. D1.

Asher, M. (1987, January 3). No postgame drug testing. *Washington Post*, p. D3.

Assael, S. (2003, February 3). Big night. *ESPN The Magazine*, p. 77.

Bayless, S. (1990). *God's coach*. New York, NY: Simon and Schuster.

Baylor Lawsuit. (1991, July 25). Former Baylor basketball player sues coach. *The Associated Press* [Online].

Bock, H. (1987, January 7). Bosworth gone after social criticism. *Associated Press* [Online].

Boswell, T. (1986, July 9). Rozelle: Hollowest of gestures. *Washington Post*, p. D1.

Bosworth, B. (1988). *The Boz*. New York, NY: Charter Books.

Bosworth Barred. (1986, December 25). Bosworth barred from Orange Bowl. *Associated Press* [Online].

Bosworth Leaving. (1987, January 5). Bosworth leaving Oklahoma. *Associated Press* [Online].

Bouchette, E. (2005, March 24). Haslett admits to using steroids. *Pittsburgh Post-Gazette* [Online].

Bregel Suspended. (1986, December 23). USC guard won't play in Citrus Bowl. *Associated Press* [Online].

Brubaker, B. (1987, February 1). Players close eyes to steroids' risks. *Washington Post*, p. C1.

Caddes, G. (1986, December 28). Bruce address NCAA steroid policy. *United Press International* [Online].

Chad, N. (1985, May 21). Howard Cosell: He still is the one telling it like it is. *Washington Post*, p. D1.

Chad, N. (1986, February 28). Cosell keeps telling it, but his reach shrinks. *Washington Post*, p. C2.

Chaiken, T. (1988, October 24). The nightmare of steroids. *Sports Illustrated*, p. 82.

Chandler, L. (1996, October 17). McNairy continues to use steroids, and NFL dreams closer to coming true. *Charlotte Observer* [Online].

Chaney, M. (2001). *Sports writers, American football, and anti-sociological bias toward anabolic drug use in the sport*. Warrensburg, MO: Central Missouri State University.

Clemson Coaches. (1985, January 20). Clemson coaches reportedly gave steroids to football players. *United Press International* [Online].

Clemson Program. (1985, March 7). Clemson begins drug counseling program. *Associated Press* [Online].

College Testing. (1984, June 14). Panel: NCAA should start testing athletes. *Associated Press* [Online].

College Players. (1985, January 22). College players used steroids. *United Press International* [Online].

Coming Clean. (1986, November 5). Coming clean about steroids. *New York Times*, p. D24.

Cooper, D.L. (1985, January 17). Athletes are losers by winning with illegal drugs. *New York Times*, p. 5 — 2.

Cosell, H., & Bonventre, P. (1985). *I never played the game*. New York, NY: Avon Books.

Courson, S. (2005, March 7). Interview with author. Farmington, PA.

Courson, S. (2005, May 1). Telephone interview with author.

Courson, S. (2005, June 22). Telephone interview with author.

Courson, S., & Schreiber, R. (1991). *False Glory*. Stamford, CT: Longmeadow Press.

D-IAA Suspensions. (1986, December 12). Three players suspended in Division I-AA. *United Press International* [Online].

D-III Suspensions. (1986, December 10). Drug tests: The kickoff. *New York Times*, p. D29.

Dan Duchaine. (1997). Dan Duchaine the steroid guru. *Quest For Advanced Condition: www.qfac.com*.

Davie Suspended. (1986, December 27). Virginia Tech tackle confirms steroids for his suspension. *Associated Press* [Online].

Deal Rumor. (1986, November 17). Steroid deal rumor irritates test supporter Bill Fralic. *The Sporting News* [Online].

Denham, B. (1997). Sports Illustrated, the "War on Drugs," and the Anabolic Steroid Control Act of 1990. *Journal of Sport & Social Issues, 21* (3), p. 1.

Denlinger, K. (1982, July 2). Teamwork is the solution. *Washington Post*, p. C1.

Denlinger, K. (1987, January 15). Makers of NCAA rules on a winning streak. *Washington Post*, B1.

Discussing Drugs. (1986, March 11). Rozelle discusses drugs. *New York Times*, p. B8.

Domowitch, P. (1986, December 14). NFL declares war on steroids. *Toronto Star*, p. E3.

Donohew, L., Helm, D., & Haas, J. (1989). Drugs and (Len) Bias on the sports page. In Lawrence A. Wenner (Ed.), *Media, Sports, & Society* (p. 225). Newbury Park, CA: Sage Publications.

Dunham, W. (1985, August 21). Steroid testing poses problems for colleges. *United Press International* [Online].

Finder, C. (2003, January 30). 1980 strong-man show portended steroids rage. *Pittsburgh Post-Gazette* [Online].

Fisher, M. (2005, July 10). Waters, steroids and a slippery slope. *TheRanchReport.com/ Scout.com.*

Football Use. (1985, December 18). Football player steroid use disclosed. *United Press International* [Online].

Ford Denies. (1985, March 12). Ford denies his assistant approved steroid use. *United Press International* [Online].

Ford Speaks. (1985, January 21). Ford says assistant coaches did not provide steroids. *United Press International* [Online].

Former Player. (1985, January 22). Former Vandy player says he used steroids. *The Associated Press* [Online].

Freeman, D.H. (1986, December 27). Sherrill lectures on steroids. *The Associated Press* [Online].

Garber, G. (2005, January 24). A tormented soul. *ESPN.com* [Online].

Goodwin, M. (1985, January 20). Drug use believed to extend beyond two schools in the South. *New York Times*, p. 5 — 9.

Goodwin, M. (1986, July 8). NFL plans random drug tests. *New York Times*, p. A1.

Holleman, J. (1986, December 26). Bosworth declares right to 'healthy' body. *The Associated Press* [Online].

Holleman, J. (1986, December 27). Bosworth professes both guilt and innocence. *The Associated Press* [Online].

Huizenga, R. (1995). *"You're okay, it's just a bruise."* New York, NY: St. Martin's Griffin.

Insurance Halted. (1986, November 21). Insurance firm halts new football policies. *United Press International* [Online].

Jackson Talks. (1986, November 14). Steelers running back discusses steroids in NFL. *The Associated Press* [Online].

Janofsky, M. (1983, August 28). Advisor suspects NFL steroid use. *New York Times*, p. 5 — 1.

Janofsky, M. (1986, March 9). Drug tests, lawsuits on NFL agenda. *New York Times*, p. 5 — 10.

Janofsky, M. (1986, December 2). Dowhower gone as Colts' coach. *New York Times*, p. B9.

Johnson Speaks. (1986, December 30). Auburn player blames pressure of college football. *The Associated Press* [Online].

Johnson Suspended. (1986, December 27). Johnson declared ineligible for Citrus Bowl. *The Associated Press* [Online].

Johnson, W.O. (1985, May 13). Steroids: A problem of huge dimensions. *Sports Illustrated*, p. 38.

Johnson, W.O., Lieber, J., & Keteyian, A. (1985, May 13). Getting physical — and chemical. *Sports Illustrated*, p. 50.

Johnson, W.O., Lieber, J., & Keteyian, A. (1985, May 13). A business built on bulk. *Sports Illustrated*, p. 56.

Kaufman, I. (1985, June 20). NCAA committee wants drug testing plan. *United Press International* [Online].

Keim, B. (1986, December 26). Bosworth admits steroid use. *United Press International* [Online].

Keim, B. (1986, December 27). Bosworth lashes out at NCAA. *United Press International* [Online].

Keim, B. (1987, January 2). Sooners, Razorbacks look for excellent 1987 season. *United Press International* [Online].

Kephart Contact. (1985, December 18). Kephart had contact with Fitton. *The Associated Press* [Online].

Keteyian, A. (1987, January 5). A former Husker fesses up. *Sports Illustrated*, p. 24.

Keteyian, A. (1989). *Big Red confidential: Inside Nebraska football.* Chicago, IL: Contemporary Books.

Klecko, J., Fields, J., & Logan, G. (1989). *Nose to nose.* New York, NY: William Morrow and Company, Inc.

Kreis Apologizes. (1985, December 16). Kreis apologizes for steroids. *The Associated Press* [Online].

Kreis Defended. (1985, January 10). Associates defend strength coach. *United Press International* [Online].

Kreis Named. (1986, August 20). Kreis named volunteer strength coach at Middle Tennessee. *The Associated Press* [Online].

Laing Wins. (1986, May 16). Laing wins unanimous 10-round decision. *United Press International* [Online].

Lamme, A.J. III. (1985, May 23). Separate college sports from academics. *Christian Science Monitor*, p. 16.

Latt, S. (1985, January 9). Coach on leave amid Vanderbilt scandal. *The Associated Press* [Online].

Latt, S. (1985, January 15). Vanderbilt institutes steroid testing. *The Associated Press* [Online].

Latt, S. (1985, February 10). Vanderbilt is steroid hotbed. *The Associated Press* [Online].

Lawmakers Question. (1986, July 11). California lawmakers question Rozelle's policy. *United Press International* [Online].

Lawyers Satisfied. (1985, November 28). Lawyers satisfied with Kreis' probation. *The Associated Press* [Online].

Letterman Show. (1987, January 13). Bosworth appears on Letterman. *United Press International* [Online].

Lieber, J. (1985, May 13). Getting physical — and chemical. *Sports Illustrated*, p. 50.

Long Tackles. (1986, July 27). Long tackles steroids. *New York Times*, p. 5 — 9.

McLain, S. (1985, January 11). Steroid expert to meet with Vandy officials. *United Press International* [Online].

McLain, S. (1985, January 12). Vanderbilt not alone in steroid problem, expert says. *United Press International* [Online].

McLain, S. (1985, September 12). Kreis asks state to give dates of alleged steroid sales. *United Press International* [Online].

McLain, S. (1985, November 27). Former strength coach sentenced. *United Press International* [Online].

McLain, S., & Lillard, M. (1985, April 20). Kreis quits in wake of indictments. *United Press International* [Online].

Mira Practices. (1986, August 21). Hurricanes linebacker practices with team. *The Associated Press* [Online].

Mixed Reaction. (1983, October 25). Mixed reaction to NCAA study. *New York Times*, p. B8.

Moore, T. (1991, July 28). Another Alzado perspective. *Atlanta Journal and Constitution*, p. E3.

Nadel, J. (1986, July 25). Howie Long says many players take steroids. *The Associated Press* [Online].

Nathan, D.E. (1986, July 7). Rozelle announces drug plan. *United Press International* [Online].

NCAA Testing. (1986, December 26). Steroid testing began in early December. *The Associated Press* [Online].

NDSU Linemen. (1986, December 5). Two North Dakota linemen suspended for steroids. *United Press International* [Online].

NDSU Suspension. (1986, December 5). North Dakota State players suspended for steroids. *The Associated Press* [Online].

Nebraska Clean. (1986, December 19). Nebraska clean in steroid tests. *United Press International* [Online].

Nebraska Purchases. (1985, December 18). Nebraska players purchased steroids. *The Associated Press* [Online].

Nebraska Testing. (1984, August 16). Nebraska football players tested for drugs. *The Associated Press* [Online].

Needs Chemistry? (1991, July 24). Who needs chemistry? *United Press International* [Online].

Neff, C. (1985, December 9). Steroid justice. *Sports Illustrated*, p. 11.

Neff, C. (1986, December 8). Reversing field. *Sports Illustrated*, p. 15.

Neff, C. (1987, January 5). Bosworth faces the music. *Sports Illustrated*, p. 20.

Neff, C., & Sullivan, R. (1985, December 23). The people helper. *Sports Illustrated*, p. 26.

Neff, C., & Sullivan, R. (1986, April 21). Anabolic actions. *Sports Illustrated*, p. 13.

Nelson, J. (1986, December 27). Bosworth and Bregel head banned list. *The Associated Press* [Online].

Nevada-Reno Suspensions. (1986, December 12). Two Nevada-Reno players suspended. *The Associated Press* [Online].

NFL Testing. (1986, November 21). The NFL plans steroid testing. *The Associated Press* [Online].

NFL Use. (1983, September 11). NFL steroid use. *New York Times*, p. B-26.

Nissenson, H. (1985, June 22). NCAA approves tough measures against cheating. *The Associated Press* [Online].

Noonan Used. (1987, May 5). Noonan used steroids to regain weight. *The Associated Press* [Online].

Not Aware. (1987, January 10). Osborne not aware any Husker used steroids. *United Press International* [Online].

Officials Guilty. (1985, June 21). Upshaw says team officials guilty as players for steroids. *The Associated Press* [Online].

Osborne Retires. (1997, December 10). Osborne retires, Byrne names Solich as replacement. *University of Nebraska-Lincoln, www.unl.edu/pr/osborne.html.*

Padwe, S. (1986, September 27). Drugs in sports: Symptoms of a deeper malaise. *The Nation* [Online].

Pasquarelli, L. (1991, July 16). Blaming steroids. *Atlanta Journal and Constitution*, p. D1.

Pfaff, D. (1985, June 21). Study: Drug use by college athletes overblown. *The Associated Press* [Online].

Players Oppose. (1986, November 28). Courson: Many NFL players oppose steroids but use anyway. *The Associated Press* [Online].

Pomerantz, G. (1986, December 31). NCAA overreacted, 49ers' Walsh says. *Washington Post*, p. C3.

President Praises. (1987, January 15). NCAA president praise steroid testing. *The Associated Press* [Online].

Provost, W. (1983, September 11). Study of All-American provides an NU shock. *Omaha World-Herald* [Online].

Richey, W. (1986, September 26). NCAA cracks down on drug use by athletes. *Christian Science Monitor*, p. 6.

Riker Dies. (2004, March 1). Walter Riker, 87; helped craft drug policies for NFL. *The Associated Press* [Online].

Riker Obituary. (2004, February 23). Dr. Walter F. Riker Jr., *OwlNet*, Columbia University.

Ritter, M. (1986, December 26). Athletes risk health and test detection. *The Associated Press* [Online].

Rosen, B. (1982, February 3). FSU player details allegations. *Washington Post*, p. D6.

Samson, D. (2004, August 29). Lincoln: Land of linemen. *Kansas City Star*, p. J6.

Schreiner, B. (1986, October 15). Nebraska coach promises fight against steroids on team. *The Associated Press* [Online].

Schuyler, E. Jr. (1986, July 7). Random testing for NFL. *The Associated Press* [Online].

Shearer, E. (1984, May 16). Curry finds cheating in college football recruiting. *The Associated Press* [Online].

Star Turns. (1987, January 4). Star turns: Drugged out. *New York Times*, p. 4 — 16.

Steroids Funneled. (1985, January 10). Steroids funneled from Vanderbilt to Clemson. *The Associated Press* [Online].

Steroid Investigation. (1986, August 28). Steroid investigation concerns two football players. *United Press International* [Online].

Sullivan Says. (1986, November 13). Patrick Sullivan says league ignores drug problems. *The Associated Press* [Online].

SWC Survey. (1985, April 22). Steroids reported at Southwest Conference schools. *The Associated Press* [Online].

Testing Announced. (1985, January 15). Vanderbilt crackdown. *New York Times*, p. B-14.

Thompson, J. (1986, December 25). Bosworth, other players knew hazards of using steroids. *The Associated Press* [Online].

Thompson, W. (2002, October 30). Super agent man. *Kansas City Star* , p. D1.

Todd, T. (1987, Spring). Anabolic steroids: The gremlins of sport. *Journal of Sport History, 14* (1), p. 87.

Tucker, D. (1985, January 16). NCAA delegates approve preseason NIT. *The Associated Press* [Online].

Tucker, D. (1987, January 6). NCAA officials tout testing as success. *The Associated Press* [Online].

Two Disqualified. (1986, December 12). Two players disqualified from Division I-AA playoffs. *United Press International* [Online].

Two Sentenced. (1985, November 27). Kreis and former pharmacist receive probation. *The Associated Press* [Online].

Use Growing. (1983, August 29). Steroid use said to grow. *New York Times*, p. C-8.

Vandy Room. (1985, January 19). Ex-judge, ex-con in Vandy weight room crowd. *United Press International* [Online].

Vandy's Fight. (1985, April 28). Vanderbilt's drug fight. *New York Times*, p. 5 — 11.

Vega, V. (1985, May 23). College athletes take more painkillers than college students. *The Associated Press* [Online].

Volsky, G. (1986, December 27). Bosworth tells of steroid use. *New York Times*, p. 1 — 19.

Voy, R. (1991). *Drugs, sport, and politics*. Champaign, IL: Leisure Press.

White, G.S. Jr. (1985, January 16). NCAA shelves drug plan. *New York Times*, p. B8.

White, G.S. Jr. (1985, June 22). NCAA approves stiffer penalties. *New York Times*, p. 1 — 1.

Wilson, A. (1985, June 20). NCAA committee proposes national drug testing program for college athletes. *The Associated Press* [Online].

Wilson, A. (1986, December 26). Barbay tests positive for steroids. *The Associated Press* [Online].

Wilson, A. (1986, December 31). Federal judge forbids Barbay from playing. *The Associated Press* [Online].

Win-At-All-Cost Attitude. (1986, December 30). Courson says winning drives steroid problem. *The Associated Press* [Online].

Wolff, C. (1986, December 26). Bosworth barred from bowl for steroids. *New York Times*, p. D7.

Yaeger, D., & Looney, D.S. (1993). *Under the tarnished dome.* New York, NY: Simon & Schuster.

Yesalis, C.E. (2005, June 16). Telephone interview with author.

Yesalis, C.E., Bahrke, M.S., Kopstein, A.N., & Barsukiewicz, C.K. (2000). Incidence of anabolic steroid use: A discussion of methodological issues. In Charles E. Yesalis (Ed.), *Anabolic Steroids in Sport and Exercise* (2nd edition), p. 73. Champaign, IL: Human Kinetics Publishers.

Zentner Speaks. (1986, December 24). Stanford's Zenter regrets steroid suspension. *The Associated Press* [Online].

Zimmerman, P. (1986, November 10). The agony must end. *Sports Illustrated*, p. 17.

Chapter 5 [Testing What? Urinalysis and policy for steroids, 1987-89]

"We are only catching the dumb ones."

Dick Schultz
NCAA executive director, 1990

As headlines in football doping persisted from 1986 into 1987, some officials touted their new anti-steroid testing policies before the American public, claiming eradication was at hand. Officials suggested urinalysis for steroids was perfected. "Testing does two things," said Ed Bozik, Pitt athletic director. "It allows you to identify the problem, and it acts as a deterrent. People will quit using drugs because they are afraid of being caught." Officials were wrong, of course.

Steroid use continued unabated in football on teams throughout the NFL and NCAA. "Today... anabolic steroids remain the choice drug of many bulk- and strength-conscious football players," reported Bill Brubaker, Washington Post, in a comprehensive analysis. "I use 'em; everybody uses," a St. Louis Cardinals veteran told Brubaker, anonymously. "Some guys are carrying around bags full of this stuff. I'll tell you one thing: steroids make you a hell of a lot bigger and a hell of a lot stronger. They make you faster, too."

The increasing performance parameters of football were obvious to anyone with a clue. "Players have gotten so large and so fast that the field has shrunk," said Saints GM Jim Finks, who played in the NFL during the 1950s, pre-steroids. "It wasn't too long ago that a 230-pounder was the biggest player out there, a lineman with very little mobility. Linebackers now weigh 230, and they're fast... there's nowhere to hide."

Hiding steroid use, however, was something most players and officials were inclined to do. An exception was Saints' center Steve Korte, who spoke openly of his use "so people will understand why we do this," he told Brubaker, during a journalistic interview on par with the Courson-Lieber story in *SI* a couple years before. "There's still a hush-hush attitude about this," Korte said. "Players feel that if somebody finds out they're taking steroids, they'll be called an artificial person."

Korte began using anabolic steroids in 1981 at the University of Arkansas, where he developed into a consensus All-America. In an experience exactly in line with Courson's, he resorted to the drugs in college after getting knocked around by larger players, along with recognizing his strength limits via more natural means. "I first used [steroids] during the summer after my sophomore year. ..," Korte recalled. "I used to watch these track and field athletes who were throwing around those huge amounts of weights day after day. ... I wasn't blind to the fact that these guys — and other people at Arkansas — were taking steroids. My goal was to become the best football player I could be, and I was looking for any kind of edge at all, as far as trying to take myself better to get to the pros. So I started taking steroids that summer and, right away, I felt a big, big increase in my strength."

Korte bench-pressed 585 pounds in college, after using. As an NFL lineman, the 6-2, 270-pounder scoffed at the False Dogma, the old talk that steroids did not enhance performance, faulty rhetoric still employed by some coaches, doctors, and sport officials. Korte discussed a steroids cycle of usage before the 1986 preseason: "I was feeling real bad. It had been a rough training camp. I felt run-down, beat-up, fatigued, susceptible." He stacked Anavar pills with injectible Deca-Durabolin for six weeks. "By the third week of the season, my joints started to feel good again," he said. "By the sixth week, my strength was much, much, much higher. ... [I]nstead of feeling real sore and weak, I was ready to go again by the next day."

At that point, Korte ceased using for the rest of the year. "Deep down inside, I felt that the less I took, the less chance I had of getting sick," he said.

Korte estimated that about two-thirds of linemen in the NFL had cycled, and he knew about 10 of his teammates to be using. Competitive pressure was constant. "Look, I don't want to use steroids," Korte told Brubaker. "But I'm a center, and any time I go against a big noseguard, like I do every week, there's a good chance he's taking them. So if I don't take them, I'm at a disadvantage."

In San Francisco, a prominent NFL figure concurred that systematic forces influenced the use of anabolics. Bill Walsh, head coach of the 49ers, discussed steroids in interviews with media. Acknowledging the drugs were "much more common than I thought a year ago," Walsh said he suspected some of his players had juiced. "I think players have used them defensively to keep up with the competition. Only certain positions would use steroids. Running backs and quarterbacks definitely would not." Walsh largely opposed steroid testing on the basis of "individual rights."

Walsh expressed a common viewpoint of NFL coaches: Athletes on street drugs were to be avoided, but not those using steroids. He confirmed the 49ers would draft a steroid user out of college. "Steroids would not bother us," Walsh said. "We feel we can educate and get rid of the problem. That's not the case with heavy cocaine or marijuana use."

Teams certainly were not shying away from Brian Bosworth, the Oklahoma All-American linebacker hit by a positive steroid result during NCAA testing for bowl games. Bosworth, amid speculation he would declare for the NFL draft, drew plenty of interest in the winter-spring of 1987.

The Philadelphia Eagles' head coach Buddy Ryan salivated over the prospect. "Really, what I'm hoping is that enough [teams] think something's wrong with [Bosworth] that he's still there when we pick. ...," Ryan said. "I'd love to have him."

Indianapolis, holding the draft's No.2 pick overall, looked good for landing The Boz, and team officials courted him through the press. "Brian Bosworth would love it here," gushed Colts GM Jim Irsay. "He would love the fans. It is a good situation." Bosworth was no question mark for Irsay. "I'm concerned about his reputation on the football field and this is tough and aggressive," he said. "He is a leader on and off the field. ... We're interested in taking the best football player available."

The writer Brubaker, meanwhile, charged that pro and college officials had for decades avoided cleaning up the doping mess, despite their recent instituting of steroid testing. NFL executive director Don Weiss said, "I don't think steroids became an issue in football until the early '80s." Brubaker responded, writing, "If steroids didn't become an issue in football until the 1980s, that is news to thousands of college and pro players, past and present, who are believed either to have used the Juice or witnessed its effects on others."

George Dostal, strength coach of the Atlanta Falcons, was more up-front than most football officials. "I hear horror stories all the time — even about high school kids using them, which gives me cold chills," Dostal said. "Who's to blame? Everybody in football's to blame. I think we all just rode the white pony too long and decided this thing was going to take care of itself. Well, it hasn't."

Players such as Korte and Bob Golic were hopeful steroid urinalysis would prove a valid preventive in the NFL, but they also reserved skepticism. "Morality-wise, it would be great if nobody used steroids — then everyone would be equal," Korte attested. "So, if they want to use testing as a deterrent for everybody and say they're going to fine us or throw us out or whatever, that's fine with me. I'll abide by the rules. I'll stop taking them. But, will everybody really stay clean? Or will some guys find a way to go undetected in these tests?"

Korte offered no information about beating steroid testing, while Golic, in quotes published by the *New York Times*, mused if new anti-doping were effective "a lot of offensive linemen [would be] playing indoor soccer next year." Golic, former linebacker in college, was switched to nose tackle in the NFL, where his weight increased from 235 to 270. "I went from a two-legged, walking, upright, thinking human being to a four-legged, crawling, sniveling beast of burden," Golic quipped, adding he had considered anabolic steroids but avoided them. Golic, 29, said he gained weight through power-lifting and massive calorie intake.

Golic expressed readiness for steroid testing by the NFL, scheduled to begin soon at the league combine for 300 college prospects. "It would make my job a lot easier," he said. "There are guys around the league that you know are using something because there is no way they could look like that. They look like somebody pumped them up with an air hose."

A former field foe of Golic differed, Gene Upshaw, executive director of the NFL Players Association, a Hall of Fame lineman. Upshaw was steadfast in asserting no steroid problem existed in the league, and he flatly opposed urinalysis of any football player, professional or collegiate.

Pete Rozelle had established an NFL steroid testing policy but wanted to improve upon it by implementing an element of surprise, *random testing* — also favored by many media, fans, and team executives such as Tex Schramm. "You need random testing so [players] don't know when it's coming," Rozelle said.

I. Exploiting Loopholes of Urinalysis

In the summer of 1987, a rather lone NCAA official affirmed that steroid urinalysis had loopholes, questioning whether it would become effective at all. Testing had neither stopped nor slowed use in college football, said John Toner, the U-Conn athletic director and chairman of the association's Drug Testing Committee. "Among football players whose schools are testing them and using our laboratories, we know that 50 to 70 percent of our athletes are using steroids," said Toner, citing surveys and tests conducted at the University of Oregon and UCLA.

One strength coach, called the allegation "ridiculous." Mark Larson, University of Colorado, said, "I think Toner is reacting to misinformation. It's somebody pointing a finger at football programs without knowing what's going on."

Another strength coach backed Toner, Oregon's Mike Clark. "Thirty to 70 percent of the members of your college football team are on steroids," said Clark, ethics committee chairman for an organization of strength coaches. "We're seeing kids go from 220 to 260 pounds in one year — and you don't have to be too intelligent to figure it out."

Timing a cycle of classic steroids for avoiding scheduled testing was simple — cease use in time for the body's clearing of detectable traces, typically a week or two for pills like Dianabol — but the hot method for beating urinalysis among athletes was undetectable substances, wholly undercover anytime, unidentifiable by current testing technology and method. Human growth hormone, for which no test existed, had been used for several years in professional and collegiate football. "Designer" steroids, undetectable and of unknown variety, had been available since the early 1980s.

Athletes employed more techniques to defeat testing, like gaining the inside word of pending tests from sources like coaches and trainers, or substituting clean urine for tainted specimens under the nose of overseers. In 1988 in Philadelphia, reportedly, a group of Eagles had their steroid-laden urine drained from bladders by an out-of-town consultant, who brought along clean urine to substitute in order to pass their scheduled tests at Veterans Stadium. Using steroids despite testing was still lost on some athletes, beginning with those few who produced positive results, but many more were educated and disciplined at circumventing urinalysis, and new tricks would always develop throughout sports.

Undetectable Substances Invade Sport

A designer or bootleg steroid, with modified molecular structure — unrecognizable to screening machinery programmed for distinct chemical signatures of patented anabolic steroids — was used by college football players as early as 1984, in Nashville, where pharmacist and avowed Vanderbilt booster Woody Wilson reportedly hawked a "super" steroid for $75 a bottle, his special concoction. At that time in NCAA football, predating steroid testing, the goal of a new molecular structure was to minimize androgenic side effects, but the primary mission was anabolic potency, an explosive synergy of formerly independent compounds.

Olympic athletes were using designer steroids for smooth-acting potency and avoiding detection. Perhaps the earliest public report of designer steroids in American sport was by Dr. Irving Dardik, U.S. Olympic Committee, who oversaw testing at the 1984 Games in Los Angeles. Dardik learned about the mysterious bootleg steroids from testing engineer Dr. Don Catlin, who directed lab analysis of samples from Olympic athletes. After Catlin's briefing, Dardik understood the urinalysis system to be fallible, and he said as much to writer Will Dunham for a *UPI* report. "There are hundreds of different types of anabolic steroids. And you can devise all kinds of variants," Dardik said. "Drugs have their own individual chemical fingerprints or thumbprints.

"By taking designer drugs, it's like putting a piece of tape over the thumbprint. ... It's a very, very big problem, and the absolute solution I'm not sure of. But people who think that drug testing is the answer, it's just not so."

Dunham consulted with Dr. Douglas McKeag, NCAA steroids researcher, who acknowledged faults persisted for urinalysis. McKeag said effective testing by any party was almost "impossible" and "not something that's even close to being practical to be used on a mass scale."

The progressing sophistication of anabolics for avoiding detection was evident in a 1988 investigative series in The *New York Times*, by writers Peter Alfano and Michael Janofsky, particularly through the story of Dan Duchaine, a cocky "drug guru" gaining fame beyond the traditional doping underground of weightlifters and bodybuilders.

"Hopefully, I'm a guiding light," said Duchaine, 36, conducting his first lengthy interview with a mainstream publication.

Doping Gurus Emerge from Shadows

Dan Duchaine, who began using steroids in the 1970s, was an early known expert on doping for performance, though not the father guru, as often credited. Alvin Roy, high priest of Dianabol in football, surely knew methods beyond merely popping pills, and Olympic athletes worldwide obviously benefited from doping technicians before Duchaine's time.

Duchaine, however, was the first to go public as rock-star guru, telling America about his unique expertise much like Timothy Leary had done with hallucinogenic drugs. In writings and interviews, Duchaine detailed his doping programs for anonymous bodybuilders, power-lifters, athletes, and movie stars. "The infamous Dan Duchaine had no scruples," a fan posted online decades later. "He told no lies. Dan Duchaine was no holds barred."

More anabolic whizzes joined Duchaine in public during the 1980s, seeking attention for their business in bookselling and personal training, if not ego, and the notables included Bill Phillips and Fred Hatfield, two Americans, and Paul Borresen, of England.

When Duchaine spoke with *The Times* in 1988, he was a convicted steroid dealer and former bodybuilder vowing to use anabolics the rest of this life. He held street credibility with users of every sort, having defied the False Dogma promoted by establishment figures. Indeed, Duchaine said anabolic substances like steroids definitely built mass, enhanced performance, and were safe in moderation under informed supervision — guidance that physicians and scientists were incapable of providing, he charged, because of their ignorance. "If you can rebalance your metabolism so that it is optimal for your sport and it does not endanger your health, then I think it's fine," Duchaine said.

A resident of Venice Beach, California, the gym capital notorious for strutting specimens augmented by anabolics, Duchaine had interviewed users for a decade to compile valid information on their methods, results, and health. "I am the expert in the country by default," he said. There was no disputing Duchaine according to Dr. Robert Voy, chief medical officer of the USOC. "He knows more than I do," Voy said. Duchaine was co-author and publisher of the *Underground Steroid Handbook*, in its third edition. He and California bodybuilder Mike Zumpano printed and distributed the first press run about 1980, an 18-page pamphlet informing readers about anabolics. The handbook became so popular that Duchaine and Zumpano sold upwards of 50,000 copies over four years, $6 each, while bootleggers distributed photocopies. Voy called the publication "a fabulous pharmacological text." A staple of the handbook was Duchaine's formal introduction of human growth hormone, HGH, to the training world.

Human growth hormone was used medically to treat dwarfism by stimulating growth of internal organs, along with expansion of skin, teeth, tongue, and skeletal mass. Natural HGH, extracted from cadavers, was scarce and expensive, costing $1,000 and more for a month's dosages. The substance was also dangerous, with some harvests infected by a latent viral disease, Creutzfeldt-Jakob, causing deaths among bodybuilders. Non-contaminated HGH also was suspect, with some researchers concluding as much as 80 percent of users developed diabetes; doctors also linked it to thyroid and liver disease, impotence, and menstrual disorders, but no one recorded clinical evidence.

Presumed dangers aside, HGH was part of Olympic training by 1980, when doctors secured and administered the substance for athletes. A physician spoke publicly in 1984, Dr. Robert P. Kerr, of San Gabriel, California, who said he was among "several hundred doctors who have been prescribing growth hormone for selected athletes." Soon after, lower-cost synthetic growth hormone became available and athletes flocked. Duchaine was excited, declaring in 1988: "I will revolutionize human growth hormone use in this country." It was already done, thanks more to steroid testing than any doping guru. Growth hormone was the rage among athletes for staying invisible under urinalysis screening. "There's a lot of dispute over whether a test can be developed for it," said Dr. Terry Todd, doping historian at the University of Texas. "It raises nightmarish problems for those who are in charge of sports."

Dr. Voy addressed the HGH quandary in his book *Drugs, Sport, and Politics*. "Today synthetic growth hormone is readily available to athletes, in spite of claims by the country's two producers of synthetic growth hormone — Eli Lilly and Genetech — that they tightly control sales," Voy wrote. "Is there a need for better control? I think so. Athletes tell me it is not a problem to buy synthetic HGH."

II. Steroids Widespread in Football, Despite Testing

In the fall of 1987, Duke University was pumped about its basketball program blossoming under head coach Mike Krzyzewski, on the verge of beginning a streak of five straight appearances in the NCAA Final Four.

On the football field, meanwhile, Duke was a laughingstock, and many players sought to change that through juicing. "We just wanted to win," defensive lineman Murray Youmans would later recall. "We were tired of losing." Youmans was among about 10 upperclassmen gathering behind closed doors to do anabolic steroids. "We gave each other shots," he told the *Charlotte Observer*. "You could get [steroids] anywhere. We got them from a bodybuilder. A doctor gave us prescriptions..."

That physician apparently was not team doctor Frank Bassett, who later said he denied steroid requests from some players, opting instead to lecture them on potential dangers. Dr. Bassett thought steroid use was obvious on the Blue Devils team. "You could tell a lot of guys were doing it, especially over the summer," he recalled. "They'd come back with these huge muscles." Duke University administrators and sport boosters also worried about football, but only for rampant losing. They dismissed any claim of widespread muscle doping. "There is no drug problem at Duke," an official said during this period.

At a rival school of the Atlantic Coast Conference, at least one coach recognized steroid use in football players. "I think some schools actually advocate the use of steroids," said Frank Costello, Maryland strength coach and former coach in U.S. Track and Field. "[We play] some teams that are flagrant, outrageous steroid users." Maryland randomly tested athletes for steroids, but officials had not disclosed results during two years of policy. Costello provided some insight. "Have there been football players at Maryland who I think have used steroids? Yes," he said.

Elsewhere, the administrators and coaches of the University of Miami, a high-profile school, and Akron University, a low radar school, were quick to deny that steroids were tainting their football programs.

Speculation swirled around head coach Jimmy Johnson's Hurricanes after football strength coach Pat Jacobs was arrested for steroid distribution as part of a national crime investigation. Jacobs was one of 34 people indicted in San Diego in connection with a steroid-distribution ring that, authorities contended, controlled up to 70 percent of the drug's illegal U.S. market serving athletes and bodybuilders.

Immediately following the federal grand jury's indictment in California, Miami administrators expressed certainty Jacobs had no steroid dealings with athletes. Moreover, "school officials doubt any of their [football] players are involved with" steroids at all, reported *The* AP. Jacobs was suspended from his position pending further investigation, and his arrest "stunned" Miami officials, said Sam Jankovich, athletic director. "But I would be even more surprised to learn any of our student athletes are involved. I'm not ruling out that possibility, but... we don't have a major problem with steroids." Jankovich said 96 steroid tests had been administered to Miami football players during the previous year, and "less than two" produced a positive result.

Jacobs was taken into custody at his Miami apartment as the indictments came down, apparently with little notice even though police reportedly found "boxes of liquid and tablet steroids, hypodermic needles and a stack of cash marked 'profits.'" A green university notebook, allegedly containing names of customers, was discovered hidden in the back of a TV set. The same day, reportedly, university officials joined with police "in tracking down the names."

United States Customs spokesman Patrick O'Brien downplayed Jacobs's associations with both the steroid network and the university, announcing the coach operated exclusive of the Canes football program. "He was a small-time guy who got caught in the wrong place at the wrong time," O'Brien said. "We have no reason to believe at this time that Jacobs was passing the drugs on to athletes."

Most Miami players interviewed by media backed up the Customs agent, but not everyone. Defensive back Don Ellis said anabolic steroids were integral to big-time college football, including for his team. "They're here, they're everywhere you look," Ellis said.

The NCAA enforcement division had no interest in probing steroid matters involving the Hurricanes, bound for a fourth national-title game in five years. NCAA investigators, in a period of chasing major schools for "improper benefits" as trivial as tee shirts, car rides, or plane tickets home for athletes, preferred to avoid performance-enhancing substances that spun tangled, public-repulsing webs, if not legal bombs, among athletes, coaches and schools.

Nevertheless, Hurricanes football, a program widely viewed as renegade, hardly appeared innocent next to Jacobs's criminal case. By contrast, the Akron allegations surprised many football fans because of Gerry Faust, the Zips' second-year head coach generally regarded as a good guy, particularly by sportswriters. Faust was famed as the failed head-coaching experiment at Notre Dame, a sympathetic character hired straight from the high-school rank. The media and fans nationwide, charmed by Coach Faust, were rooting for him to succeed at Akron University, an outback of Division I football.

Steroids did not discriminate among football teams, large-school or small-school programs, coaches "good" or "bad." In spring 1987 at Akron, the student newspaper *Buchtelite* quoted an anonymous source alleging that at least six Zips football players used steroids the previous season, Faust's first for the school. The source, without providing names, also said personnel in the athletic department knew about the drugs.

University president William V. Muse immediately denied the charges, contending players had not used steroids but a commercial "weight-gaining substance" derived from protein. Faust, through a prepared statement, denied any knowledge of steroids on the team, promising to suspend any player known to be associated.

The Buchtelite reported Faust had at least heard of a potential problem, according to strength coach Pat Ciccantelli, who recalled informing the head coach of four players he "speculated" could be users. "It was just over-cautious action on our part," Ciccantelli said. "The players denied any steroid use in front of me and Coach Faust." The *Cleveland Plain Dealer* also quoted an anonymous source, who speculated that the Zips, had they made the Division I-AA playoffs, would have had several players suspended over NCAA steroid testing. "Steroids are available," the source said. "They've been seen in the dorms. There's a black market for them."

Muse appointed a university committee to conduct an internal probe, and three months later, the primary result was a recommendation for the school to drug-test athletes. In-house urinalysis, the nine-member panel believed, would prevent any talk or use of steroids in the future, and President Muse promised to appoint a second committee to examine the feasibility of testing. They said no evidence was found of Akron football players employing muscle dope. "We simply couldn't substantiate any of the allegations of NCAA rules violations, or the allegations of the use of steroids," said committee co-chair Robert Dubick, associate provost and dean of student services. "From our study, the allegations made by *The Buchtelite* were proved inaccurate or third-party at best."

Steroids apparently had been in Faust's former program, Notre Dame, where players were continuing to juice under successor head coach Lou Holtz, as future reports would substantiate. Holtz, after winning with tainted programs at Arkansas and Minnesota, had come to Notre Dame smelling a national championship. Holtz cleared house in the Irish program, casting out waves of Faust recruits, replacing them with his own, and the killer attitude for championship football took over in the program. Players had to be aggressive for Holtz, ready to waste opponents and even each other in practice — and anabolic steroids, of course, physically served the mindset. Holtz would get his national championship.

During the 1988 football season, Miami had the attitudes and physiques to win the national title, but there came one more roadblock to the summit: two starters, junior offensive tackle John O'Neill and senior linebacker George Mira, Jr., were suspended in December through NCAA steroid testing before the No. 2-ranked Canes met No. 1 Oklahoma in the Orange Bowl. Each player tested positive for Lasix in his system, a diuretic banned by the NCAA for its ability to mask steroid use, and Mira was a repeat for such headlines. The year before, Miami police had found steroids in his truck following a disturbance on campus, but Mira and his father, George Mira, a former Hurricanes and NFL quarterback, said the steroids belonged to someone else. No charges were filed.

Mira and O'Neill challenged the NCAA suspensions in court, scrambling for reinstatement in time for the Orange Bowl. They waged a brief, unsuccessful court battle, stirring media attention frowned upon by the game's opposing coaches. Both Miami's Jimmy Johnson and Oklahoma's Barry Switzer blamed individual players for a "negative image" dogging their teams, and the media gave lip service, posing no questions to the contrary. Presumably, there was no institutional culpability whatsoever, and these iconic coaches were not accountable.

"This year was very positive, all year, until [this Mira-O'Neill] incident," Johnson said, overlooking the steroid-distribution arrest of his former strength coach, Jacobs. "Unfortunately, anytime something happens, it brings out the dirty laundry."

Switzer continued his surliness about Brian Bosworth, one of three Sooners suspended for steroids the year before, and by now the coach completely blamed the athlete. "A media egomaniac," Switzer said of The Boz. "He affected the public perception of our team. I'm disappointed that one guy gave us that image."

Soon the coaches found solace on the sidelines of the big game, the Orange Bowl, where TV cameras framed them as leaders of young men. Johnson wore the final smile, as Miami beat Oklahoma in the Orange Bowl, 20-14, for the school's second national championship in five years.

NFL Tests for Steroids, Condemns Use, and Employs Juicers

In January 1987, the NFL introduced its steroid screening as part of scheduled drug testing on prospective rookies at the league combine in Indianapolis. In coming months the public learned of the results, and at least one big name was caught in the sweep.

Among the 300 college players attending the talent evaluation, 20 tested positive for steroids, six for marijuana, one for cocaine, and one for alcohol. Gil Brandt, Cowboys player personnel director, credited colleges for intervention. "[T]he colleges are becoming much more aware of the drug problem and doing a much better job of eliminating the problem," he said. An anonymous NFL team official, advocating random testing, was skeptical of announced testing. "Players who get caught are either very stupid or so heavily into it they can't get off it," he said. "The players are getting smarter."

Cowboys officials were none too concerned about their No.1 draft pick's testing positive for steroids, Danny Noonan, Nebraska All-American defensive tackle. Noonan, 6-4, 280, told media the steroids were meant to restore weight lost during an illness, and Dallas GM Tex Schramm was not worried: "We have always been satisfied that [steroid use] would not be any problem with Danny Noonan," he said. Other franchises held the same sentiment about confirmed users, including Cleveland, which selected Duke linebacker Mike Junkin as its No.1 in the draft. The fifth pick overall, Junkin had tested positive for steroids at the combine.

In the coming months, the NFL moved to scheduled steroid testing of veterans during pre-camp physicals, although without labor agreement on a policy. No penalty was involved and no player names would be made public in the testing, implemented by Rozelle alone; later, the commissioner revealed 6 percent of veterans had tested positive for steroids. The 1987 regular season was marred by a players' strike in which the drug policy was not considered pivotal by either the management or the union, at least publicly, and by the next year officials were pulling together their anti-steroid act, denouncing the drugs. Beyond the talk, actions spoke differently.

At the league combine in February, scouts relished a rich selection of linemen coming out of the colleges, gigantic and athletic. They drooled over Dave Cadigan, 6-5, 285 pounds, All-American offensive tackle from USC. One of the biggest amid 330 players, Cadigan proved the strongest in strength tests. He was also among 10 prospects in Indianapolis who tested positive for anabolic steroids, but that did not deter the New York Jets from making Cadigan their No. 1 pick, selecting him eighth overall in the draft.

Meeting with media in New York, Cadigan and the Jets officials downplayed his steroid use as experimental and not even beneficial — Cadigan claimed that he actually lost weight and speed because of the drugs, which he said he used for six weeks after concluding his college career. "I want to clarify it because I don't want to be stereotyped as some sort of steroid head," he said. Cadigan also revealed he had wanted steroids for competing against other prospects; he had witnessed performance gains in users, including teammates in college. "I've been playing football since I was 8 years old," Cadigan said. "I've dedicated my life to football. I'm not going to fall behind. I'll do almost anything to succeed. ... I'll do anything to be the best lineman in the NFL or the best lineman I can be. If that's taking steroids and [if] in fact they worked, I'd use them." Cadigan emphasized he passed 10 steroid tests during college football, and he and his father studied the drugs five years before he tried them. Pat Cadigan, a former Boston College defensive tackle, was his son's "leading cheerleader," said a USC official. Jets draft director Mike Hickey knew about Cadigan's test result before selecting him. Hickey would not comment much, but he inferred steroids did not increase Cadigan's size and strength. "Sometimes there's a look to a guy who's on steroids, and he didn't have it," Hickey said.

Elsewhere in the league, Raiders physician Rob Huizenga knew steroid users were everywhere, including many on his team. Huizenga knew Raiders surgeon Robert Rosenfeld prescribed anabolic steroids for some players, including skinny quarterback Marc Wilson, who told Huizenga he spurned the drugs. In addition, team owner Al Davis was not worried about steroids or amphetamines when discussing user players with Huizenga.

The Raiders were only symptomatic of the problem. Despite holding a wild reputation for partying, this franchise represented status quo around the NFL in drugs for performance enhancement. "It was true that [in 1988] the National Football League regarded the drug problem as merely a public relations snafu. ...," Huizenga later wrote in his book memoir, contending that officials had "an ambivalent position on anabolic steroids" and "lack of a position on amphetamines."

Typically, NFL officials would not acknowledge potentially hazardous or liable steroid practices in the league, but a few were bolder, like Tex Schramm in Dallas, who would outright scoff at the suggestion. When the Raiders' Howie Long was quoted about rampant abuse, the powerful GM derided the player's perspective as "gross imagination". Schramm said Long's Raiders might be a bunch of users, but his Cowboys were clean like a vast majority of NFL teams. Schramm claimed health concerns about steroids scared away most contemporary players.

Schramm's Cowboys were not clean of steroids. This organization had hired strength coaches Alvin Roy and Bob Ward, both users themselves, and generations of players had abused steroids. Moreover, team officials had no qualms about drafting or scouting confirmed users, including Noonan and Ben Johnson, disgraced Canadian sprinter. Schramm supported the concept of random urinalysis for drugs — but for street narcotics, not steroids. Behind closed doors, Schramm condoned steroids for his players, according to Cowboys retiree Charlie Waters, a safety during the team's Super Bowls of the 1970s. "Back when we were playing, and recreational drugs were becoming popular, Mr. Schramm made an announcement to the team," Waters told Mike Fisher, Dallas sportswriter and broadcaster, in 2005. "They handed out a sheet with all the little nicknames for all the drugs, and then Mr. Schramm said, 'The drugs we use to enhance the game of football are OK. These drugs we use for recreation are not OK.' It was a strange way of looking at it," said Waters, who also coached in the NFL and NCAA. "Mr. Schramm was certainly naïve, and not aware of all the ramifications of what he was saying. His point was that you can take things if they enhance your play, as long as they're not a danger to your health — except, of course, players don't worry about the future. They want to perform now."

Steroids in Prep Football: 'No Big Problem'

High-school football players had used anabolic steroids for decades, but most coaches and athletic directors contacted by the media in the mid-1980s said the drugs were rare or non-existent at their schools. Many said anti-steroid education was in place for teen athletes. "Interviews with more than 35 Washington-area coaches, players and administrators indicated that the steroid problem has yet to filter down to the high schools on a level that would be considered a major problem," reported Donald Huff, *Washington Post*.

"Our kids aren't quite that sophisticated to deal with steroids. I doubt if most of them know what they are," Frank Park, athletic director at Spingam High, told *The Post*. "We are more concerned about the [street] drugs."

Ken Poates, football coach at W.T. Woodson High, said, "I think anytime you see some youngsters lifting weights and getting bigger, the rumors concerning steroids begin. We've had a few kids who really pump iron and work hard. I know they work hard because we watch them and can see them get bigger. I don't think it's from steroid use. Of course, there's no way you can prove kids use them but we don't have any evidence of any steroid use. We don't make a big deal of telling the kids not to use them because it's relatively new. Steroids is just a part of our 'don't use this and don't use that' talk. Hopefully, kids understand that and nothing else should be said."

Claudia Dodson, chemical abuse official for the Virginia High School League, said, "Right now, our state hasn't shown much in the way of steroid usage. Our workshops include information about steroids but we don't separate it from the other drugs. Steroids are just part of our entire education package."

"I'm not in favor of drug-testing athletes," said Charles Stebbins, health administrator for the National Federation of State High School Associations. "One, it's costly; two, there are legal ramifications; and third, what happens when you get the results? I don't think it's a good idea at any level. If you develop a sound program with workshops, seminars [for athletics personnel], you can achieve good results."

Some coaches interviewed by *The Post* had seen or heard of steroid use. "Peer pressure is hard to handle and some athletes succumb to it. ...," said Mark Gowin, Gonzaga High football coach. "But I don't think we've reached the point where we need drug testing yet." Bill Holsclaw, football coach for Woodbridge High, said, "Sometimes you have some kids in your program who want to get bigger and they think steroid use is the way. And many times, college kids who use steroids come back and tell the younger players that's the way to get bigger and stronger. In college, there is probably more pressure on them to use. We monitor our kids very carefully here. ... Right now, we aren't worried about steroid use because the problem hasn't presented itself in our athletic program."

Scattered reports did indicate a steroid problem in prep football, such as allegations by police in Atlanta and an NFL physician in New Orleans. In Texas, the *Fort Worth Star-Telegram* interviewed current and former prep athletes who used muscle dope in the 1980s. "There are so many other drugs in high school, why not steroids?" said Darrell Melton. "You've got your kids that are really sports-minded, and it is a way to enhance their athletic ability." Gary Engasser said he tried Dianabol but ceased after reading of possible health risks. "If I knew there were no side effects I would be on them quicker than ever," he said. James Coffman, recent prep graduate, said he obtained steroids through a prescription from a doctor. In other reports, Florida state officials "heavily suspected" steroids at a wrestling championship meet for large schools. On Long Island, New York, "people would be naïve to think" steroids were not in school sports, said Bill Piner, Nassau County athletics official. "I wouldn't limit the use of steroids to football players," Piner said. "Any young people interested in weight lifting and increasing their body size and weight would be exposed to them."

In Toronto, Canada, the steroid question was raised when college football scouts converged on the area for its "bumper beef brigade" of line prospects at high schools. "They [steroids] exist, I know that as a fact," said Clark Tatton, a hot recruit. "If you want them, they're easy to get. I've never touched them."

III. Rozelle Takes Final Spin With Steroid Policy

Pete Rozelle always could withhold information, adroitly, but he was masterful in 1988, concealing the fact that he was leaving the National Football League. This would be the mythic commissioner's final full year, but he was keeping that to himself. At this point, Rozelle just wanted to retreat for home, California, to retire there with his wife Carrie and simply have, he would say, "some fun before it's too late."

Heading the NFL was no longer fun, not for Rozelle at age 62. Major problems hung on the league, some for the decade, including antitrust lawsuits, an alienated players union, a divided owners group, and drugs. Rozelle was coming to accept that he could not much tidy the NFL's house before leaving.

Time had changed so much from a January day in Miami, 1960, when a 33-year-old Rozelle hid from reporters in a hotel men's room, peeing, puffing cigarettes, combing his hair, repeatedly washing his hands, biding time until a roomful of bickering NFL owners finally hired him as commissioner. Then he went in that smoky room and busted them up, cracking, "I can honestly say that I come to you with clean hands."

By the late 1980s, Rozelle was tired of living the role of football icon in New York City, of playing a caricature of himself for the NFL, smiling, laughing, back-slapping. Behind closed doors, where Rozelle could twist arms with the toughest, he hardly wanted to deal with owners as a group anymore. Once the supreme organizer of ownership consensus on matters, Rozelle had seen his power plummet across the league. Now he was hard-pressed to mobilize enough owners to get anything done. Indeed, a youthful faction of owners, the "New Breed," defied Rozelle at their every opportunity.

Rozelle could not control the steroid issue in the least, not even sources spewing openly from within his league — players, coaches, and other personnel yakking away to the press. In public Rozelle had for years downplayed the problem of drugs, contrary to the NFL's inside information of widespread abuse shared among clubs and his office, according to the records of a 1986 arbitration hearing closed to media. Rozelle had bungled on drugs, beginning with his trying to suppress and ignore the issue decades before. "Drug-Test Policy Is Bedeviling Rozelle," the *New York Times* headlined in 1988, atop one of its many articles on sport performance enhancement. Among substances abused in the NFL, steroids and other dope were established and only escalating, having impacted countless competitors throughout football, schoolboys notwithstanding. Drugs were an aging problem, with ghosts of the past starting to surface consistently, the latest Charlie Krueger, a former 15-year lineman in the league who won a $2.36 million judgment against the 49ers. Krueger had sued the franchise for the 49ers' personnel administering drugs to him after 1963, including more than 100 cortisone shots to the left knee, which was destroyed — prevailing medical opinion held that pain-blocking injections for a weight-bearing joint should not exceed three or four in a lifetime.

Moreover, much to Rozelle's chagrin, he himself had hired a league drug advisor who could not keep quiet in public. The candidness of Dr. Forrest Tennant, a Californian, was rare among NFL officials, and appreciative reporters pounced, particularly for his comments on anabolic steroids. Tennant, operator of drug clinics and a UCLA lecturer, had assumed the position of the league drug advisor after agreeing with union and league management to make no public statements about the league.

Tennant violated that pre-nuptial immediately, at his introduction in summer 1986, when he told reporters the NFL had a "serious problem" with anabolic steroids and the drugs were known to have impacted "numerous" injury cases throughout football. To Rozelle's displeasure, the nerdish Tennant babbled in the presence of live microphones and note-takers, spouting quotes far outside the league protocol. Rozelle would testify in court that he and other NFL officials "very forcefully" instructed Tennant he was "to be seen and not heard."

Rozelle, maestro of image, could hardly believe what he was seeing and hearing of Tennant. The doctor once said, "If you lined up 10 people and let me examine their eyes, I'll do as well as a urine test in naming the drug users." He said cocaine abusers were easily identified by their manner of dress. Tennant also discussed in detail, with a Boston newspaper, the cases of six Patriots players and street narcotics, enraging them and the players union. Dr. Tennant's straightforwardness was admirable, the Raiders' Dr. Huizenga would recall, "but sometimes he was too open."

Tennant was at it again in the summer of 1988, in the wake of the Krueger case about cortisone injections by a 49ers physician, publicly promoting his steroid-addiction research while also popping off about a steroid "epidemic" plaguing all sports. Then Tennant revealed details of the forthcoming testing policy Rozelle had not finalized. Steroid testing was a volatile topic between Rozelle and the players union, and Tennant was supposed to steer clear rather than spark trouble.

Perhaps in response to Tennant's latest headline, a Rozelle memo was leaked to the media, his message to franchises about new steroid policy. The biggest change was a positive result now could lead a player to disciplinary action, possibly suspension. In addition, Rozelle almost publicly affirmed the NFL had a serious steroid problem, the closest he would ever come, writing of "widespread misuse... throughout much of the sports world, including football." Suddenly, Rozelle disavowed his former stance that steroids could be justified for injury rehabilitation: "The NFL Physicians Society declares there are no legitimate medical purposes to prescribe steroids for NFL players. ...," his memo stated. "The league no longer merely condemns the use of the substance. It is prohibited in any quantity for any purposes."

Overall response to Rozelle's latest policy was lukewarm, and a few sportswriters ripped him. "Hard to believe the NFL is seriously interested in cleaning up its steroid problem," commented Jack Sheppard of the *St. Petersburg Times*, ridiculing the penalties riding in part on judgment by team doctors. "Rozelle later admitted he does not plan to suspend any second-time users," Sheppard noted. "This is a policy intended to deter?"

Inside the league, team physicians wondered how they would enforce Rozelle's proposals, measures fraught with legal and professional landmines for them. Cowboys GM Tex Schramm had his own ideas about drug policy. Specifically, Schramm wanted random urinalysis, which Rozelle had tried to mandate for street drugs in 1986, only to be struck down by an arbitrator favoring union objections. Random urinalysis remained a popular idea for battling drugs, espoused by many athletes, coaches, media, and medical experts. "I support Pete and what he is trying to do," Schramm said, "but the way we are doing it won't even get us to first base."

Rozelle felt the cracks in his support, especially the vocal criticism of Schramm, normally his great ally, but he regrouped on drugs, trying to tighten proposals and rally enough owners to back him against Upshaw and the union. Meanwhile, bad press on steroids in football continued to mount.

The Los Angeles Times polled 1,000 NFL former players on league issues, and 440 responded, with their overall views on doping flying in the face of league officials. They rebuked management's rhetoric that always placed systematic drug problems in the past, the stock line most recently heard from Schramm. In reality anabolic steroids were rampant across a dangerous NFL environment. Russ Bollinger, offensive lineman for the Rams from 1983-85, used steroids because the sport was "a street fight," he said. "If somebody brings a club, you bring a club." Former players in the poll also were frightened by the unnatural weight gains of steroid users, believing users' lives could be shortened.

Elsewhere, *Washington Post* sportswriter Bill Brubaker produced another damning exposé on the NFL and Rozelle, after obtaining confidential documents on the closed hearing from a league source. "NFL Commissioner Pete Rozelle [testified that] clubs have a 'conflict of interest' in administering their own drug programs 'because they want to win,'" Brubaker reported. "Rozelle also admitted that in [media] interviews he had attempted to 'diminish the nature' of player drug use even though he believed it was a 'serious problem.'"

Jan Van Duser, NFL director of operations, echoed Rozelle's stance in the arbitration testimony, during a three-hour interview with Brubaker. Van Duser said the NFL took over drug testing in 1986 to eliminate shenanigans by teams determined to keep certain players on the field, despite positive results for drugs. "There were clubs that did not address their drug problems as well as they might have," Van Duser said, "either through putting football considerations first or just not knowing enough about the problem. What we heard from clubs was this: 'We would be happy to do everything that's needed in a drug program provided we know that the team we're playing next week is doing the same thing.'

"What they didn't want to do is to have their top player taken off the field by their own actions when they knew that the team they were playing — their biggest rival — might not do the same thing. [Some clubs] might sweep the problem under the rug in order to keep a player who was not only a drug user but also a very good football player out there."

Van Duser joined other NFL officials in saying no one knew the prevalence of drugs, street narcotics or steroids. He said the league office was now taking charge in bona fide testing and prevention, so the outlook was promising.

Critics disagreed, including from within. "Some N.F.L. owners and players say that the policy is doomed to fail because it does not deal with the issue decisively," reported Thomas George, *New York Times*. "Some say that the league should assign a full-time, year-round drug officer to each team, and others say suspensions should be stiffer, possibly for one year."

Outside pro football, astute observers saw more doping in major sports. "Testing is a joke," said Dr. Fred Hatfield, the Los Angeles psychologist and former power-lifter who had used steroids and sold books. Hatfield noted many undetectable chemicals were already employed throughout athletics. Maryland strength coach Frank Costello, a former champion high jumper, estimated that as much as 90 percent of athletes in power competition had cycled on steroids. "The temptation is so great with all the emphasis on winning," Costello said.

Rozelle stood rigid in public, always qualifying use as "isolated" in his league. In October 1988, acting on the steroid scandal of the Olympics, Rozelle announced confidential steroid urinalysis of 1,600 players the previous year had produced positive results from 97 of them, or 6 percent, and founded the league practice of misrepresenting testing data as accurate measures of usage. "Everybody says half the league is on steroids," Rozelle said, "but I think this is a clear indication that it's not that big a problem."

Acting in concert with Rozelle, Minnesota Vikings GM Mike Lynn declared the league was innocent as charged and steroid eradication was in sight. "The public perception was that it was a major problem in the NFL," Lynn said. "That [6 percent of positives] is way low, and within a few years no one will be using steroids. In a few years this league will rid itself of [use] by its players."

Rozelle announced another policy twist on steroids, generating more headlines: Starting in 1989, players testing positive a second time definitely would face suspension, for 30 days. Rozelle criticized the players union, again, for lack of cooperation in the issue, and he returned to rhetoric about his just coming to understand muscle doping. "I've felt for a year that we should include steroids in our drug policy, but we've spent that time educating ourselves," Rozelle said.

Sports columnist Ira Berkow did not believe it. "Rozelle's recent decree sounds as though he had only recently learned of the steroid problems. ...," Berkow wrote for *The New York Times*. "[T]here has been a flood of such information developing in mass-circulation periodicals for more than 30 years."

Some in law enforcement were cynical of Rozelle, particularly his claim of isolated steroid use in the league. "It's an affront to anyone who thinks about the problem," said Phillip Halpern, assistant district attorney in San Diego, citing his sources' information of widespread use in football.

Dr. Robert Voy, chief medical officer of the USOC, said his Olympic sport faced reevaluation of in-house urinalysis for steroids, and the NFL needed to do likewise. "You can't have a sport test itself and be trustworthy," said Voy, who also had worked in football. "It's like the fox guarding the henhouse. You can't depend on it." Olympic testing had failed thus far, Voy claimed, noting evidence.

Rozelle disregarded the scientific reality that he could not police muscle dope in football, or anywhere else. He would retire soon and meanwhile keep the good public front, proclaiming on national television the NFL drug policy was "the strongest" in American sports.

Many media went along, typically. "Mr. Rozelle deserves commendation for his actions against drugs," The *Pittsburgh Press* editorialized. "It serves to cleanse the NFL of hazardous-substance abuse and sends a warning to athletes on down the line to get off drugs or never start using them."

IV. Steroid Scandal Dogs NCAA, Colleges, Tainting Image

College officials felt good about the football-steroids situation, and the year 1988 began benignly where the issue was concerned. In April, football fans laughed over steroid allegations about Columbia University players and coaches, a program infamous for its current losing streak exceeding 40 games, an NCAA record. Naturally, the joke went that even steroids could not help Columbia.

Soon, however, college football and steroids returned to the not-so-funny pages. That summer Oklahoma University officials sweated an impending autobiography by Brian Bosworth, co-written by Rick Reilly, and their fears were realized upon the book's release in August. The Boz, presently in the NFL, detailed many allegations about OU football under 16-year head coach Barry Switzer, including abuse of anabolic steroids and cocaine, illegal cash payments, and off-field violence.

University administrators gave little comment on the book, for good reason: Switzer's program was already under NCAA investigation for alleged recruiting violations. Even the athletic department was short on vocal supporters for the embattled coach. Switzer got no immediate help from athletic director Donnie Duncan, who had nothing to say about Bosworth's book, promising to comment after reading it but setting no timetable. Switzer declined comment initially, as did Bosworth himself.

Then NCAA investigators announced their intent to review the book's contents, and a blitz of denial broke from OU, led by men's basketball coach Billy Tubbs and taken up by players past and present, denouncing Bosworth and his allegations. "When you are family, you don't air your wash out in a book or a newspaper," Tubbs said: "I don't think Bosworth is in a position to write a book about himself — you've got to do something first before you write a book."

Several former Sooners criticized Bosworth harshly. "I'd like to tell Boz to stop embarrassing us," said Derrick Crudup, former Sooner and Raiders rookie. "He's embarrassing the school and he's embarrassing all of us. I got a lot of harassment from my teammates about that story. I don't think there's anything to what he wrote. I can't say I believe any of it." Ex-teammates largely dismissed Bosworth's charge of widespread steroid use among Sooners in the mid-1980s. "If it happened, it was a very isolated incident," Jon Phillips, a Phoenix Cardinals lineman, said of his time at OU. "I don't know if the public realizes it, but Oklahoma has one of the most extensive drug-testing programs in the nation." Former Sooner Steve Sewell, running back for the Denver Broncos, said Bosworth's talk about steroids "was overblown." Former Sooner Sonny Brown, trying to make the Oilers, said, "Maybe that stuff went on, but I never saw any of it." Paul Migliazzo, whom Bosworth had called his best friend on the team, qualified the allegations as "fabricated."

Switzer emerged after a couple days with ominous words for the tell-all author. "It's a tremendous price we both are paying," said Switzer, who would resign the following spring. "I know it now and he will know it in the future. Because he doesn't realize how people here now feel about it, the attitude they've taken toward him." Switzer said Bosworth was motivated by profit, fame. "It's [a book] as seen through the eyes of one person," the coach said. "There are other players here who saw it differently. The problem is they're not selling a book."

In Kansas City, Chiefs defensive end and former Sooner Jeff Tupper tried to rip Bosworth without reading the book. Tupper said he was "pretty disgusted" by its charges. "From what I've heard, the things he's saying about the school are not directly related to the University of Oklahoma," Tupper surmised. "They were isolated incidents, and he's trying to exploit them as part of the university and part of the heritage of the school, which doesn't fit." Pressed to be specific, however, Tupper found himself having to agree with Bosworth on several points. "Some of the things in the book happened," Tupper conceded, "and I'm sure due punishment was served when they did happen."

Tupper ended up confirming steroid use on the team, though he said athletics personnel were not involved. "In the group that followed mine, a lot of guys were using steroids," Tupper said. "As common as aspirin, no, but readily available, yes... The kids weren't getting them from the school. The weight coach was dead set against them." Tupper staunchly defended his former coach, Switzer: "I don't think Barry should be held responsible for kids 19, 20, 21 years of age... They ought to be held responsible for their own actions." Tupper accused Bosworth of "just acting as a storyteller, trying to play the rebel without a cause again, and he's doing a great job of it. He'll make a million dollars off this book, I promise you."

The book did make bestseller lists, and Bosworth, used to controversy, certainly smiled on his way to the bank. The Boz stood by his allegations, ignored his OU critics, and continued making money off his image, even as injury snuffed out his NFL career.

Elsewhere, in South Carolina, a former player was not so fortunate in leveling steroid allegations against his old school. Tommy Chaiken, paid $4,500 by *Sports Illustrated*, told his own muscle-doping story as a Gamecocks defensive lineman, though he knew going in the money was no reparation for what he had experienced and would encounter after publication.

Every party involved was impacted adversely by Chaikin's harrowing tale. For the first time, football coaches representing a university would be criminally charged for providing steroids to players, forcing NCAA Enforcement into its first probe of steroid allegations. Anabolic drugs were but one of the problems in South Carolina football from 1983 through 1987, during Chaikin's career in Columbia a decade after Steve Courson. The team had winning seasons but also impropriety by players and coaches, on and off the field. Drug abuse fueled Chaiken and many more players, including steroids and growth hormone for their performance, and alcohol and cocaine for partying. Chaikin barely escaped careening into personal disaster, and college players nationwide could identify.

The time-honored practice of denial in such cases included refocusing blame onto the whistle-blowing athlete, and South Carolina officials took the PR tactic against Chaiken, but only briefly. Quickly, the public deduced Chaikin's allegations were accurate and grasped he was different than Bosworth. "Oh, yeah, I take responsibility for my actions," Chaikin wrote for *SI*, continuing:

I'm headstrong and I've got a temper. I can't blame others for my mistakes, certainly not for making me take dangerous drugs. But I still think of myself as someone who started out as just a normal guy, a hard worker, a studier, a kid who loved sports. And I feel part of the trouble comes from things outside of me — the pressures of college football, the attitudes of overzealous coaches and
our just-take-a-pill-to-cure-anything society.

Chaikin's lengthy first-person narrative for *SI* was co-written by Rick Telander and released in mid-October 1988, amid the hysteria around sprinter Ben Johnson. The account was unprecedented, a college football player detailing steroid abuse involving coaches. The backlash echoed throughout the game, especially for major schools.

Chaikin recalled turning to muscle doping after spring practice his freshman year, 1984. He began with an ambitious purchase for college football; HGH along with steroids from a dealer. Already an extraordinary weightlifter and rock-hard specimen, a 210-pounder able to bench-press about 375 and squat more than 400, Chaikin anticipated the anabolic effects to break through his natural barriers.

In eight weeks of cycling on steroids and growth hormone, he gained lean mass to reach 235 on the scale. He bench-pressed 400 pounds for the first time and went higher, to 420, while increasing his squat to above 500. Everybody noticed at summer practice, especially juicers and at least one coach, Chaikin said. Dangerously, he staked his self-worth in football, and muscle doping changed his life for the game. Dramatically, though not miraculously, Chaikin was no longer a meat-squad player, yearning to merely dress out for a game. Anabolics worked, quickly, diabolically, remodeling the youth into a star nose-guard of college football.

The coaches' approval of steroid use on the Gamecocks was unyielding, Chaikin revealed. Their statements about doping were typically positive, veiled or otherwise, like praise directed him for "working hard." In the weightroom, coaches always glorified the new or heavier juicers, heaping praise for their unnatural gains in size and strength. The coded, obvious point to players was simple to comprehend: Get bigger, faster, stronger.

By 1985 roughly half the South Carolina players were on steroids, Chaikin estimated, or about 50 of the 100 practicing with the team — about the number of guys who saw game action. Chaikin and juicing teammates traded the goods, swapped information for better results, and injected the stuff, including into each other. His body, on cycle and boosted by manic workouts, held scant body fat although swelling to as large as 270 pounds. He retained quickness and speed. Strength-wise, Chaikin bench-pressed as much as 500 and leg-squatted 650 to 700.

Chaikin's physical makeover through anabolics was not unusual in football, despite his 30 percent hike in body mass. However, he encountered health issues while so enormous, such as spiking blood pressure, a swollen liver, and, during a game, an angina episode or pre-heart attack condition, with chest pains, dead-arm numbness, and chills; his jersey had to be sliced off for an emergency ride to hospital.

Moreover, emotional darkness besieged Chaikin, and he believed anabolics were the cause. Certainly, Chaikin's essential personality reversed on steroids and growth hormone, switching from an easygoing teen to a raging, violent young man, dangerous to himself and others. Never a street fighter, Chaikin was "huge," reveling in physical confrontation. The physicality of football alone could not appease him. Crazily, gleefully, he started brawls on and off the field, throwing punches at teammates on a whim, for example, as coaches watched, doing nothing. Frightening incidents seemingly had no effect on Chaikin. His idea of fun had warped, especially living around the football dorm known as "The Roost." Once, Chaikin brandished a shotgun to greet a pizza delivery boy, terrifying the teen; then he laughed.

As tough as he was, Chaikin could not subdue strange urges and thoughts coming to grip him. Chaikin hit bottom mentally in the summer and fall of 1987, his senior football season, even though he took just one shot of steroids during that period. Strong anxiety attacks brought on paranoia, feelings of insecurity, and doom and detachment. He isolated himself in his dorm room, avoiding friends, missing classes, and thinking of suicide.

Football was the only motivation Chaikin had left, but he imploded there, too, midway through the season. The raucous crowd of a Gamecocks home game sent him into a severe panic, and he left the field on his own in the third quarter, quietly removing his pads and sitting down on a bench. Afterward, coaches allowed Chaikin to see psychiatrists, but the counseling and prescribed medications were ineffective.

Finally, Chaikin suffered a horrendous experience while trying to attend a morning class, hallucinating and losing control of bodily functions as he fled. Back in his room, he locked the door, loaded rounds into a .357 Magnum, and pointed the pistol to his head. Teammates kept vigil in the hallway until Chaikin's father arrived to coax him out and take him home. At Bethesda, Chaikin spent a week in a mental ward.

Chaikin returned to South Carolina in the spring of 1988 to complete his undergraduate degree in English, but he did not resume football or steroids. On a visit to the football complex, Chaikin watched the Gamecocks pump iron, the noisy room crowded with juicers slamming weights. He called out to an old line mate bloated on drugs. "Look in the mirror, man," Chaikin challenged. "All you're going to see is my reflection."

"I don't give a damn," replied the young man. "It won't hurt me, Tom. It just affects you a whole lot worse than it affects other people."

The following October, however, the issue hit everyone in the Gamecocks program through Chaikin's published story, "The Nightmare of Steroids." *Sports Illustrated* was a premier agenda-setter in the world of sport, and the negative response rocked all of South Carolina. The matter enveloped Columbia, with university officials and football coaches issuing denials, excuses, and no-comments — familiar in these parts, where steroid allegations had surrounded Gamecocks football for years.

The University of South Carolina president James Holderman, in a prepared statement, utilized precise terms to focus blame on the individual, saying the institution "deeply regrets the personal tragedy of Tommy Chaikin." Holderman stressed that he himself had disposed of an athletic director just the previous spring, over then-allegations and criticism blasting the department's urinalysis program for athletes.

The college president portrayed the drug problem in school athletics as officially resolved. "Since early this year, the university has taken a variety of positive steps to strengthen our drug testing and wellness program and assure as far as possible such a tragedy [as Chaikin's] should never reoccur here."

Football coaches tried to avoid comment, although Chaikin had made specific charges against two in particular: Jim Washburn, Chaikin's defensive-line coach and the assistant who recruited him, and defensive coordinator Tom Gadd. As the story broke, neither man made substantial comments nor seemed anxious to answer the allegations. Gadd apparently avoided the media that first night, at least, while Washburn would only say that a statement was in preparation. Head football coach Joe Morrison, who Chaikin charged had condoned his steroid use, also declined comment. Another coach Chaikin named did speak, former Gamecocks strength coach Keith Kephart, reached by reporters at his new post with Texas A&M. Kephart said he tried "to head off some possible problems" at South Carolina, adding that the coaching staff was anti-steroid.

University officials and coaches who downplayed Chaikin's allegations found themselves outmatched, however, against a tidal wave of counter-publicity across the nation. Chaikin had support from two sportswriters of heavy influence, Telander and *Washington Post* columnist Tony Kornheiser. Telander, opining on back page of the *SI* edition featuring Chaikin's story, framed his perspective on his own past in college football. "I saw the drug age sprout and send out tentative shoots; Tommy and his peers have grown up entangled in the whole sprawling, thorny mess," Telander wrote. Kornheiser placed the blame squarely on the football system. "Let's not be naïve," he declared. "There's tremendous pressure on athletes to get bigger, stronger, faster quickly. This pressure comes from the coaches as well as the players. Players want to win jobs, coaches want to keep them. The pros and the major colleges have winked at steroid use for years. It's about winning, which translates into money."

Gamecocks players were mixed in their responses to Chaikin's story, particularly on the allegation of widespread doping in the program. Their division fell fairly evenly, with former players largely in support of him and current Gamecocks largely opposed.

Current quarterback Todd Ellis vehemently denied he had considered using steroids, per Chaikin's recall of the past. Likewise, Ellis maintained that steroids had been eradicated throughout college football, contrary to Chaikin's contention that the problem remained huge. "I don't blame *Sports Illustrated*," Ellis said. "I blame Tommy for it being a false statement and him trying to get a little more attention." Ellis claimed drug testing had "completely knocked out" steroid use in college football. "I've got friends from Notre Dame... all over the place, and they say it's just not used anymore," Ellis said.

Defensive end Kevin Hendrix and linebacker Matt McKernan defended their coaches, contending that none condoned steroid use on the team, and both implied Chaikin was bitter at the program. They said urinalysis was impossible to beat, but McKernan, fence-riding, also was empathic of players who doped to compete. "People on the street don't understand why [players use]," McKernan said. "In some cases, you take them or you don't play. The trouble with steroids is they work. They've helped a lot of people in the short term. If you're a college football player not playing, you're miserable."

Three former Gamecocks linemen backed Chaikin. "His statement's probably pretty accurate," said Deron Farina, who confirmed using steroids. "There was a lot of pressure to take [steroids]. They [the coaches] never directly come out and tell you to, you just understand what they want. They stressed the weightroom so much." Ricky Daniels denied using steroids but said Chaikin's estimate that about half the team did in 1986 was "pretty close to accurate." Former center Woody Myers readily discussed his use as a Gamecock — his college career had ended in 1987, when he tested positive for steroids and was banned from the Gator Bowl. Myers said the environment of major-college football had led him to steroids, which increased his body weight from under 200 to almost 290 at South Carolina. Myers contended steroids were easy to obtain, and if he were to play football again, he said, "[I] would use them again."

The anticipated press releases by coaches, meanwhile, consisted of their denial.

"We have never condoned the use of steroids or any illegal substance," head coach Morrison said in his statement. "If there was any use of steroids, it certainly was done without our knowledge. We have tried to educate and certainly have discouraged the use of any illegal substances." Washburn, the D-line coach, refuted Chaikin's claims in a separate release: "I have never been abusive in my coaching techniques, and I think my players know that." Washburn stated he treated players as his own children. "As for steroids, I am totally against them and I never encouraged Tom Chaikin to use them."

South Carolina athletic director King Dixon backed the coaches at a news conference they did not attend. Asked if he believed Chaikin, Dixon did not answer directly. He said his department properly handled steroids. Soon after, university president Holderman concurred with Dixon, telling media the school had taken preventive steps against steroids. Holderman said Morrison's job was not in jeopardy. "Both Morrison and Washburn — and I believe them — say they knew nothing about this kind of thing," Holderman said. "They did not condone it. They did not encourage it. I have to accept that as fact, and I do. The University of South Carolina feels it's a tragic set of circumstances regarding Tommy Chaikin, and that doesn't mean we're prepared to take all the responsibility for the problems in Tommy Chaikin's life. I don't think we should have to."

The public diatribes of university officials were not convincing enough. An outside investigation of the scandal had begun, primarily because law enforcement did not yet accept the university's version of steroids and Gamecocks football. Not this time.

High-profile reports on steroids had implicated the football program before, like Courson's story about South Carolina in the 1970s, when a coach pushed Dianabol to him and the team physician prescribed it. In more recent history, there was the report of strength coach Kephart having telephoned steroid dealer Tony Fitton in the early 1980s, prior to his second arrest. That information became public in 1985, and Kephart, when asked for comment, said he contacted Fitton to learn more about steroids so he could better counsel the Gamecocks players against using. In a different interview, Kephart acknowledged the probability of steroid use on the Gamecocks and said coaches would "highly recommend… it be done under a doctor's supervision." Local gossip swirled of Gamecocks on muscle drugs, with tipsters contacting police and media.

Now, as Chaikin's story drew a national spotlight, regional authorities made their move, announcing that a grand jury in Richland County would hear the case of steroids in South Carolina Gamecocks football. The witnesses would include basically everyone named in media stories around Chaikin. "We're going to take every step to determine his credibility," said James Anders, federal attorney in the local circuit. "If he is telling the truth, we're going to go toward prosecution." Anders vowed anyone involved would be pursued, player, coach, or otherwise. "I view it as most serious," said the prosecutor.

The grand jury began hearing witnesses in December, and it returned indictments the following spring, April 1989. By then Morrison had died of a heart attack and his coaching staff had moved on to other colleges, but four of the former assistants faced misdemeanor charges in connection with the distribution of steroids to Gamecocks football players: Washburn, defensive line coach, age 39; Tom Kurucz, tight ends coach,

42; Gadd, defensive coordinator, 42; and Kephart, strength coach, 44.

The indictments accused Washburn, Kurucz, and Gadd of conspiring to "provide money to certain players and athletic personnel of the university for the purchasing of steroids for use by athletic personnel." The U.S. attorney overseeing the case, Vinton Lide, said some coaches were steroid users. The indictments stated Kephart and unidentified others "would administer the steroids to each other to improve athletic performance and to enhance physical appearance." A fifth man was charged with felony distribution, John Carter, of Maryland, identified as Chaikin's alleged source for steroids in Bethesda. Former players and graduate-assistant coaches were not charged with crimes. "My philosophy from day one was that these student athletes were victims," Lide said.

That summer Washburn, Kurucz, Kephart, and Carter each pleaded guilty to reduced charges, and the four were sentenced to probation and halfway houses, where their stays would range from three to six months. Attorneys for each complained media reports had overblown their clients' involvement with steroids in Gamecocks football. The lawyers accused former players Chaikin and others, granted immunity for their testimony, of having committed more serious crimes.

The lawyers claimed their clients had been ruined, but most of the coaches continued working in college football. Washburn, for example, remained in his new job at Purdue, after having been hired by head coach Fred Akers. The fourth former Gamecocks coach won acquittal of his charges, Gadd, whose role in the scandal was described as "minimal" by his attorney. The coach, however, certainly was no stranger to steroid use among football players in his charge.

During Gadd's trial, facts came to light about steroid distribution to athletes at the University of Utah in the late 1970s and early 1980s, when he was an assistant football coach at the school. Utah officials began providing steroids to selected players after noticing athletes on other teams were "unnaturally big," Gadd testified. Utah athletic director Chris Hill, speaking following Gadd's aquittal, confirmed existence of the old steroid program in his department, but defended it. "The university took a sensible approach," Hill said. "They opted to watch over the kids instead of ignoring the problem and possibly let it get away."

After the trial, Gadd went home again — back to Utah, as defensive coordinator for Utes football, rehired by Hill. The athletic director told media he was thrilled Gadd was found innocent of steroid charges in South Carolina. "We were with Tom all the way and he explained everything to us," Hill said. "That's not an issue. In our eyes, Tom is innocent and we don't discipline people who are innocent."

Tommy Chaikin, meanwhile, was hardly considered innocent around South Carolina, where his motives for going public were held in question. Chaikin, speaking during limited interviews following the *SI* article, said a prime factor for telling the story was his inability to forget, look the other way. Chaikin knew more young players were following his football path into muscle doping, and he felt compelled to act. There was no hidden agenda, Chaikin said, denying money and vengeance as driving forces. "I didn't want to see anyone get in trouble," Chaikin said.

A motive, Chaikin said, was to portray reality, how far college football had gone with anabolic substances. "A freak show," he said. Chaikin said his focus was not on South Carolina alone for steroids, but on the entire football institution. "I just feel [coaches in general] need to take a more personal view toward the athlete, and not look at them as a commodity," Chaikin said. "My personal view is that the NCAA should take a lot of time and effort and look at what the coaches are doing. ... I don't want the public to look at me as a martyr. I just want the public to look at me as a human being, an athlete just like everybody else who ever played an athletic sport, who just got caught up into it, and became obsessed with winning."

A couple months after Chaikin's exposé, bowls games began in college football, and several All-American players discussed anabolic steroids for an article by Hubert Mizell, *St. Petersburg Times*. Most said or implied they did not use the drugs. Heisman Trophy winner Barry Sanders, Oklahoma State tailback and devout Christian, said winning drove athletes to juice more so than amorality. "Just because they're users, it doesn't make them bad guys," Sanders said. "They just want success too badly. To me, football is just a game. Use what God gave you, work hard, and take what comes." Marv Cook, Iowa tight end, said, "I just want to be myself, with nothing artificial inside me. But for some, when steroids are run under their nose, they see an express ride to success. The price usually doesn't matter to the greedy."

Several players told Mizell steroids were prevalent in college football. "There's a heck of a lot of steroid use," said Mark Stepnoski, Pitt offensive tackle. "People my age aren't prone to worry about it." Mark Messner, a 244-pound defensive lineman for Michigan, said: "I've played against obvious steroid users. Guys who should be my weight come at me at 270 or 280, because they've blown themselves up with steroids. I take great offense. It's outright cheating. I wish steroids could be killed some way and somehow." The chemical arms race raged at the line of scrimmage, according to Anthony Phillips, 287-pound offensive guard at Oklahoma. "Everybody keeps wanting to be bigger and stronger," he said. "If the enemy is bigger, a true competitor can think he's got to do [steroids] to keep up."

V. Courson Under Siege Personally, Publicly

As rough as times were for Tommy Chaikin in 1988-89, the period was worse for Steve Courson, the other former South Carolina player speaking openly about muscle doping in football. For Courson, living became a siege.

As 1988 wound down, developments threatened to madden Courson's mind if not extinguish his life. A grave health problem challenged Courson to make internal changes, to finally move beyond his destructive youth. Externally, the sport-doping dilemma engulfed him. As a messenger of hard truth, Courson was made the symbol of the degenerate jock, branded as such by football and cast in the role by the media. "I was faced with survival in more ways than one," Courson said later. "Survival politically, physically, and spiritually."

Nothing had been easy for Courson since his *SI* confessions in 1985 and subsequent ouster from the NFL. Among setbacks, Courson's agent had lost $500,000 of his through bad investments, squandering what was left of his football fortune. The former All-Pro was broke, living in cheap apartments and unable to afford health insurance. He was disillusioned with football and doubtful about the society worshipping it. "The whole time [as a player] that I basically kept my mouth shut, took those drugs and performed, I was glorified for it, hugely rewarded for it," Courson said in 2005. "But as soon as I called out the reality behind the myth, all of a sudden everything changed. And it was just a matter of being a man and speaking the truth. I could barely cope with that."

Disenfranchised with football in his early thirties, Courson drank frequently, heavily, losing days and weeks in bars. He chugged beer and downed hard liquor, competing to drink more than anyone. In addition, as a fledging pro wrestler and power-lifter, Courson continued to cycle on anabolic steroids, once or twice a year in large dosages. The curtain was closing on Courson's false portrayals of living large through football, physique, and partying. Turmoil and danger stalked him, beginning in September with a feat in weightlifting, normally his greatest pleasure.

Courson bench-pressed 605 pound to win a power meet, a plateau reached by few lifters on earth. That night Courson reveled in victory, glory, like the old days, and he looked ahead with a familiar athletic zeal and desire to become the best in power-lifting. He started plotting his training — and drug program — to top the world bench-press record of 705.

The next morning, he awoke feeling differently, a bitter aftertaste of mind. Yes, he had benched 600 for the first time, won a big meet, enjoyed some spoils, but fallout guilt left him low-down in spirit. Courson realized that conquest through artificial means, steroids, could no longer gratify him; it may never have. The young man wondered whether his true football calling was only beginning, with a higher challenge coming to claim his focus: The Issue, doping in sport, particularly in American football. He was excelling, as usual, but on brain power.

In media stories on steroids, Courson was typically cast as the former NFL lineman alleging widespread abuse, but he was maturing into much more. He was rapidly filling a void in the debate as a scholarly critic beyond the scientists and physicians. Still two years shy of a college degree, Courson could compete in the topic of muscle doping with any scientist or sociologist. Courson may have been initiated by his own steroid use, but intelligence and drive for learning made him a budding expert, even if the media routinely denied him the credit.

Continuing his work on a book about steroids in football, Courson had canvassed the country for information, checking libraries for press articles and valid research. He also had stayed inside athletic circles for firsthand word. He knew, for example, that many NFL players still used steroids, including friends like Mike Webster. They timed intake of patented pills so their bodies cleared of any substances in time to meet testing standards, or they simply employed low-dose testosterone, undetectable in itself. Moreover, synthetic HGH was the underground hit, with no test available. Courson closely studied track and field for doping by coaches, physicians, and athletes versed in testosterone, growth hormone, and designer steroids, among muscle substances invisible to the limited eye of urinalysis technology. Courson understood sport doping to be immense, with no effective prevention available. Even a partial solution was out of the question, he realized, despite the talk and show of sports federations.

Scholarship was his saving grace, most importantly for Courson, against destructive interests like getting wasted on alchohol. Courson's experience, intellect, and respect for truth were a rare combination for the doping issue. His life was worthwhile. Just as Courson benched 600 and fell into soul-searching, the steroid tempest cranked up around the Olympic Games in Seoul, or, specifically, around an individual, Canadian sprinter Ben Johnson, who tested positive for stanozolol following his world-record dash in the 100 meters. Courson lately had avoided most media contacts, but he dove back into the steroid argument, amid what one writer dubbed the "Johnson effect." Courson fired away by mail and fax, forwarding letters and commentaries to newspapers, magazines, and broadcast outlets.

Widely quoted once again, Courson shone for his real-world perspective on sport doping, but media and the public generally were not agreeable. Courson's take on Johnson rang highly unpopular: He largely blamed the system rather than the sprinter, who in this case was labeled "disgraced" or "shamed" by sportswriters. "In that Olympics, Ben Johnson was a sacrificial lamb for all of them, no doubt," Courson said. "He heightened the issue to the boiling point, more so than ever before. I remember seeing the media behave, as far as how they were treating him, how they vilified him. And from the standpoint of a former athlete who had already talked about this publicly, it just made me angry."

Courson, through extensive review of articles on track and field, knew performance-enhancing substances were pervasive in Johnson's sport; fresh insider quotes around the Seoul Games affirmed the conclusion. American track stars Edwin Moses, Carl Lewis, and Evelyn Ashford said drug use was rampant and an accepted practice. A sprinter from Sierra Leone, Horace Dove-Edwin, stated, "Everybody uses drugs." The *New York Times* interviewed experts who collectively estimated about half of the year's 9,000 Olympic athletes used performance enhancers. Dan Jenkins, a convicted steroid dealer and former sprinter for Britain, said a group of American athletes visited him for schooling on undetectable substances. "A bunch of guys. . . came to see me; they wanted to know what's up," he said. "I know of 12 or 13 other things they can't catch." Dr. Robert Voy, USOC chief medical officer, corroborated, saying, "The athletes are ahead of us and have stuff we don't even know about; I know that for a fact. We are not deterring use at all, as far as anabolic steroids are concerned. We have to come up with better analytical programs and with better technology."

Reports of systematic abuse and culpability were the minority, however. Perspectives such as Voy's and Jenkins' were published but not repeated. The fantasy of sport held firm, across self-indulgent America and the planet, allowing the federations to escape once again. Athletes alone were portrayed as the problem, once again. Johnson suffered the reaction of the world against him. His positive result for steroids negated both his gold medal and world record of 9.79 seconds in the 100 meters. He lost an estimated $10 million in endorsements and faced a two-year ban from competition.

Courson, a lonely contrarian, was compelled to speak out on behalf of Johnson, whom he regarded as a symptom of doping, not a cause. In a larger aim, Courson sought to deflate the burgeoning movement toward "random" testing for steroids by major sports. He understood doping was just an image game for organizations, anyway, especially the NFL, where drugs for both size and pain were imperative. Courson believed that league officials were not concerned about players' health, and they needed no new tool of control, especially random urinalysis. "Because I was doing the research on my book, I understood drug testing would never work," he said. "Then I understood that basically the NFL wanted to jerk the players around with this, just something else that they held over their head. ... Well, I had a bunch of friends still playing the game, Webbie included, who needed those drugs to continue to make their living."

Courson believed few players wanted to use steroids, but they had no choice in a sport marketed as mass entertainment. Doping fit the equation for athletes as well as organizers. "From the beginning, I've viewed this not so much as an ethical issue," he said. "To me, it was more a training issue of science. It's always been that, the way I looked at it. ... Being introduced to those drugs by a [college] team physician, you know, it was legal and no big deal. I said, 'If the doctor has no problem in prescribing it, there's not really an issue here.'"

The overriding evil of sport doping, Courson believed, was the hypocrisy of a culture refusing to acknowledge certain realities about its beloved games. Americans always squawked about wholesome values, but they lived by winning at all costs, seeking gratification through any means necessary. Why should anyone expect more of athletes, particularly those negotiating the bloody path of football?

Other critics concurred with Courson, notably Dr. Norman Faust, director of medical ethics at the University of Wisconsin. "We cannot plausibly argue that we prohibit professional football players from using steroids or amphetamines because of concern for their health," Faust wrote for the Hastings Center Report, "when the sport itself permanently disables a high proportion of participants." In a media interview, Faust dismissed organizers' transparent posturing about steroids. "Pete Rozelle worries about steroids, but not roughing the passer or hockey slashing," he said. "Sport itself is much more harmful than steroids... The claim that drugs are unnatural is incoherent to me. Nothing in sports is natural, from running shoes to slimy bathing suits to special diets to Gatorade."

In the steroid debate of autumn 1988, as stories of Ben Johnson were joined by Chaikin's allegations about college football, Courson fought the prevailing notion of random urinalysis as the answer. He espoused the only option at hand for helping athletes: public acknowledgment of their drug use so physicians could control it. Since there existed widespread, unpreventable doping in games, Courson reasoned, why not monitor competitors for steroids and other enhancers? Then, at least, systematic usage might be tracked and capped by doctors in an intervention strategy known as risk reduction.

Editors at *Sports Illustrated* disagreed with Courson but eagerly enlisted him for a commentary to garner reaction. They titled the piece "Steroids: Another View" and placed it on the magazine's back page, prime-time exposure, where Courson predicted failure for NFL testing. "There is great controversy — and hypocrisy — about steroid use in sports," Courson wrote, continuing by slamming the NFL's historical apathy and society's willingness to blame athletes alone for the drugs. "What's a nose tackle supposed to do when he knows his coach expects him to weigh 295 pounds and bench-press 600 pounds?" Courson called for a new "realistic" approach considered radical, *soft doping* by athletes, unfathomable for most leaders of public opinion, politicians, and pundits. He proposed America should sanction steroid use for adult sport under medical supervision.

The response was swift in the denunciation of Courson. In Tampa Bay, where some still reviled him for steroid honesty, sports columnist Hubert Mizell suggested the former Buccaneer was a publicity freak. Mizell implied lunacy fueled Courson's claim that pro football could not return to pre-steroid days. "If the NFL accepts that," the scribe fumed, "the league should become fodder for a federal grand jury."

Two decades hence, as the modern NFL continued to wallow in drugs and deny it, Courson chuckled. "I mentioned the potential of medically monitoring the situation, and, man, that made me a major target... for crackpots on both sides of the issue," he recalled. "I guess the thing I didn't understand was the fact you can't monitor something that the whole culture wants to pretend does not exist. ... I think I tripped a wire in the media more than [the citizenry]."

Actually, given *SI's* enormous audience, Courson had expected his commentary to make waves, bring grief upon him. "Even before I started dealing with the media here, I kind of knew what they were going to do. And that was kind of depressing, knowing that it was coming and there was nothing I could do about it — and knowing I didn't really have any answers [for doping], either."

Courson could not fret long over the backlash to his message. Two weeks after *SI* ran the commentary, in late November 1988, his life took a terrifying turn. Warning signals had begun in October, when Courson, weighing about 300 pounds with low body fat, experienced difficulty holding down food and drink. Something else, he became winded easily in wrestling workouts. By mid-November, his stomach had bloated and he was vomiting daily. He was lethargic but unable to sleep, and he could not cease hiccupping. Lacking health coverage, Courson hoped the illness was a virus or stomach disorder, and he avoided seeing a doctor. Growing sicker, he had no choice.

At friends' urging, Courson drove himself to a Pittsburgh hospital the day before Thanksgiving. Graying in color, hardly able to sit upright, Courson's pulse hit 200 beats per minute; his blood pressure was 80 over 50. An ER physician figured Courson would be dead by morning. Doctors immediately placed him in intensive care, where he rested four days before beginning a battery of tests. Courson provided caregivers his complete history of injuries and substance abuse, the primaries alcohol and anabolic steroids — which he would not use again.

A cardiologist delivered the diagnosis: Courson, 33, suffered from cardiac disease, cardiomyopathy, enlarged heart too flabby to pump blood normally. Doctors concluded he probably needed a heart transplant, or he likely would die within three to five years. Courson's name was added to a waiting list.

Did steroids cause the cardiomyopathy? Courson, the disciplined student of medical research and son of a nurse, knew no conclusive study existed to answer the question. He suspected enlarged body mass and alcoholic binges could have contributed as much as anabolic steroids. Webster urged Courson to keep private his medical problem, for the public would blame him harshly, but news broke a few months later. A copy editor wrote the headline "Avid Abuser Now in Line For A New Heart," and the media debated whether steroid-abusing athletes like Courson should receive organ transplants. In Pittsburgh, a radio personality slammed him on-air, declaring, "Courson did this to himself. He knew the risks."

Courson Gains an Ally in Yesalis

Monday evening, January 2, 1989, the problem of teens and steroids was examined on The MacNeil/Lehrer NewsHour, a PBS television program based in Washington, D.C. Guest panelists included Steve Courson, from Pittsburgh, and Dr. Charles Yesalis, from Penn State University, author of a landmark study on the topic. Before airtime, Courson wondered about Yesalis, especially on the question of blaming systems for steroids along with individuals. Courson, advocating systemic blame, was accustomed to uninformed attacks from so-called experts, but he had a different sense about Yesalis, whose published research and quotes he respected. The show bore out his hunch.

Yesalis said steroid use had reached epidemic proportions in America and no effective preventive was employed anywhere. He spread blame, citing users, parents, officials, and society at-large. Yesalis decried the lack of research and the sport organizers who stonewalled study proposals. He did not exaggerate verified health risks of steroid use, despite close questioning from Robert MacNeil, the *NewsHour* host. "The short-term effects in adult males are transitory, meaning when you go off the drugs, everything returns to normal," Yesalis said. "We do not know what happens with repeated or prolonged use. Unfortunately, using these drugs is like trying to eat one peanut or potato chip. Many people just keep coming back and using more and more. So we're at a considerable disadvantage in dealing with this problem, given this absence of information on the long-term effects."

In addition, Yesalis agreed with Courson that steroid urinalysis had achieved nothing in sport, though the doctor did believe that unannounced, year-round testing could make a difference. Yesalis, an avid weightlifter and former strength coach, really endeared himself to Courson when the ex-athlete encountered a tough question from the host. MacNeil posed to Courson: "[W]hat kind of advice do you give teenagers who may ask you about [steroids]?"

"That's one of the most difficult problems that I face," said Courson, who opposed usage by children. "I frequent gyms and I train with the weights, and I get a lot of questions. ... Number one, if you tell them not to do the drugs, some of these people will not have the ability to compete at the level they want to compete at. But you can't tell them to do [steroids] because of the health risks involved. That's a decision they can only make themselves. What I try to tell them, [I] warn them about some of the side effects and say if you're going to do it, do it under a doctor's supervision..."

There was momentary pause, quiet, and MacNeil turned to Yesalis: "Is that good advice, Dr. Yesalis?"

"I think it's very reasonable advice," Yesalis replied unflinchingly. "Sometimes the best you can do with young kids is to get them to postpone their decision to use the drug. Short of that, you try and get them to take very, very low doses under a doctor's supervision... [G]iven the choice of using a drug in a black-market situation or using it under a doctor's supervision, the latter is a better alternative."

Courson had found a comrade.

VI. Politicians Grab Spotlight of Steroid Hysteria

As the world trained attention on steroid abuse in sport, with deposed Canadian athlete Ben Johnson as Exhibit A, bureaucrats reaped political hay in countries including Australia, Canada, and the United States. Popular opinion demanded punishment of offending athletes like Johnson, and politicians capitalized, grabbing headlines for staging hearings that hardly approached protecting young athletes from drugs. In addition, the political dog-and-pony shows went far in perpetuating the myth of urinalysis as a prevention for doping.

The politicians did impress most journalists and sports fans, who wanted to believe government hearings fostered legitimate solutions. "Athletics has done away with its [dirty] carpet. ... Everywhere, there is a Johnson effect," reporter Neil Wilson wrote from Canada. "Americans, Britons, Soviets and Germans have all been touched by the scattergun of its investigations." The writer was primarily referring to athletes, the usual suspects, and the simplistic rationale of urinalysis as savior. "Sport has gained invaluable intelligence in its fight against the junkies," Wilson stated, predicting random testing was at hand and unbeatable.

Athletes naturally absorbed the heaviest fire for steroids, but Johnson's coach and physician took bullets, too, among select officials worldwide. Called to testify in the Canadian inquiry headed by Charles Dubin, a provincial chief justice, coach Charlie Francis and Dr. Mario "Jamie" Astaphan did not pander for mercy through false contriteness. Fully cognizant that the blame would stop with them, instead of rising further to track-and-field organizers, Astaphan and Francis spoke reality.

"If there was any athlete not on [steroids at Seoul], they were probably from Sri Lanka or Timbuktu or some other godforsaken place," the caustic Astaphan told the media. The doctor derided wistful thinking about eradication, promoting instead the strategy of risk reduction. "The IOC knows how widespread steroids are in every sport — amateur and professional," he said. "[Steroids] should not be banned. There should be specific provisions placed on them to prevent their abuse, then everyone can get back on an equal footing." Astaphan decried "scare tactics" about health and the myth of amateurism, its influence on official evasion. "In professional sports there's a lot less bull and hypocrisy. Steroids are used all through the National Football League. It's part of the game."

Francis was calm, straightforward, engaging on the witness stand, answering questions with conviction. "We're awash in a sea of denials," the coach observed. "People have to recognize what's going on, admit the levels of performance are not possible without performance-enhancing drugs, and get on with the process of trying to make some changes."

Francis recalled Johnson's coming to him in 1977, a shy, impoverished 15-year-old recently emigrated from Jamaica. Refuting claims of Johnson as an athletic fraud by rivals, Francis described him as a natural wonder who nevertheless had to resort to anabolic drugs. "If he wanted to compete, it's pretty clear that steroids are worth a meter [of speed] at the highest levels," said Francis, a former Olympian. "I think he understood his competitors were on them."

Already suspended from coaching by sports officials, Francis testified of counseling Johnson on steroids prior to the athlete's first use in 1981. Astaphan added injections of growth hormone and vitamin B-12 to Johnson's drug regimen in 1984, and three years later he set the 100-meter record, 9.83 seconds. Francis said Johnson's doping remained undetected in 17 post-race tests prior to Seoul.

Johnson himself maintained he never knowingly took any banned performance-enhancer, but another Canadian sprinter under Francis, Angella Issajenko, said, "That is the standard procedure — when a athlete gets caught, you deny." Issajenko testified Canadian athletes would not have broken their conspiracy of silence if government had not investigated. "We were such a close-knit group — and we had a big secret — and if it hadn't come to this, we would have all gone to our graves not even telling our parents."

Issajenko, 30, and Francis, 40, named more than a dozen athletes in the scandal, and she described her coach as "like a brother." After Seoul, she said, the two had spoken regularly on the phone, but not to concoct tales for the inquiry. "We decided we would come here and tell the truth," Issajenko testified.

In America, track and field drew criticism in an inquiry conducted by the Senate Judiciary Committee, but the politicians were different for football officials under questioning, allowing the benefit of the doubt. This curious double standard of America, damning Olympic or other sports for drugs while always allowing football to sneak by, was historical. "It's really unfortunate that track and field gets the black eye from the steroid issue. ...," Steve Scott, U.S. Distance runner, said during this period. "You look at the NFL and at collegiate football players, and you can't tell me that those guys get that big naturally."

Several football officials were saying exactly that, repeatedly, including Pete Rozelle and NFL coaches who made statements without rebuke at the May 9 hearing in Washington. Senator Joe Biden convened the football hearings, as politicians seemed bent on accommodating football figures rather than calling them out. Biden lavished praise on Steelers coach Chuck Noll and was highly complimentary of Chiefs coach Marty Schottenheimer, who politicians worried might miss an early flight home.

Biden was "very pleased" by the appearance of commissioner Rozelle, whom he once had battled over the issue of franchise relocation. Rozelle recently had announced his retirement, effective when league owners could determine a successor, and on this day politicians would gush in his presence. "Some have said that the NFL has not done enough about [steroids]," Biden said, "but I think it is commendable that one of the most significant and, as it turns out, one of the last major public appearances of this extraordinary man with an extraordinary career has been to come and speak out on this problem. Twenty-nine years as commisioner, and now [Rozelle is] culminating that career with a significant contribution. Commissioner, I know that the sports history books will look very kindly upon you, and if you are able in your final days of your tenure to commit the National Football League to ridding pro football of drug abuse, including steroids, you will be making a contribution not only to pro football but to all of your fellow countrymen." Biden saluted Rozelle for building the NFL "into a major institution in this country," for claiming regard as America's greatest sports administrator, and for winning election to the Pro Football Hall of Fame. "And we are delighted to have you back here," the senator told Rozelle. "And if you would like to proceed with an opening statement, we would welcome it."

Rozelle appeared forthright this time before Congress. "Thank you very much, Mr. Chairman, members of the committee....," he began. "Seven weeks ago I announced new procedures in the NFL's effort to combat anabolic steroids. NFL players now face the possibility of missing a large portion or all of the 1989 season if they use these drugs. As is true under our policy on cocaine and other so-called street drugs, we will not hesitate to remove those who use steroids from participation in professional football."

Rozelle described his latest steroid policy as "more comprehensive," and he stuck to his line that the league only recently had determined how to effectively treat the problem. He said steroids posed health risks for players, violated fairness of competition, and set a dangerous precedent for kids.

Revising simple history, Rozelle claimed the league was clueless about steroids until the 1970s, and he directly blamed power-lifters and bodybuilders for the drugs' influx into football, ignoring history's documented involvement of coaches, trainers, physicians, and franchises. By 1983 the league was committed to educating players about the "discouraging trend" of steroids, Rozelle said. "We believe that our... educational efforts have been a deterrent to many players who otherwise might now be using steroids."

Skewing testing data, Rozelle declared the invalid urinalysis methodology of 1987 and 1988 "indicated a solidly documentable steroid use by 6 to 7 percent of NFL players." Rozelle, nervy and secure with his receptive politicians, disputed claims of widespread use, including those from within the league, calling such charges "largely anecdotal or speculative." Rozelle did allow he could not "guarantee that our testing has detected or will detect every steroid user in the NFL." Rozelle espoused tougher penalties and random testing to rid his game of steroids, while still referring to his newest rehash of scheduled testing as "the first systematic and pervasive approach to combating steroid use among athletes in major team sports."

During Biden's cross-examination, Rozelle relented a little on his usage figures. "I thought it may be, it may be higher," the commissioner said. The senator also wondered about the possibility of league sanctions against former college players who tested positive for steroids prior to the NFL draft, as had been the case for dozens of draftees in the past two years. In addition, the Dallas Cowboys had considered a tryout for Ben Johnson. Rozelle reasoned that the athletes were unsigned when testing positive, and the NFL probably could not levy sanctions.

Biden was equally nice to Chuck Noll, in part because of a thoughtful act by the coach in 1972, when the senator's family endured a terrible car accident that killed his wife and daughter. Noll had his Steelers team sign a football for each of Biden's sons hospitalized after the crash, and the grateful politician did not forget, relating the story once again at the hearing. Years later in 2005, Noll would ignore Courson's tragic death, making no effort to contact his former player's family, but in 1989 neither the coach's persona nor testimony was subject to question by politicians. Biden gave him his glory.

"Coach...," Biden addressed Noll, "you are the second winningest coach, I need not tell you, in NFL history and the only coach in the NFL to have won four Super Bowl championships. ... I will be forever indebted to you and your 1972 Steelers football team. At any rate, I thank you personally... and thank you for what you have done for the sport. Now, if you have an opening statement, please proceed."

Noll proceeded with several nonsensical comments. Noll had been an assistant coach alongside Roy at San Diego in 1963, but he blamed Olympic coaches and lifters — one of whom he hired as a Steelers strength coach, Lou Riecke — for infecting the NFL with steroids. Noll said steroid use was often unrecognizable and the drugs produced little or no benefit for athletes, at least in his sport. "Steroids, although they provide weightroom strength, do not provide playing strength," Noll asserted. "When I am talking about strength on the field, the ability to survive contact. ... It is counterproductive to be dependent on the pill or to think you can get something out of a bottle." Noll described one unnamed player of his who tested positive as "rather thin, almost emaciated by pro football standards." Instead, he said, many weight-trained athletes could indeed add 30 pounds of muscle in one year without steroids, because of their massive eating and "large families."

Biden asked Noll whether coaches proven to know of players' use should be penalized. Noll replied coaches had no way of knowing for sure, only "speculation," then he rambled about testing until gently redirected by the senator: "But that is really not my question," Biden said. "My question is: If in fact — I know in your case you did not know — but if in fact a coach encouraged a player or condoned a player's use of anabolic steroids, should there be a sanction against that coach?"

Noll: "I have nothing against that, no. I would be for that."

The Steelers had just drafted known steroid user Tom Ricketts, a 6-foot-4, 300-pound tackle, from the University of Pittsburgh, where he roomed with defensive end Burt Grossman. Both tested positive for steroids at the NFL combine, but both became first-round picks, with Grossman drafted by the Chargers. Their new employers in pro football told the media that each had used prescription steroids to heal injuries. Biden asked Noll, "Did you take Ricketts' positive steroid [result] into account when you drafted him number one?"

"Very much so," Noll replied. "We have done that with many players and have downgraded them as a result. ... [W]e had the young man in and talked to him, and he said, just as he said in the paper, that what he had taken was for the rehabilitation and the testing. And obviously, when you deal with anybody who has been involved in any kind of drug things, we treat that very suspiciously. But after much consideration, I think we were satisfied that that was the case and there wouldn't be any in the future because we told him he would be tested."

"You basically believed his story," Biden stated, deciphering for Noll.

"That's right." The Steelers had no interest in players "we consider hard-core steroid users," Noll said, without detailing how the franchise reached such conclusions, after contending increasing mass was no reliable evidence.

Senator Biden suggested Noll and Chiefs coach Schottenheimer were courageous for appearing before the committee, where they risked being "put on the spot." Senator Strom Thurmond, of South Carolina, asked Schottenheimer, a former NFL defensive end, if he believed "some teams that are aware of steroid abuse have allowed it to continue despite its effect upon the players, society, and the integrity of the game?"

Schottenheimer: "Senator, I am of the opinion that in the National Football League today there is no evidence that management supports in any way the use of these anabolic steroids."

Thurmond: "Do you think that management is doing all it could? Is it going over and beyond the call of duty, so to speak, to take steps to try to prevent the use of steroids?"

Schottenheimer: "I believe that the process is clearly under way, Senator, in that regard. As I suggested earlier, there are alternatives to steroids [for gaining size], and that educational process, in my mind, must be made available to players so that they can realize what they consider to be their optimum skills as players."

Schottenheimer and Noll, in concert with Rozelle, characterized as exaggerated the statements of player witnesses to come, Falcons tackle Bill Fralic and former Steelers-Bucs guard Courson, who both alleged widespread steroid abuse among NFL linemen. Likewise, the coaches and commissioner agreed there should be no federal legislation in the steroid issue. "I think that it is up to us to try and clean our own house of this problem first, initially," Rozelle told inquiring senator Charles E. Grassley, Iowa.

Regarding prescription use of steroids for injury rehabilitation, Rozelle changed completely from a few years previous. "There would be no [legitimate medical] reason," Rozelle told Grassley. "If we found it in the National Football League, there would be a trainer without a job for awhile, I will tell you that much. ... I think that we have to do all we can to save them, save the individual athlete from the consequences of lengthy steroid use. And I think we owe it to our sport to get rid of steroids so that these role models will not cause young athletes in high school and college to take up steroids."

Biden moved toward concluding the panelist session, for which no oaths of truth were required, by explaining "this was not intended to be confrontational but informational." He had one last question for Noll, a tough one regarding the administering of pain-killing injections and pills in the NFL.

In the period, Courson alleged players were pressured to use painkillers by Steelers coaches and trainers, and All-Pro defensive lineman Joe Klecko said the same of his former team, the New York Jets. The practice was wide open across the league, as numerous public reports since the 1960s corroborated, along with teams' records of drug dispensing. Noll appeared oblivious, however, when Biden broached the issue of erasing pain for performance, widely known as "blocking" injury.

Biden: "If an athlete has a serious muscle pull, or a problem with his shoulder, the team doctor will shoot him up, and he will be able to play this game. Is that fact or fiction?"

"From our standpoint, that is fiction," Noll began. "Pain is analyzed to a great deal of, you know, our doctors, what is the pain there? Let me put it that way. I am not saying that shots for pain have not been given, but they are not given just to get rid of pain. If pain is there indicating that someone should not play, then he is not going to play. If killing that pain will cause further injury, then it is not the way we want to go. If it is something that is minor, then that is done. But pain-killing just for that is not done."

Now Biden was incredulous, of Noll. He asked again whether players were pressured to take shots.

Noll: "You know, in my experience, I do not think we have ever had anybody do that. ... We have had people not play in championship games because that kind of thing would have caused further injury and harmed them, and we are not interested in doing that."

After Rozelle and coaches cleared the hearing room, with Schottenheimer presumably on time for his flight back to Kansas City, the next witness panel entered: Gene Upshaw, NFL players union executive director, Fralic, and Courson. The primary points Fralic and Courson would make were already publicized, but Upshaw flip-flopped on his view of doping in the past. Four years previous, Upshaw told *Sports Illustrated* he neither knew a user nor believed a problem existed for the league. Now the former 16-year lineman contended steroid use was widespread in all games, including football, because of systematic forces.

"I first must say that it is virtually unanimous why steroid use is pervasive in sports. ...," said Upshaw, who was fighting NFL urinalysis of players. "And it has to do with something that Senator Thurmond said... it has to do with pressure. There is the pressure to earn money; there is the pressure to keep a job; there is pressure to keep ahead of competition; and there is pressure to win."

Upshaw, long-trying to negotiate a new collective bargaining agreement with Rozelle, lauded NBA drug policy because it was "a jointly agreed-to program," though lacking steroid testing. Upshaw noted modern football mandates of "Bigger is better" and performing through debilitating injury — "As players, we all recognize that," the union leader said — requiring pharmaceuticals that coaches like Noll claimed were a mystery to them.

The ever-accelerating arms race of weight training swept up players and coaches alike, according to Upshaw, speaking with clarity on doping like never before in public. "You have a young player... that is trying to break into the NFL, and he is seeking that weight advantage to win a roster spot on the team. You have the established starter who is trying to become dominant on the field, and that might be a reason for that particular player to use steroids. And you have an older player who is hoping to gain strength and hold on to [his job against] the new breed that is coming into the league."

Regarding a player's uphill battle for gaining weight, strength, and speed, Upshaw disagreed with Rozelle, Noll, and Schottenheimer, their claim that options existed besides muscle substances. Upshaw, fully aware of the athlete's dilemma, noted coaches need say nothing directly about doping. Steroid use "really comes down to the pressure, keeping up with the Joneses," Upshaw said. "It is something that is there. And no one has to tell you that you are not as strong as the guy that is in front of you, and if you want to make this team, you need to gain some weight."

Upshaw accused management of "image" priorities regarding muscle doping, and expressed empathy with every man in football, all levels, each hamstrung by an epidemic impossible to change on his own. The health problem was "institutional," he said, and tied to societal ethos. "It comes about by the win-at-all-costs attitude. It is an awful lot of pressure put on a club owner, an awful lot of pressure put on a coach, which eventually gets down to the player because it all turns on the player. Can he play on the field? The coach is under pressure because he has to keep his job, and if he has a young talent, a guy out there that is right on the verge of becoming a superstar, and he needs that little extra push, quite naturally; there are ways to do it. And it is not by taking all the vitamins in the world and eating all of the food you can eat. There are other ways. And it is no salvation for the college coaches. We have several in the room, and they are under a lot of pressure. It is all of our collective problem."

Following Upshaw's earnest opening statement, he was questioned about his turning 180 degrees in public about steroids.

Biden: "[I]n 1985, in a *Sports Illustrated* article, you said, and I quote, 'I never knew any guys who took steroids. There's no black market of steroids. I don't think steroids are a problem in the NFL.' Do you still think that is true?"

Upshaw: "I said that? Are you sure?"

The reply befuddled the committee chairman, who let the matter drop and opened the floor for Fralic, the Falcons tackle. "I thank you for this chance," Fralic told the committee, "and I hope your investigation will lead to ridding athletics in our society of steroids. I believe steroid use is rampant among the NFL, and that includes my own team. It is rampant in colleges, and it is rampant in high schools. Everybody is blind to it because they choose to ignore what is happening in the world of steroids. It is time to stop ignoring the problem and to open the eyes of the naïve. Steroid use in football represents a vicious cycle. I know there are many players in high school, college, and the NFL who want to stop using steroids. But they cannot or will not because they do not believe they can be competitive without them. ... Obviously, coaches at every level turn their back to the steroid situation. High school coaches are trying to build an impressive record for their resume or to build their status within a community. College coaches face tremendous pressure to win. Pro coaches are judged only on one basis, their win-loss record. The cycle keeps repeating itself, and a monster problem is growing. NFL owners cannot grasp this problem. They have not been living in the middle of the steroid madness. They cannot see their friends affected by it. The recent NFL draft is a great example of how teams will look the other way when it comes to steroids."

Courson Spells Out Reality, Politicians Ignore Him

Steve Courson, figuratively battered by doping in football if not seriously ill of it, was fairly cynical by the time politicians asked him to testify in 1989. Courson understood Washington, D.C., the land of smoke and mirrors. The old saying was right-on: The halls of lawmakers provided a chance at justice, but no guarantee, not with these people. Similarly, a political committee may have *no hope* of solving a problem, nor would really try, staging instead a public show featuring the appealing, ineffective quick fix. Therefore Courson, in going before Congress on May 9, after the politicians fawned over Rozelle, Noll, and Schottenheimer, already knew what the latest "solution" would be for steroids in football: random testing, however lousy.

Courson did take comfort knowing he would speak honorably, and he was heartened by Upshaw's words, suddenly so sincere. In addition, Courson was proud of Bill Fralic, the Falcons' young All-Pro lineman, for confessing his own steroid use and coming to Capitol Hill in patriotic fashion.

While Fralic impressed everyone, however, Courson knew the young man also played into the hands of management regarding a perceived solution. Fralic, without fully doing his homework, told politicians random testing was the answer, and he claimed a large majority of NFL players supported the method.

Courson would not play along. Granted, he had come to Washington a sympathetic figure, a formerly powerful athlete now awaiting a heart transplant, struggling to climb stairs or lift small barbells. He was sickly, slow, 80 pounds lighter than when diagnosed six months before. However, when Senator Arlen Specter attempted to wrap the steroid hearings by touting random testing as the solution by consensus, Courson firmly objected, a fighter still to reckon with.

"I am not in favor of random testing," Courson told Specter. "I will give a reason why, and it is based on a scientific reason. It is because the present testing methodology is not capable of cleaning the sport."

Specter, of Courson's homestate Pennsylvania, glared. "Is not the present methodology capable of making a factual determination when someone has used a steroid?" asked the federal policymaker.

"Correct," Courson replied, clarifying for the senator. "In other words, I think the

Olympic sport is a very good teacher of this. The mass spectrometer gas chromatograph, which is state-of-the-art testing, has had its problems in cleaning the Olympic sport. And I do not think, with present capabilities, that testing is going to work."

Courson recited the list of documented factors — published in a recent newspaper commentary of his, including low-level testosterone — that rendered urinalysis ineffective for preventing muscle doping. "The human growth hormone, which is one of the newest sports-enhancer drugs used by modern athletes today, is virtually undetectable, and it is a very dangerous drug. Also, water-based [patented] steroids, if stopped three weeks before testing... more or less go undetected. Also, rearrangement [by design] in the steroid molecular structure and masking drugs can confuse testing. This I see, as the biggest crux in the problem, is trying to use testing as an answer. ... [U]nless I am mistaken from all the research I have done, to my knowledge, there is no testing methodology that today is 100 percent efficient."

Flustered, Specter attempted only limited bantering with the studious Courson before switching attention to Fralic's assertion as the final word, that most NFL players viewed random testing as an appropriate solution.

Courson was ignored, the spiral of denial in charge. Shaky random urinalysis had overcome truth as the order of the day. Fralic was privileged by powerbrokers as the authority on testing over Courson, and even anointed superiority on the football field — Biden gushed to Fralic he was a "great" player. Courson just felt the pols' contempt, as messenger debunking their hopeless plan for preventing muscle substances in football.

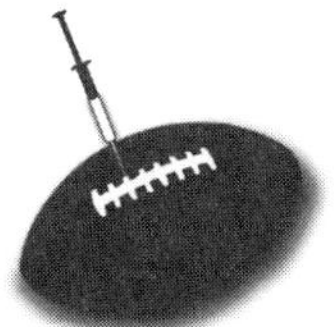

REFERENCES

1984 Survey. (1986, August 30). NCAA did survey on drug use in 1984. *The Associated Press* [Online].

30-Team NFL. (1987, January 24). A 30-team NFL might be only two years away. *The Associated Press* [Online].

49ers Pay. (1988, June 2). 49ers pay Krueger $2.36 million for injuries. *United Press International* [Online].

49ers' Use. (1986, December 28). Walsh: 49ers use steroids to meet competition. *United Press International* [Online].

97 Players. (1988, October 7). Rozelle says 97 players tested positive in 1987 steroid urinalysis. *The Associated Press* [Online].

Aides Indicted. (1989, April 20). 4 ex-football aides indicted in South Carolina steroid case. *New York Times*, p. D25.

Akron Panel. (1987, July 22). Akron panel investigates steroid allegations. *The Associated Press* [Online].

Akron Testing. (1987, July 22). Akron U. to test athletes for drugs. *United Press International* [Online].

Akron Use. (1987, April 17). Akron football players reportedly used steroids. *United Press International* [Online].

Aldridge, D. (1988, October 20). Chaikin tells more, South Carolina coaches deny condoning steroids. *Washington Post*, p. B6.

Alfano, P., & Janofsky, M. (1988, November 19). A guru who spreads the gospel of steroids. *New York Times*, p. 1 — 1.

Altman, L.K. (1988, November 22). For new specialists in drug detection, athletes set fast pace. *New York Times*, p. C3.

Anderson, D. (1986, July 8). New dimension in drug issue. *New York Times*, p. B7.

Anderson, D. (1988, July 10). New drug epidemic. *New York Times*, p. 8 — 6.

Anderson, D. (1989, March 24). Pete Rozelle: Integrity's Clean Hands. *New York Times*, p. B7.

Anderson, H. (1987, June 10). NCAA won't investigate Miami for steroids. *United Press International* [Online].

Astaphan Speaks. (1989, March 23). Johnson's doctor said every Olympian takes steroids. *The Associated Press* [Online].

Barnes, M. (1989, January 10). Runner says double standard benefits football. *United Press International* [Online].

Barrett, M. (1989, March 7). Johnson's coach advises officials on testing. *United Press International* [Online].

Berkow, I. (1988, October 28). Rozelle and fool's gold. *New York Times*, p. A22.

Bethesdan Bargains. (1989, June 20). Bethesdan bargains in steroids case. *Washington Post*, p. E2.

Black, B. (1989, June 22). Utah athletic director thrilled Gadd's acquitted of charges. *The Associated Press* [Online].

Blum, R. (1988, December 15). Sports commissioners discuss issues. *The Associated Press* [Online].

Bock, H. (1987, March 22). NCAA testing draws praise, questions. *The Associated Press* [Online].

Bock, H. (1987, June 28). Big money, big pressure. *The Associated Press* [Online].

Bock, H. (1987, December 31). Orange Bowl has annual drug sideshow. *The Associated Press* [Online].

Bosworth, B., & Reilly, R. (1988). *The Boz: Confessions of a modern antihero.* New York, NY: Charter Books.

Bosworth Chaos. (1988, August 7). Bosworth details chaos at Oklahoma. *Washington Post*, p. C6.

Brubaker, B. (1987, February 1). Players close eyes to steroids' risks. *Washington Post*, p. C1.

Brubaker, B. (1988, September 15). NFL official says some teams let drug users play before crackdown; league moved into enforcement to eliminate 'conflict of interest.' *Washington Post*, p. B1.

Brubaker, B. (2008, June 3). Telephone interview with author.

Buddy Wants. (1987, January 8). Buddy Ryan wants Bosworth. *The Associated Press* [Online].

Catlin, D. (2007, February 17). E-mail correspondence to author.

Chaikin Recounts. (1988, October 18). Chaikin recounts widespread steroid use for Gamecocks. *The Associated Press* [Online].

Chaikin, T., & Telander, R. (1988, October 24). The nightmare of steroids. *Sports Illustrated*, p. 82.

Chandler, L. (1996, October 17). McNairy continues to use steroids, and NFL dreams closer to becoming true. *Charlotte Observer* [Online].

Chargers Confirm. (1989, April 25). Chargers confirm top pick used steroids. *The Associated Press* [Online].

Cole, B. (1988, October 20). Grand jury to study ex-USC player's drug claims. *Columbia State*, p. 1A.

Columbia University. (1988, April 20). Columbia University investigates steroid allegations about football team. *The Associated Press* [Online].

Coming Clean. (1986, November 5). Coming clean about steroids. *New York Times*, p. D24.

Courson, S. (1988, November 14). Steroids: Another view. *Sports Illustrated*, p. 106.

Courson, S. (1989, May 6). Steroids and modern sports. *Pittsburgh Post-Gazette.*

Courson, S. (2005, March 7). Interview with author, Farmington, PA.

Courson, S. (2005, March 27). Telephone interview with author.

Courson, S. (2005, April 7). Telephone interview with author.

Courson, S. (2005, May 1). Telephone interview with author.

Courson, S. (2005, June 5). E-mail to author.

Courson, S. (2005, June 7). Telephone interview with author.

Courson, S. (2005, June 22). Telephone interview with author.

Courson, S. (2005, June 26). Telephone interview with author.

Courson, S. (2005, November 1). Telephone interview with author.

Courson, S., & Schreiber, L.R. (1991). *False glory*. Longmeadow Press: Stamford, CT.

Dan Duchaine. (2004). Dan Duchaine the steroid guru. *Quest For Advanced Condition: www.gfac.com.*

Denlinger, K. (1986, December 10). NFL's rule book is overridden by talent, equipment. *Washington Post*, p. D1.

Disciplinary Action. (1988, July 19). Players using steroids subject to disciplinary action. *United Press International* [Online].

Domowitch, P. (1986, December 14). NFL declares war on steroids. *Toronto Star*, p. E3.

Donaghy, J. (1988, December 28). Ben Johnson scandal top story of 1988. *The Associated Press* [Online].

Dunham, W. (1985, August 21). Steroid testing poses problems for colleges. *United Press International* [Online].

Dunham, W. (1987, January 31). NFL injuries rise, insurers get tough. *United Press International* [Online].

Dunham, W. (1989, March 23). Lews says more Olympic medalists used steroids. *United Press International* [Online].

Dunn, M. (1989, July 9). He was one of professional football's mightiest men. *The Associated Press* [Online].

Edwards, C. (1990, January 28). Northwestern will investigate steroid allegations. *The Associated Press* [Online].

Elderkin, P. (1987, January 26). Rozelle faces thorny issues during last years of long NFL reign. *Christian Science Monitor*, p. 20.

Eskenazi, G. (1988, April 27). Jets' top pick says he took steroids. *New York Times*, p. D26.

Fans Concerned. (1989, November 30). Football fans concerned about steroid use. *United Press International* [Online].

Faust Says. (1987, April 17). Faust says he would suspended known steroid users. *The Associated Press* [Online].

Fewer Test. (1988, March 9). Fewer NFL prospects test positive at combine. *The Associated Press* [Online].

Fisher, M. (1989, August 5). 49ers tackle Barton says 80 percent NFL linemen use steroids. *Gannett News Service* [Online].

Fisher, M. (2005, July 10). Waters, steroids and a slippery slope. *TheRanchReport.com/ Scout.com* [Online].

Fitton Contacted. (1985, December 18). Kephart sought information from Fitton. *The Associated Press* [Online].

Friend, T. (1989, July 23). NFL experiences changing of the guard; commissioner search resembles 1960 process. *Washington Post*, p. C8.

George, T. (1988, September 20). Drug-test policy is bedeviling Rozelle. *New York Times*, p. A25.

George, T. (1988, October 26). N.F.L. tightens steroids policy. *New York Times*, p. B13.

George, T. (1989, March 23). Stunning owners, Rozelle says he's retiring. *New York Times*, p. D23.

Gillespie, B. (1989, August 10). Coaches will be sentenced. *Columbia State*, p. 2B.

Gillespie, B. (1989, August 11). 3 former USC coaches get detention in steroid case. *Columbia State*, p. 1A.

Gillespie, B., & Heffner, T. (1988, October 19). Ex-player says USC coaches knew steroids used. *Columbia State*, p. 1A.

Goldberg, D. (1988, July 20). NFL getting tougher on steroids. *The Associated Press* [Online].

Goldberg, D. (1988, October 1). NFL teams consider Johnson. *The Associated Press* [Online].

Goldberg, D. (1988, October 25). Two steroid positives could mean suspension. *The Associated Press* [Online].

Goldberg, D. (1989, March 22). NFL classifies steroids worse than cocaine. *The Associated Press.*

Grogan, D.W. (1987, February 9). An incurable killer strikes three ex-49ers, and an anguished victim doubts it's a coincidence. *People*, p. 94.

Grossman, D. (1986, October 16). Metro has bumper crop of beefy football stars. *Toronto Star*, p. H14.

Grossman Experimented. (1989, May 17). Grossman admits experimenting with steroids. *The Associated Press* [Online].

Hamm, L.M. (1988, October 19). Chaikin wants other athletes to avoid steroids. *The Associated Press* [Online].

Hanley, C.J. (1988, September 27). Olympic athletes seek performance from drugs. *The Associated Press* [Online].

Heffner, T. (1988, October 20). Ellis says Chaikin's statements false. *Columbia State*, p. 1D.

Hendel, J. (1987, August 22). Drug problems exist despite NCAA tests. *United Press International* [Online].

Herman, S. (1987, January 27). Prospects to be tested for steroids by NFL. *The Associated Press* [Online].

Hopefuls Fail. (1987, March 6). Twenty-nine NFL hopefuls fail drug test. *United Press International* [Online].

Huff, D. (1985, July 7). Drugs in the high schools. *Washington Post*, p. D11.

Huffman, S., & Telander, R. (1990, August 27). 'I deserve my turn.' *Sports Illustrated*, p. 26.

Huizenga, R. (1995). *"You're okay, it's just a bruise."* New York, NY: St. Martin's Press.

Idaho Career. (1989, July 21). Idaho football career ended by steroid use. *United Press International* [Online].

Janofsky, M. (1989, March 23). Unexpected choice transformed N.F.L. *New York Times*, p. D29.

Janofsky, M., & Alfano, P. (1988, November 21). Victory at any cost: Drug pressure growing. *New York Times*, p. A1.

Jaworski Works. (1987, May 6). Jaworski works out with the Dolphins in his latest camp stop. *St. Petersburg Times*, p. 8C.

Jenkins, R. (1988, August 8). Now the NCAA wnts to read Bosworth's book. *The Associated Press* [Online].

Jenkins, R. (1988, August 9). Switzer disappointed with Bosworth's book. *The Associated Press* [Online].

Jenkins, S. (1988, August 11). Switzer disputes Bosworth. *Washington Post*, p. C1.

Jenkins, S. (1989, March 22). Athlete's steroid adventure ended, but impact has not: Upheaval lingers at South Carolina. *Washington Post*, p. A1.

Jenkins, S. (1989, April 20). Five indicted in Chaikin case. *Washington Post*, p. B1.

Jennings, J. (2004, August 27). Pro football is brief, but life is eternal, says Derry pastor. *Blairsville Dispatch* [Online].

Johnson, W.O., Lieber, J., & Keteyian, A. (1985, May 13). Getting physical — and chemical. *Sports Illustrated*, p. 50.

Junkin Positive. (1989, May 7). Junkin tested positive for steroids prior to 1987 draft. *The Associated Press* [Online].

Jury Investigates. (1988, December 19). Grand jury investigates steroids in South Carolina. *United Press International* [Online].

Keim, B. (1986, August 21). Mira: Steroids in truck belonged to friend. *United Press International* [Online].

Keim, B. (1987, December 25). Mira will miss Orange Bowl. *United Press International* [Online].

Keim, B. (1987, December 26). Despite court order, Mira won't practice with Hurricanes. *United Press International* [Online].

Kershler, F. (1989, February 26). Why our sporting image is under siege. *Sunday Mail* [Online].

King, L. (1990, July 16). Former NFL drug advisor. *CNN* [Online].

Kornheiser, T. (1988, October 22). Thinking big with needles and pills. *Washington Post*, p. D1.

Lambert Says. (1989, August 5). Lambert says you can succeed in pro football without steroids. *The Associated Press* [Online].

Lederman, D. (1989, June 28). Steroid program for athletes confirmed by U. of Utah. *Chronicle for Higher Education*, p. A26.

Lederman, D. (1989, June 28). Switzer quits as Oklahoma football coach after a winter of turmoil. *Chronicle of Higher Education*, p. A25.

Lyons, R.D. (1984, June 14). Athletes warned on hormone. *New York Times*, p. D23.

MacNeil, R., & Lehrer, J. (1989, January 2). Pumping poison. *The NewsHour*, transcript [Online].

Macnow, G. (1991, December 29). Use of steroid alternatives growing. *Houston Chronicle*, Sports p.9.

Martinez, J. (1987, May 22). Miami strength coach implicated in nationwide ring. *The Associated Press* [Online].

McCartney, S. (1990, January 11). NCAA adopts tough new drug testing regulations. *The Associated Press* [Online].

McDonough, W. (1988, September 18). Owners get testy on drug policy. *Boston Globe*, p. 63.

McDonough, W. (1988, October 9). Steroids a problem. *Boston Globe*, p. 76 McDonough, W. (1989, March 23). The Rozelle resignation. *Boston Globe*, p. 66.

Miller, R. (1988, October 12). Ohio State players reportedly test positive for steroids. *The Associated Press* [Online].

Mizell, H. (1988, December 18). All-Americans decry steroid use. *St. Petersburg Times*, p. C1.

Molinski, M. (1987, October 19). Olympics scientist praises NCAA tests. Mortensen, C. (1989, May 6). Fralic to testify before Senate that steroid use in NFL is rampant. *St. Petersburg Times*, p. 6C.

Mossman, J. (1988, August 6). Broncos' Reed tests positive for drugs. *The Associated Press* [Online].

MSU Allegations. (1990, March 22). MSU officials: Allegations of widespread steroid use are false. *The Associated Press* [Online].

NCAA Tests. (1988, August 31). NCAA tests show third of players used steroids on some teams. *The Associated Press* [Online].

NCAA Results. (1988, August 31). NCAA test results on steroids. *The Associated Press* [Online].

Nelson, G. (1989, June 11). Courts are needed to ease players' pain. *St. Louis Post-Dispatch*, p. 1D.

Newspapers Say. (1988, November 16). What newspapers are saying. *United Press International* [Online].

NFL Use. (1988, October 8). Steroid use in the NFL. *New York Times*, p. 1 — 52.

Noonan Used. (1987, May 5). Noonan says he used steroids to regain weight. *The Associated Press* [Online].

Peters, K. (1989, January 11). Phillips, A., & Thompson, L. (1988, September 27). **Experts surprised, not shocked.** *Washington Post*, p. D10.

Player Defends. (1988, October 5). Women's Olympic basketball player defends Johnson. *United Press International* [Online].

Player Ineligible. (1987, December 19). Player ineligible. *New York Times*, p. 1 — 50.

Pomerantz, G. (1986, December 31). NCAA overreacted, 49ers' Walsh says. *Washington Post*, p. C3.

Pomerantz, G. (1988, June 26). Krueger's court score puts doctors on spot. *Washington Post*, p. D13.

Possible Link. (1987, February 6). Possible link between fertilizer, disease needs investigation, expert says. *The Associated Press* [Online].

Possible Use. (1988, October 22). Kephart told to keep Morrison posted on possible steroid use. *The Associated Press* [Online].

Precede Atlanta. (1988, July 19). Precede Atlanta. *The Associated Press* [Online].

Raffo, D. (1988, August 17). Rozelle defends Manley's suspension. *United Press International* [Online].

Reinwald, P. (1988, October 1). Most area high school football coaches favor drug testing. *St. Petersburg Times*, p. 1C.

Reminick, J. (1989, February 12). The steroid subculture. *New York Times*, p. 12LI-10.
Rhoden, W.C. (1988, October 2). Varying standards on steroid use. *New York Times*, p. 4 — 9.
Ribadeneira, D. (1988, October 31). The growing threat of steroids. *Boston Globe*, p. 39.
Robinson, M. (1989, May 10). NFL players, coaches testify about steroid use before Senate committee. *The Associated Press* [Online].
Rozelle Years. (1989, October 27). Through the years with Pete Rozelle. *USA Today*, p. 8C.
Scoppe, R. (1988, October 24). Morrison heard steroid rumors in 1985. *The Associated Press* [Online].
Sheppard, J. (1988, July 24). Two ex-Bucs may have to settle for seconds. *St. Petersburg Times*, p. 8C.
Sheppard, J. (1988, October 26). NFL cracks down on steroid use. *St. Petersburg Times*, p. 1C.
Sherman, J. (1987, December 31). Mira, O'Neill fail in bids for reinstatement. *United Press International* [Online].
Sherman, J. (1988, April 26). Jets' first-round pick briefly used steroids. *United Press International* [Online].
Shipley, A. (1999, September 24). Drugs: A family tradition? *Ottawa Citizen* [Online].
Shurr, M. (1988, October 21). Holderman backs coach, new drug policy. *Columbia State*, p. 1A.
Slater, J. (1987, April 9). Colts expect to sign top draft choice. *United Press International* [Online].
Steelers Knew. (1989, April 25). Steelers knew top draft pick tested positive. *The Associated Press* [Online].
Steroid Secret. (1989, March 15). Canadian sprinters would have kept steroid secret. *The Associated Press* [Online].
Steroids Helped. (1988, October 5). Steroid helped winning for Arizona State. *The Associated Press* [Online].
Students Admit. (1986, April 27). Fort Worth area high school students admit using steroids. *United Press International* [Online].
Sussman, S. (1989, March 2). Johnson's coach said sprinter used steroids. *The Associated Press* [Online].
Sussman, S. (1989, April 2). Canadian inquiry has much ground to cover. *The Associated Press* [Online].
Telander, R. (1988, October 24). A peril for athletes: The author is shaken by a story about steroids. *Sports Illustrated*, p. 114.
Telander, R. (1989). *The hundred yard lie*. New York, NY: Simon and Schuster.
Tennant Trouble. (1986, July 15). Tennant in trouble over loose talk. *United Press International* [Online].
Texas Users. (1990, April 1). 25 Texas players reportedly used steroids since NCAA ban. *The Associated Press* [Online].

Thomas, R.M. (1987, January 19). An awful mystery. *New York Times*, p. C2.

Thompson, L. (1988, September 13). What constitutes an 'unfair' edge? *Washington Post*, p. Z16.

Todd, T. (1987, Spring). Anabolic steroids: The Gremlins of sport. *Journal of Sport History*, p. 87.

Toner's Allegations. (1987, July 3). NCAA official says half of football players use steroids. *The Associated Press* [Online].

Tracking Johnson. (1988, September 29). Schramm: Cowboys would give Johnson tryout. *United Press International* [Online].

Troy, T. (1989, April 3). Athletes call for stern steroid measures. *United Press International* [Online].

Tully, M. (1989, February 9). Sports and drugs. *United Press International* [Online].

Tupper Dislikes. (1988, August 11). Tupper dislikes Bosworth's book. *The Associated Press* [Online].

United States Senate, Committee On The Judiciary. (1989, April 3, May 9). *Steroid abuse problem in America, focusing on the use of steroids in college and professional football today* (Serial No. J-101-12). Washington, D.C.: U.S. Government Printing Office.

USC Player. (1985, May 10). Former USC player says he used steroids in college. *United Press International* [Online].

Use Accepted. (1988, October 2). Drug use accepted practice for world-class athletes. *The Associated Press* [Online].

Utterback, B. (1987, September 2). Battle against steroids picks up steam. *Pittsburgh Press*, p. B1.

Vandy Room. (1985, January 10). Ex-judge, ex-con in Vandy weightroom crowd. *United Press International* [Online].

Voy, R. (1991). *Drugs, sport, and politics*. Champaign, IL: Leisure Press.

Wallace, W.N. (1987, January 1). Golic is strong point for Browns. *New York Times*, p. 1 — 19.

Washburn Remains. (1989, April 19). Washburn remains in job at Purdue. *The Associated Press* [Online].

Wilbon, M. (1988, October 26). NFL plans to act against steroids. *Washington Post*, p. C1.

Wilbon, M. (1989, March 23). Rozelle to retire from NFL. *Washington Post*, p. A1.

Wilson, N. (1989, May 2). Athletics takes its purgative. *The Independent* [Online].

Wilson, A. (1988, July 21). Korte calls for mandatory testing and stiff penalties. *The Associated Press* [Online].

Yaeger, D., & Looney, D.S. (1993). *Under the tarnished dome*. New York, NY: Simon and Schuster.

Zucco, T. (1989, April 11). A body built by steroids. *St. Petersburg Times*, p. 1A.

Chapter 6 [Random Urinalysis]

Doping, policy in football, 1990s

"In general, I think a lot of fans could care less. Football is like a religious experience. People have to have it. If steroids are a part of it, I think people think, Well, that's OK."

Bill Fralic
NFL lineman, 1990

Leaving New York early one morning, I broke for home by car, escaping the great metro as it slept. Flying through Brooklyn's southern outskirts before dawn, the lights of Manhattan distant, I hauled ass on the Shore Parkway, gunning for turnpikes in Jersey and Pennsylvania. And there alone in the darkness, Brooklyn, I had to pause, to think about Lyle Alzado.

Brooklyn was Alzado's home turf, dearly beloved he swore passionately in interviews, though mostly left behind by the time he died in 1992. I shot along the parkway at 70, 80 mph, peeking up shadowy streets and alleys, considering the high-rises and row buildings, homes and businesses modest, cramped, competitive. Brooklyn teemed with football legends, including native icons Lombardi and Paterno, but I was trying to sense something of a gridiron antihero, circa pharmaceutical era, or spirit of the boy who became *Alzado*, jungle physique, nutty athlete, Hollywood wild man, and, finally, tragic symbol for us all.

I was not short on stories to begin; the man was no media star by accident. During a lengthy pro-football career he parlayed into endorsements and acting, Alzado provided storylines constantly, telling good ones at least, often becoming big copy himself. The hulking Alzado talked a lot about Brooklyn, and media devoured, if not wholly bought, his themes of love, hate, toughness, redemption, all set amid this grizzled flatland of lore. "The way I grew up is the way I grew up. That part of it's the truth," Alzado said as a Raider, adding, "I play off it a little bit."

"Alzado was an unbelieveable character in every sense. ...," recalled C.W. Nevius, a San Francisco writer. "It seemed no one knew where the hype ended and the man began." Alzado's street theatre played well in the NFL, where he hyped games with the feigned viciousness of a TV wrestler. Contorting his face into rage, eyes glowering, veins popping, Alzado spewed vile comments about the opponent of the moment, the whipping he would inflict. During Super Bowl week 1984 in Tampa, Alzado berated Washington's massive offensive linemen, reducing them to wimps in his stories, talking how he'd dominate. The attendant cluster of sportswriters scribbled furiously, recording Alzado's pseudo war declarations, and suddenly he lost his poker face, laughing uproariously. "All these outrageous things I say, like no one can kick my butt," he said. "Do you actually believe that?"

Alzado did grow up a scrapping son among six siblings, of a mother abandoned by their father, herself fighting to sustain the family in the notorious Brownsville section of Brooklyn, which later produced the boxer Mike Tyson. Alzado had come up a promising ring fighter too, known around the city, and he likewise employed fists for survival on Brooklyn streets, among weapons. Tyson could relate: "I couldn't understand how a white guy could be from my neighborhood," the heavyweight champ said in 1990, "but then I met him."

Alzado starred in football at Lawrence High on Long Island, growing to 6-foot-3 with good speed, but weighing only 190. College recruiters didn't flock around Alzado, and the teen's only decent scholarship offer fell through because of a growing rap sheet with New York police, he would recount. Next he was rejected by a junior college in Texas and landed in South Dakota, small-time college football at Yankton College. Alzado threw punches at his first practice, brawling with new teammates.

Alzado was a tough young guy, but required chemical aid for his football dream, and he began using Dianabol in 1967 at Yankton — NCAA Division II — a time and place where "no one had ever heard of a steroid," a former teammate would recall. Alzado did not cease anabolics for 24 years, until facing mortality. "He had his mind set on playing professional football, he focused on it, and he accomplished it," Bill Bobzin, Alzado's old coach at Yankton, said in 1992. "He earned everything he achieved." The old teammate, Roger Heirigs said Alzado "definitely bulked up, but he lived in the weight room."

A big, ripped, athletic lineman in pro football, Alzado's laurels included All-Pro, twice, AFC Defensive Player of the Year in 1977 for Denver, and a Super Bowl title with the Raiders in Los Angeles. His overall career, for D-line statistics and winning with three clubs, amounted to borderline Hall of Fame.

For major saleable persona, pop-culture celebrity on and off the field, Alzado played his violent-lunatic shtick to the hilt, not always acting, of course, with dark moods and physical outbursts problematic in his life. Alzado rode the caricature of juiced psycho into TV commercials and poorly scripted movies and shows, but he was gone at age 43, leaving heavy debt and having believed abuse of muscle drugs caused his fatal brain cancer, without clinical evidence and to the rebuke of scientists.

Dying in Oregon, far removed from the glitz and glamour he craved in youth, Alzado was buried in a private ceremony. By then, most football brethren had isolated him too, effectively washing their hands of his admitted, detailed doping to play the game. Formerly close associates from college through the NFL stayed mum about Alzado's abuse — and, for many, their own — and sportswriters readily forgot his allegation of continued widespread doping in football.

Everyone ignored a critical historical fact about Alzado, when he beat the NFL's heralded new "random urinalysis" for steroids in 1990, utilizing undetectable growth hormone under a personal drug guru who had a pharmacist.

My car moved out of Brooklyn, crossing the Verrazano Narrows to Staten Island, and I glanced back northward at Manhattan, the famed bright lights, once seductive for young Alzado, a kid reared across East River without much, beyond a full heaping of willpower. "In my mind and heart, I believe I can do those things," Alzado had remarked of lofty goals. "In my soul, I don't know. It's what I dream. It's what I think. Nobody can take that away from me." Crossing that New York bridge at 40-something myself, past the age of Alzado at death, I was relieved to be in my common car bound for home, Missouri, and wife and children who loved me. I never would have been *Alzado*, but I might have been like him.

"Football is exalted and consumed on a grand scale, apparently without reservation," Gwen Knapp wrote for the San Francisco Examiner in 1997. "But adoring the game doesn't preclude loathing its consequences. The NFL, for those who really know it, should be a guilty pleasure."

"And unlike eating red meat or smoking, the sport doesn't threaten the consumer's health at all. The risks belong entirely to someone else. To someone paid handsomely for absorbing hits, to someone with Reebok and Nike fighting at his feet. ... Lyle Alzado went to his grave prematurely, insisting that steroids had brought on his brain tumor. He played some great football, for himself, for the Raiders, for us. If he thought, in the end, that he had made a bad bargain, what are we to think?"

I. Officials Blame Athletes, Establish Random Testing

For Dick Schultz, NCAA executive director, the shoddiness of steroid testing for policing college athletics was impossible to deny by 1989. "I'm concerned that we might only be catching the dumb ones when it comes to steroids," Schultz said that spring, speaking in South Carolina and promoting random urinalysis to solve muscle doping in football and other collegiate games. "The only way to know for sure is strictly unannounced, unscheduled drug testing."

The NCAA executive director's call for random testing sounded good, coming in conjunction with a hearing in Washington, where Penn State football coach Joe Paterno described a pervasive steroid problem. Schultz talked much about reform of NCAA sports, a return to morality for collegiate games — he had to, in the face of mounting negative publicity for his association, including member schools' blatant mishandlings of young people in areas such as recruiting, academics, and drugs. "We're not minor leagues for the professionals. Our business is education," Schultz said. "We need to have coaches and athletes returned to their proper position as role models."

Coaches took a hit from the NCAA executive director, but the lion's share of blame for NCAA problems fell on young athletes, according to Schultz. The ills would be repaired soon, Schultz promised, though none were really the fault of organizers in charge of college athletes nationwide. The problem, he contended, remained that static isolated minority of athletes who were products of society, not the games they played. "A handful of people can create an image that all of intercollegiate athletics is bad," Schultz said. "We have athletes not graduating. We have athletes who are not bona fide students. We have athletes who were illegally recruited. They are in the minority. Yet, it casts a cloud over everyone. Stressing education, Schultz asserted major schools in particular were "not here for national championships, Rose Bowls and Fiesta Bowls."

Extravagant sport was exactly the consumer's demand of the NCAA, however, and Schultz and Company knew it. They feared their product was tainted for mass marketing by the end of the 1980s. Collegiate sports had "taken a pretty good beating in recent years on the national level," said Tom Osborne, Nebraska football coach, who primarily blamed parties beyond the NCAA, especially media, for sensationalizing problems. The public perceived college sports as "not very wholesome," Osborne said. "There are so many reform movements because of the image college athletics has." Osborne had recently downplayed allegations and questions raised by an exposé book on his program, *Big Red Confidential: Inside Nebraska Football*, by Armen Keteyian. The book contained significant steroid allegations involving several players of the 1980s, including stars, but Osborne denied widespread use for his Cornhuskers and college football in general.

A former coaching rival differed from Osborne's outlook. "Everybody's taking [steroids]," said Barry Switzer, who had resigned at OU over NCAA violations. "Oklahoma, Nebraska for years did it. No one thought anything about it. ... [N]o one was getting hurt." Switzer believed street narcotics to be dangerous, not muscle hormones. "You're not robbing 7-11s, you're not murdering someone to get steroids," he said.

Differing with the ex-coach, many NCAA officials and delegates thought steroids to be harmful, at least for product image, and they addressed the issue once again at the 1990 national convention in Dallas, where "random, year-round testing" was approved for football players in Division I. The NCAA earmarked $1.6 million for the new policy, cost easily covered by the association's billion-dollar entertainment monopoly in football and men's basketball.

The measure's PR finish was smooth, but actually the NCAA would screen less than half of D-I football players for steroids and not year-round, just during August camps and the academic year. Any athlete testing positive would face harsher penalties, which officials claimed would prove a strong deterrent. "The punishment must be more persuasive than it has been," said Ed Bozik, University of Pittsburgh athletic director, who a few years previous touted steroid testing and education as effective deterrents, in a period when Pitt linemen tested positive as pro picks.

Meanwhile, in the NFL, new commissioner Paul Tagliabue was attacking the administrative mess left by Rozelle, including ongoing court cases, hostilities among owners, standoff with labor, and a variety of outdated policy. Tagliabue, a youthful former college athlete and NFL lawyer of 20 years, was intent on unifying league factions for moving forward as one.

The steroid issue was an immediate priority for Tagliabue, controversy needing to be quelled, but it would be handled his way. The schmooze tactics of Rozelle were over in this office, of little use for attorney Tagliabue in heading the modern NFL. Vast power and huge money were the stakes, and more tact was essential. Court litigation had buried Rozelle, exposed his inadequacies, but Tagliabue was prime for his job in that swamp.

Tagliabue's approach to steroids, capitalizing on the public drumbeat for random testing, would mend the NFL image bruised for the lack of a firm drug policy, one agreed upon by management and the players union. A critical result of the new policy would be league control of information, thanks to Tags' entreating Upshaw and the union to join him on the steroids issue, rather than oppose. No longer would the outflow of information regularly fuel steroid headlines about the NFL, as was the case of Rozelle's latter tenure.

The release of inside information on steroids did continue into Tagliabue's reign. Athletes and coaches still courted trouble in interviews, playing dumb about the problem or crying "injury rehab" when exposed by testing, and league drug advisor Dr. Forest Tennant remained too loose in his comments on steroids. But negative press about muscle doping in the NFL narrowed quickly under Tagliabue, who worked toward establishing random urinalysis while enjoying public support. Joe Biden, Washington's foremost politician working the issue of doping in sport, declared for Tagliabue that steroids "simply won't be tolerated" anymore by NFL management. Fans overwhelmingly blamed players, not the league, and virtually every sportswriter was ready to move on and enjoy the games, to focus again on the goodness of the NFL spectacle.

Most importantly, the league was growing into the highest-valued content in sports entertainment, and the media were realizing high revenues in business synergy with the product. Close ties with the NFL and Tagliabue were to be treasured by the rich and powerful of America, especially the power brokers of television, radio, newspapers, and magazines.

In March 1990, Tagliabue saw to the "resignation" of Tennant, then he made his big move for hearings in Washington, introducing his so-called random urinalysis, featuring terms such as computerized selection and "year-round" testing. Steroid use in pro football, Tagliabue said, created competitive pressure, threatened players' health, and posed dangerous examples for kids. "We do a grave disservice to our young people if we fail to move aggressively," Tagliabue, former D.C. lawyer, testified before a congressional subcommittee involved in adding anabolic steroids to the Controlled Substances Act. "We do not want to encourage young athletes, still in their formative years... to emulate professional athletes by using steroids to increase their size and strength." Tagliabue expressed confidence he would eradicate steroids in the NFL, without producing any hard evidence in support, then basked in public applause.

And that was that, seemingly. Random urinalysis was widely accepted as the end for steroids in American football; both the NFL and the NCAA enjoyed immediate returns with fans and the media, for new policies on tissue-building dope; and equally significant, each organization asserted control of drug information, ranging from rules enforcement to public relations.

News about football was sounding good for the 1990s. A bandwagon swell of optimism, fervent enthusiasm, was building for America's thrilling blood sport of choice — including media conglomerates who shelled out billions to Tagliabue for TV rights to the NFL, along with paying exorbitant fees to the NCAA.

Football was fashionable like never before in the culture. Women joined men as fervent, spending fans, and a new wave of stadium construction was in progress.

Billions in public funds helped erect palatial facilities coast-to-coast, in turn yanking up gate and luxury-box receipts for private football enterprise.

The product could not be swiped completely of doping's taint, however. Not as incidents continued nationwide, including players and coaches caught with and talking about muscle substances, steroids and growth hormone. Nothing would change, reminded critics such as Steve Courson, until the entire culture resolved to fight the problem. "We, as a society, as long as we base the hiring and firing of coaches on winning and losing, are not part of the solution. We are part of the problem," Courson said in a speech to athletes at Furman University. "We, as a society, do not want to accept what elements of our sports world do on Saturdays and Sundays for us to be entertained."

Courson labeled the NFL steroid policy "a sad joke," declaring urinalysis was no solution. "Anyone who believes that the 13 positive tests [in 1989] are an indication of the size of the anabolic steroid dilemma in pro football still believes in the tooth fairy," he said. "No athlete can be honest about their drug use without committing career suicide. They have to maintain the conspiracy of silence."

NCAA and Colleges Stake Moral Ground, But Juicing Continues

Never failing to humor America was the satire of college football, hilarious storylines of blatant corruption casting dumb-ass jocks as essential characters, masquerading as students. Comedians capitalized on this basic football theme for generations, including the Marx Brothers in *Horse Feathers*, their riotous film classic of 1932.

College officials, meanwhile, thought the gags were getting old by end of the 1980s, as real-life misdeeds in NCAA football and other sports were beyond preposterous. College officials opened the 1990s posturing about cleaning up the mess, once and for all, and they spoke "reform" with the frequency of a chant. The concerted NCAA response was due largely to critics increasing in number and variety. Academics, students, athletes, journalists, lawmakers, and sports fans voiced complaints, as did advocates for women's rights, minorities, and crime victims, among groups and individuals.

"I discovered that people with very different interests and views of intercollegiate athletics could wear a ['Smash the NCAA'] button with sincerity," wrote Edward G. Lawry, a professor of philosophy and former college athlete, commenting for the *Chronicle of Higher Education*. Lawry, an Oklahoma State faculty member who lightheartedly produced and distributed a few of the buttons, soberly dismissed NCAA reform, labeling it impossible given the association's inherent scheme of combining education and amateurism with the pursuit of lavish financial incomes.

Tennis great and sports activist Arthur Ashe blasted the college reform movement as failing young athletes. "To me, most of the NCAA's actions show that it would rather tinker with the real problems than tackle them," Ashe commented for the *Washington Post*.

On the issue of performance-enhancing substances, enthusiastic NCAA officials touted new random testing, but experts Dr. Charles Yesalis and Dr. R. Craig Kammerer shot down urinalysis in a co-commentary for the *New York Times*. "There is no guarantee that tests will be administered or reported properly, and even if they are, it has been proven that testing cannot catch all substance abusers," Yesalis and Kammerer wrote, listing types of muscle dope for avoiding detection. "In summary, the principal problem of drug testing in sport is predominantly one of false negatives. Many users of performance-enhancing drugs appear to have continually bested the testing process; it does not appear that this will change in the near future."

A panel of three college athletes, speaking for their under-represented peers, discussed drugs with the NCAA Presidents Commission. The athletes saw pervasive forces as systematic and societal, and they sought effective prevention for drug use they described as "everywhere" in the sport-academic environment.

Brendan Kinney, a free-lance writer and former college football player, discussed reality's trumping morality in his sport, for *The Times*. "The obsession with success on the field is common and accepted by all who play," Kinney wrote. "Also accepted, and just as common, are the various means of obtaining success, including steroids." Kinney was a Cornell recruit, briefly, before injuries halted his playing career. "The players are made to achieve an awesome physical condition. Bigger, stronger, faster, are the watchwords. ... I have never been explicitly pushed by a coach or a doctor, but the pressure of keeping up with the competition was always there."

Yet NCAA officials maintained that steroid use remained isolated in their football, for three decades running. In legal parlance, their stance meant no acknowledgement of environmental influences for steroids, and therefore no potential liability. The minimizing or denial of institutional culpability about steroids was evident in the NCAA's first investigation involving the drugs at a member school, South Carolina, where the Committee on Infractions wrapped up the Enforcement Division's probe by concluding no major violations occurred in Gamecocks football — despite the criminal convictions of coaches determined to have encouraged use and purchased the drugs for players. Stark truth had even forced the university to reverse field: Administrators initially denied Tommy Chaikin's allegations but later had to confirm the basis of his story, admitting "widespread experimentation" by football players under the direction of coaches from 1983 to 1987.

In July 1990, the NCAA Committee on Infractions announced only minor violations had occurred in Gamecocks football, stunning sportswriters close to the case. "Really, for the life of me, I can't figure it out," said Rick Telander, co-author of Chaikin's account for *Sports Illustrated*. "It doesn't matter that a player almost died? That three coaches urged players to use illegal drugs? If that doesn't merit some kind of public embarrassment [for the university], it's hard to say what big-time college football is all about. ... Now the table is set for this to happen all over again."

By this time, Telander had resigned his job covering college football for *SI* and had written a book damning the NCAA system, accusing it of "child abuse." A former college football player, Telander was weary of watching schools wriggle off the hook in scandal after scandal. "Who screwed up here?" Telander asked rhetorically of the South Carolina situation, in an interview with *The State* newspaper of Columbia. "Do you point the finger at nobody? Clearly the coaches were wrong, but whose bidding were they doing? Is this again an indictment of a system that is out of control? Maybe that is the case; the whole ball of wax is out of control."

It appeared that way with muscle doping, among the ills of NCAA football. By the early 1990s, college players were huge and getting larger, and many universities were hit by steroid evidence or allegations, including Washington State, San Jose State, Texas, Northwestern, Michigan State, and Notre Dame. Everywhere, of course, coaches and school officials absolved themselves before the media, denying any responsibility.

Washington State football coach Mike Price said his staff was unaware of steroid use on their team, until several players tested positive in the NCAA's random urinalysis. Some players had made enormous weight gains in short periods, including a veteran lineman who added 30 pounds during one spring, but coaches were oblivious, according to Price. "We're doing everything we can to curtail steroid use at Washington State," he said. "We talk to our players monthly."

The use of steroids and amphetamines by football players at San Jose State led to the firing of coach Claude Gilbert, but no higher-ups were held responsible, among administrators associated with the program.

Prestigious Northwestern University, the small private school near Chicago and Telander's alma mater, was hardly immune to steroid controversy. Trying as it was to compete in Big Ten football, former defensive lineman George Harouvis alleged Northwestern had a majority of players who used anabolics at least once during his two years in the program, and many beat urinalysis tests. Athletic director Bruce Corrie acknowledged problems existed with urinalysis for steroids, despite his department's unannounced testing. However, a two-month, in-house investigation turned up only "isolated" use, and "experimentation," on the football team, according to officials. University president Arnold R. Weber issued a press release, reading in part: "While we cannot rule out the possibility that there might have been an individual player or players who experimented with steroids [in high school or at Northwestern], there is no evidence that there was or is widespread steroid use by members of the football team or systematic efforts to evade drug testing, as was alleged."

Another university taking itself seriously, Notre Dame, was jolted by steroid shenanigans around Fighting Irish football. The Notre Dame program enjoyed near-mythical status again, having won a national championship under Coach Lou Holtz, and the university had scored an unprecedented independent TV deal worth $37 million, selling game rights for five years to NBC. Then former offensive lineman Steve Huffman emerged a spoiler during the 1990 preseason, alleging steroids were widespread during his time at Notre Dame and Holtz "had to have known," for an *SI* story co-written by Telander.

Huffman wrote he did not use steroids and was criticized for lack of strength — he could bench-press only 300 pounds while Notre Dame coaches demanded 400 — and he charged that two assistants "suggested" steroids for him. Huffman, a Texas native whose brothers included linemen in college and the NFL, said about half the Irish team's lettermen used steroids at least once, with the highest rate among linemen. Huffman said he was acquainted with steroid dealers on the team, having seen quantities of pills and liquids in players' rooms, along with used needles. Motive for the story was "a rebuttal" to Holtz, Huffman said, after the coach had branded him a "quitter" in a book about the 1988 championship season. Huffman was paid $5,000 by the magazine.

The response was public lashings of Huffman by Holtz, Irish players, and Notre Dame officials. Again he was labeled a quitter, but now guilty of sour grapes. "I unequivocally deny Steve Huffman's allegations," Holtz said. "I think I have done everything I possibly can to deter the use of street drugs and steroids." Players and team physician Dr. James Moriarity acknowledged only isolated use on the team. "Tests indicate Notre Dame does not have blatant steroid problems," Moriarity said. "There's no question our athletes know our feelings on steroids. We don't tolerate them."

Outside Notre Dame, Holtz gained the support of Nebraska coach Tom Osborne, who could be counted upon to rebuke a college player alleging systemic steroids at any school. "Many of us in athletics are fairly defenseless against certain types of things where the sources are unnamed, or the person has a built-in bias," Osborne said from Lincoln. "You get into a defensive posture and, no matter what you say, you're presumed guilty."

Another veteran coach, Joe Paterno at Penn State, expressed hope that *Sports Illustrated* was acting responsibly with Huffman's story, but he would not quickly dismiss the allegations. "I think we still have a big problem with steroids," Paterno said of college football and society. "I could not tell you we don't have anybody [at PSU] who has used steroids." Paterno said some assistant coaches in college football likely encouraged players to use steroids, and he griped about other schools' refusal to sign steroid-testing pacts before playing Penn State — Notre Dame, for example, had ignored such a request from PSU the previous season. "It worries me a little bit, but you have to go on the assumption that people are testing on their own and acting in good faith," Paterno said. "But then you hear about somebody going to the NFL and testing positive for steroids, and you wonder what's going on."

The public had not heard the last about steroids under Holtz in South Bend, a topic destined to resurface in the near future.

At the University of Texas, meanwhile, officials downplayed steroid headlines cropping up around Longhorns football. Trouble began in spring 1990, when the *Austin American-Statesman* reported 25 Texas players had used steroids since testing began in 1986. The newspaper cited several players as sources, most unnamed, saying the team included steroid dealers and urinalysis could be circumvented. University officials immediately discounted allegations, saying any use was isolated and no internal investigation would be conducted. Officials lauded their in-house, random urinalysis for steroids, declaring just four male athletes had tested positive in four years. "These results demonstrate that the university has been successful in deterring drug use by athletes," said Edwin Sharpe, UT vice president for administration. "We are proud of our record, especially when you consider that we are living in a drug-prone society."

Texas football players continued with steroids or related substances. Six months after the *American-Statesman* story, police found a vial of epitestosterone in the vehicle of a Longhorns lineman. The chemical was not illegal, but doctors and NCAA officials said it was commonly employed to mask traces of anabolic steroids and to boost testosterone levels. Doping expert Dr. William Taylor said epitestosterone could be injected one hour before urinalysis and the athlete would pass. Frank Uryasz, NCAA director of sports sciences, said, "Athletes are very savvy, and this is just another example of it. We're always faced with the problem that athletes know what to use and when to use it." The athlete and his lawyer claimed the chemical was a painkiller for an injured shoulder, but experts said it was useless in that capacity. Texas athletic director DeLoss Dodds, pleading ignorance of epitestosterone on the part of the school administration, said he might investigate if the NCAA provided more information about the chemical.

Steroid abuse apparently remained problematic in Longhorns football, at least through the 1990 season, according to *The Dallas Morning News*, when as many as 25 players used despite random urinalysis by three bodies in the school, the Southwest Conference and the NCAA. Newspapers, citing unnamed sources, hand-writing experts, and a player's arrest record, reported steroid dealings continued on the team, including sales of forged prescriptions, and at least two star linemen were known users. Athletic director Dodds threatened action against certain players, but, again, school officials made no plans for a comprehensive investigation.

Michigan State officials had little choice but to review their football program for steroids, after media speculation blew up around mammoth offensive tackle Tony Mandarich, who added as much as 50 pounds of mass at the school. By spring 1989, Mandarich had repeatedly denied steroid use — and passed drug tests — when he appeared on an *SI* cover shockingly buff at 6-6, 315 pounds, clad only in shorts, sneakers, and a ball cap. Mandarich ran 40 yards in 4.65 seconds, broad-jumped 10 feet, and bench-pressed 225 upwards of 40 reps — his max reportedly was 600 — thrilling NFL scouts who labeled him the greatest O-line prospect in history. *Sports Illustrated* headlined the balding 22-year-old as "THE INCREDIBLE BULK." Telander, assigned to the story, called him "a creature."

Rebuking steroid accusations was George Perles, Michigan State football head coach, who denied Mandarich was a user. The coach attributed the player's leaps of size and strength to increased lifting and eating. Perles, a former Steelers assistant, also evoked the explanation of genetic wonder, telling media that Mandarich weighed 13 pounds at birth in Canada. "This is a different player," Perles told a skeptical Telander. "We'll never see another." The Packers picked Mandarich second overall in the 1989 NFL draft, behind only UCLA quarterback Troy Aikman, chosen first by the Cowboys, and, after a highly publicized holdout, Mandarich signed the richest deal ever for a lineman, $4.4 million over four years.

Steroid suspicion clung to Mandarich, however, and in March 1990 the *Detroit News* quoted former college teammates alleging he had not only been a user at MSU but a supplier on the team. Mandarich was part of a larger probe by *The News* into rumors of steroids in Spartans football under Perles. "The newspaper... found widespread steroid use during the 1987 season and that the problem, while it may have abated, is by no means gone," reported *United Press International.* Several Spartans beat steroid testing by both MSU and the NCAA, players alleged. The newspaper reported players injected each other with steroids, regularly discussed the drugs, and shared an underground pamphlet detailing chemical combinations for maximum potency.

Perles caught heat from Gary Hostetler, father of a player who transferred from MSU. Hostetler charged that Perles made unreasonable strength demands of players and failed to prevent steroid abuse in the program. Hostetler, a police officer in Ohio who played pro football in Canada, said he once called Perles because his son, Lance, was struggling to get playing time at offensive center. "George says, 'Well, he can't even bench-press 400 pounds,'" Hostetler told *The News.* "I said, 'Do you know how hard that is?' He [Perles] said, 'We have 13 or 14 players who can bench-press 400.' I said, 'He can play football.' George said, 'Not 'til he's stronger.'"

Michigan State officials immediately denied the accusations, declaring they had no knowledge of widespread steroid use in football or any other sport on campus. University spokesman Terry Denbow said the accuracy of such allegation was "highly unlikely," and he blamed individual athletes for "a few isolated specifics." Dr. David Hough, sport medicine director, said the school had determined only a handful of athletes used steroids, through testing and "reasonable cause" methods such as observing behavior changes or personal problems. "We can pick them out — we're getting better at it," Hough said. "The numbers are not that large."

Perles categorically denied knowing of use on his football team. "No. No," he said. "I'm honest, I answer them all honestly. N-O, no, underlined, period. Truth." Perles, stressing players' health to be his foremost concern, acknowledged that a college coach whose job depended on winning could look the other way from steroids. "It might be tempting," he said. "I hope to God it's not on my conscience or any of the other coaches in [the Big Ten]. I don't think it would happen in our conference."

Denbow said an MSU coach found to be ignoring steroid use would be fired. The university opened an internal investigation of its steroid testing and oversight, headed by athletics administrator Robert Wilkinson, who promised "a fair and thorough review." Wilkinson also said MSU officials essentially dismissed, already, the notion of a systematic problem in the football program. "Some recent media accounts, it is clear, have raised in the minds of some the possibility of 'widespread steroid use,'" Wilkinson stated. "As we have said, there are allegations afoot that we feel encourage inappropriate generalizations based on a few isolated specifics." Perles said any problem rested with media who disliked him personally, and Mandarich emerged after a couple weeks to deny the latest allegations against him.

Eight months later, Michigan State announced its probe uncovered no evidence of widespread doping. "We know that there is some steroid use, but it is very, very small," said James Studer, assistant vice president for student affairs. "We're very confident that MSU has a low usage. It's not anywhere near the national average."

NFL Tagliabue Battles Distasteful Doping Image

Paul Tagliabue's NFL program of random analysis for steroids sputtered ahead during the spring of 1990, in the face of continued doping and allegations involving the league. Dr. Forest Tennant was on the loose, making media rounds to allege widespread doping following his hasty departure from Tagliabue's new NFL. In Pittsburgh, the Steelers once again drafted a prospect who had already tested positive, third-rounder Craig Veasey of Houston, and coach Chuck Noll parroted his excuse from Ricketts' case the previous year, claiming Veasey had used the drug merely for injury rehabilitation. "It wasn't a long-term thing," Noll explained. "It was a mistake. I'm satisfied with [Veasey's] story." Noll referred to a Steelers policy of intolerance for hard-core users, however broadly defined, and sportswriters did not press the coaching legend for specifics.

Elsewhere, the league image got scraped in Tampa, with Tagliabue's testing freshly in place, where police arrested Bucs lineman Carl Bax in a fast-food parking lot for acquiring hundreds of steroid tablets from an undercover detective. Bax's coach, Ray Perkins, was not worried. "I see it as somebody making a mistake, and we all make mistakes," Perkins said. "I believe Carl when he says he never put a steroid in his mouth or has never used steroids."

The press reported the items once, generally, then overlooked them, allowing each to flicker out. Indeed, this was a burgeoning era for decidedly upbeat football coverage, even for the American media, and the NFL and Tagliabue were becoming darlings for writers. A popular pack theme, rehashed in stories across America, was the smashing success for new commissioner Tagliabue. In succeeding the frazzled Rozelle, "Tags" was acclaimed as progressive, decisive, shrewd, visionary, especially for his instituting of random urinalysis. Tagliabue talked up his steroid policy, impressing people with phrases like "computerized selection," and he latched onto Bill Fralic, the notable All-Pro against steroids in the league, to tell media this young athlete's aims were his own. The policy packaging was dressed up in every possible way under Tags, such as a new title for Tennant's successor, Dr. John A. Lombardo, who was presented as the NFL's "first steroid advisor," relegating Tennant obsolete as the former "drug advisor."

Tagliabue made the highest promise — eradicating steroids from the NFL — while speaking during Lombardo's unveiling. Whenever a rare reporter suggested systematic pressure for a player's using, Tags employed classic pass-the-buck rationale, deflecting blame downward to college and prep football, where he said the problem was reportedly "extensive." The commissioner conceded any use was cancerous, bound to affect other players, if not drive them to doping. "The pressure is great if some players use, for all players to use," Tagliabue said. "The side effects concern us. The combination of medical effects, risks, and competitive problems led us to strengthen the testing program. We recognize there will be efforts to mask use. We think we can deal with that."

Muscle doping continued bedeviling the NFL under Tagliabue, however, during the commissioner's honeymoon period with the media. Random urinalysis hardly stopped muscle doping; the use of growth hormone was "epidemic" for preseason testing 1990, Raiders doctor Rob Huizenga would later report, and more evasion tactics were available to players, like low-level testosterone. Tags' drug policy would wobble in public for a few years, through events that threatened its perceived credibility.

The year 1991 brought the NFL a dose of doping criticism, inspired by the Alzado furor, the attempted suicide of an active player who tested positive for steroids, and a track-and-field star's wooing by football scouts — despite his steroid past. Public-relations trouble brewed that spring, when NFL teams could not resist sniffing around Randy Barnes, the 300-pound shot putter suspended from world track and field over testing positive for a steroid. Tryouts were offered Barnes, and the 24-year-old displayed requisite talent on paper — athleticism, power, bulk — though he had not played football since high school. The 49ers signed him to a free-agent contract as a defensive lineman.

Critics piped up at the NFL about Barnes, steroid hypocrisy, then a major headliner struck: Lyle Alzado cranked up the debate, suddenly revealing his cancer and decades of muscle doping. In the final days of June, Alzado opened a blockbuster media tour, his visage and words blaring across television, newspapers, and magazines. Gravely ill, Alzado was alarming in appearance and compelling in story. He moved about slowly, unsurely, having dropped about 60 pounds from a rippling 280 to gaunt and bony. At 42 Alzado was sickly in the face, rapidly aged, wearing bandannas to cover a head shorn bald after chemotherapy left his hair falling out in clumps. The former football star spoke about his steroid abuse, the winning, fame, money, and now inoperable brain cancer, life experiences he believed linked one to another.

Alzado declared he sought neither vengeance nor attention, only the chance to testify publicly of drug evils he had lived, especially for children's sake. A friend, Dr. Huizenga, believed him. "Lyle had been off steroids for three months," Huizenga would write. "No more tantrums. No more out-of-control fits. He was turning into a nice guy."

"My dreams are different now than they once were. ...," the stricken Alzado told Maria Shriver on NBC, in prime time. "It's just a workingman's dream. To work, to have a nice car, a nice house. You know, to live decently. To treat people decently."

"To live," Shriver said.

"Yeah," Alzado replied. "To live is more important than anything."

The Wednesday afternoon of July 3, 1991, millions saw Alzado on ESPN, the "Up Close" interview show hosted by Roy Firestone. "How tough is it...," Firestone began gently, "to talk publicly?"

Alzado let out a sigh, new bride Kathy at his side. "Well... It's, it's a little frightening," Alzado answered, Brooklyn accent. "I don't know, wanta... I don't wanta indict anybody. I just don't know how quite this sounds... I don't want anybody to be hurt by it anymore. Either I'm dying, or something [is] obviously, obviously, very wrong with me. I don't want anybody to haveta go through what I'm going through. If I had to make the decision to be part of pro football for 16 years, if I had to... take the steroids that I took, the growth hormone for my comeback, and all the other stuff that I did — I wouldn't give up my life for it."

"And I don't think that the kids that walk on the beach that are built by steroids, the athletes that compete in pro football, pro basketball, pro baseball — I don't think that they should have to make the choice... I'm not doing this for my own benefit. I'm doing this for the benefit of all my friends, all of the people I played with."

As Alzado's interview aired on ESPN, his face adorned the cover of *Sports Illustrated*, with the caption 'I LIED,' in reference to his years of denying or evading the fact he abused muscle substances. He remembered virtually no steroid talk around the Denver locker room in the 1970s, playing for the Broncos, but by the end of the decade at Cleveland, Alzado was referring dealers to inquiring teammates on the Browns. After his trade to Oakland in 1982, Alzado understood the problem was wide open, pervading the league. "A lot of the guys on the Raiders asked me about steroids," he stated in *SI*, "and I'd help them get what they needed. A lot had their own sources."

Alzado criticized NFL testing — "I passed with flying colors" — and charged that football coaches and officials really avoided steroids. "Did the Raiders coaches know I was taking stuff no matter what the test said?" he posed. "It was just like it was when I was playing with the Broncos and Browns. I think the coaches knew guys were built certain ways, and they knew those guys couldn't look the way they did without taking stuff. But the coaches just coached and looked the other way."

While most press focused on Alzado's disputed contention the drugs caused his cancer, he also alleged steroids and growth hormone were widespread in football, that a large majority of NFL players were users. "Almost everyone I know. They are so intent on being successful that they're not concerned with anything else. ...," he wrote in *SI*. "Ninety percent of the athletes I know are on the stuff. We're not born to be 280 or 300 pounds or jump 30 feet. Some people are born that way, but not many, and there are some 1,400 guys in the NFL."

Alzado's claims drew support from Dr. Tennant, former league drug advisor. "With the levels of anabolic steroids that some of these guys are taking, I do not see how some of these fellows will not develop cancer," Tennant said, without proof. "Alzado is not the first steroids user to develop cancer. He's just the first famous person. He's a signal. He's going to be the first in a long line of these people with cancer."

Football's muscle-doping debate was officially renewed, hot as ever, with essential questions summed up by Robert Lipsyte of the *New York Times*: "Is Alzado, who admits to having lied in public for years about his drug use, telling the whole truth now? Is the NFL finally sincere in its anti-drug posture? Are steroids really a great risk? Why shouldn't athletes have the right to go beyond healing medicines and expensive machinery to enhance their performance?"

Tagliabue declined comment, but his spokesman Greg Aiello defended NFL policy as effective for eradicating steroids. "The fact that we have random testing year around is clearly indicative of the position of the league and the owners in the league," Aiello told *The Times*. "We want steroids out of the league." Dr. John Lombardo, Tennant's replacement as NFL drug advisor, said random urinalysis would eventually stop steroids. "Are there going to be people who beat these tests? Probably," Lombardo said. "But we're in for the long haul. When you're not testing at all there is a green light to take whatever you want. Testing at least closes some windows. And when the windows begin to close, soon no windows will be open at all." Lombardo said he had reports that NFL players presently were "getting smaller."

Jim Finks, New Orleans GM, declared an early end to the war, that anabolic steroids were already wiped out by testing. "Zip," Finks replied to the question of use. "And I don't think I'm being naïve."

In Washington, Redskins coach Joe Gibbs agreed, saying the steroid problem was "over with, as long as we keep testing." Redskins defensive lineman Eric Williams said steroid use in the NFL was just a fad, although once widespread as Alzado described. "I tell you it's non-existent now," Williams attested. "The hip thing now is to be clean." Former Redskins lineman Dexter Manley said steroids were "sort of a common thing" of the NFL in the previous decade, including on Gibbs' teams, but he thought random urinalysis was cutting the problem now.

Reporters pursued comment from Howie Long and other Raiders, former teammates of Alzado in Oakland. "Collectively, the players' concern is for Alzado. ..," Michael Martinez reported for the *New York Times*. "Individually, they insist they have no knowledge of teammates using steroids." Long, the All-Pro defensive end, was defiant of any suspicion about the Raiders. "This is one of the most natural teams in the NFL," he said. "And I'll tell you why: Because [owner] Al Davis always drafts the biggest guys in the league." Long, on-record for years as denying personal steroid use, said of Alzado, "I don't think his intent was necessarily to drag down the Raiders, Browns or Broncos. I think Lyle, in his heart of hearts, is trying to prevent someone else from doing what he did. I'll tell you this, too: People here aren't sitting around talking about steroids."

Linebacker Jerry Robinson shrugged off the steroid spotlight's glare on his team, deeming it more excessive attention based on reputation. "People always think there's a black cloud hanging over the Raiders... People associate us with badness. ...," Robinson said. "Same thing with steroids. Steroid use has been around a long time, but now,

because a former member of our team admitted to using them... it might get associated with our team."

Former Raiders coach Tom Flores confirmed he knew Alzado used steroids at Oakland in the early 1980s. "The extent of it, however, I didn't know," Flores, the Seahawks president, told the *Seattle Times*. "You knew he was, because the doctors informed me. Lyle and I never really got into it in any depth, because the doctors had done that. ... If I had known the extent, which none of us did, I would have sat on him a lot harder." Flores recalled he once confronted Alzado at Oakland. "He was self-injecting [steroids]," Flores said. "I did grab him once and told him that he was being very blatant about it. I told him he should back off. ... I look back at that now and wonder what could you have done? You can't baby-sit them. You can't take them by the hand. Back then we didn't know exactly what the dangers were. We were all very naïve."

Officials did not want to know, according to Tennant, NFL drug advisor from 1986 to 1990. "To even suggest that anabolic steroids were a problem, you were condemned," the doctor said. "They even went so far to say the athletes had a right to take steroids."

Former Cowboys strength coach Bob Ward, like Tennant, believed steroids remained beyond control for the league. Ward had left the Dallas franchise in 1990, around the release of Skip Bayless's book *God's Coach*, which contained information of steroid use by Ward and some Cowboys under former coach Tom Landry. "I'd be a fool to say steroids weren't being used by the Cowboys when I was there," Ward said. "That's all I want to really say about it. But I think basically we still have a major problem around the league."

Other football insiders discussed steroids during the Alzado controversy of July 1991, a handful of players both active and retired.

Eagles lineman Bruce Collie revealed he used in college at Texas-Arlington and later as member of San Francisco's Super Bowl teams, 1989 and 1990. "It was a way to get bigger and stronger and do it fast," said Collie, 6-6, 275 pounds. "I passed all the urine tests and I never had a problem with it, controlling it. Fortunately, I got off them before it became a problem."

The *Atlanta Journal and Constitution* surveyed 20 Falcons veterans about Alzado and steroids. The Falcons were known for having users in the past, at least, following headlined confessionals by Fralic and former lineman Joe Pellegrini. "At some point, most of us in the game face that steroids crossroads," Atlanta lineman Chris Hinton told sportswriter Len Pasquarelli. "But Alzado crossed the road and never came back." Lineman John Scully noted NFL users were measuring their intake versus Alzado's 20-plus years of abuse, as a way of justifying their own. "Personally, I don't think it's going to have a big effect on current users," Scully said. "You have to figure that a person using steroids lives his life by rationalization anyway." Nose tackle Tony Casillas, who had admitted use as a college player for Oklahoma, wanted to see more medical research, and defensive end Mike Gann, who grew up an Alzado fan in Colorado, said he had not realized the lengthy history of steroids in the NFL.

Fralic, meanwhile, no longer had faith in random testing for eliminating muscle doping from the NFL. "I still know people who are doing it," Fralic said, "and I don't know of any way to keep them from doing it."

Retired Raiders cornerback Lester Hayes, a former teammate of Alzado, believed performance pressures of the NFL would ensure drugs' longevity in the environment. He said he first noticed steroids' pervasiveness in the early 1980s. "There were a few cornerbacks involved," said Hayes, who denied using, "but most of the guys who eventually became T-1000 terminators were offensive and defensive linemen, tight ends, and linebackers. ... [Y]ou'd realize that what you're seeing isn't a gift from God but a gift from Satan. When these guys get around 40, that's when steroids start to rock their worlds. It seems like every year I see another offensive or defensive lineman that I know who is in his late 30s or early 40s who doesn't have much time remaining on God's green earth."

As Hayes made his comments, NFL player Terry Long was struggling to maintain his life at age 32, and steroids underscored his anguish. Long, a short but massive offensive guard for the Steelers, had become the only player to test positive during 1991 training camps. Upon learning of the result, he twice attempted suicide at his Pittsburgh home and was hospitalized. Terry Long refocused steroid attention on the Steelers and coach Chuck Noll, but no one with the franchise nor the NFL was saying much about the case. The 5-11 Long, known for prodigious strength, had gone from 160 pounds in high school to 280 with the Steelers.

Noll declined comment about Long specifically, reportedly "citing concerns over privacy." Noll and assistant coach Joe Greene contended that teams and the league were doing their best at policing steroids, but the problem boiled down to individuals. "You can't do any more," Noll said. "You're handicapped by legality, by laws, by unions, by everything else. All you can do is instruct, but it's up to the individual." Greene, a former Steelers All-Pro lineman, said, "These are grown men. They make this choice of their own volition."

Alzado and Long elevated media criticism of the NFL to a peak for steroids, but at least one sportswriter, fresh on the national scene, was willing to blame players entirely for the problem. Peter King represented the new breed of football writer for *Sports Illustrated*, corporately owned and moving toward marketing relationships with NFL Tagliabue. In-depth steroid exposés or analyses focusing on football were shelved for this magazine, and King took the lead on Alzado and Long, ripping them in a short commentary titled "One More Lesson."

King questioned why anyone would use steroids in the contemporary NFL. "Long's sad story again demonstrates the irrational nature of the steroid abuser," King wrote. "Even had he lost his job to [rookie Carlton] Haselrig, there was still a place for him in the NFL." Relying on Coach Greene's word, or questionable science, King charged that "with the volumes of information now available about the dangers of steroids... Long had no excuses for using the drugs."

A few weeks later, Tagliabue finally addressed Alzado's claims of health risks and widespread use of steroids. The commissioner said the allegations troubled him because of the former player's condition and because systematic pressures were part of the past, "behind us in the National Football League." Tagliabue said now random urinalysis was reducing steroid use.

A testing expert disagreed, contending the NFL program was only increasing the number of false-negative results, or instances of users beating urinalysis. "If I wanted, I could have every NFL player up to his eyeballs in steroids and the league would not catch one of them," said Dr. Mauro DiPasquale, an author on doping in sport who had introduced urinalysis to power-lifting.

Moreover, a large majority of the 506 NFL retirees polled by a newspaper, 77 percent, qualified steroids as still a serious problem for the league. "The coaches and management don't [directly] endorse it; they just kind of turn their heads," said Mike Raines, 40, who played defensive tackle in the NFL, USFL, and CFL. "Anything that enables a guy to perform better or at all, they condone. That goes for any pain medication, any anti-inflammatories, to steroids.

"Whether a guy can play in the NFL is based on how fast he runs the 40, his vertical jump and bench press. Believe it or not, that weighs heavily on whether a guy makes the team, gets a tryout, is drafted high or low. It's ridiculous."

An anonymous ex-Steelers lineman was quoted in the poll conducted by *The Atlanta Journal and Constitution*. "I'd like to see the game played by guys that are [natural], but the league is going to have to put a lot more bite in their policy," he said. "They're trying to tickle the ears of fans: 'Hey, we're trying to get this straightened out. We suspended this guy and that guy.' The players association, too, is going to protect the players."

II. Football Sidesteps Scandals on Muscle Drugs

Despite the Alzado-NFL fracas and despite muscle-doping allegations against numerous NCAA universities, American football navigated smoother waters with the issue as 1991 concluded. The public had tired of such coverage, millions of fans were ready for some football, and all but scattered sportswriters were dropping the topic of anabolic steroids. In addition, organizers' policies featuring random urinalysis and penalties were good for image by effectively silencing active athletes and coaches from speaking publicly, beyond their repeating the new stock line that any problem was over.

Just a few doping waves remained, and football could really hit clear sailing. First, in 1992, Steve Courson's book, *False Glory*, had to be ignored, basically — "People can't be naïve enough to think this will go away," he said — and Alzado had to die, rather quietly — "Nobody learns," lamented Sam Rutigliano, former Browns coach.

Those items out of the way, football officials worked next to deflect a pair of potential PR torpedoes: the arrests of two NFL linemen for quantities of steroids and growth hormone, and a book's tarnishing of the hallowed Notre Dame under coach Lou Holtz.

DEA Agent Alleges Trafficking by Players, But NFL Denies

On January 5, 1993, a federal grand jury in northern Georgia indicted Eric Moore, New York Giants offensive tackle, and Mark Duckens, Tampa Bay defensive lineman. Each was charged with three felony counts: conspiracy to possess anabolic steroids with intent to distribute, possession of anabolic steroids with intent to distribute, and possession of human growth hormone with intent to distribute.

Moore and Duckens, informed of the indictments by NFL security personnel, were arraigned January 12 in Atlanta, where each pleaded innocent to the charges and were released after posting recognizance bond. Both 27, Moore and Duckens were pro veterans and brothers-in-law, having been teammates on the Giants in 1989, and friends and associates praised them for good character. For years, both players had passed random urinalysis by the NFL — including after their alleged $15,000 purchase of steroids and growth hormone in January 1992.

The indictments were part of an ongoing investigation that targeted anabolic drugs entering the United States from Mexico, and a DEA informant had fingered Moore and Duckens. Authorities described the informant as a former football player who fitness-trained athletes in Atlanta; reportedly, he had been arrested in the spring of 1992 at Hartsfield International Airport in Atlanta, possessing steroids purchased in San Diego, where a network of Mexicans said to include children smuggled the drugs from across the border.

The informant led authorities to believe several NFL players were involved, a possibility discussed by DEA special agent Garfield Hammonds, Jr., on January 13, 1993, in Atlanta. "Let me state that the indictment and arrests of Moore and Duckens clearly demonstrates that the NFL players are still using and trafficking in steroids and human growth hormones," Hammonds said. "This investigation is continuing. We anticipate the arrest of other NFL players. ... [Moore and Duckens] were dealing in such large amounts, you can assume that they were distributing as well as using. I can't see them stockpiling."

Denial was immediate from NFL officials in New York. "We strongly disagree with [Hammonds'] off-the-cuff comment...," said Joe Browne, league spokesman. "We don't know what Mr. Hammonds is referring to when he talks about more arrests. We also believe that his blanket indictment of steroid use among NFL players is uncalled for, and there is a large body of evidence that clearly indicates that steroid use in the NFL has dramatically decreased in recent years due to our year-round random-testing program.

"Team doctors, trainers, and players themselves readily support our beliefs. We're realistic enough to know there will always be problems when you have 1,500 players in the league, and we're not naïve enough to believe that we are 100 percent problem-free in this area or can expect to be that way in the near future."

The NFL's united front on steroids counted a new face, Upshaw, the union executive director and ex-adversary of management on the issue. Formerly a tough critic of the league drug policy, Upshaw had flip-flopped since Alzado's fatal illness, particularly on steroids. "We have the strongest testing program in sports, and to say it's widespread among NFL players, I just don't agree...," Upshaw said. "You can see it in the locker room. Guys have shrunk; they haven't gotten larger."

People surrounding Moore and Duckens suggested the indicted players did not even use steroids. Johnny Parker, Giants strength coach, said muscle doping had never been problematic for the team, and he vouched for the 290-pound Moore, who had gained 100 pounds since high school. "I have complete confidence Eric Moore doesn't use drugs," Parker said. "I would be surprised if any of this is true."

Tampa Bay coach Sam Wyche likewise downplayed Duckens' involvement. "I'm still not sure anything has happened," Wyche said. "I've heard and read too many things about me that I know weren't true. Lots of people are wrongly indicted, too." Wyche, representing a team with a second steroid bust in three years, claimed steroids had been a passing fad and users were easy to identify. "I don't suspect any use on the Bucs," he said. "Usually, just being around it over the years, when it was more popular than it is now — now it's not popular at all — you could spot a user just by your instincts... No,

I don't suspect anyone and haven't suspected anyone. Neither have any of the other [Bucs] coaches and trainers, who would spot it right away. Maybe you can mask the test, but it's pretty hard to mask the effects, the signals of steroids."

Agent Hammonds, following NFL rebuttals, was not available to reporters for a short period. In his next public statements, Hammonds offered a general number on the drug quantities Moore and Duckens were charged with receiving, staying firm in his suspicion of networking. "It wasn't one or two hits," he told the *New York Times*. "There were several thousand units seized. That would lead a reasonable person to believe that the drugs wouldn't be intended for one person. In law enforcement, if you find a person in possession of a kilo of dope, you have to assume it's not for one person's use. It's intended for distribution."

The DEA agent backed off his talk about additional players' involvement. Hammonds said the drugs were delivered in Atlanta, but no Falcons players were involved, and he conceded the probe's focus was going nowhere in the NFL beyond those charged. "As far as I'm concerned, the only two teams that are implicated are New York and Tampa Bay, and then only so far as it concerns those two players," he said.

Tagliabue waited two weeks to comment on Moore and Duckens, during press conferences on Super Bowl weekend in Los Angeles, and the commissioner was predictable in characterizing the arrests as an isolated incident. In three years of random urinalysis thus far, roughly 15,000 tests, the NFL had suspended a total of four players for steroid-positive results.

"We are confident our testing program is very effective and reliable," Tagliabue said. "We know it is a deterrent. We think steroid-free is something we may never get to. ... You are not delighted when there are arrests. This is the second time [since 1990] players have been allegedly involved. ... We are optimistic the problem is under control. We don't think there's a substance problem in the league."

Tagliabue acknowledged no reliable test existed for human growth hormone, but use of the drug was "isolated, not endemic" in the NFL. He noted some experts even wondered whether the drug worked well for building muscle. "There are questions about the effect of those hormones on performance enhancement," he said. "We continue to monitor them." Media were skeptical but reserved harsh judgment, and, following the Super Bowl, Tagliabue did not enter public discussion lingering around Moore and Duckens.

The Raiders' Howie Long addressed anabolics a final time as a player, entering his 13th NFL season. "I think steroid use is down quite a bit... growth hormones are a factor now," he said. "It's undetectable. It's the ultimate football drug. I don't know how prevalent it is, because I don't know how available it is. I know it's very expensive."

Football players were not giving up drugs for performance enhancement, according to former Redskins lineman Dexter Manley. "Here's the thing: Everything is so competitive," he said. "It's like when people want to speed on the highway, so they buy radar detectors. ... People on these steroids use these growth hormones to outdo the cops."

Undetectable doping was the reliable way for NFL players to beat random urinalysis, critics said, despite reports some athletes resorted to methods such as switching urine, employing a catheter, or waiting to be tipped-off for a test. In addition, the standard combination invisible to testing technology was growth hormone and low-dosage testosterone. An NFL player only had to keep his testosterone-epitestosterone ratio below 6:1, compared to the average human ratio of 1:1. A newly released dispenser of testosterone, the skin patch, helped users stay under radar, along with inexpensive T-E readings available privately through commercial labs. Testosterone testing was "totally flawed," said Dr. Mauro DiPasquale, urinalysis consultant at the University of Toronto. "The 6:1 ratio is a joke."

Nothing had changed about muscle drugs in pro football, critics said, as league policy remained inept. "I don't think NFL testing has lowered usage," Penn State expert Dr. Charles Yesalis told New York sportswriter Barry Meisel, for a series in *The Daily News*. "I think it has dropped the dosage [players] use." Drug guru Dan Duchaine, claiming clients in football he would not name, said, "It is in the testosterone part of the drug test that the most cheating is going on, especially in sports like professional football, where testosterone is the drug of choice."

Doping author and critic Dr. Robert Voy once felt helpless working on the side of testing, as medical officer for the USOC during the 1980s, when he knew thousands of athletes worldwide utilized a cornucopia of undetectable drugs. Voy's honest doubts at the time, expressed in public, had led to his resignation from the job. Now, as an independent critic, Voy believed nothing had changed. "Anabolic steroids are still tremendously popular among a high number of athletes," he said, "for one simple reason: They work."

Whether sport doping was maintaining or growing, public discussion was declining, writer Meisel observed, and Yesalis agreed. "When I was being interviewed five years ago, I said this was a very secret issue," Yesalis said. "It's 10 times more secretive now." Steve Courson also saw inside football information cut to trickles since random testing. "The only thing that's changed in the situation is the problem has gone further underground," he said.

And, really, who cared?

Scant attention was paid the Moore and Duckens cases as they concluded in the summer of 1993. Duckens, who would not return to the NFL, avoided trial by completing a drug-treatment program. Moore pleaded guilty to a reduced charge, misdemeanor possession of steroids, and was sentenced to probation by U.S. District Judge Marvin H. Shoob, who said, "I recognize [anabolic drug use] is not an uncommon practice in both college and professional sports." The NFL suspended Moore for the first four games of the regular season.

"Have I used steroids?" Moore said, addressing a reporter's question. "I know what steroids are, let's leave it at that. I've never tested positive for drugs or steroids in any NFL test." Moore said his associating with the wrong people had caused the trouble.

'Tarnished Dome' Book Enrages Loyalists of Notre Dame, Holtz

A single book stung America's merriment with college football in 1993, *Under The Tarnished Dome: How Notre Dame Betrayed Its Ideals For Football Glory*, by Don Yaeger and Douglas S. Looney. The investigative story chronicled steroid abuse and other ills in the program of Lou Holtz, a cultural favorite among coaches, and reaction was vitriolic, instigated in part by religious leaders of the fabled Notre Dame.

University officials avoided interviews, but one did surface to read a prepared statement pledging support of Holtz. "Notre Dame emphatically denies the premise of the book...," said E. William Beauchamp, executive vice president. "Coach Holtz has done the three things Notre Dame asks of any coach: He has lived by the rules, his players have graduated, and he has fielded competitive teams."

Palpable public contempt focused on the book's authors and former Irish players who made allegations. Angry folks included many sport media who struck back at Yaeger and Looney, questioning the book's motive and blowing off allegations as so-what news, whether true or false. Commentators in print and broadcast argued that steroids pervaded big-time college football, not to mention tyrannical coaches and rules violations. They labeled any critics naïve, of Holtz and Notre Dame.

Why single out Notre Dame in the moral slop of major NCAA football? With 106 schools wallowing, all told? Why pick on Holtz?

Minneapolis writer Patrick Reusse stated America already understood the harsh life of a college football player, contending the culture had known since at least Gary Shaw's book *Meat On The Hoof*, which exposed brutalities of Texas football under coach Darrell Royal. "It wasn't croquet they were playing 25 years ago. Still ain't, baby," Reusse commented, macho but safe in his seat at a football game.

Holtz enjoyed strong support from Minnesota, where as coach of the Golden Gophers he had broken NCAA rules, according to Yaeger's and Looney's book. Veteran sportswriter Sid Hartman encouraged Holtz to sue the book's publisher, Simon and Schuster. Hartman blamed athletes for the trouble, not the coach he had known for three decades, whom he described as "honest... not a phony or self-promoter." Again, Hartman cried, *everybody does it* in this game. "You could write the same book about Nebraska, Michigan, Miami, Alabama or any of the college football powers," the scribe claimed, "because you could get the malcontents — the players who are recruited and don't play hard — to rip the respective school and football coach."

College football's classic good-time announcer on ABC, Keith Jackson, famed for his "Who-o-oa, Nellie!" cry, suddenly went beyond yarns and clichés to display a cold perspective on the game. Jackson, lauded for knowing every young player's hometown down to the tiniest burgs, was nonplussed about anyone's exposure to serious drug use. He shrugged off muscle-building dope in college ball. "I've read the book and I didn't find a damn thing I didn't know," Jackson told *USA Today*. "Taking steroids is not very significant, because virtually every lineman since World War II has taken some body-building aid. It's just that lately overdoses have proven harmful."

Television representatives at NBC stood behind Notre Dame, the network holding an exclusive football contract with the university as well as multi-million-dollar broadcast rights. Dick Ebersol, president of NBC Sports, said, "From my look at the book, I personally see it as a lot of rehashed bunk." Announcer Cris Collinsworth, a former college and pro receiver, said, "That book's absolutely a joke. I hate it when people come out with trash like that. Something that nasty could have been written about any big-time football program in the country."

The excuse of rehashed bunk was no reassurance about college football, but it was popular among athletic officials nationwide, lending their support to Holtz and Notre Dame. Arkansas athletic director Frank Broyles was one, as were Akron coach Gerry Faust and Stanford coach Bill Walsh. "[Holtz] stands for the best in college athletics," Walsh said. "My feeling is he would never allow steroids, never allow cheating by his coaches. ... He doesn't have the trait of deception." At Florida State, coach Bobby Bowden told his staff the controversy could be about them, "just as easily as Lou Holtz." Bowden shuddered at the thought; he said football coaches had "all been guilty" of striking, grabbing, verbally abusing players, and, presumably, encouraging steroids directly or indirectly. "The things Lou Holtz is accused of are something we've all probably done one time or another," Bowden said. "As coaches we don't think anything of it. Maybe we were wrong, and we're going to change."

The book's authors and their few supporters contended Notre Dame deserved the allegations because it assumed a higher moral plane in college football. "Notre Dame spends millions of dollars telling us they're different," Yaeger observed. "Maybe the story is their hypocrisy." Sportswriter Keteyian, author of the book about Nebraska and Tom Osborne, said, "Sure you'll find [problems] in every college program. "The difference is that Notre Dame has always said it's different — and it's profited from being different. This book shows Notre Dame has made some serious concessions to its image to deal with the realities of big-time football."

Keteyian blasted the common claim the book was old news, suggesting most media were mere accomplices to the university's evasion tactic. "I think it's a first-rate job of reporting, and Notre Dame is trying to shift the argument from reporting to the reporters...," Keteyian said. "People do a disservice to the profession we're in when they pop off without reading the book. I read it three times. We at [ABC] *Nightline* took it apart piece by piece, and it held up. ... Excuse me, but I haven't read any other on-the-record comments lately about player abuse, widespread steroid abuse, intolerance for injury and lower academic standards for Notre Dame."

Yaeger and Looney had interviewed more than 80 former Irish players, and the authors requested a public discussion of allegations with university officials beyond Beauchamp. That did not happen, but Looney got phone calls at home from upwards of 2,000 angry Irish fans, since someone at the university released his unlisted number.

"From one standpoint, it makes sense when there is no [official] response," Looney said. "If there had been anything wrong in the book, Notre Dame would have been all over that in a New York moment."

In New York, *Times* sports columnist Malcom Moran criticized the university. "Notre Dame has the right to reject the premise of a book...," Moran wrote. "But the current institutional strategy of stonewalling the questions the book raises about the price of its football success, ignoring its contents, treating it as pornography and keeping it off the shelves of the bookstore, has not created Notre Dame's finest hour." Moran tied the fierce denial to the school's lucrative myth of pristine football, but "the truth is that Notre Dame cannot operate in a vacuum."

The Notre Dame faithful, however, were determined to enjoy the 1993 season, and millions more football fans were happy to join them, as Holtz and his scrappy Irish marched to an 11-1 record, narrowly missing a shot at the national championship. The societal celebration surrounding Notre Dame football — from fans to heart-warming TV features to a glorious *SI* cover captioned WE DID IT! — seemed exaggerated for dousing the inflammatory book. Perhaps Football America was protecting the college game as a whole, everyone acting as apologists for pulse-point Notre Dame.

Chicago writer Jay Mariotti was not buying. He knocked the culture "which more than ever wants to view sport as fantasyland" and decried that no supposed watchdog party, including the NCAA or media, held Notre Dame and Holtz accountable. University officials were allowed to simply ignore the allegations, to issue a paper denial and turn their backs. Maybe that pointed to a deeper malfeasance, for society as whole.

"In a former America, that would be perceived as running away from a problem," Mariotti surmised. "In today's America, it is known as a shrewd tactic."

III. Sportswriter Lonely in Public Issues

As the 1980s concluded, my work as an investigative sportswriter was under way and promising, or so I thought.

Actually, my budding specialty as a journalist — public issues of sport and particularly those involving football — had seen its short shelf life. Media editors and executives at mainstream newspapers, magazines, and broadcast outlets already had enough of investigative journalism in sports. Some realities in America were just bad for media business, especially systematic ills in games that people regarded as wholesome and advertisers guarded zealously.

Thusly, barely 30, I was not an up-and-comer in the business but a dinosaur, unwittingly swept under by a tidal wave of "civic journalism," the PR name for corporate media's pandering to audiences, giving readers and viewers what they want. My philosophy of "traditional journalism," providing citizens facts they need to know, regardless of who gets pissed, was largely dead.

Far out of touch with contemporary, publicly owned media, my avowed intent to probe and publicize football reality completely violated the industry's newly dominant business model. Media executives and stockholders were counting on a football-fantasy content — the classic, fan-friendly themes such as Oriard's Necessary Roughness, Football Hero, Coaching Genius, Patriotism and Social Event — to key their financial profits in the decade and beyond. The reporting of widespread doping in football, the pervasive use of drugs for performance, was a definite no-no for the new popular press.

This was the 1990s, decade of consumer self-indulgence to the point of heavy debt, and the NFL under Paul Tagliabue would grow into a world-elite name brand, packaged and presented virtually tamper-proof by American media, football's loyal, de facto partner since the Victorian Age. College football and prep football saddled up for the entertainment ride, too, on media large and small.

By 1996, I found myself adrift as a sports journalist. Along the way, reporting on issues, I'd been slandered with actual malice by one sportswriter and ignored by the multitude of others. I was driven out of one job just as I received an investigative-reporting award, because my newspaper was taken over by a chain with no use for my kind; indeed, the libelous sportswriter was one of "theirs." Immediately upon learning of my newspaper's sale, to whom, I resigned and walked out, perhaps before they fired me.

I felt pretty sorry for myself, but I'd either learn to play the special game of sports in popular press, at least sometimes, or learn how to survive on fringe as a critic, risking lunatic classification. The latter was scary to consider, but I followed, haltingly. I was as good as anyone at producing the good, happy sport tales for America — "traditional slogans, cliches, sacred cows, and ritualized trivia," observed critic George H. Sage — and continued for a while to capitalize somewhat, claiming a modest income from a regional sports show on radio and scattered free-lance writing. I held my sacred cows like anyone negotiating the old sport-media complex, protective of certain individuals, but I would not look away from systemic problems impacting athletes and society. Eventually I contemplated new jobs for income, as a husband and father who wasn't producing much, and to family relocation.

Having gained some success as a self-published book author, I decided to pursue a good companion occupation in college teaching, which I could "believe in" still. I needed a master's degree for the job, minimally, and was accepted by the Graduate School of Communication at Central Missouri State University. After eight years in my beloved southeast Missouri, often struggling financially, I moved my family to Warrensburg and entered graduate studies in the fall semester of 1996.

My thesis research focused on print media's coverage of anabolic substances in football, and the analysis revealed the scope of doping and a sportswriter's role in the mess. The lessons were hard to take, particularly for having to acknowledge my own *multiple* roles of culpability, ranging from former user player and perpetrator coach to journalist who ignored doping. Moreover, I was still enough the football fan to have staged Super Bowl parties at my house, not to mention having parked at the TV Monday nights to watch big games I always forgot. In opening my thesis study, I wrote:

This study emerged out of the author's personal background in college football and sportswriting; in both fields, the author encountered realities conflicting with the ethical missions the institutions claim to practice. As a college football player and student coach, for example, the author was exposed to the phenomenon of anabolic steroid use by athletes in the National Collegiate Athletic Association, an organization which supposedly stands for fair play and the well-being of participants. Likewise, while working in sport media — an aspect of journalism as a "public trust" — the author saw reluctance by reporters and editors to address topics that negatively impact the sports world, including racism, NCAA rules violations by college programs, and performance-enhancing drugs like steroids. The author acknowledges personal culpability in both problems introduced here: I used muscle-building anabolic steroids as a small-college football player in 1982; later, as a sportswriter, I compiled football stories in which I ignored signs of anabolic drug use, including print and radio features on mammoth adolescent boys who were college prospects. The author last worked in daily sport media in 1995.

The thesis study also showed me how little I had known about football doping, before entering grad school. During the 1980s and early 1990s, I had collected articles and books regarding the subject, the issue's biggest headliners such as Courson, Bosworth, Chargers history, Chaiken, Mandarich, NCAA data, Fralic, Senate hearings, Alzado, and Notre Dame. Yet much more had gone down in football doping around the country, and not until the latter 1990s, thesis research by instant electronic means, did the big picture emerge for me through online databases such as Lexis-Nexis. No wonder clueless thought reigned on football muscle doping. Prior to the establishment of simplified, easily accessible search modes on the Internet, many events portraying the problem's enormity escaped Americans, whether football players, organizers, politicians, sportswriters, critics, fans, or non-fans.

The research also deflated a hope I held going in — that improved random urinalysis in NFL and NCAA football would solve the problem. Unfortunately, I discovered the idea was naive. Still too many loopholes existed for urinalysis, practically rendering nil the chance it could ever be refined to the point of battling widespread doping in sport — particularly in any game involving big money, prestige, and upwards of two million participants to monitor, the vast majority kids.

Talk of eradicating muscle drugs through urinalysis was folly for the ignorant, or the tool of propagandists following an agenda.

IV. Heyday: America's Suspended Belief in Sport

In 1998, baseball's Mark McGwire was some 260 pounds of virtual muscle, but he was the full embodiment of America's quandary over muscle doping in their beloved sports, games and heroes. The culture could not get enough of celebrating Big Mac, a virtual comic-book hero come alive after his packing on at least 25 pounds of lean mass in his mid-30s — then swatting 70 homers in a season to obliterate legends like Maris, Ruth, Mantle, and Mays.

However, many sporting people knew something was wrong. "Does it all add up?" Armen Keteyian posited for *Sport* magazine's August issue, writing of modern performers and doping in general, a few weeks before another scribe would spy the infamous bottle of "andro" in McGwire's locker at Busch Stadium. "You catch yourself staring," Keteyian wrote, "mentally multiplying size and speed and strength times genes, factoring in a wicked workout schedule and muscle-boosting products like creatine. ...

Are we watching a new superhuman breed of athlete, almost aberrant in mass and velocity, grow naturally before our eyes? Nothing artificial? No drugs? No steroids?"

Keteyian had recently covered the summer's "Doping in Elite Sport" conference, an invitation-only gathering of experts and insiders in Los Angeles, where the consensus conclusion was the problem remained epidemic and institutionalized, despite urinalysis testing, with a wealth of evidence in support. "And we see it, yet we don't," Keteyian intoned, chiding the suspended belief of collective American conscience, for sport mythology.

The culture did not care, not in its exploding lust for sport entertainment during the 1990s. Looking the other way was essential for enjoying every great story, increasingly routine, and especially the quick legends like Big Mac. The trend was perpetuated by sport media, capitalized upon. *Sports Illustrated* editorialists seemed resigned: "It may be time that we at SCORECARD [section], self-righteous solvers of sport's problems, say it as well: We give. Uncle," Steve Rushin wrote, after firing a fleeting salvo at invalid drug testing of the NFL, NCAA, and Olympics. "Somebody, give us a towel."

Actually, the magazine had long relented on doping, joining the happy crowd as substances revved-up athletes and games. Most *SI* staff writers readily went along with the fantasy ride, not asking about drugs, not telling. Indeed, Rushin may have been the minority at *SI*, the magazine already the leading media bandwagon for Big Mac, a strutting, smiling, talking windfall. *SI* produced six covers glorifying McGwire in 1998, including the year-end "Sportsmen of The Year" issue, for which the Cardinals superstar happily shared the award and photo shoot with "Slammin' " Sammy Sosa, Cubs slugger and ballyhooed good buddy of Big Mac.

The magazine, despite Rushin's words, readily defended McGwire for his use of androstenedione, once that revelation broke in St. Louis. Medical literature classified androstenedione as an anabolic steroid, and Major League Baseball's complete lack of a drug policy left wide open the abuse of performance enhancers from steroids to speed. Andro was a legal "dietary supplement" by government definition, under 1994 deregulation, and really no one cared, crowed sportswriters drunk on Big Mac.

America detoured only slightly over McGwire and andro, with fans and media pausing briefly on their fairytale. Quickly, any doping allegations against McGwire were deemed irrelevant, innuendo at best, and critics were told to shut up. Society wanted its magic with the man, regardless. "Like one of his Herculean home runs, the drug controversy around Mark McGwire seems to be going, going, gone," observed Brian Derwin and Jay Weiner, for the *New York Times*.

Baseball, its fans, and America would pay in years ahead, as fraud permeating McGwire and his feats would become clear. People would learn that as fast as hype could elevate athletes to heroic icons, truth about drugs could lay waste to contrived images, thus confronting the internal values of everyone.

Moreover, countless athletes had been influenced, young and old, including baseball's greatest all-around player, Barry Bonds, an insecure personality who vowed to hit the juice himself, so he could top the power numbers — and public adulation — of McGwire and Sosa.

V. SUPER TEAMS, SUPER SIZES ESCAPE SCRUTINY

For what remained of the 1990s, Americans insisted on halcyon sport, a peace for enjoying their games, football foremost, and media had no objections. Sportswriters gave a free pass to baseball's dopers, as they had looked away from football juicers since Alzado. In American mainstream athletics, football players were the obvious poster boys for muscle doping through steroids, growth hormone, and more substances.

Media had their explanations for ignoring football doping in the 1990s. The NFL and NCAA persistently denied a systematic problem, for example, and everyone in football had clammed up. The public could not care less, so journalists need not worry. The majority of sportswriters simply assumed nothing was going on anymore, as far as anabolic drugs in football, because of random testing.

Nevertheless, plenty was happening during the 1990s that national media failed to connect to doping in football. Despite new steroid laws, obtaining anabolic substances became easier, as illicit dealers moved from gyms to cyberspace and a controversial supplements measure made muscle dope legal and available in stores and online. In other developments, the sizes of players rose far above 1980s parameters, incredibly, with athletic 300-pounders proliferating at all levels, preps to pros. In clinical research, scientists concluded anabolic steroids produced significant gains in mass and strength, and quickly, but not a page of valid data emerged to support mere weightlifting and diet as capable — the typical claim of athletes and coaches that media accepted at face value. Gaping loopholes in urinalysis became public information by definition, documented repeatedly by a host of experts; in contrast, no significant advance occurred in the technology, such as a reliable test for growth hormone. News items of the decade also included health problems afflicting or killing active and former football players — some ex-pros filed lawsuits — and the revelation that the NFL was capable of burying positive drug results, as was the case with 16 players during a three-year period.

Media definitely ignored the drug specter following new Super Bowl teams. In the past, allegations clouded winning by the Steelers, Cowboys, and Raiders, among clubs. During the 1990s, first the Cowboys then the Broncos drew doping attention, two teams combining to win half the decade's Super Bowls.

In 1993, former Cowboys defensive tackle Danny Noonan discussed steroids with Barry Meisel of the *New York Daily News*. Noonan had tested positive at the 1987 NFL combine, before Dallas made him the draft's 12th pick overall, and his steroid use continued "off and on," he said, during five seasons with the Cowboys. He played for two head coaches in Dallas, both Super Bowl winners, Tom Landry and Jimmy Johnson. During Landry's era, steroid use was documented on the Cowboys and league-wide, and nothing changed in Johnson's tenure despite NFL urinalysis, according to Noonan, who competed in the league as large as 6-4, 290.

"In the pros, I never got any feedback at all [on steroids]," Noonan said. "As long as you got the job done, I'm not sure how much they really wanted to know. Jimmy [Johnson] came in in '89, and they had some real tough testing. With Jimmy, though, he couldn't have cared less. The bottom line is, you win, you play well, you get your job done." In the year Noonan was drafted, "75 to 80 percent of the linemen were taking them, especially defensive," he estimated. "A lot of the guys who came out [of college]... were heavy into it."

Noonan's quotes were not widely disseminated, and another provocative item about the Cowboys raised no concern about doping. By Super Bowl 1994, the team was publicly connected with Bill Phillips, supplement salesman, bodybuilder — and former self-promoted steroid guru who claimed to have changed. Phillips was billed as an "anti-steroid crusader" now, an advocate of clean, healthy living. Phillips promoted and sold Met-Rx, a supplement endorsed by coaches and players like strength coach Mike Woicik of the Cowboys, amid that franchise's run of three Super Bowl championships in four years. Woicik pushed Met-Rx and more company supplements to Cowboys players, and he advised about a dozen on the use of ephredrine, he told Bill Brubaker, *Washington Post.*

Phillips, proceeding to build fabulous wealth in the industry of "dietary supplements," told reporters of his recent conversion from steroid user and author — his 1991 how-to-use book *Anabolic Reference Guide* was a top moneymaker — to becoming a straight entrepreneur of good nutrition. Phillips, however, could not sever ties to the sport-doping underworld, not as a businessman fully in tune with the athletes' demand for performance enhancement, a huge commercial market he helped establish. Phillips' popular magazine *Muscle Media 2000* published steroid advertising and PED stories available nowhere else, including how-to information and review of new substances, along with columnists such as Dan Duchaine, doping guru and convicted dealer.

Yet Phillips, an American success story in his latter 20s, personified credibility with most media. Keying his rise was a talent for securing celebrity clients that included major Hollywood stars, leading men and women. In the NFL, Phillips aligned with the Cowboys, then the Denver Broncos in his home-state Colorado, where his business empire exploded on the acquisition of an unknown little supplement company, Experimental and Applied Sciences, or EAS.

At Denver, Phillips gained a glittering local endorsement group in the A list of Broncos stars: quarterback John Elway, tight end Shannon Sharpe, running back Terrell Davis, and linebacker Bill Romanowski. Phillips signed the foursome right before they led the Broncos into prime-time national exposure — two straight Super Bowl victories — so in media interviews they wore EAS gear, stylish caps and turtlenecks, and swore by the company's supplements and training techniques. The Phillips strategy would force NFL thinkers into revising licensing and copyright policy. Broncos stars claimed impact performance improvements under the tutelage of Phillips, assisted by his brother Shawn, a fitness trainer known for his "abs," and EAS revenues shot to $170 million annually. "I wish I could say that we were geniuses," Phillips said in 1998. "But it was pretty much just being in the right place at the right time."

Elway was the crowning symbol for the company, with his success story of a physical rebound after health struggles in his mid-30s. Injured and out of shape, Elway hooked up with Phillips, according to the EAS narrative, *then* forged his NFL legend, going from goat to great in the Super Bowl to cap his Hall of Fame career. "It was an important time for Elway," Phillips said later. "He really focused on his exercise and his nutrition those last two years. Otherwise, there was no way he would've been able to keep up, and he admits that."

Sharpe, formerly skinny, and Romanowski, known for his companion tackle box packed with "supplements," ardently supported EAS and Phillips. Everyone's gains were steroid-free, of course. "Trust me. I get tested five or six times a year," Sharpe said. However, testing apparently did not prevent Romanowski's muscle doping at Denver, where the 6-3, 245-pound linebacker used steroids and growth hormone, according to statements by his wife, two teammates, and a personal trainer. "Romo" did not fail an NFL urinalysis with the Broncos.

Phillips would not be implicated by Romanowski's doping — that distinction would fall on another Broncos associate of the period, Victor Conte, head of BALCO laboratory in the California Bay Area. Conte had met Romanowski in the mid-1990s through Remi Korchemny, the linebacker's speed coach. In Denver, Romo introduced Conte to Broncos teammates, and the BALCO president designed "mineral programs for all the guys," as he would recall.

The NFL cracked down on the EAS-Broncos relationship, shooing away Phillips as he sold his company for a reported $245 million. Conte remained a regular figure around the Super Broncos and other teams, counting about 250 NFL players as clients, reportedly, for his BALCO supplement ZMA, comprised of zinc, magnesium, and vitamin B6. [Following a federal raid on the BALCO lab near San Francisco in 2003, Conte said he had introduced the designer steroid THG to Romanowski at Denver in 1999. Thus the NFL obtained the chemical signature of THG for its testing library, and in 2003 Romanowski was one of four Raiders who tested positive for the anabolic, previously undetectable. Later, Conte and Korchemny pleaded guilty to charges stemming from the BALCO case.]

Any suspicion of Denver doping lapsed quickly. For media, the Super Broncos were a fresh NFL legend, especially Elway, and mountains of content spewed in testament, video, audio, print, and online. Champions Elway and the Broncos assumed their high plane in American sport mythology, uncontested.

Football media and fans gave a symbolic wink elsewhere, too, over the sizes of contemporary players at all levels. During the first 60 years of NFL competition, 300-pound players were a rarity, amounting to less than 20 total. A few dozen emerged during the 1980s, and in the 1990s, the first decade of random urinalysis, the NFL's number of 300-pound players increased by about 1,000 percent, to almost 300 in number. In 1990s NCAA football, major-college lines swelled to average 300 pounds, and lines at many smaller schools approached the standard. Blue-chip recruits coming out of high schools typically approached or topped 300. Packers defensive coordinator Fritz Shurmur said enormity was required in the modern NFL. "No question about it — this has become a game on the line of scrimmage of 300-pound men. And if you are just 300 pounds [on average] across there, you are pretty small," he said.

Moreover, the giants were athletic. "The NFL has become obsessed with big guys over 300 who can still run a 4.7 or 4.8 [40-yard dash]," said Redskins offensive tackle

Joe Jacoby. In Green Bay, Packers trainer Pepper Burruss observed that a player with size had to maintain athleticism. "A 300-pound football player and a 300-pound person on the street, Joe Six-Pack, are two different 300-pounders," Burruss said. "These are well-conditioned athletes." A professor of physics at the University of Nebraska, Dr. Timothy Gay, would review historical size and performance data of the NFL, calculating the average offensive lineman gained more than 100 pounds in eight decades, from 1920 to 2000, while increasing foot speed upwards of 70 percent.

Oblivious were the vast majority of football writers, or at least they acted that way. By the latter 1990s, the word "steroid" was not often associated with football in media content — highly rare, in fact, were specific mentions, much less full exposures of the problem, relative to the massive pulp of gridiron content gorging America. Some writers practiced vague allusion to steroids, leaving audiences to read between the lines. Steve Wilstein, *Associated Press*, noted the spiral of silence surrounding football's increasing sizes and muscle dope, the culture's denial for making the link. "It's just a matter of… biotechnology, nutrition, training and, shhh, steroids," he wrote.

Leigh Montville of *SI* happened onto some possible doping material in an otherwise happy sort of interview with veteran NFL quarterback Doug Flutie, who recognized the rise in performance levels upon returning to the league in 1998. After dominating Canadian football for eight seasons, Flutie, 35, signed with Buffalo, and that summer he openly worried about the continual arms race among players, their perpetual competition for more size, more strength, more speed, always pushing higher the parameters. "You know, I see these young guys at the Bills' training facility…," Flutie told Montville. "They're 22 years old, 23, and football is their life. I was just like them at their age. They're taking all this stuff, trying to get bigger and bigger, add more muscles. You get older, you have a family, you see what matters." Flutie was no rookie at speaking out about football's problems. He had shaken Canada near the end of his CFL career, for example, by declaring that the league "legitimized" steroid use among players.

Montville, however, did not clarify the context of Flutie's remark about Bills players' seeking size and strength; the writer failed to make clear whether the quarterback meant muscle doping or not. Likewise, the lengthy, detailed feature did not mention steroids or pertinent history, Flutie's controversial stance on the drugs in Canada, where he had been pro football's highest-paid player.

The forceful silence on football doping stood rigid in 1999, when Chiefs star linebacker Derrick Thomas broke ranks during a *Sport* magazine survey of pro football players. Regarding problems facing the NFL, Thomas answered, "Without a doubt, No. 1 is steroids." Thomas' words did not go beyond *Sport*. In his adopted hometown of Kansas City, where football content was hawked year-round by newspapers, radio, and TV — and Thomas was the worshipped figure "D.T.," charismatic, warrior leader of the Chiefs — his national steroid quote went disregarded, ignored. Routinely, Kansas City editors and reporters made multi-media headlines of utterly trivial events and personalities surrounding Chiefs football, but they treated D.T.'s frankness about NFL muscle doping as no news.

Sportswriters naturally balked at connecting drugs to football's increasing sizes. Generally, players and coaches had their "explanations," and the media multitude repeated the excuses without question, however outlandish or improbable. "Steroids are down. Glutamine is up. And creatine is still king in the football player's cupboard.... The NFL and NCAA have cracked down hard on illegal substances," *Denver Post* scribe John Henderson proclaimed during the 1999 football season, drawing his information strictly from coaches, players, and supplement marketers. Henderson, in compiling his highly subjective analysis, might have checked backgrounds for his interviews, one source in particular — E.J. "Doc" Kreis, the former Vanderbilt strength coach who keyed that football program's steroid scandal of the early 1980s, along with a steroid-dispensing pharmacist friend in Nashville.

Kreis had moved on nicely from Vanderbilt — and his misdemeanor conviction for distribution — by remaining in NCAA athletics. He returned quickly to big-time college sports, hired by the University of Colorado as the strength and conditioning coach, and continued to elevate performance results for young athletes. During the 1990s, Buffalos football was among CU teams that won national recognition, and Kreis became one of the NCAA's best-known athletic trainers, enjoying commercial success for ventures outside the university. He promoted supplements from manufacturers such as Colorado-based EAS, owned by Bill Phillips.

The new age's supposed non-steroid formula — food intake, supplements, and manic training — was publicly sold by Kreis associate Jeff "Mad Dog" Madden, the University of Texas Longhorns strength and conditioning coach determined to produce huge players, in his own image. Madden, an enormous man who once benched 600, had played football at Vanderbilt and trained under Kreis, and the two later worked together at CU and in a lucrative side business. In 1998, Madden joined an up-and-coming head coach at North Carolina, Mack Brown, who brought him to Texas. "I've got over 100 players in the NFL, and they all come back to me in the summer," Madden told *SI*. "I can take players where they can't take themselves."

Gulping creatine, an amino acid, and pounding iron reportedly did the trick for players at Florida State, home of huge lineman under Bible-thumping training coach Dave Van Halanger. Same storyline at Nebraska, where long-time strength coach Boyd Epley directed a staff of 35 employees who trained Cornhusker athletes in all sports. At Wisconsin, Badgers team physician Greg Landry said a player could legitimately add as much as 75 pounds of muscle in five years — on just creatine, eating, lifting, and running; no steroids or other hormones were required. Everywhere in college football, phenomenal lean-mass gains by waves of young athletes were routinely attributed to creatine, eating, training.

Reportedly, the formula of high calories plus heavy lifting also had swept the NFL, though the media hardly questioned the tested credibility of quotes posted from players and officials. "It's safe to say that steroid use is pretty much gone," said Ralph Tamm, Broncos offensive lineman. Gil Brandt, the old Cowboys talent scout, said testing had minimized use by pro players. "I just think that the kids' eating habits are better," Brandt hypothesized. "They get better nutrition at the college training tables and they work out more."

Media stories avoided answering basic questions, particularly how "natural" supplements and exercise could so dramatically impact body mass, strength, and speed. "Very beneficial to athletes when taken correctly," Broncos receiver Shannon Sharp said of EAS products, for example, without elaborating. "Should be for highly skilled athletes, not to be toyed with. … Carefully supervised. Very misunderstood."

"Fat" athletes were a favorite football excuse for increasing sizes, and insiders and media alike repeatedly offered an example in Nate Newton, the Cowboys' 333-pound offensive guard, who welcomed his role in discounting any steroid problem. "When I came into the league, I looked around and saw all these guys with perfect bodies playing in the offensive line…," Newton said. "I would think, 'How can all those guys be built like that.' Then [commissioner] Paul Tagliabue said, 'Hey, no more steroids.'" Newton claimed he was All-Pro because of massive eating — his unnatural strength and athleticism had nothing to do with it — and he implied success for any lineman now meant the same.

Cliff Christl, a sportswriter who gathered data on football sizes, was skeptical "fat" could explain history's increase. Christl observed that "what's amazing is that many of the 300-pounders of today don't even appear fat," writing for the *Milwaukee Journal Sentinel*, where he and graphics artist Enrique Rodriquez painstakingly researched sizes through NFL history. "There are still some fat guys. But they don't play like fat guys."

In fact, roly-poly bodies remained the exception in the NFL. As always, speed and agility, along with bulk *built for quickness*, were imperatives. "Now, all of a sudden, the guys who are playing these games are 325 pounds and they're running 4.75 40s and benching 525 pounds," said Dr. Pierce Scranton, former Seahawks surgeon and book author. Shurmer noted the wave of 300-pound defensive linemen, all fast, that evolved to meet the ever-accelerating bulk of offensive lines.

California kinesiology professor Robert Girandola was sure of what he was witnessing in football: the continued abuse of steroids and other muscle dope. "I don't think it's magical," Girandola said. "There are so many anabolic products out there, it would be naïve to think that people are not going to take something." A marginal NFL rookie said essentially the same, after testing positive for a steroid during league urinalysis at Vikings training camp in 1997. The seventh-round draft pick, Artie Ulmer, a 6-2, 239-pound linebacker from Division II Valdosta State, heard "that a lot of players do it," said Phil Williams, his agent. The rookie had heard steroids "helped you get through camp and that you wouldn't get caught," Williams said. "He did it. He got caught." The agent, asked about Ulmer's future with the NFL, said, "Artie's a good kid. He's a country boy who was told something. It's his responsibility and his mistake, but he was told that a lot of people are doing it [and] you won't get caught. He realizes now it was wrong and he regrets it."

Football officials insisted, however, that doping was controlled. "The players testify to the fact that steroid use has gone down dramatically since the introduction of year-round testing [in 1990]," said Greg Aiello, NFL spokesman. Players union executive director Gene Upshaw said, "I don't agree that any player in the National

Football League is forced to take any substance to continue playing football. I just don't agree with that at all." Dr. John Lombardo, head of NFL testing, said "unbridled" steroid use was a problem of the past.

Media largely went along, and for whatever debate that flickered, football enjoyed plenty of supporters who held the ear of the media. "In the old days nutrition was often overlooked because of the rampant use of performance-enhancing drugs," said Phillips, supplements salesman and disavowed steroid guru. "Today things are different. I don't know of a single pro football player who uses anabolic steroids." As for any athletes like Ulmer, caught and branded for doping, sportswriters stuck to the notion of blaming the individuals only. "The NFL is clearly making an effort to catch cheaters," Mike Freeman wrote for the *New York Times*.

Nancy Armour, *Associated Press*, was certain of whom to blame for doping in the NFL, writing that "no matter what happens, the ultimate responsibility rests with the players."

A Decade of Football Doping Closes in Silence

In November 1999, a single commentary posted online ripped through the quietness shrouding doping in American football. The piece, written by critic Andrew Taber for *Salon.com*, made a mockery of mainstream media, or the thousands of everyday outlets in television, radio, newspapers, and magazines that denied the existence of the problem and marketed the game as family entertainment.

Taber identified a contrived, conventional fantasy in talk about random urinalysis as a deterrence. The writer attributed misguided, universal support for urinalysis to "the steroid backlash of the late 1980s." Recounting congressional hearings chaired by Senator Joe Biden and the passing of anti-steroid laws, Taber concluded nothing had changed in the decade since. "The drugs have saturated sports and seeped into high school gyms, turning records at all levels of sport synthetic," he wrote.

Taber noted the recent death of Walter Payton, the NFL's all-time leading rusher who succumbed to liver cancer at age 45. The hot question, discussed privately around football and beyond, was whether anabolic steroids had contributed to Payton's disease. Speculation about Payton and doping was off limits for the popular press, however, beyond a few reports that noted his physician denied a possible link. *Sports Illustrated's* coverage of the football legend's misfortune, for example, did not mention "steroid."

Again, Taber violated media taboo by going right to the topic. "Like Florence Griffith Joyner's mysterious demise in 1998, Payton's death from bile-duct cancer this month will never conclusively be pegged on steroids...," he wrote. "Pat Connolly, a former [Olympic athlete and coach], suggests that Payton's recent passing has to be regarded as suspicious. 'For every person who knows about steroids or has used them,' she says, 'the first thought that passed through our minds when we heard of Walter's liver problem was that it might be steroid-related.'"

Mainstream media and consumers were not interested in Taber's commentary, and charges by the issue's few independent experts were generally quelled as well.

Dr. Charles E. "Chuck" Yesalis, the Penn State epidemiologist, was accustomed to media censor of his charges on football doping. Sportswriters loved to quote Yesalis on the subject of steroids in track and field, which served as an historical whipping post for the issue, but the scientist's criticisms of football typically did not make print or broadcast. Sportswriters even balked at stating the established fact about urinalysis, its documented ineffectiveness against muscle doping.

Yesalis said the accelerating scale of sizes, strength, and speed in athletes correlated exactly with the advent of anabolic steroids and introduction of more muscle substances over time. Yesalis, who had interviewed numerous elite competitors while compiling his lauded histories on performance enhancement, noted the world's biggest and strongest specimens pre-steroids were Olympic lifters and throwers weighing 220 to 230 pounds. In the 1960s, Olympic and football athletes used steroids to push the size bar to 245, 250, initially. "Then, as I see it, guys started taking multiple cycles and higher dosages… and coming in at 275, 280," Yesalis said. "And now, over the last 10 to 15 years, as growth hormone and [insulin growth factor] have been added, you're getting over 300 pounds, easy."

Regarding football, Yesalis' friend and collaborating critic Steve Courson was indicative of the accelerating scale. In the early 1970s, Courson employed only weightlifting and eating to reach a maximum 230 pounds of lean weight, along with bench-pressing 400. Then a therapeutic cycle of Dianabol upped his mass to 260 and his bench to about 500. In the 1980s, Courson stacked or mixed steroids to approach 300 pounds in body weight and topped 600 on the bench. By 2000, however, Courson would have been too small for starring as an NFL lineman, because he did not advance into anabolics such as growth hormone. "Steve in his time was a legend of strength in the NFL," Yesalis said. "But if he went on the field today, in his prime playing weight of 285, he wouldn't be remarkable."

As obvious as the NFL was for drugs, Yesalis said, he was disappointed by NCAA football, its muscle doping, and more personally too as an informed faculty member of a major university. Yesalis' stomach could boil in angst at merely reading tales of college players' incredible gains in size and strength, like the linebacker at Kansas who added 55 pounds in mass, or the lineman at Missouri who packed on 45 to bench 500, or the former skinny scrub at K-State turned star on the O-line, after his 75 new pounds.

On and on the stories came, repeated every year from colleges, revolving young faces. The tales of wonder boys grated on Yesalis for their stating it was possible to gain significant mass, power, and agility through honest means. "That's just absurd," declared Yesalis, drawing on both his epidemiological research of doping and his thousands of hours in weightrooms over decades, lifting and coaching. Beyond excuses for increasing sizes, other NCAA rhetoric bothered Yesalis, particularly the line about isolated steroid use heard from athletes, coaches, hired medical personnel, and other officials.

Wrong again, Yesalis responded, declaring there could be no middle ground. A sport had practically no use or it hosted a real problem, and especially upper-level football, a physical, bloody confrontation with tangible rewards riding on the outcome. Yet he resisted placing the lion's share of blame on organizers. This culture craved the superhuman athlete, real or not, and paid handsomely for the escapement. "We love the entertainment so much, you know," Yesalis said. "It *is* the old bread and circuses of Roman days. "*What if* the NFL completely got rid of all drugs? I think we'd be looking at linemen, lean, 220 to 230 pounds; running backs at 170, 180; linebackers, 190, 200. I suspect some of the speed would go down... What would happen to the marketing and value of the NFL? What would happen to the market share on television?

"They [organizers] have figured out the fans don't care. If the public really didn't like it, if the public were grossly outraged about it — meaning if they turned off their television sets — you can darn well be assured something would change. But, again, the NCAA and in particular the NFL, they realize their fan base doesn't care."

Jason Whitlock was a rather lone sportswriter for portraying football doping as pervasive and hopeless in 2000. "You'll never get rid of steroids in sports. There's virtually nothing the major sports leagues can do to slow the use of 'roids. There's too much fame, fortune and ego on the line," wrote the *Kansas City Star* columnist, a former college lineman. Whitlock said most football players accepted steroids, users or not, and so did coaches. "I'll never forget how proud the Ball State strength coach was when a known steroid user broke the school's bench-press record. The player abused steroids throughout his four-year career, and no one ever said a word to him or any of the other users." Whitlock dismissed anyone's moralizing or posturing about a solution. "We can grind our teeth and get upset about steroid use all we want, but it's not going to stop," he wrote.

"I'm not suggesting that the NFL quit testing. What I'm suggesting is that it's useless for major-league baseball to begin testing. Athletes know how to beat the test. And the leagues really have no interest in suspending their big-time stars."

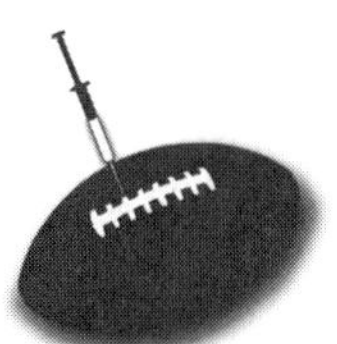

REFERENCES

A Way. (1994, January 25). Introducing a way to get kids off steroids. Business Wire, Inc. [Online].

Abrahamson, A. (2005, October 18). BALCO founder gets 8 months in steroid scheme. Los Angeles Times [Online].

Admitting Steroids. (1991, August 19). Defensive tackle admitting he used steroids. The Associated Press [Online].

Agent Says. (1993, January 16). U.S. agent says two players had large amounts of drugs. New York Times, p. I31.

Almond, E. (1995, January 23). Drug testing in NFL under microscope. Los Angeles Times, p. Sports—1.

Alzado Dies. (1992, May 14). Former All-Pro Lyle Alzado dies, claimed steroids killed him. The Associated Press [Online].

Alzado Funeral. (1992, May 15). With Alzado funeral. The Associated Press [Online].

Alzado, L. (1991, July 3). Television interview with host Roy Firestone [transcript]. ESPN.

Alzado, L. (1991, July 8). 'I'm sick and I'm scared.' Sports Illustrated, p. 20.

Alzado, L., & Edwards, W. (1991, July 29). Fourth down and long. People, p. 52.

Alzado Says. (1991, June 27). Alzado says brain cancer caused by steroids. The Associated Press [Online].

Anderson, D. (2001, April 22). The NFL gets 'big' in the draft and keeps getting bigger every year. New York Times, p. 8—3.

Archer, T. (1998, July 18). Muscling into mainstream. Cincinnati Post [Online].

Armour, N. (1999, December 20). Players, teams learn the hard way that supplements aren't so simple. The Associated Press [Online].

Ashe, A. (1990, January 20). NCAA propositions itself over 42. Washington Post, p. D1.

Asher, M. (1993, January 15). DEA agent: Number of NFL players arrested in steroid case could grow. Washington Post, p. C5.

Assael, S. (2007). Steroid nation*. New York, NY: ESPN Books.

Baker, G. (1996, November 2). Steroids muscle in on spotlight. Ottawa Citizen, p. 2.

Baum, B. (1992, May 16). Alzado buried in private ceremony. The Associated Press [Online].

Bax Test. (1990, May 19). Bax takes drug test, tries to clear name. St. Louis Post-Dispatch, p. 2C.

BeDan, M. (1999, August 25). EAS chief to direct new branch. Rocky Mountain News, p. 2B.

Bhasin, S.; Storer, T.W.; Berman, N.; Callegari, C.; Clevenger, B.; Phillips, J.; Bunnell, T.J.; Tricker, R. ; Shirazi, A.; & Casaburi, R. (1996). The effects of supraphysiological doses of testosterone on muscle size and strength in normal men. New England Journal of Medicine, p. 1.

Bill Phillips. (2006, March 6). Bill Phillips (author). en.wikipedia.org [Online].
Blaudschun, M. (1993, September 10). Thunder being shaken from Notre Dame sky. Boston Globe, p. 82.
Blaudschun, M. (1993, September 17). Holtz has been exposed, now let's call off the dogs. Boston Globe, p. 87.
Bock, H. (1990, April 25). Tagliabue appoints Lombardo as NFL's first steroids advisor. The Associated Press [Online].
Bock, H. (1993, January 29). Tagliabue feels league has no steroid problem. The Associated Press [Online].
Bonfatti, J. (1989, August 30). Rookies' dreams sidetracked by steroid positives. The Associated Press [Online].
Boswell, T. (1990, January 27). Quick to the defense. Washington Post, p. D1.
Bowles, J. (1991, June 29). Former NFL drug czar supports Alzado's claims. The Associated Press [Online].
Brooks, B.S., Kennedy, G., Moen, D.R., & Ranly, D. (2004). Telling the story: The convergence of print, broadcast and online media (2nd ed.). Boston, MA: Bedford/St. Martin's.
Brown, B. (1993, September 7). Irish eyes not smiling about book. USA Today, p. 1C.
Brubaker, B. (1995, January 22). In NFL, supplements complement. Washington Post, p. D1.
Burwell, B. (1993, August 6). League deserves praise for rethinking drug policy. USA Today, p. 7C.
Canavan, T. (1993, July 31). Moore knew what to expect from NFL. The Associated Press [Online].
Chaney, M. (1998, October 2). Big Mac steps up to the plate; steroids awareness steps back. Kansas City Star, p. C7.
Chaney, M. (2001). Sports writers, American football, and anti-sociological bias toward anabolic drug use in the sport. Warrensburg, MO: Central Missouri State University.
Chaney, M. (2001, January 28). Despite drug testing, players get heftier. Kansas City Star, p. B9
Chaytor Admits. (1996, October 28). Chaytor admits to steroid use. The Associated Press [Online].
Chemical Found. (1990, December 10). Chemical found in possession of UT player used to mask tests. The Associated Press [Online].
Cialini, J. (1989, August 29). Eagles lose Solt to steroids, reduce roster. United Press International [Online].
Cialini, J. (1989, September 27). NFL reinstates Solt, Douglass, 9 others. United Press International [Online].
Coach Helped. (1991, July 28). Ex-Pitt coach helped order testosterone-increasing plant extract. The Associated Press.
Cole, B. (1990, July 27). Verdict means new era to Dixon. Columbia State, p. C1.

Collie Used. (1991, July 31). Eagles' Collies says he used steroids. The Associated Press [Online].

Conte, V., & Assael, S. (2004, December 13). BALCO owner comes clean. ESPN The Magazine [Online].

Cote, E. (1989, August 8). NFL drug counselor says steroids No. 1 problem for athletes. The Associated Press [Online].

Cougars Positive. (1991, June 15). Cougars tested positive for steroid use. The Associated Press [Online].

Cour, J. (1989, May 10). Knox favors random testing. The Associated Press [Online].

Courson, S., & Schreiber, L.R. (1991). False glory. Stamford, CT: Longmeadow Press.

Courson Steroids. (1990, September 21). Courson began taking steroids at South Carolina. The Associated Press [Online].

Christl, C. (1998, August 16). Supplements and diets have helped transform image from fat to fit. Milwaukee Journal Sentinel, p. 1.

Dan Duchaine. (2004). Dan Duchaine. www.afac.com [Online].

Daubenmier, J. (1990, March 27). Perles looks for silver lining. The Associated Press [Online].

Denial Again. (1990, April 4). Mandarich again denies steroid use. The Associated Press [Online].

Denlinger, K. (1992, May 15). Alzado dies at 43. Washington Post, p. C1.

Denlinger, K. (1984, January 18). The ultimate Raider opens fire. Washington Post, p. D1.

Derwin, B. (1998, September 20). A uniform drug policy needed for all sports. New York Times, p. 8—15.

Doctor Pleads. (1992, June 2). Doctor pleads guilty to trafficking in steroids. The Associated Press [Online].

'Dome' Author. (1993, September 9). 'Dome' author talks about book reaction. The Associated Press [Online].

Dominic Speaks. (1989, September 2). Dominic speaks on steroid positive. The Associated Press [Online].

Douglass Denies. (1989, August 29). Douglass denies steroid use. United Press International [Online].

Duckens Program. (1993, August 25). Duckens likely to enter a drug program. New York Times, p. B6.

Dunham, W. (1989, August 28). Judge blocks union on NFL steroid suspensions. United Press International [Online].

Dunham, W. (Hughes plans assault on steroid-pushing coaches. United Press International [Online].

Eberhart, J.M. (2001, March 11). More than a musclehead. Kansas City Star, p. I6.

Edwards, C. (1990, January 28). Northwestern will investigate steroid charges. The Associated Press [Online].

Eskenazi, G. (1989, August 24). Taking a stance against steroids in the NFL. New York Times, p. D23.

Eskenazi, G. (1991, May 20). Barnes, a shot-putter, gets NFL tryout. New York Times, p. C2.

Fans Concerned. (1989, November 30). Football fans concerned about steroid use. United Press International [Online].

Fainaru-Wada, M., & Williams, L. (2003, November 16). Romanowski got banned hormone, wife told sheriff. San Francisco Chronicle, p. A1.

Fainaru-Wada, M., & Williams, L. (2006). Game of Shadows. USA: Gotham Books.

Farmer, S., & Wharton, D. (2002, January 29). Weight matters. Los Angeles Times, p. 4—1.

Farrey, T. (1990, October 14). Negotiating his way—Tagliabue brings attorney's touch to NFL's top job. Seattle Times, p. C1.

Farrey, T. (1991, September 1). America's new national pastime. Seattle Times, p. C1

Fecteau, A. (1995). NCAA state action. Seton Hall Journal of Sport Law, 5, p. 291.

Fish, M. (1991, September 29). Steroid stigma affects even retired players. Atlanta Journal and Constitution, p. F1.

Fish, M. (1993, September 26). Steroids riskier than ever, part one. Atlanta Journal and Constitution, p. A1.

Flutie Flak. (1996, October 29). Flutie catches flak for allegation about steroids. Toronto Star, p. B1.

Forbes, G. (1999, December 10). Suspensions prompt union meeting on drugs. USA Today, p. 8C.

Forged Prescriptions. (1991, March 7). Texas players identified as authors of forged prescriptions. The Associated Press [Online].

Freeman, M. (1991, July 14). In NFL's fight against steroids, new technology is half the battle. Washington Post, p. B9.

Freeman, M. (1993, July 31). NFL suspends Moore for four games for steroid possession. New York Times, p. I29.

Freeman, M. (1993, August 8). NFL is told how players cheat on drug tests. New York Times, p. B9.

Freeman, M. (1998, May 31). NFL gets serious on supplements. Milwaukee Journal Sentinel, p. 13.

Freeman, M. (1999, August 30). Tapes show that NFL looked the other way on drug tests. New York Times [Online].

Freeman, M. (1999, September 5). Uneasy lies helmet with Broncos' logo. New York Times, p. 8—10.

Freeman, M. (2000, August 27). Drug policy loophole revealed in an appeal. New York Times, p. 8—11.

Gano, R. (1989, August 29). Packers tackles suspended 30 days. The Associated Press [Online].

Gano, R. (1999, February 2). Payton has rare liver disease. The Associated Press [Online].

Garrison, B. (1993). Sports reporting (2nd ed.). Ames, IA: Iowa State University Press.

Georgatos, D. (1991, July 13). Barnes an athlete without a sport. The Associated Press [Online].
George, T. (1990, May 20). Owners meet to confront new and old issues. New York Times, p. 8—5.
George, T. (1993, June 27). The force is with them. New York Times, p. 8—2.
Girard, F., & Dye, D. (1990, March 22). Lawmaker and MSU officials call for investigations. Detroit News [Online].
Glauber, B. (2005, September 25). After recent deaths, NFL and its players worry about weight. Newsday, p. B6.
Glickson, G., & Thomas, R.M. (1988, November 28). The Mandarich diet. New York Times, p. C2.
Goldberg, D. (1990, March 16). Changes in the Paul Tagliabue era. The Associated Press [Online].
Goldberg, D. (1990, May 31). Tagliabue said Tennant's failing was in presentation. The Associated Press [Online].
Goldberg, D. (1991, July 6). NFL opens camps with full steroid testing program for first time. The Associated Press [Online].
Greenberg, B. (1999, December 18). Researcher links Mark McGwire, increased steroid use among boys. The Associated Press [Online].
Harig, B. (1993, September 9). Bowden: Coaches beware. St. Petersburg Times, p. 6C.
Harrah, S. (1990s). Dan Duchaine unchained. Elite Fitness News [Online].
Hartman, S. (1993, September 10). Holtz has backers around these parts. Minneapolis Star Tribune, p. 2C.
Hasen, J. (1984, September 27). Alzado defends role in 'violent game.' United Press International [Online].
Henderson, J. (1999, October 24). NFL Sunday. Denver Post, p. L1.
Hickey, P. (1993, January 31). Expansion fiasco proves that CFL failed to do its homework. Montreal Gazette [Online].
Holtz Accused. (1993, August 31). Holtz accused of condoning abuses. United Press International [Online].
Holyfield, J. (1991, January 16). MSU panel finds no widespread steroid use. The Associated Press [Online].
Huffman, S., & Telander, R. (1990, August 27). 'I deserve my turn.' Sports Illustrated, p. 26.
Huizenga, R. (1994). 'You're okay, it's just a bruise.' New York, NY: St. Martin's Press.
Indoroids. (2003, November 10). Steroid use among the athletes. BodyBuildingPro.com [Online].
Itule, B.D., & Anderson, D.A. (1987). News writing and reporting for today's media. New York, NY: Random House.
Jets Waivers. (1989, September 26). Amoia and Riley waived by Jets. The Associated Press [Online].

Kelley, S. (1991, July 10). Call this chapter of Alzado story sad. Seattle Times, p. H1.

Keteyian, A. (1989). Big Red confidential: Inside Nebraska football. Chicago, IL: Contemporary Books, Inc.

Keteyian, A. (1998, August). Mass deception. Sport, p. 26.

Keteyian, A., & Jennings, P. (1997, January 22). Former player sues NFL for drug dependency [transcript]. ABC World News Tonight [Online].

Kindred, D. (2001, August 12). Bodies so powerful, yet so vulnerable. Los Angeles Times, p. 4—2

King, L. (1990, July 16). Former NFL drug advisor. CNN.

King, P. (1990, July 9). 'We can clean it up.' Sports Illustrated, p. 34.

King, P. (1991, August 5). One more lesson. Sports Illustrated, p. 15.

Kinney, B. (1990, August 26). Wearing the scars of football. New York Times, p. 8—1.

Klis, M. (2005, October 14). Romo juiced while a Bronco. Denver Post, p. A1.

Knapp, G. (1997, September 16). Football is a guilty pleasure. San Francisco Examiner [Online].

Kornheiser, T. (1991, July 16). Another test for the NFL. Washington Post, p. E1.

Kravitz, B. (1993, November 13). Seeing red over green: Irish purity is pure blarney. St. Louis Post-Dispatch, p. 3C.

Kubat, T. (1992, September 15). Legs like redwood trees and arms like oak trees. Lafayette Journal-Courier [Online].

Lane, W.E. (1993, October 1). Walsh takes pains not to antagonize Holtz. The Associated Press [Online].

Lapchick, R.E. (1986). Fractured focus: Sport as a reflection of society. Lexington, MA: Lexington Books/D.C. Health Co.

Lawry, Edward G. (1991, May 1). Conflicting interests make reform of college sports impossible. Chronicle of Higher Education, p. A44.

Layden, T. (1998, July 27). Power play. Sports Illustrated, p. 61.

Lederman, D. (1991, March 13). Big sports programs are out of control, most say in survey. Chronicle of Higher Education, p. A33.

Legwold, J. (2005, October 13). Romanowski comes clean on steroid use. Rocky Mountain News [Online].

Lesko, R. (1997, August 19). NFL suspends Vikings' Artie Ulmer. The Associated Press [Online].

Lewis, D. (1994, March 2). 'Engineered food' pumps up firm. Rocky Mountain News, p. 42A.

Lipsyte, R. (1991, July 12). The cancer in football and pro wrestling. New York Times, p. B13.

Litke, J. (1989, September 28). Douglass back on bubble with Bears. The Associated Press [Online].

Litke, J. (1992, September 23). NFL preaches bigger is better. The Associated Press [Online].

Litke, J. (1999, January 29). Getting bigger, stronger and faster—for free. The Associated Press [Online].

Litsky, F. (1993, January 14). Giants' Moore facing felony steroid charges. New York Times, p. B11.

Litsky, F. (1993, January 15). DEA says more players are at risk. New York Times, p. B9.

Littwin, M. (1998, August 27). Product's promotion very questionable. Rocky Mountain News, p. 2C.

Long Positive. (1991, July 25). Steelers' Long tests positive for steroids. United Press International [Online].

Lowitt, B. (1993, January 15). Wyche surprised by steroid charges against Duckens. St. Petersburg Times, p. 6C.

Lowitt, B., & Topkin, M. (1993, January 14). Duckens indicted on steroid charges. St. Petersburg Times, p. 1C.

Magee, J. (1999, October 31). The 300-pound lineman, once a rarity, is now the norm in the NFL. San Diego Union Tribune [Online].

Maly, R. (1990, August 23). Osborne strongly defends college football. Des Moines Register [Online].

Mandarich Passes. (1989, September 13). Mandarich passes steroid test for Packers. United Press International [Online].

Manoyan, D. (1999, November 2). Payton, 45, NFL's top rusher with 16,726 career yards, dies of rare liver disease. Milwaukee Journal Sentinel, p. News 1.

Maraniss, D. (1996, December 10). In NFL, the beef goes on. Washington Post, p. C1.

Mariotti, J. (1993, November 12). Why is America afraid to check under the dome? Chicago Sun-Times, p. 123.

Martin, D.S. (1989, September 14). Penn State asked opponents to submit players for testing. The Associated Press[Online].

Martinez, M. (1991, July 28). Black and silver and controversy all over. New York Times, p. 8—1.

Martzke, R. (1993, September 2). Bradshaw's wish: Chiefs-49ers finale. USA Today, p. 3C.

Martzke, R. (1993, September 9). Irish receive support from unlikely places. USA Today, p. 3C.

Marvez, A. (1998, May 28). NFL eyes nutritional substance. Rocky Mountain News, p. 1C.

McCartney, S. (1990, January 11). NCAA takes evolutionary steps. The Associated Press [Online].

McDonough, W. (1989, May 11). He knows of steroid danger. Boston Globe, p. 77.

Meisel, B. (1993, October 31). The muscle hustle. New York Daily News, p. 86.

Meisel, B. (1993, November 1). Cheating & beating a flawed system. New York Daily News, p. 48.

Meisel, B. (1993, November 2). Steroid stories. New York Daily News.

Melani, D. (2000, December 5). Experts weigh in on programs that promise taut bods in a few weeks. Rocky Mountain News [Online].

Mihoces, G. (1991, August 28). Tagliabue rules out pay-per-view until '94. USA Today, p. 10C.

Mihoces, G. (1992, May 15). Alzado dies of cancer. USA Today, p. 2C.

Miklasz, B. (1996, December 2). Telephone interview with author.

Montville, L. (1998, June 22). Passing time. Sports Illustrated, p. 58.

Moore, Duckens. (1993, January 13). Moore and Duckens indicted in steroid charges. The Associated Press [Online].

Moore, T. (1991, July 28). Another Alzado perspective. Atlanta Journal and Constitution, p. E3.

Moran, M. (1993, September 14). How to make Notre Dame's dome shine. New York Times, p. B11.

Morrissey, R. (1995, January 10). Drug suspicions still dog football. Rocky Mountain News, p. 17B.

MSU Probe. (1990, March 22). MSU to probe steroid drug testing. United Press International [Online].

MSU Refutes. (1990, March 21). MSU officials refute report of widespread steroid use by football players. United Press International [Online].

Murphy, A. (1993, November 22). Round 1 to the Irish. Sports Illustrated, p. 12.

Murphy, A. (1998, May 25). Taking his medicine. Sports Illustrated, p. 56.

Muscle Media. (1996, May). Muscle Media 2000 Magazine. www.getbig.com [Online].

Nadel, J. (1985, August 1). Alzado has image of tough guy with loose screws. The Associated Press [Online].

Nadel, J. (1993, August 26). Howie Long one of first to scream about steroids. The Associated Press [Online].

NCAA Manual. (1989, March). 1989-90 NCAA manual. Overland Park, KS: NCAA Publications.

Newman, B. (1990, July 26). South Carolina avoids major punishment for steroids mess. United Press International [Online].

Newton, D. (1990, July 27). SI's Telander dismayed by decision. The State, p. C1.

Nevius, C.W. (1992, May 16). Alzado stayed in character to the end. San Francisco Chronicle, p. D1.

NFL Doesn't. (1993, January 15). NFL does not believe it has steroid problem. The Associated Press [Online].

NFL Policy. (1991, August 21). NFL's policy helps cut use of steroids, but testing often inaccurate. The Associated Press [Online].

NFL Survey. (1999, February). National Football League players survey. Sport, p. 34.

No Probe. (1990, April 3). Texas not expected to probe reported steroid use. United Press International [Online].

Nordiques Coach. (1990, June 1). Last-place finish costs Nordiques coach his job. USA Today, p. 13C.

Northwestern President. (1990, March 8). Northwestern president says steroid use isolated, not widespread. The Associated Press [Online].

Not Serious. (1989, July 5). Magazine says NFL problem not as serious. The Associated Press [Online].

Notre Dame Denials. (1990, August 24). Huffman discusses Notre Dame's fervent denials. The Associated Press [Online].

Oates, B. (1993, January 30). Tagliabue vague about drug issues. Los Angeles Times [Online].

O'Brien, R. (1993, January 25). Question of substance. Sports Illustrated, p. 9.

O'Hara, M. (1990, March 14). National Football League takes stronger stand at eliminating steroids. Detroit News [Online].

Ostler, S. (2001, September 9). The big, the bad, and the baddest. Chronicle Magazine, p. 16.

Ostler, S. (2005, October 17). Romo's words don't ring true. San Francisco Chronicle [Online].

Pasquarelli, L. (1991, July 16). Blaming steroids. Atlanta Journal and Constitution, p. D1.

Paterno Concerned. (1990, August 22). Paterno concerned about steroids. United Press International [Online].

Pearlman, J. (1999, February 22). A hard burden to bear. Sports Illustrated, p. 28.

Polish, J. (2002). Joe Polish interviews Shawn Phillips. www.thegenuisnetwork.com [Online].

Posnanski, J. (1997, August 10). What happened to the fun and games? Kansas City Star, p. C1.

Quotelines. (1989, August 31). Quotelines. USA Today, p. 10A.

Rabun, M. (1993, January 29). NFL expansion on schedule. United Press International [Online].

Rabun, M. (1994, January 27). Steroid ban benefits Nate Newton. United Press International [Online].

Raffo, D. (1990, March 14). NFL expands drug testing. United Press International [Online].

Raffo, D. (1990, March 16). Tagliabue takes control at NFL meetings. United Press International [Online].

Reilly, R. (1998, September 7). The good father. Sports Illustrated [Online].

Reilly, R. (1999, February 1). Lip shtick. Sports Illustrated, p. 40.

Richman, H. (2000, September 22). Hungry for success. Kansas City Star, p. D18.

Reusse, P. (1993, September 9). Holtz book a wakeup call only to Rip Van Winkle types. Minneapolis Star Tribune, p. 1C.

Rhoden, W.C. (1990, January 11). NCAA stiffens drug penalties and expands testing in football. New York Times, p. A1.

Rhoden, W.C. (1992, October 29). Call it the lock of the Irish. New York Times, p. B17.

Rivera, G. (1992, January 22). Now it can be told [transcript]. Investigative News Group [Online].

Robinson, A. (1991, July 26). Long was distraught about impending suspension. The Associated Press [Online].

Romanowski, B., Schefter, A., & Towle, P. (2005). Romo: My life on the edge. New York, NY: William Morrow.

Rushin, S. (1998, August 10). Throwing in the towel. Sports Illustrated, p. 17.

Samson, D. (2004, August 29). Lincoln: Land of linemen. Kansas City Star, p. J6.

Schwartz, J. (1993, September 10). Giants Moore draws probation and a fine. New York Times, p. B16.

Scoppe, R. (1990, February 19). South Carolina reports to NCAA on 'steroid scandal.' The Associated Press [Online].

Scoppe, R. (1990, February 21). South Carolina report lacks definitive answer on steroid users. The Associated Press [Online].

Scoppe, R. (1990, July 26). South Carolina football program escapes sanctions. The Associated Press [Online].

Scruggs, K. (1993, January 14). Officials: 2 NFL players 'pawns' in steroid ring. Atlanta Journal and Constitution, p. E1.

Shultz Says. (1989, May 10). Schultz says NCAA can't get a grip on steroids. The Associated Press [Online].

Simers, T.J. (1999, August 31). NFL-Gate: Execs, lies, videotape. Los Angeles Times, p. D1.

SJS Program. (1990, June 12). Study finds drug abuse in SJS program. United Press International [Online].

Slater, J. (1990, August 22). Holtz denies steroid allegations. United Press International [Online].

Smith, T.W. (1991, July 3). NFL's steroid policy too lax, doctor warns. New York Times [Online].

Smith, T.W. (1991, July 29). Teammate's troubles cloud Steelers camp. New York Times, p. C1.

Spain, Z. (2007, May 16). 2 cents. Florida Times-Union [Online].

Spear, B. (1992, July 7). Telephone interview with author.

Spindler Disputes. (1990, April 24). Spindler disputes positive steroid test. United Press International [Online].

Stack, J. (1990, May 14). Eye openers. St. Louis Post-Dispatch, p. 2C.

Star Player. (1991, March 19). Star player accused of falsifying drug test. United Press International [Online].

Starkman, R. (1996, November 3). How widespread a problem is steroid use among athletes. Toronto Star, p. C12.

Steeler Choice. (1990, April 29). Steeler draft choice tested positive for steroids. United Press International [Online].

Stellino, V. (1991, July 21). Manley says steroids used more by whites. Baltimore Sun, p. 7F.

Steroids Attitude. (1996, May 19). Steroids still fuel win-at-any-cost attitude. St. Louis Post-Dispatch, p. 3F.

Stinson, T. (1999, January 27). Broncos tread fine line. Atlanta Journal and Constitution, p. 11F.

Stroud, R. (1991, August 1). Versatility is key to Bax's survival in Tampa Bay. St. Louis Post-Dispatch, p. 1D.

Taber, A. (1999, November 18). 'Roid rage. Salon.com [Online].

Tackle Suspended. (1990, October 25). Texas coach suspends reserve tackle. The Associated Press [Online].

Tagliabue Congress. (1990, March 23). Tagliabue tells Congress testing will help rid steroid use. The Associated Press [Online].

Telander, R. (1989). The hundred yard lie. New York, NY: Simon & Schuster.

Telander, R. (1989, April 24). The big enchilada. Sports Illustrated, p. 40.

Tench, M. (1991, September 1). The curse of steroids makes it a testing time for the NFL. The Independent [Online].

Testing Defended. (1990, March 12). Michigan State defends drug testing program for athletes. United Press International [Online].

Texas Denies. (1990, April 11). Texas denies steroid use among athletes. United Press International [Online].

Texas Players. (1990, April 1). Twenty-five Texas players used steroids since 1986 ban on the drugs. The Associated Press [Online].

Thomas, J. (1988, April 24). Berkeley High grad Moore could go near top of draft. St. Louis Post-Dispatch, p. 6G.

Thomas, J. (1990, September 11). K-State 335-pounder is more than just a novelty. St. Louis Post-Dispatch, p. 5C.

Thomas, J. (1993, January 14). St. Louisan indicted in steroid case. St. Louis Post-Dispatch, p. D1.

Tucker, D. (1990, June 27). NCAA Presidents Commission always has clout, sometimes lacks answers. The Associated Press [Online].

Underwood, J. (1990, December 30). Keep the college bowls, but clean up the mess. New York Times, p. S9.

Utterback, B. (1987, September 2). Battle against steroids picks up steam. Pittsburgh Press, p. B1.

Vaughan, K. (1998, June 28). EAS bulks up with creatine, Broncos. Rocky Mountain News, p. 1C.

Vaughan, K. (1998, June 28). Supplement star shoots for silver screen. Rocky Mountain News, p. 15C.

Vaughan, K. (1998, June 28). NFL jury still out on creatine use. Rocky Mountain News, p. 17C.

Vecsey, G. (1993, January 15). All muscles not the same, rats prove. New York Times, p. B9.

Vint, T. (1989, September 2). Osborne says book isn't all bad. The Associated Press [Online].

Weir, T. (1993, November 10). Notre Dame myth outshines The Book. USA Today, p. 3C.

Whelan, B. (1999, May). The drug problem is worse than ever! The Iron Master [Online].

Whitlock, J. (2000, August 24). There's no stopping steroid use. Kansas City Star, p. D1.

Wieberg, S. (1989, February 10). Sooners tackle adversity. USA Today, p. 1C.

Wilstein, S. (1994, January 26). Gap between football linemen and sumo wrestlers blurs. The Associated Press [Online].

Wishart, N. (2002, July 2). Workout wizard. St. Louis Post-Dispatch [Online].

Witosky, T. (1990, January 14). College athletes face increased penalties for steroids. USA Today [Online].

Wolper, A. (1997, December 27). Worship on the sports page. Editor and Publisher [Online].

Wyman, T.P. (1990, August 22). Lou Holtz denies widespread steroid use. The Associated Press [Online].

Wyman, T.P. (1990, August 24). Two years ago Holtz was hailed as another Rockne. The Associated Press [Online].

Yaeger, D., & Looney, D.S. (1993). Under the tarnished dome. New York, NY: Simon & Schuster.

Yesalis, C.E. (2001, January 17). Telephone interview with author.

Yesalis, C.E., Ed. (2000). Anabolic steroids in sport and exercise (2nd edition). Champaign, IL: Human Kinetics.

Yesalis, C.E., & Coward, V.S. (1998). The steroids game. Champaign, IL: Human Kinetics.

Yesalis, C.E., & Kammerer, C. (1990, February 4). The strengths and frailties of drug tests. New York Times, p. 8—10.

Yost, P. (1989, August 28). About two dozen NFL players test positive. The Associated Press [Online].

Zagaroli, L. (1990, March 13). Michigan State officials say drug guidelines work. The Associated Press [Online].

Zucco, T. (1989, August 30). NFL needs to come clean, discontinue flawed steroid tests. St. Petersburg Times, p. 1C.

Chapter 7

Football Word

Communication of football doping; construct spiral of denial

"Out There, the 'people we fly over,' as network executives refer to so-called Middle Americans, think Joe Namath is larger than life Why? Because we told them so. And now, no matter what happens, even if the press changes its mind, we're stuck with our monster."

Robert Lipsyte
sportswriter, 1975

A fresh sportswriter I was in 1987, and one challenged to meet my obligations under press ethics and law — lessons I had skipped in college. Clueless of proper boundaries, I groped for understanding, especially coming from my former campus universe of jock life and coaching.

At baseball spring training in Florida, my journalistic dilemma was about reporting details, or not, of an athlete's more private life. Working up a feature on Mets wonder Dwight Gooden, the New York media sensation and a young pitcher I followed as a fan, I questioned whether his off-field affairs should make headlines. Yeah, Gooden was starting to screw up, fathering a child out of wedlock, scuffling with a policeman, shouting at a rental-car agent in an airport: But whose business was all that?

A famed broadcaster provided guidance, Bob Costas, during an interview for the story. Costas, an acquaintance of mine from St. Louis, said everything newsworthy involving public figures must be reported, especially on celebrity ballplayers who reaped fortunes from the media spotlight. Gooden in baseball, Jordan in basketball, Montana in football, Gretzky, hockey — each really made his millions in the fame game, the cultural popularity contest conducted by media, not athletic competition.

Teaching me as much as commenting, Costas explained that any superstar of sport would play just for fun, no money, if not for media's spinning up gold around games. In support, Costas referenced historical points on sports writing, pulling notes instantly and precisely from memory. The industry had evolved, he said, from mythologizing a Babe Ruth to more modern shifts such as info-digging on athletes, the signature of the *New York Daily News* scribe Dick Young, and investigative reporting on public issues, *Sports Illustrated's* forte since the 1960s.

Media made sport into prime pop culture, entertainment of enormous value, and Costas, though empathic of the 22-year-old Gooden, said celebrity athletes must accept bad press with the good, if accurately reported. "It's an extraordinary circumstance for him to be placed under; it is very difficult," Costas said. "But I think it's fair in a sense that it's to be expected."

Costas described a giant scene in Manhattan, covering one side of a building and visible for blocks: a mural of Gooden in action, Mets colors blazing. "I guess that this is the price — that kind of pressure and attention — it's his price to pay for his performance and the rewards," Costas said. "The contract he signed with the Mets, the lucrative endorsements and the other attention, I'm sure he enjoys that. So it's just the other side of the coin."

Costas made well his argument, leaving a right impression with me, and fortunately for my story on "Doctor K" Gooden. Published in suburban St. Louis, the copy was still biased in the athlete's favor — especially after an editor tacked on a gushy ending — but at least I made no apology for him. Soon after, the Costas lesson deepened for me, upon the news that Gooden had entered drug detoxification; my story retained credibility, and I had Costas to thank. The helpful broadcaster's advice was a beginning step toward realizing my role as a journalist, my *duty* as member of the *free press*, the only private enterprise afforded constitutional protection in America.

Therefore, it was personally regrettable, five years later, to end up haranguing Costas about doing *his* job. By then I had left daily media in part over ethics, or the unwillingness of sportswriters and editors to address the systematic ills of athletics, and Costas was among journalists nationwide who drew my ire on the issue of football doping. I implored him by letter to investigate and report, but he would not.

"Matt — I'm in a bind," Costas replied by postcard. " I'm impressed by your reasoning & your passion. I would like nothing better than to do <u>real</u> sports documentaries & reporting. My present commitments constrict me. Worthy though it is, I haven't got the necessary time to tackle this issue now independently, & [NBC's NFL] pre-game formats and approach don't allow for it. A year or so from now, I'll be doing different things. Please stay in touch. Bob Costas." Only a few months before at the summer Olympics, Costas and NBC loudly accused Chinese female swimmers of doping, based on rumor and speculative evidence, the women's physical changes and performance increases. Yet, back on American soil, NBC gave a free pass to football players, the most obvious juicers in the world of major sports. Other U.S. media acted same during the 1990s, including *Sports Illustrated*, which chased Irish swimmer Michelle Smith for doping suspicion while ignoring gargantuan football players at home, pro, college, and prep.

I understood, relatively speaking. When a public issue struck sport, the media really were about hatin' the player, not the game, despite claims of allegedly tough writers and commentators. Costas, after all, *could not* touch the story of muscle substances in football for NBC, and at least he was honest with me. Ninety-nine percent of sports journalists I hammered privately, for their laxness on football doping, would not answer. They could not, having to choose between acknowledging hard truths or spewing bullshit, in response to me.

Neither disappointed nor surprised, I knew the restraint Costas felt about word on steroids and growth hormone in football. The topic was one to avoid in *my* circles, too, from college and prep football to media and grid fandom. Virtually nowhere could I find someone to engage me on football's muscle doping; always, it seemed, I ended up talking to myself. Whenever I babbled to friends about 'roids or HGH in football, just watching a TV game together somewhere, I got a few nods askance and nothing else.

Their eyes stayed fixed on the tube, ears trained to inane announcers. Seemingly, no one wanted to hear about this special problem, nor see it, speak it — a social phenomena that broadcaster Howard Cosell explained as "inexorable force working against revelations of truth about sports in America."

The squelching of information about football doping was exerted rather simply, via mass media or across a family room, and imperative for protecting the image of the revered institution. And it was a familiar communication dynamic in history, evident in other times, domains, and issues, often described in phrase or metaphor such as *information control*, *sin of omission*, *conspiracy of silence*, *elephant in the room*, *taboo subject*, *Loose lips sink ships*, or *When in Rome, do as Romans do*. For my football analysis, the term *spiral of denial* was in deference to media analyst Elisabeth Noelle-Neumann, author of Spiral of Silence, the theoretical force of public opinion. Communication critic Stanley Cohen, author of the acclaimed *States of Denial*, established Spiral of Denial as theory, but admittedly I was oblivious until the final week of this manuscript's preparation. Even without reading Cohen, relying only on brief critiques, I presumed to grasp precisely his spiral of denial. Football had taught me the model like nothing other, regarding drugs, violence, and other game ills.

So who and what were behind the denial spiraling about muscle substances in American football? The collaboration was no conspiracy, initially at least, but an outgrowth of the modern game's bonding with specific technologies: television and pharmaceutical drugs. Post-World War II, American football became highly conducive to mass entertainment and drug use as well, and the former was not enhanced by ugly truths of the latter.

As the Golden Age press once glossed over violence, to ensure survival of the game and its lucrative content, modern media so ignored football's drug addictions, particularly to avoid upsetting the children's market, which in turn pushed their parents' patronage. In general, the feeding of team games as virtue to generations of American youth had stimulated growth for both media and sport, according to analysts such as Koppett, Lipsyte, and Oriard. The standard media approach, absurd and necessary, meant painting games and athletes as moral beacons of an amoral universe.

The net result for football's doping, then, was to chill speech on amphetamines, painkillers, and especially muscle substances, developed over time among parties committed to sustaining the game: players, organizers including coaches, lawmakers, fans, and the media.

Of all, however, the press had to leave the eternal football party, sober up about drugs, and get to work on effecting positive change, before hope was eclipsed. Studies showed news media had to become *the* critical agents for impacting change. Iconoclastic journalists would have to drive reform in any such issue: war, civil rights, doping in favored games. To ignite a turnabout, reporters, photographers, editors, and producers would have to thoroughly investigate, and therein lay the abominable conflict of interest over drugs in football.

Sport media's essential existence was not about exposing a repulsive problem in football, despite journalistic protocol, but instead about weaving pleasant gridiron mythology, their mode since the Victorian Era. The accurate reporting of this game's doping reality would translate into very bad business for the American media, violating the historic economic synergy between football and the popular press — the foremost example of the sport-media complex.

"Newspapers, radio and television… have prudently presented sports as entertainment," observed author James A. Michener. "Consequently, one of the happiest relationships in American society is that between sports and the media. This interface is delightfully symbiotic, since each helps the other survive." Some critics blessed the arrangement during the 1980s, pardoning TV networks in particular. "Big Television and Big Sports are interlocked in a common interest," Ron Powers, Pulitzer Prize-winning media analyst, wrote for *Inside Sports* magazine. "TV's mission is to make sports as attractive a package as possible — so as to catch an audience for delivery to advertisers. By what perversion of human nature should those same Big Sports Departments be expected to turn around and act as adversary watchdogs upon activities of their business partners?"

No perversion, but constitutional duty, cried critics calling for press action on athletics, for increased attention on public issues involved. Cosell railed against the media's role in the sport spiral of denial, for vital reasons, he said, tied to the culture's being. "Only rarely does one ever read or hear about how sports in the current era inextricably intertwine with the law, the politics, the sociology, the education, and the medical care of the society," Cosell wrote in his 1985 autobiography, *I Never Played The Game*. "The world of sports today is endlessly complex, an ever-spinning spiral of deceit, immorality, absence of ethics, and defiance of the public interest." Cosell qualified television, the medium that made him a cultural icon, as "all garbarge," and he was contemptuous toward sports content in general, broadcast, wire service, or print. Sports were known as media's Toy Department, but critics like Cosell warned the merry presumption was faulty and dangerous.

Sportswriter Robert Lipsyte, whom Cosell admired, concurred. Lipsyte viewed sports as potentially the "deadliest" news content, and he characterized modern America's sport obsession as a "concentration camp" for children and "emotional Disneyland" for parents.

I. NFL Rides Media to Become Money Monolith

When Pete Rozelle retired as NFL commissioner in 1989, some league officials worried about going on without him. "It would be nice if we could get another commissioner like Pete Rozelle — someone who could come into this league young and do a bang-up job for 30 years," said Tex Schramm, Dallas executive. "But that is not going to happen. There is only one Pete Rozelle."

The legend himself, however, was bullish on league futures. Rozelle, shrewdly cognizant of the continuing impact by its partner media, knew the NFL would deepen market saturation through new mediums like cable TV and satellite, if not computer.

"The next 30 years we'll see as much growth and change as ever before," he said. "I don't think the last 30 will compare to the next 30 years." Paul Tagliabue saw to that, and Rozelle lived long enough to witness astonishing NFL growth under his successor. Eventually, the NFL's Tagliabue earned the moniker "megalith," only 17 years post-Rozelle.

American football was monolithic by the 2000s, accounting for roughly one-tenth of sport's business in the world, with the collegiate and prep games exploding along with the professional. Football created — or orchestrated, critics alleged — a full cultural experience every autumn.

The NFL alone commanded upwards of $6 billion in revenue for the year 2006, boasting prime global recognition and wielding influence over media, government, consumers, non-fan taxpayers — American life in general. The NFL left nearest competitors far behind, Major League Baseball and the NBA, while burying the NHL, hardly considered a major sport anymore. *The Washington Post* called the NFL "the richest and most highly rated professional league in the United States… a major force in popular culture, with its imprint stamped on video games, music and fashion."

League owners were initially drawn to Tagliabue for his legal skills and Washington connections, but his business acumen hugely benefited them. A ruthless negotiator, Tags stared down powerful TV networks, ignoring their complaints of financial losses on NFL games; he sent NBC packing in 1998, for example, until it came crawling back, seven years later. Tags was 3-for-3 in homeruns for TV negotiations during his tenure, scoring record broadcast packages every time. "Known for pursuing its corporate goals aggressively, the NFL is viewed by some as a tough — even bullying — negotiator," *The Post* observed. "Its huge popularity gives it leverage in deal-making and in enforcing strict rules on how its business partners portray the brand."

One media client described the NFL image as "not a negotiable thing," an unwritten rule apparent in the league's banning of local TV cameras from sidelines. League spokesmen explained the move prevented any "unauthorized" game footage, even if shot in stadiums largely bankrolled by tax dollars. The league controlled as much as possible, down to the appearance of players, who conformed to uniform dress codes, wearing that NFL-licensed apparel correctly, or they paid fines.

The president of CBS Sports, Sean McManus, fell in line for the NFL: "From my seat in television sports, the more you look at the landscape, the more the NFL continues to distance itself from every other sport in terms of ratings, in terms of interest, in terms of magnitude of the game," he said prior to the 2003 Super Bowl. "It seems to me the NFL is becoming more and more dominant." Furthering the point, McManus said the league was "becoming not just the dominant *sports* programming on television, but in a lot of ways the dominant *television* programming of all types."

The league began new TV contracts in 2006 that would command $24 billion over six to eight years, from among NBC, CBS, Fox, ESPN, and DirecTV. The bonanza meant each of 32 NFL franchises started collecting about $100 million annually from television alone, up from about $90 million previously.

The NFL also mobilized its own television network, in a tough response to

Comcast's balking at the league price of $500 million per year for a Thursday-Saturday package. Reportedly low-balled by a Comcast counteroffer of $400 million, Tagliabue did not blink, according to the *Los Angeles Business Journal.* Those games were simply placed with the NFL Network, the league's own cable- and direct-TV apparatus in need of bait for carriers, anyway. Rich Eisen, NFL Network broadcaster, crowed about the monopolistic power play. The added games made the NFL Network "even stronger," said Eisen, formerly of ESPN. "The cable operators who have said we weren't worthy of distribution now have to consider what subscribers want. The NFL is the gold standard." Its own TV network was but one example of the league's self-contained sport-media complex, which also included NFL Radio and NFL.com, its highly popular Web site.

Elsewhere, pricey league offspring included NFL Mobile, the product of a $600-million agreement with Sprint Nextel, providing shows, audio, and text downloads via cell phones, and Tagliabue mentioned the possibility of live game feeds for the medium. The NFL, anticipating audience trends, was ready to capitalize as viewers moved away from mere stationary TV to access live content on the Internet and hand-held wireless. In video games, editions of the single title *Madden NFL* had sold some 50 million copies since 1989, and the "07" version released in 2006 grossed $100 million its first week.

Journalists could not account for the sponsorships or deals cut by the NFL, and franchises and officials did not clarify the list, if they knew in any given week. In the 2000s, bounty on NFL trademarks sprang from a myriad of sources, including: $300 million from Coors, as the official beer; $120 million from Viacom, AOL, and SportsLine.com, for operating the NFL site; $120 million from Invesco Funds Group, for naming rights to Denver's new stadium; and $250 million from Reebok for apparel. The league was cutting into the billion-dollar market for "fantasy football," and realized $700 million from Houston businessman Bob McNair, expansion fee for his new franchise, which in turn promptly banked $17 million in "personal-seat licenses" sold to fans over the Internet.

The league's Midas touch flourished in traditional revenue streams, including the income at stadium sites such as gate and concessions. A million fans converged at stadiums nationwide on NFL Sunday, snapping up every ticket at premium prices and entering assorted money traps. They pulled cash and spent it, an army of walk-in consumerism, and franchises drew fortunes from inflated pricing for parking, food, beverages, merchandise, and more.

Understandably, in early 2006, the vast majority of NFL owners were sorry to see Tagliabue announce his pending retirement. Values of income and capital holdings had skyrocketed under his leadership. Thanks to an aggressive tactic by Tagliabue, virtually every taxpayer in America had contributed handsomely to ownership's wealth. He had seen 17 new stadiums erected and five existing lavishly renovated, costing billions in public funds. Highly effective had been a stock strategy by NFL Tagliabue: threatening to leave cities that balked at funding stadium construction. Some metro municipalities, by "saving" NFL football for the present, assumed debt that would carry for a century.

Paul Tagliabue had critics, including a few owners he clashed with, but he was extraordinarily effective in his job as NFL commissioner, 1989 to 2006. "Pro football has been the No. 1 sport in America for years, but under Paul's leadership, the NFL has become the dominant sports league in the world," told Alex Spanos, San Diego owner, to the *Kansas City Star*. "His vision has helped the league stay on the forefront for a new generation. The NFL's TV and media packages are second to none. The league has taken full advantage of new technologies and the Internet. The league added more fans around the world through NFL Europe and [its] American Bowl games.

"Bottom line: He oversaw the greatest period of growth in league history and was able to maintain labor peace at the same time, which to me was his greatest accomplishment. Both the owners and players as well as the fans are enjoying the rewards of his leadership."

The media had to be just as grateful to Tag's NFL, most assuredly client TV networks. The Super Bowl, for example, was seen by half of Americans while the broadcast maintained a massive share of at least 40 percent of households, raising advertising rates to exceed $2 million for a 30-second spot. "The NFL is the premier sports property in the world, bar none," said Dean Bonham, consultant. Neal Pilson, former CBS president, called the Super Bowl a "unique and rare" property with a "permanent hold on the American Public."

In a case study of NFL mania for businesses, personnel at CBS prayed — openly — for regaining game rights in 1998, then rejoiced when they won the AFC contract, a less desirable package composed primarily of second-tier markets. "Some have been moved to tears," McManus reported from headquarters in New York. "There have been a lot of hugs, a lot of high fives, a lot of stories, a lot of smiles. Everyone in the hallways is beaming. It's a great day for this network."

Fox had driven up bidding for NFL rights, starting in 1993 with a then-unheard-of $2 billion. Tagliabue scored big in his first television negotiations, and Fox continued paying extravagantly despite declared losses on NFL advertising, including a write-off of $387 million for 2001. "It is the perfect sport for television," said Artie Kempner, Fox director of NFL games. "There are natural timeouts and stoppages in play so you can show replays and get the commercials in without missing any action. [And the] fact the games are a week apart allows for a tremendous buildup." Announcer John Madden wondered if NFL content was not reaching over-exposure, but, he said, "No matter what they do, they can't really screw it up."

Executives at NBC once walked away from escalating rates for the NFL, with sports chairman Dick Ebersol griping about the broadcasts as overpriced. But NBC gladly reentered NFL bidding in 2005, coughing up $3.6 billion to win a six-year deal. Apparently, NBC had come around to embrace the industry view of the NFL as a loss leader of programming, driving up numbers for other shows in audience and share. "When you have the NFL on your network, you have viewers looking for you and tuning you in," Bonham said. "You're selling advertising, and you're making money." In Kansas City, the NBC affiliate welcomed back NFL programming. "It's a really huge deal for the network and for us," said Jack Harry, local sports anchor. "It's all about identity in our business and nothing identifies you more than the NFL. Now we're a player."

The media treasured its business with football, and society generally sanctioned the relationship, but critics thought it rotten. *Los Angeles City Beat* columnist Donnell Alexander derided the sport-media complex behind NFL success, in a commentary titled "Winning Ugly," with the sub-head: "American football is fabulous product, but players, owners, and the sports media are tangled up in a soul-robbing corporate sack dance."

Alexander noted the media frenzy over Randy Moss and marijuana, the All-Pro wideout's discussion of his use and the resultant avalanche of coverage — dated news, since Moss was known for smoking weed as far back as college. Nevertheless, reporters fixated for days on one athlete's pot smoking, constituting media hypocrisy, according to Alexander. "That would be the very same collection of reporters that looks every which way but at the subject when the issue is heavy drugs in pro sports," Alexander charged, continuing:

> Here's how it jumps off: The NFL is so far up inside ESPN that the two exchange media executives and on-air personalities like Hollywood swingers. So deeply getting down that, a couple years back, when ESPN dared air the fictional drama Playmakers, which speculates on what goes on in locker rooms, the league… forced the network to cancel its highest-rated scripted show ever. Cold bitch-slapped the Worldwide Leader in Sports like, don't even think about shining light on what goes on 'round these parts.

Undeniably, TV owed its existence, in part, to its lucrative business with football, so networks were the easy targets of media criticism for overlooking the ills in the game.

Newspapers and magazines were just as culpable though, with a longer history of "sanitizing" football reality to fit public taste, per Courson's description of gridiron mythology. Newspapers and magazines, which Oriard identified as original hosts of the sport-media complex in America, had been incestuous with football since the 1870s. Print media were addicted to football content, according to modern insider analysts like Lipsyte, and Cosell, and generally they were the same as television, prone to protecting a sport rather than policing it. "Newspapers frequently contain strong criticism of a team's management or performance," Koppett wrote, "but never any opposition to its existence."

Cosell was harsh on TV colleagues for shallowness on football, especially the "Jockocracy" of ex-NFL players occupying jobs, but he ripped print media, too. During the 1980s, Cosell insinuated that the NFL was centrally more powerful than government, and every medium was to blame. "Take the *Boston Globe*," Cosell said, "which had the courage to publish the Pentagon Papers, but for three weeks, [until after a Super Bowl], they hold a stinking drug story about a stinking football team. Something's very wrong in this country."

Lipsyte had grown up lukewarm about sports in New York, but following his college graduation in 1957 ended up a sportswriter for *The Times* where "all the news fit to print" actually was not printed. Local sports teams and athletes always caught breaks from the esteemed publication, like Yankees stalwarts Mickey Mantle and Yogi Berra, both of whom Lipsyte found to be crude and rude in person, verbally abusive with media and fans. *Times* management insisted on a stock mythology of The Mick and Yogi, the happy portrayals preserving them as heroic, fun figures. Editors would not publish Lipsyte notes about Berra's real persona as a profane jerk, nor Mantle's cursing him — "Go fuck yourself," said the superstar to the young sportswriter — because such negative references drew complaints from readers and sports officials. The public would not tolerate such casting of Mick and Yogi, truth be damned. The implicit mission for the *Times Sports*, therefore, was the same as at any paper in America — "placid rivers of ink...," Lipsyte recalled, "because no one in the Sports Department wanted to rock the boat and no one from Outside cared."

Years before, cultural critic Sut Jhally established the term "sport-media complex," for the alliance of sports with media and other institutions like government, education, and healthcare. Lipsyte fashioned the label *SportsWorld*, the title of his acclaimed 1975 book. "SportsWorld is a grotesque distortion of sports," Lipsyte explained. "It has made the finish more important than the race, and extolled the game as that William Jamesian absurdity, a moral equivalent to war, and the hero of the game as that Henry Jamesian absurdity, a 'muscular Christian.' It has surpassed patriotism and piety as a currency of communication, while exploiting them both."

Lipsyte observed that no one escaped SportsWorld in America; children, even, were classified as athletes or spectators by puberty, and writers entered "the fray" at their peril. And Lipsyte himself strove to be a *journalist* in sports, an objective reporter of the good and bad; he refused to shy from tough topics. "Lipsyte was concerned about public-policy issues — violence, racism, drugs, unions, etc.," Cosell recalled. "He was perceptive and dead honest, unafraid to probe for the truth." Naturally, Lipsyte clashed with then-NFL commissioner Pete Rozelle, who expected a media that he could control. Once, in a conversation with Cosell, Rozelle said of Lipsyte: "He's not a sportswriter, Howard. He doesn't write about the games."

Lipsyte eventually gave up sportswriting on a full-time basis, before his time, leaving the daily worship of games to the bowing scribes and ruling Rozelles.

III. MEDIA DENIAL: NO KILLING GOLDEN SPORT

Inspired by America's sports gluttony of the 1990s, the *New York Times* revamped and increased its coverage of games and players, for better appeasing readership and advertisers, if not certain power brokers about town. Just a few years previous at the paper, sports news rated low in focus and was considered for dropping altogether, reported Kelly Bishop Seymore for *Mediaweek*. A fresh sports approach at *The Times* would mean hiring new editors, writers, and technicians, employing state-of-the-art graphics and color, and prominently placing a fatter section within the paper's fold, among other changes. "And," Seymore noted, "[the sports upgrade] will be backed by one of *The Times*' most aggressive marketing campaigns ever, with television and radio ads and a sponsorship on broadcast television coverage of New York Mets games." Reaction was ho-hum from *Times* competitors, who viewed the publication as finally joining media's lucrative capitalization on sports. "All *The Times* is doing is catching up with the rest of the world. We have nothing to fear," said Jim Willse, *New York Daily News* editor.

Certainly, the media's sport market was an America less concerned with pondering reality than gulping fantasy, in bigger bites, and, entering the new millennium, sport mythology tasted sumptuous to consumers. The newspaper industry, fighting to survive against TV and onrushing new media, geared-up its sports *coverage*, if not sports journalism, then declared positive returns. At least one veteran sportswriter was unimpressed, Frank Deford, who saw little but "tip sheets" in modern newspaper sections. "It's all about who is going to win, why they're going to win, insider stuff, and it's all very much the same. Everybody covers the same few sports," Deford said.

Newspaper sales personnel were not concerned with this journalistic critique from folks like Deford. They coveted content for revenue. "Whether you are in a circulation war or not, you maximize sports events," Linda Sease, marketing executive for the *Denver Rocky Mountain News*, told *Editor & Publisher* in 1999. "We took a formula from last year and made it even better." Around Denver and the Super Broncos, the NFL product was the specific formula for making better bottom lines for media. "A Bronco game sells the newspaper; people want the newspaper," confirmed Tom Philand, the *Denver Post's* manager of advertising and marketing.

The hook of pro football worked for newspapers everywhere. Major dailies in NFL cities pulled in audience and advertisers through pulp football content and promotions, and newspaper representatives unabashedly confirmed business ties with the league at Atlanta, Tampa, Miami, Dallas, Denver, St. Louis, Minneapolis-St. Paul. In Jacksonville, national ad revenue for the *Florida Times-Union* hit eight figures in the latter 1990s, and executives credited the expansion Jaguars franchise. "Some advertisers target the... NFL cities," said Carl Cannon, publisher.

Those ad clients included the NFL itself, which spread money around to papers like the *Kansas City Star*, reportedly receiving about $500,000 annually from the Chiefs franchise for advertising. Magazines were no different in their relationships with the NFL, and some were bound as directly as television, likewise disregarding a journalistic conflict of interest.

The formerly veritable *Sports Illustrated* had taken the full plunge by the 2000s, constantly promoting its partnership with the NFL. The magazine once hounded Rozelle for NFL problems, especially doping, but now rolled in bed with the league. On magazine promotions throughout multiple media, the *SI* logo stood alongside the instantly recognizable NFL trademark, the red-white-and-blue shield with a football sailing through stars. An editor pledged "Total Football" in his sales pitch to readers, while the so-called football expert Peter King became a reflection of the modern *SI*. King, the NFL beat writer promoted heavily by employer Time Inc., hardly mentioned the word "steroid" in conjunction with the league for 15 years, 1990-2005, while producing enough magazine copy for several large books on football. The magazine had come to disappoint former staffer Deford. "Parts of *SI* now read like a teen magazine," he said. "Now they have whole sections — a hugely popular section, I might add —

about fantasy football. They are not even writing about real sports."

The company targeted the very young, too, using football as an enticement to attract small children and their parents. Direct-mail solicitations for *Sports Illustrated For Kids* were adorned by the magazine's logo set right beside the NFL's, in correspondence labeled on the enveloped as "FOR FAMILY USE ONLY."

It was a given of American capitalism: Media's business with big sport largely nixed journalistic probing into public issues, even when apparent, such as McGwire and Sosa in baseball, their summer of 1998, with America holding in suspended disbelief. "In fact, investigation with stories such as this is sometimes actively discouraged because sports editors don't want to kill the golden goose that gave them so much space and status," charged Barbara Walder, a New York sportswriter commenting for *Newsday*. "It's also much easier and more fun to celebrate than debunk. That's why, in part, sports reporters are often seen as second-raters — unserious journalists covering unserious events. It's also in part why... sports sections are seen as mostly simple-minded stats and scores." Walder, echoing Lipsyte, complained of editors' carelessness for journalistic application to the sports section. "The news bosses, whatever their Walter Mitty fantasies of playing center field, generally see sports as beneath them, and leave sports sections to their own devices," she wrote.

Bill Tammeus, veteran writer and editor for the *Kansas City Star*, roasted editorial decisions governing all sections of a newspaper. He blamed editors for demanding "mindless junk about our celebrity-infatuated culture," and though Tammeus did not specify, he could have swiped at his own publication. *Star* executives and editors regarded NFL football as premier content for stories and visuals, and especially the hometown Chiefs. Perhaps no other local entity gained front-page placement like Chiefs football, and the team dominated the sports pages and other sections throughout the year, even baseball season. Nothing — no singular subject of government, education, business, religion — claimed column inches in *The Star* like football, particularly the Chiefs as a news centerpiece.

"Sports has become a big business in a skeptical, celebrity conscious age," noted David Shaw, the *Los Angeles Times* media critic, "and many newspaper editors, long-accustomed to thinking of sports as the 'toy department' of journalism, are struggling to figure how best to cover this change."

Business ties and politics aside, more obstacles lay in way of enterprising sports reporters in the pursuit of public issues. Of immediate concern was expending the time and resources for working such an intensive topic. Media editorial and sales hawked sports in an unprecedented fashion, but, paradoxically, sports staffs and resources generally dwindled in the industry's print sector. Newspapers and magazines hemorrhaged for loss of audience and advertising to TV and new mediums, so investigative sport reporting did not fit the modern print model on several levels.

Sportswriters already carried heavy assignment loads, typically working across six days a week, sometimes seven, morning and night, trying to keep pace with editors' commitment to serving up gobs of entertainment. Sports content amounted to relatively little in local historical value, composed of infinite statistics, trivial human interest, exaggerated headlines, photos, and graphics — or the repeating cash themes featuring revolving names and games. Print managers, catering to corporate ownership that took over newspapers and magazines down to the smallest of markets, deemed the mythical sport content as vital for the survival of entire publications. The contrary topic of muscle substances in football did not serve company profits, so an enterprising reporter could have expected little time allotted by editors, beyond regular duties, if even allowed to pursue the fire-hot issue at all. And the specialty of investigative sports reporting was almost non-existent, with a half-dozen or so journalists nationwide, total, in all media.

"Generally speaking, newspapers are struggling as an enterprise," said Bernie Miklasz, St. Louis sportswriter and broadcaster. "So do you have the manpower and the time to free up a reporter to pursue something of that magnitude? I think the answer is no. A lot of editors would tell you no." Traditional journalism in practice was hardly realized by sports staffs, writers and editors alike, leaving ethical guidelines loosely applied. When serious problems confronted sport media, regarding athletes, coaches and institutions, the urge was to look away, and everyone did so routinely.

Football officials stonewalled notoriously, aggressively controlling information in an everlasting effort to mold and maintain a positive public image. If nothing else, they wielded a scary, persuasive prospect against reporters — the threat of denying access to teams and players. For the sportswriter who did not play along with the sport institution, who resisted the official word on a serious issue, the threat of access denied applied. "If you piss people off, they shut you out," said Gary Jacobson, the *Dallas Morning News*, about baseball personnel and doping.

While athletes and coaches wanted a compliant media, vigilant fans of football impacted coverage too. Many fans were frightfully committed, in fact, to fighting negative stories about their beloved teams and players, regardless of factual misdeeds. If coverage on doping in football adversely affected a revered team and coach, writers and editors anticipated an outcry from the fans with blinders on, enraged. "It's just tougher and tougher to work such stories," said Miklasz, a veteran analyst. "It's the last thing people want to hear."

IV. Fans in Denial: Consuming The Freak Show

"Football media — and fans — essentially ignore the use of anabolic drugs by players, according to a host of critics," began a passage of my graduate thesis, a study of print press coverage on the issue from 1983 to 1999. "Pennsylvania State University epidemiologist Charles E. Yesalis, a longtime researcher, writer, and editor on drug use for human performance, doubts football in the NFL and NCAA could enjoy its immense wealth today without the entertainment value drugs bring to the action in terms of athletic feats and violence. 'Fans want to see bigger-than-life people doing bigger-than-life things,' said Yesalis. 'They want a freak show.'"

Bona fide doping reform of American football would have altered the freak show, diminished the product, for fans and media, who shared values for how the game was to be played and presented. A columnist made the point with wit, Bruce Keidan, *Pittsburgh*

Post-Gazette. Keidan seemingly ripped sports fans for their crude tastes, including bloody NFL action featuring "steroid monsters on the field." The sportswriter griped about fans as "a motley lot if I've ever seen one," then drove the punch line: "And heaven help me, I'm one of them."

Media, not fans, created American football as a mass spectacle, and media had to sustain the game despite problems. Media were essential to both football product and market, nurturing each component simultaneously. Media were the close kin of football organizations, in the sport-media complex, and likewise of fans, in the marketing of the game. The bond was historic between fans and writers of American football, essential since the beginning. Media and fans protected The Spectacle against enemies like early abolitionists, who tried but failed to outlaw football over injuries.

Later, football fans and media together rationalized the game's abuse of performance-enhancing drugs as incidental, nothing significant to worry about, though some media took exception. In 1986, Sandy Padwe, a sports investigations editor at *SI*, charged that "in the anything-goes world of athletic competition, no one cares about how players excel, as long as they excel." Commenting for *The Nation* magazine, Padwe wrote, "To be consistent, the press and fans should be as concerned about athletes' use of painkillers or performance-enhancing drugs as they are about cocaine."

Football fans did not hear Padwe. They were too busy accessing modern football, and in an overindulgent style, from big-screen home theaters to big-vehicle camps for "tailgating" and expensive seats in palatial stadiums. Down at the field, football players moved about as gods, if only as replaceable pieces on this grand stage of pop culture, and the media celebrated everyday fans in stories and visuals. The Golden Press had first drawn people to football through stories and engravings of the game as a social event, but modern media, employing dazzling multi-medium capabilities, so publicized and glamorized gridiron fandom that the pastime became elevated into American fashion, or true religion.

Across the nation in autumn, symbols and colors of football teams decorated buildings, residences, vehicles, humans, and their animals. Weekly rituals revolved around football, for homes, schools, businesses, and, yes, churches, where people rehashed previous games, anticipated the next, or watched them play out on big screens over prayer and meal. Emotionally, many fans exalted or anguished with their favorite team's fortunes, in their daily lives, rising or falling with its victory or defeat.

Many fans sought to affix a select morality to football, condemning elements like drug use, fighting, vicious hits, antiheroes, and "obscene" content, while at the same time ignoring or missing the game's base attractions of male violence enhanced by drugs, a social event established on alcohol, and sexual atmosphere of the entire scene. In Kansas City, complaints rose over a coach's foul tantrums on TV, his angry expressions and cursing lips caught on camera without audio. A mother called it "R-rated" content during what she termed "family" viewing on a Sunday afternoon, a football game.

Nationally, thousands of NFL viewers reacted to skin flashes by a pair of female celebrities. Singer Janet Jackson exposed a breast during a Super Bowl halftime on CBS, causing moralistic hysteria that pulled in opportunistic politicians; and actress Nicollette

Sheridan dropped her shower towel before *Monday Night Football*, in a promotion with Terrell Owens, player villain, for both ABC's sagging MNF ratings and the hit show *Desperate Housewives*.

After the Jackson fiasco, NFL commissioner Paul Tagliabue appeared shocked, calling the incident "offensive, embarrassing and inappropriate." But Miklasz was skeptical, writing for *The Post-Dispatch*: "What is the Super Bowl and the annual broadcast if not classless, crass and, in some instances, deplorable?" Miklasz commented, firing at complaining parents as well as seemingly contrite officials of football and television.

The writer recounted that infamous Super Bowl halftime, when previous to Jackson's boob drop the audience saw rapper Nelly grab his crouch, chanting "So take off all your clothes," and heard Kid Rock sing of drugs, booze, easy women. "That's why the NFL's hypocrisy is so amusing," Miklasz wrote. "The league isn't opposed to raunchy behavior… as long as it doesn't go too far, of course. The NFL is enthusiastic about using sex to promote the sport. NFL cheerleader outfits seem to shrink every year. The new NFL Network frequently runs promos showcasing scenes of dancing, scantily-clad cheerleaders. And the league signs on with sponsors who peddle sex or crudity."

The huge majority of football fans, meanwhile, did not care about the controversies, other than to joke. They just loved The Spectacle, everything it represented, and willingly lavished their time and money as proof. By the 2000s, football fans were a cross-collection of American people, male, female, affluent, middle class, poor, and of virtually every ethnicity. Football dominated other games in popularity, named as the favorite in a 2006 poll by 34 percent of participants, followed by basketball, 14 percent; baseball, 13 percent; and soccer, 4 percent. Football was the real national pastime, for decades. "I think the game in some ways sums up the American experience," said Neal Pilson, former president of CBS sports. "I think a lot of people see their daily lives and the history of the country in the NFL because the game is also linked to the personality and the attitude of the country. There's a high degree of teamwork, an emphasis on toughness."

Randy Vataha, former college and pro player, said of football allegiance: "It's the game itself. Baseball has almost no following in high school or college. Basketball has made great strides... But football has always had it." So powerful was the allure that many parents strongly encouraged — or pushed — tackle football for their children, boys and girls, and there were heartbreaking outcomes. Every season kids died playing football — including two in one week for the same Texas youth league — but the games continued. Many parents of the dead told media their children would have wanted the games to go on.

Parents contributed to more problems. Studies of child steroid users concluded parents were top sources for the drugs, and anti-steroid lecturers encountered resistant parents at schools — or those seeking how-to information for performance enhancement. "After the talks, I would have parents and kids come up to me and ask if I could help them find a more advanced drug regiment that they might be able to use safely," said Dr. Clifford Ameduri, a New York writer and speaker, and former powerlifter. "I was appalled. Their urge to succeed was so great that they had completely disregarded the health risks and the moral issues I had raised. I became so disenchanted that I stopped lecturing in high schools and colleges." Parents who sought to live through their children were part of the football world of fans.

Fans experienced vicarious sensations, watching football. In Kansas City, an adult Chiefs fan wrote of feeling "like you had an impact on the game." Another was reverent about the Sunday atmosphere at Arrowhead Stadium. "Think about it," he wrote. "On a normal day, when you're at work, or at home, how often to you get to express extreme emotion?" Fans gambled on football, heavily, as another way of feeling a personal stake in games. A professional odds-maker estimated annual totals of gambling at about $500 million legally and *$20 billion* illegally, not including fantasy leagues. Office gambling pools keyed the draw of women into football consumerism. Since the 1980s, the NFL had enjoyed tremendous growth in female followers, their retail clout jibing perfectly with league marketing from merchandising to gate and television.

Politicians reveled in football at every chance, "the worse kind of jock-sniffers," said critic Chuck Todd. And while male politicians were avowed NFL fans, or acted the part to please voters, the U.S. Secretary of State put a female face to the rule in the 2000s: Condoleezza Rice could talk football as well as she could real warfare. Rice loved to declare her NFL allegiance and lived it with a personal history of dating or showing up around the game's men. In Washington she enjoyed a State Department lunch with a hot contemporary face, Giants running back Tiki Barber, and she was mentioned as a possible NFL commissioner, successor to Tagliabue. Reluctantly, Rice declined to enter the candidate pool to replace Tags; she already held an important job. "There's a lot of political consultants who'd rather work in sports and lots of political writers who'd rather write about sports," Todd said.

Girls and women, just like boys and men, watched the NFL for the violence, fun, and sex. "So how can any self-respecting, feminist-leaning woman be a fan?" posed Barbara Huebner, *Boston Globe* sportswriter, a confessed follower herself, in December 1996. The playoffs and Super Bowl, Huebner observed, would compel females everywhere to "join the guys around the television set during the next month and watch untold hours of a game that celebrates the very same qualities that many of us loathe in society." Football trumped all other sports for excitement, and many females torn inside could not resist. "Women are disturbed by football even when they like it, and I speak as a passionate football fan who is profoundly disturbed by it," Sally Jenkins, sportswriter and author, told Huebner.

Feminist critics abhorred the modern football females, naturally, and male researchers were concerned. Jackson Katz, who mentored in violence prevention at Northeastern University's Center for the Study of Sport in Society, told Huebner: "If you're not conflicted by football in this culture then you're not thinking critically about it. We have a responsibility to think about ways the various institutions of society contribute to problems we all recognize. … [Both genders] are complicit. Morally, we cannot evade that."

Most females did not cringe in the least. They wanted a good time from the

NFL and found it, obviously, making up 40 percent of the TV audience, with "family" enjoyment touted as their major motivation. "That's the core DNA of the NFL," claimed a league official. "It brings families together."

Critics, in turn, ridiculed tin organizers and pretentious fans.

"Steroid-crazed lunatics in pads can't wait to go helmet-to-helmet, turning themselves into human spears," commented Wayne M. Barrett. "Nothing sells better than violence, except, of course, excessive violence."

"Now, all grown up and soft in the middle, we pay others to play…," intoned sportswriter Andrew Herrmann, addressing adults, "so that we may live vicariously through someone else's 'good hits.' Football has become America's favorite pastime primarily because it feeds our bloodlust. … The rules are set up to allow maximum violence while keeping the gladiators alive to fight another week." Sportswriter Jim Souhan stated, "Football is the ultimate in institutionalized violence, edited and dramatized to make the perfect TV melodrama."

Whatever the amoral ingredients stirring the football spectacle, many fans insisted on maintaining cherished legends of the game, factual basis notwithstanding. The Cowboys' Tom Landry, for instance, had to be the dignified, genius coach, the rugged Christian model — not the master of manipulating people, co-opting success from others, and the shallow man unable to answer for his players' problems like steroids, which he could dismiss as "bi'ness." In Packerland, quarterback Brett Favre and defensive end Reggie White had to be Super Bowl conquerors, not the veteran players facing health issues that impact their lives. In college football, national championships for Ohio State, Notre Dame, Tennessee, Texas, and more had to be about heartwarming team stories, not about winning at all costs, of corrupt entertainment machines exploiting young athletes.

When fans had to address muscle doping in football through the faces of culprits exposed, steroid-using players and even steroid-dispensing coaches, a favorite storyline was about personal redemption, real or portrayed. For the man who got caught and wanted to stay in the game, player or coach, his quickest route back was playing into the good graces of the public — and the game — by acknowledging old guilt and displaying a fresh attitude for doing things *the right way*. Truthful or not, excuses and explanations did not matter much anyway. Apparently, the vast majority of football fans — and non-fans — did not care how the game managed itself. Neither wished to think about it.

"The last thing the public wants to read about on the sports page is drugs, politics, antitrust suits, or questions about racism and sexism and colliding cultures," editor Padwe observed, enduringly. "The more drug stories that appear in the papers or on TV, the angrier the public gets. Fans regard such stories as a personal affront, an invasion of sacred territory, a defilement of the temple."

V. The Power of Denial, College Football

The irony struck me, entering the athletic director's office at my alma mater, Southeast Missouri State University, on a Monday morning in October 1989. I came as a young journalist with damaging information about my former college football program, allegations of NCAA violations by the team for which I had played and coached a few years before. But there was more. I could not miss the large gymnastics poster on the AD's wall, featuring *my wife*, in her recent past as an All-American athlete for the school.

The AD was new at his job in this university, and I wondered if he knew I was married to that photogenic young woman on the wall: affirmative, I would discover rudely. I, naïvely, had hoped this meeting could be cordial, but the new AD — a latter-40s dude who strove to look sharp, talk smart, dressed in suit and tie with silver-flecked, coifed hair — was truly agitated with me, and preparing to show it.

The word was out on campus and around Cape Girardeau, an old river town on the Mississippi: I had dirt on SEMO State football, under its unscrupulous, winning head coach of two seasons, and that meant potentially larger trouble. The university was trying to move up in athletics, petitioning the NCAA for leaving Division II and entering Division I, and it sought to avoid sanctions for major violations in any sport.

Moreover, the AD and I had already discussed this coach and the football program, one month before, after dozens of scholarship players had fled along with every assistant coach, *and* after I'd heard, on the sly, solid information about several improprieties, including falsification of records to siphon cash. Yet the AD assured me everything was fine, with a straight face. The football program was on solid ground, only in transition, he said then, and absolutely run on ethical terms.

We both knew that was not the case, so when I finally requested the meeting to discuss "important information," he knew what was coming to a head on SEMO football. His spies were updated on my snooping, and he'd apparently heard the same allegations before they reached me. In the meeting, the athletic director took handwritten notes as I specified the first batch of charges: football coaches' diversion of $700 in university funds into cash, recruiting impropriety, and illicit team practices. By the end of my spiel, the AD gritted his teeth and squeezed his pen. Now he revealed his foremost concern: Who were my unnamed sources?

He wanted to know about the insiders funneling me information. He asked me to reveal them! Taken aback, I told the athletic director to focus on the allegations, to find what he could there. I promised him my newspaper would not publish a story for 24 hours.

Now he directed his eyes to the poster on the wall, at my wife, and smirked behind his graying mustache. My wife was proud of this university, where she had served as a shining student-athlete, lettering in gymnastics four years and twice an All-America for teams that finished third, third, second, and second in Division II. She graduated from this school with a B average and campus-wide respect for her integrity.

This athletic director probably knew little of my wife, beyond her gorgeous physical stature in photographs, but he did not hesitate to denigrate her character and her legacy for the department he was charged to represent. "Matt…," he began smugly, ready to get dirty, "if you heard someone said someone else was screwing your wife, wouldn't you want to know who was saying that?"

His insult was biting and utterly false of anything implied about my wife. I ignored it, had to. I declined to reveal my sources, again, but I had been officially welcomed to the football spiral of denial, college style, by this suit making quadruple my salary as a small-town reporter.

Since my time in college football for this school, as player and student coach, I had *tried* to respect people in charge of our program's welfare. Supposedly, these were capable authorities in higher education, with the utmost concern for young athletes. I should've known better already, arriving with plenty of reason to be cynical, but I'd held out some hope until that athletic director — monumental asshole. I was 29 and finally accepting how monstrously fucked up this game could get. I'd never trust such people again. Playing college football, I had my body ripped into pieces, but by reporting on its problems, I was truly educated to the sport's darkness, its hooliganism supported by society.

I absorbed more cheap shots for my journalistic probe into SEMO State football, but because the program was small potatoes, of zero popular appeal, I only dealt with ornery officials and boosters, local yokels. Had I reported on a major football program, rabid fans would've come after me, from across a state. Had I, say, reported serious problems like drugs in Mizzou Tigers football, our state's symbolic college team, the University of Missouri in Columbia — people would've been *really* pissed. "Especially in college towns, if a reporter's too aggressive in his or her reporting, that can mean real grief," Miklasz said in St. Louis, years after my SEMO scrape, discussing with me the mental strain of tackling a topic like muscle drugs in football.

It was December 1996. Football was the rage in America, and Bernie, with football expertise keying his rise among the new breed of sportswriter-TV analysts, was upfront discussing muscle drugs in the sport, including his honest critiquing of media coverage on the problem. By then I was gathering information for my graduate thesis at Central Missouri State. Bernie was a sportswriter friend, and I appreciated him for contributing to the study. The two-hour interview would be memorable for me. Bernie's points were outstanding and he was completely honest — increasingly the only type of interview I preferred conducting, journalistic or academic.

Yeah, now I was judging sportswriters like Bernie, in the haughty name of academia, but he was speaking for me, too, describing perils of the scribe daring to rake the muck of athletics. I had been there myself and become intimidated at times. Besides, Miklasz reasoned, media couldn't shoulder the moral load for football doping, among all parties involved. Not when those other participants — athletes, coaches, administrators, and fans — vociferously opposed the damaging exposure of the problem.

Virtually impossible was the prospect of obtaining solid information from football organizations, collegiate and professional, Miklasz said. The commitment to secrecy from within football effectively stonewalled media, along with many fans, from learning much about doping.

Miklasz had discussed doping off-record with football insiders. "Teams can't even detect it," he said, "or they don't bother to detect it. I've heard it said many times in the past, to paraphrase: To really test it the way it should be tested, it would cost all kinds of money. It would be cost-prohibitive. In other words, the teams are looking the other way to an extent, and their efforts are only going to go so far until it becomes cost-prohibitive." Moreover, Miklasz posed question: What if a reporter got a scoop on muscle doping in college football? Then what?

He noted sportswriters who suffered "absolute abuse" for investigations at major colleges. "I mean, reporters are human beings, and, yeah, they may get a tip on steroids, but to get that story into print and to get it into fruition? I mean, the hell they'll have to go through? And the reluctance perhaps from editors on top of it? I do think — and some people may say this is cowardly or unprofessional — but I think maybe some journalists do question really whether it's worth the effort... for all the abuse and all the hell they'll have to go through before that story even makes it into print?

"Then when it *does* make it into print, you're going to be called a liar. You're going to be called a scoundrel. You're going to be called disloyal to the state university. You're going to have your life threatened. You're going to be told to leave the state. You're probably going to need a bodyguard every time you go on campus, go into an arena. Is it really worth it? And I'm not giving an answer here, but do you understand why [writers] would ask themselves that question?"

Miklasz said he believed in journalistic duty for sportswriters, but within human reason. "I'm someone who takes pride in working hard," he said, "but it's a less rewarding profession in a lot of ways than it used to be, in the fact that you've got people doing more work for less pay, putting in longer hours, becoming more estranged from their families... And you're asking them to take on stories that are probably going to make their life hell on earth? People who are honest with themselves say, 'Geez, why would I wanta' do this?'"

Rick Telander did not blame fellow writers for passing on stories of steroids in football, even though he had taken up the challenge himself, numerous times, including probing around colleges for *Sports Illustrated* in the latter 1980s and early 1990s. As *SI's* senior writer of college football, Telander pursued dirt at South Carolina, Michigan State, Notre Dame, and elsewhere, confronting witnesses for information and stirring controversy, plenty of it, for himself and the magazine. Telander, a former college football player, typically followed leads provided by athletes who trusted him with their volatile stories, including Tommy Chaikin at South Carolina. Texts of social impact were the result.

An author of several books, Telander wrote the 1989 expose *The Hundred Yard Lie: The Corruption of College Football and What We Can Do to Stop It*, with the expressed mission to inspire positive change. Yet Telander did not expect that to happen, and by 2006 he viewed problems as having intensified in college football, especially the abuse of performance-enhancing substances. He still hammered NCAA football and more sports on a myriad of issues, as a columnist for the *Chicago Sun-Times*, but he understood why other writers wouldn't bother. "Every now and then, you get a bunch of lame-ass professors up in arms," Telander said, on actual responses to investigative sports writing. "They're the most harmless group in the world because they have no clue about the real world. And they'll get all excited, and they'll have some committees meet. *It means nothing*. [Faculty] get trampled by the [football] boosters every day. That's a no-brainer, like the Soviet Union against Chad or something. So I'm not going to spend my life beating my head against the wall for an issue that people don't particularly care about. I know where I stand. I made it very clear. So, I'm at peace."

Telander had been wishing for decades to make a break of sorts on sport, to leave most of the diabolical crap behind, at least, in writing, but the calm he sought was elusive. As Telander interviewed for this book, he personally rallied media support for Mark Fainaru-Wada and Lance Williams, the embattled reporters sentenced to prison for their refusal to reveal confidential sources in the BALCO investigation.

The example of Fainaru-Wada and Williams stood ominously for journalists with designs on investigative reporting. Any substantial work on football doping, for example, would rely on help from unnamed sources, insiders providing facts and leads. Leaks of information would be critical, ranging from off-record interviews to industry documents and government records — and legally perilous, within the blossoming exercise of restraining investigative news media, regardless the truthfulness of their information.

The courts had always held trump card on closed government records, the power of subpoena to uncloak leaks, and by the mid-2000s, federal prosecutors were jumping on journalists who protected confidential sources. Unfortunately for Fainura-Wada and Williams, their high-profile work based on the sealed testimony of BALCO athletes appearing before a grand jury — documents that drove their historic reporting for the *San Francisco Chronicle* and likewise their best-selling book *Game of Shadows*, focusing on Barry Bonds — caught attention of government officials.

More legal pressures came to bear on the contemporary sportswriter, for taking on in-depth topics such as the collegiate mess. Athletes, their families, coaching staffs, and university administrations exercised heightened restrictions on health information, and colleges zealously guarded other records, invoking "student privacy" and even "academic freedom" to keep problems under wraps. In steroid matters on some campuses, even family members could be kept in the dark. Factual information the reporter might obtain in other ways also invited trouble in litigious America, such as secret phone recordings of wrongdoing.

Yet some writers pressed on, and for those with requisite qualities and resources for probing doping in football — the necessary intelligence and resolve, start-up information, editorial support, time and legal counsel — the next step was rigorous, extensive background study. Volumes of scientific literature had to be read and understood, as did dozens of non-fiction books or research by doping experts and football insiders such as former players and coaches. Press articles had to be harvested electronically and manually, in searches through thousands of texts since the 1960s, while the extensive doping information on the Internet required testing for credibility, fact. Reading and rereading, the reporter had to pinpoint valid information versus inaccuracies, all the while recording notes. Almost unavoidable were confusion and frustration, especially following breaks in the study process.

Finally, the reporter would be ready to conduct interviews, but when on-record sources narrowed to football players, coaches, and officials, the journalist really hit walls.

When the subject was anabolic steroids and growth hormone, with discussion and names meant for publication, institutional denial or spin placed a stranglehold on solid information from within.

Apparently, student journalists hit the steroid wall at Northern Illinois University in early 2006. Responding, as journalists should, to the rising national story of doping for performance enhancement, the festering questions for sports and society, staffers of the *Northern Star* at NIU dutifully canvassed campus for evidence of anabolic steroids among athletes and general students. After dozens of on-record interviews, the student reporters had little but blanket denial, the variety of "not here," "not me," "not my friends." Yes, people *knew* of steroid use for performance enhancement, but always *elsewhere*, not NIU. "I can say with 99-percent confidence that no NIU athlete is on steroids," strength coach Matt Mangum told the student reporters.

Things got interesting after the paper published a three-story series of scant findings. Staffers were startled to encounter new information sprouting across campus, literally, in conversations they overheard. In a subsequent editorial, "Steroid investigation shows danger in apathy," the *Northern Star* stated:

> An eight-week search for sources willing to speak openly about their knowledge of steroid use at NIU turned up no concrete evidence of athletes or other students using the drugs. Though people speculated others used the substances, nobody admitted to the Star about using the drugs themselves.
>
> Yet, after the [first] issue was on racks for less than a day, people spoke freely about the who and where of steroid use, unaware of the Star reporters and editors [present].
>
> Though the speculation of these readers is hardly the substantial evidence of NIU steroid use that the Star was looking for, it does lead us to believe people are more accepting of these drugs than we, national sports writers or public service [writers] could have ever imagined.

By then, college football's stifling of facts about muscle doping was traditional and effective, by design or otherwise, throughout the NCAA, the NAIA, and the NJCAA, at least as far as anything for public record. Nebraska coach Tom Osborne exercised the artful dodge through the 1980s, talking around a succession of steroid headlines for his program. Football America allowed Osborne to wave off an investigative book in 1989, *Big Red Confidential: Inside Nebraska Football*, by Armen Keteyian of *Sports Illustrated*. "We probably spend as much time here trying to do it right as we do in trying to win games," Osborne said, downplaying facts and strong allegations of program misdeeds in the book. "You can either believe that or you don't. I don't have any control over that."

Nebraska did have the right to feel picked on, if not innocent, for its label as the NCAA epitome of muscle doping. In the same period, widespread abuse was acknowledged for the NFL and major universities, and the problem was likewise apparent at lower levels, small colleges, junior colleges and many high schools. Undoubtedly, every football power had steroid abuse in the period, and many were hit by sound allegations, but the vast majority did escape media and public scrutiny.

Flimsy or guarded responses were the unwritten NCAA rule, top to bottom, leaving the media in the dark. Legit information was scarce, beginning with players and coaches, and highly conscientious journalists struggled. The typical reports ended up either based on official fluff, or writers had to pressure football sources, with whom they worked daily, for tough truths no one wanted to reveal. Or journalists resorted to a final option, reporting nothing, working hard for no end result.

"You still don't know what's going on out there with steroids, and that's the most difficult problem for a journalist," Miklasz said. "Unless a player breaks down and tells someone in media what's up, how is anyone in media supposed to know? You can have the most honorable journalistic instincts ever given a reporter, but how exactly are you supposed to find out? Just because a guy is suddenly bulging with muscles, how do you prove steroids?"

Telander fumed in his book: "Lying is so prevalent in sports now, particularly when it comes to admitting drug use… that to trust someone regarding his own drug usage is to be… a fool. Was Tony Mandarich telling me the truth when he said he'd never used steroids? I don't know. And I'm only willing to do so much to find out. " In spring 1989, when Telander researched Mandarich for an *SI* cover story that rattled readers, the sportswriter got stonewalled on steroids throughout Big Ten football and beyond. A coach and a player who spoke anonymously did dump on Mandarich for the drugs, but each stopped short of what he surely knew about the college game at-large, his team, and himself.

Nothing had improved about the situation two decades later, when dubious statements remained standard from coaches and players. Notre Dame head coach Charlie Weis adopted the old institutional quotes for football doping, anywhere, anytime: *Steroids were bad then, but not now*. Weis offered his rationale — accepted at face value by a South Bend scribe — why the drugs no longer plagued college football. "The bottom line is… there's such a deterrent for these [players]," Weis said. "They've gotten scared away from that mentality, and I think that's a good thing. In the '80s, [doping] was rampant. As kids have gotten more education, they realize they could lose their scholarship if something happens."

Many sportswriters were buying, if not dumbly believing. During the 2000s, media stories abounded that basically supported NCAA doping prevention as legitimate. At the University of Texas, a 235-pound linebacker gained 40 pounds of mass to become a star lineman through "patient" lifting and nutrition, according to the player and his coaches. At the University of New Mexico, a linebacker said he had heard of steroid use in high school, but as for college football, he described steroids as "almost mythical to me." At the University of Tennessee, a football trainer classified the player displaying signs of steroids as "quite rare…. usually a walk-on athlete trying to make the grade." At the University of California-Davis, an assistant football coach reported the program "doesn't usually attract the type of athlete [who] would use steroids," according to a writer's paraphrase. Urinalysis for steroids in NCAA sports was a success story, according to athletes, coaches, and officials at schools like Texas-El Paso, New Mexico State, Ohio

State, St. John's, Stony Brook, Duke, North Carolina, Yale, Nevada-Las Vegas, Iowa State, Northeastern, Columbia, Hawaii, and Boise State.

Positive steroid results did occur in NCAA football, but only roughly two dozen annually, per about 10,000 players tested. In the event of a positive steroid result made public, coach and athlete routinely stuck together in minimizing information that "got out," even with the player facing a one-year suspension or team dismissal. Moreover, for positive-result situations where neither silence nor denial was exercised, the coach-athlete duo produced a ridiculously familiar storyline, a certifiably stock theme practiced in football nationwide, professional as well as collegiate: *The steroid user made a mistake, and he's sorry, everyone's sorry. And the team, meanwhile, has no steroid problem.*

Elsewhere in stories on college football during the 2000s, steroid snafus were quickly tidied up, including slip references to the past. In a press conference at UCLA, head football coach Karl Dorrell referred to "steroids" at Nebraska decades before, when he played against Osborne's Cornhuskers as a Bruins receiver. "All I know is they were a whole lot bigger than we were," Dorrell recalled, chuckling. Soon after the remarks, UCLA sports information director Marc Dellins said Dorrell was only joking.

On the national level, NCAA releases on drugs strove for consistency and coordination. Back in the 1980s, a few NCAA officials broke ranks and stirred controversy, alleging a pervasive problem with performance enhancers, particularly John L. Toner, then-chairman of the drug-testing committee. By the 2000s, however, headquarters churned out benign in-house statements, research data and urinalysis results that collectively portrayed muscle doping as restricted to the usual suspects, *isolated individuals*, the obscure, ever-present, never-expanding breed of user.

Frank Uryasz, sole contractor of the multi-million-dollar random testing for the NCAA, stuck to association rhetoric in 2006, discussing steroids and other muscle builders at his business in Kansas City. Uryasz had been the NCAA's youthful "director of sciences" in the 1980s, holding but an undergraduate degree from the University of Nebraska. In 1999 the association moved its headquarters from Kansas City to Indianapolis, and Uryasz stayed behind, branching off into his own testing business that benefited immediately, hugely, by gaining the NCAA anti-doping contract.

In meeting with this author, Uryasz acknowledged the existence of undetectable substances in growth hormone, low-dose testosterone, designer steroids, and insulin growth factor, along with the ready availability of drugs for athletes in college football. Uryasz acknowledged that players of my era experienced "fairly high exposure to anabolic steroid use." Sure, I'd been there. Now NCAA players were much larger, with no scientific evidence other than drugs to account for increasing sizes — yet Uryasz said urinalysis was reducing use in college sports, including football.

I noted the NCAA's declared steroid mission of three primary objectives: to ensure fair competition for athletes; to eliminate systematic pressures on athletes encouraging use; and to ensure the health and safety of athletes. In a 1994 decision by the California Supreme Court, the NCAA's self-declared interest for safety of athletes and fair competition tipped the court's "balancing of interests," defeating a lawsuit by Stanford athletes claiming testing constituted unreasonable search. I asked Uryasz whether steroid urinalysis had accomplished those NCAA goals, safety and fairness for athletes, mandated by the court. "I'm sure it's done that," he replied.

I noted complaints that the NCAA policy amounted to the fox guarding the henhouse, with steroid testing and information controlled internally. In case of a positive result, the public did not get many details because media were prevented asking pertinent questions of the athlete, coaches, and officials. I questioned Uryasz about transparency in the process: How could journalists accurately convey what happened? "Well, people need to understand that educational institutions are subject to student privacy," Uryasz said, though I wondered how that law would stack up against an adult athlete's confirmed illegal use of a prescription drug.

Uryasz said full disclosure would risk testing's abolishment, presumably through court judgments in suits by athletes. He insisted constructive discussion on doping was commonplace in the NCAA, but behind closed doors and only among officials or appointed panels, like the safeguards committee he served on. He said he also benefited from private conversations he had with athletes and coaches. "These dialogues are happening all the time within the NCAA," Uryasz said, "and perhaps we all should do a better job of letting the rest of the world know we're having these discussions and they're real, and they're driven by a concern for the kids.

"It does concern me when people think the organizations are operating in a vacuum and are not having discussions, or doing things to prevent their programs from being strong deterrents."

Not surprisingly, lack of NCAA openness was a familiar charge by critics. Murray Sperber, the professor at Indiana University who wrote scathing books on collegiate sport, alleged a "P.R. veil" was constructed by officials who saw to every detail, down to association-approved language such as "student-athlete" for players and "sports-information directors" for publicists. In commentary for the *Chronicle of Higher Education*, Sperber wrote: "Ever since it was founded in its modern incarnation just after the Second World War, the N.C.A.A. has emphasized damage control and public relations over fundamental reform and thoughtful reflection, particularly in Division I football and basketball." *The CHE* backed up Sperber, editorializing about the NCAA mode of profiteering on entertainment worth billions. The NCAA was experiencing "more and more trouble reconciling its existence as a commercial sports league with its attempts to be an educational enterprise," the publication charged.

Officials perpetuated the denial of doping that spiraled about NCAA football, a cocoon of protection, but media and fans held up their end too. Aggressive, vigorous apologists for Notre Dame and Lou Holtz were classic examples in 1993, and sycophants for college football held sway on public opinion into the next decade. A student columnist at Columbia University praised the NCAA steroid policy in 2005, lauding the public disregard for the issue. A UNLV sports editor was ill-informed, condemning the contemporary public focus on sport doping and claiming no "big problem among college or high school athletes." A writer at Iowa State, oblivious to testing's fallibilities, stated without attribution, "The NCAA has a strict, extensive list of banned substances that would make it difficult for any athlete to skirt around."

Professional media could be as shallow in their research and writing. "Boise State football players must prove this year that they earned their bulging muscles the old-fashioned way," *The Idaho Statesman* stated flatly, giving lip service to school officials who touted their testing as improved. Boldly, in spring 2006, NCAA officials *recycled* hoopla by putting a fresh spin on the stale policy, implying they were just instituting "year-round" testing of athletes — a program approved 16 years previously. Media bit on the hook without confirming the history. "NCAA Cracks Down on Steroids Use," Honolulu TV station KGMB headlined on the old development.

Virtually no one worried about the NCAA spin, despite polls that showed Americans saw problems such as drugs and amoral exploitation of young athletes. Truth, in fact, could draw public reaction — against the messengers. "Think it's difficult to cover topics like alleged war crimes and wiretaps without alienating readers? At least in those cases, only half the country is angry with you," noted Mike Finger, sportswriter in San Antonio. "That's child's play compared with dishing dirt on college football programs, or on steroid scandals, or on any other behind-the-scenes sports story that every fan should be aware of but that no fan wants to hear about."

Oriard observed that a program's winning galvanized an indestructible mystique, shielding teams at schools like his alma mater, Notre Dame. There was more to the power of football spectacle, namely cultural ritual. "I think sports bring people together," said Deford. "I think there are very few things in our heterogeneous culture that do that." Jim Delaney, Big Ten commissioner, said, "Essentially, [sports are] a very important part of higher education, whether that's right or wrong. It's unique to America. And it ain't going anyplace."

Neither would doping go away, particularly for football, and contemporary college officials — along with media — could not blithely ignore the reality, warned a former NCAA expert on drugs, John Toner, who during the 1980s served a term as NCAA president and also chaired the committee that established drug testing, among other related duties for the association.

In a 2006 interview, Toner disagreed with critics' consensus opinion regarding the primary motive for NCAA silence about football doping: Legalities, he said, outweighed every other internal concern, marketing image notwithstanding. "We could not comment. We did not get into [public] discussions," said Toner, living retired in Georgia. "As I look back now, if we had then the empirical evidence we have now, we could have made the public understand how much larger a problem it was, than a 1 or 2 percent positive testing [report] that we were publishing. ... But in the position that the NCAA or USOC or any of the international [federations] find themselves, [testing] has to be defensible in the court of law. That means you keep your mouth shut in all the gray areas."

"And I feel as though we failed, in our own interests of protecting ourselves legally. We had to be certain we were right. You can't afford to be wrong, and the worst thing you can do is gossip about it," Nevertheless, Toner had always wished more information could be shared from within NCAA football about muscle substances. He believed the anecdotal information was imperative for airing, the confessionals, hearsay, and the like.

"I think if the public got to know some of these things that we don't publicly state, there would be a wave of agreement that, one, the problem is much bigger than we previously thought; two, it's of scurrilous nature to the point that you either use them or you don't [compete]," he said.

No doubt at least some contemporary personnel in NCAA sports agreed with Toner, but rarely did anyone step out from the mannequins to speak. Michigan State head strength coach Ken Mannie was an exception, publicly alleging a serious doping problem. "Anyone who hasn't lived in a cave for the past 30 years is well aware of the proliferation of performance-enhancing drugs in every sport," Mannie wrote for *NCAA News*. Following revelations of the BALCO scandal, which brought an overdue spotlight to undetectable anabolic substances, Mannie admonished policymakers of every type for head-in-the-sand complacency. "The exposure of the designer steroid conspiracy should serve as a wake-up call to all coaches, administrators, parents, the governing bodies of high school associations, the NCAA, professional sports, and state and federal lawmakers," he commented on *www.naturalstrength.com*.

Even those droning NCAA releases contained anti-spiral nuggets, such as findings from the association's annual anonymous survey of athletes about steroids. In 2005, while self-reported use was unbelievably low, including 2.3 percent among football players surveyed, almost one-quarter of admitted users were "certain" their coaches knew. In addition, 17.8 percent of admitted users reported receiving steroids from athletics personnel, their coaches, trainers, and doctors.

College media were the proverbial sheep on sport doping, but some writers stood out for their perspective. Virginia Tech sportswriter David Covucci ripped America's hypocritical expectation for "clean" sport; everyone cheats at everything, he reasoned, so performance-enhancement for athletes should be condoned too. Moreover, testing was invalid for prevention. "Face it — there is no possible way to stop anyone from using the cream, the clear or the cow steroid Bonds took," Covucci opined for *The Collegiate Times* in Blacksburg. "There's an expectation that testers will catch up to cheaters and that's just not true."

At UC-San Diego, student columnist Nicky Buchanan criticized cultural pressures for doping in sport and society, along with citing "leniency" in NCAA testing as an enabler. "While watching ESPN or Fox Sports, it's difficult to see the 6-foot-plus guys with veining muscles bulging from their jerseys and not wonder how many of them are shooting or popping," Buchanan wrote for the campus *Guardian*. "People need to speak out, not only for the health of the users but for the protection and integrity of sports as a whole. Or perhaps we don't really care as much as we say?"

VI. The NFL: Standard-Bearer For Denial of Doping

While football colleges and conferences enjoyed a powerful influence on the football word, the NFL and franchises set the standard, exerting their calculated, comprehensive PR offensive upon a receptive America. The NFL objective was not only to sell content but to control information, and the mission was carried out at every level of multi-media, small to large markets, in print, radio, TV, online, satellite, and cellular. Negative events did occur, consistently as always, from player violence to drug abuse, for this was pro football. Unlike other sports of the new millennium, the NFL fires were contained, tamped out, before swelling into serious image problems. Bad news seemingly never stuck to the league.

The NFL could thank its "executive vice president in charge of Teflon," cracked sportswriter David Steele, the *Baltimore Sun*, in 2006. "There has to be someone with that title in the league offices, right?" Steele, a veteran in chronicling malfeasance of athletics, continued:

> This has been the Year of the Knucklehead in America's favorite sports league, but its position remains utterly unchallenged, while every other sport pays for player misbehavior in dollars and credibility.
>
> How? If this is a forgiving nation, why hasn't it forgiven baseball for McGwire, Palmeiro and Bonds (and, maybe, Clemens)? If it's the land of second chances, when does the sport of Sprewell and Artest get its second chance?
>
> Are autumn Sundays in front of the plasma screen so sacred that looking the other way is that easy? Why is every other sport held to a different standard than this one? What is it about the NFL that has earned it a singular benefit of the doubt?

Journalists knew this peculiar force, the non-irritant coating of football spectacle, and some explored the strata of the shield's mesh over the bloody NFL. The main PR gears turned in league headquarters in media hub Manhattan, according to a consensus finding, and significantly, the commissioner's office, where Rozelle and successor Tagliabue ruled for nearly a half century combined.

Lipsyte referred to "pro football's colossal public relations machine" under Rozelle, who manipulated the media by charm or strong-arm. Cosell wrote, "Never in my lifetime in sports has anyone commanded and controlled the media like Pete Rozelle." The commissioner enjoyed business confidants in television, a "partnership," Cosell charged, and "almost ironclad" command of newspapers and magazines.

Later, executive charm was bereft under Tagliabue, but the NFL control of messages was stronger than ever. The league's lasting clout with media signified an "ability to do things that no other professional league can do," marveled author John Feinstein, who described Tagliabue as "professional sports' Last Don." As Tagliabue retired in 2006, the league and franchises clamped tighter on information, including limiting access to practices and locker rooms and denying game-day video and audio for media who did not pay rights fees, a development analyzed by sportswriter Randy Covitz of the *Kansas City Star*. David Elfin, president of the Pro Football Writers Association of America, told Covitz: "My nightmare scenario is 10, 20 years from now, you will not be able to cover the NFL unless you pay a rights fee. As the NFL Network gets established and the teams' Web sites get established, and you have the whole ESPN machine, anybody who is either not working for the team or not paying a rights fee is not getting great access." Andrew Lackey, professor of business journalism at Arizona State, said, "We know the

NFL wants to govern everything it does. Any business can try whatever it wants, but they have to realize they're part of a public trust and have a responsibility to the public."

The NFL withheld doping information and dodged outside suspicion unlike any other major sport, declared Steele, among a host of writers ridiculing public hypocrisy over baseball. "Oh, yes, steroids and other enhancers," Steele intoned. "Strictly baseball's issue, in the eyes of no less than the U.S. Congress. ... Yet if any sport ought to flunk the eyeball test on doping, it's not baseball or track or cycling — it's pro football."

Looks somehow did deceive in this case, because the culture instead accepted an outlandish story — no systemic doping existed in football — the NFL had fashioned since steroids first confronted Rozelle. The theme was central to NFL rhetoric on football drugs, however illogical or unbelievable, and faithfully followed basic, time-proven claims repeated when needed by administrators, coaches and players:

- Any use was always isolated, restricted to a tiny minority of individual cheaters.
- Any use was always an athlete's whole fault, a personal mistake.
- Any widespread use for the NFL was always in the past.
- Any continued widespread use was always at the colleges and high schools.
- Any report of systemic abuse was always exaggerated.
- Effective urinalysis was always just implemented, closing former loopholes.
- Upgrade in steroid policy was always coincidental to negative criticism.
- Ineffective prevention was always in the past.
- Current policy was always the most comprehensive.
- The most effective anti-steroid education was always underway.
- League mission was always fair competition, good health, positive role-modeling.
- And, finally, the top goal was always complete elimination of muscle substances.

A journalist trying to report in the issue could have merely chosen from among those NFL excuses, without attempting interviews, because typically there was no deviating for an inside response on anabolic doping. Pro football began constructing the rhetorical model of doping denial under Rozelle, despite his public bungling, and it became institutionally ingrained — guiding public response for colleges and high schools — before NFL Tagliabue's glorious run and into the 2000s.

In 1989 and 1990, the league levied suspensions against about a dozen active players for positive steroid results, including three rookies at Buffalo. "They made a mistake," said Bills GM Bill Polian, who concluded the athletes had been "tempted by street-corner pharmacists, and the bodybuilders, and the gym rats." In New York, the Jets waived two backup players suspended by the league. "They are nice young men, and we hope they'll get the help they need," said Joe Walton, Jets coach. "I hope they get straightened around and have productive, healthy lives." When two Green Bay linemen were suspended, Packers coach Lindy Infante was "quite shocked," he said, adding, "I don't think either of the players are on [steroids] now or were on it just prior to training camp." Miami lost a lineman to steroid suspension, and coach Don Shula said, "The only important thing to me is that he gets it done the right way. It's got to be an honest game." Shula said the case was isolated on his team. Ditto in Philadelphia, where Eagles coach Buddy Ryan expressed surprise over a lineman's suspension. "I'm disappointed for our whole football team," said Ryan, who once coveted steroid-tainted Brian Bosworth. "I don't understand how steroids help a guy anyway, but some apparently feel the need for them." Eagles owner Norman Braman said media coverage critical of the player had encouraged the drug use. Seahawks coach Chuck Knox entered the sport's steroid discussion, saying, "This is not a problem that is peculiar to the National Football League. It starts in high school."

Tagliabue made a priority of establishing random urinalysis *and* consistent, company rhetoric of denial for the 1990s. By the time of Alzado's death, Tags reigned in Upshaw and the players union about steroids and growth hormone, everybody spoke from the same playbook, and America went along blissfully. At the franchise level, management, coaches, and players sounded the same on doping, whenever they would comment, with an aim to shift or deflect blame toward user athletes and outside influences. Always, a confirmed user made a mistake, said NFL voices, and if widespread use of drugs still existed, it occurred at the colleges and high schools.

The refrains to media carried forward, squawks from NFL personnel on cue about steroids or HGH, obeying their rhetorical model, squelching meaningful information. In New York, a lineman's positive test result was his "mistake," said Jets coach Bill Parcells. In San Francisco, the 49ers were "disappointed" about a player's suspension, said coach Steve Mariucci. "He feels he made a mistake." In Nashville, during a state hearing on steroids, Titans strength coach Steve Watterson suggested steroid use was largely confined to "wannabe athletes" who obtained drugs in health clubs. "We need to look at this more globally," he said. "It's more of an [individual's] image problem than a sports problem." Also testifying was NFL labor-relations lawyer Adolpho A. Birch III, who directed concern toward society, including teen girls on muscle dope and the faddish employ of "steroids" as a preposition in language, such as "Apollo on steroids." Birch posed, "Is that a good thing?"

The NFL decried muscle doping, but reporters saw teams pursue track-and-field athletes suspended in their sport for steroids, looking for the next Bob Hayes. Olympic sprinter Ben Johnson and shot-putter Randy Barnes drew interest from NFL teams, following their suspensions, and a 2000s example was British sprinter Dwain Chambers, who tested positive for THG, the designer steroid from BALCO. Afterward, Chambers tried out for the NFL Europe League. "I am very keen to see him in action… to find out what he can do with an American football in his hands," said Tony Allen, international director of player development.

The large majority of suspended football players stayed in the game, with coaches and management often acting as apologists and character witnesses. When police busted NFL players for steroid quantities or paraphernalia, coaches typically said they doubted the players used muscle drugs, much less distributed them. In 2004, the Patriots signed lineman Dana Stubblefield after his own positive test for THG. Later, line prospect Luis Castillo tested positive for androstenedione at the league combine, but the Chargers selected him as their No. 1 pick, 28th overall. "Over time, when he's tested, this will go away," A.J. Smith, San Diego GM, said of Castillo. "He did cut a corner and made a mistake. But this is a good kid with solid character. It's a shame to let that go by the board."

At Denver, Broncos owner Pat Bowlen liked to tout supposed moral fiber in his players, including during the 1980s, when he said steroids were not an issue on his team. Yet, in 2005, the Broncos signed problem athletes such as NCAA refugee Maurice Clarett and Todd Sauerbrun, the All-Pro punter banished from Carolina following steroid revelations involving him and Dr. Shortt. Previously, Denver signed safety Lee Flowers after he tested positive for steroids with the Steelers. Bowlen explained he believed in second chances for people. "I'm very high on character, we've made that clear, I think," Bowlen said. Broncos coach Mike Shanahan discussed Sauerbrun, saying "you have to look at it on a player-by-player basis." A year later, Sauerbrun tested positive for ephedra, a banned amphetamine-like performance-enhancer, and Shanahan reacted as though surprised. "I told him that I was very disappointed in him," Shanahan said. "We took a chance on him." Denver officials had little to say about another former player, Bill Romanowski, and doping allegations and confirmations surrounding him.

Of course, the league readily employed silence on drugs. Steroid events inspired "no comment" from many franchises, including Dallas, Kansas City, Atlanta, Carolina, Washington, and the New York Giants.

Sportswriters could expect no help from players, as far as ascertaining the reality of doping in the NFL; modern reporters basically did not consider them as open sources. Player outspokenness on steroids and growth hormone was essentially over after the 1980s, since drug policy effectively restricted anything but official lines. Even Bosworth and Romanowski, two supposed anti-voices of modern football, guarded their comments about muscle doping in the NFL. Obviously, organizers preferred players did not speak on the topic, especially individuals who tested positive, were arrested, or otherwise implicated.

The overwhelming quiet of athletes about muscle enhancement — or their fluffy statements on-record — bemused critics who knew what was up. "These non-denial denials should come with FAQs," wrote Rick Maese, the *Baltimore Sun*, jeering alibis of dopers exposed in several sports. Maese cracked, "I used to think prisons housed the largest group of men who are overly eager to proclaim their innocence." Selena Roberts, the *New York Times*, commented, "A firm denial has lost its credibility when every culprit claims innocence. ... The hypocrisy seems pathological among the stars." Don Hooten, steroid activist, said, "Denial is a standard characteristic, whether you're dealing with a pro athlete or a kid."

A pro athlete realized financial security from silence on doping, user or not, observed sportswriter Greg Wyshynski. "You hear the occasional player speaking out of turn," Wyshynski wrote, noting "the code" that dominated Major League Baseball. "But everyone else is either using or playing with a user, and despite whatever anger they have towards this 'cheating' they keep their traps shut. Million-dollar contracts have a funny way of neutering nobility."

Whistleblowers or "real men" were rare in competitive arenas like athletics, lamented columnist Mary Sanchez, the *Kansas City Star*. "Rank and titles are often gained because you know how to follow the rules, written and unwritten," she wrote.

"But true leaders are willing to stand up for ethical behavior, even when it would be easier to look the other way."

Steve Courson spoke up while still a player, frankly discussing steroids in the NFL during the mid-1980s, including his own use. In 2005, Courson wrote he always viewed liar athletes as "pathetic" but conceded his own honesty had incurred "society's wrath," so he understood anyone's denial. Lyle Alzado lied about drugs as a player, but before dying admitted to having abused anabolic steroids and growth hormone to star in pro football. Secrecy literally buried doping in the NFL, Alzado said in 1991, one year removed from the game and facing less than a year to live. "If somebody needed something, then I would tell them where to go and they would get it. And it wasn't talked about after that," Alzado said. "And I think it wasn't talked about because nobody liked to admit the use of something to enhance their performance." After Alzado, the majority of NFL players steadfastly refuted the existence of a doping problem, led by union executive director Gene Upshaw.

President George W. Bush, during his 2004 State of the Union address, remarked of inadequate drug prevention by football and other sports, and Upshaw reacted as if insulted. "I was very upset we were painted with the same brush as baseball when it comes to steroids," Upshaw said. "I could never embrace what [the president] said, and hopefully, I'll have a chance to clarify that with him." Upshaw acted boldly, but his stance was weak. Bush's remark rode on a groundswell of evidence strongly pointing to doping pervasiveness throughout sports, especially pro football.

Tagliabue also rebuked critics such as the president, although deftly, in contrast to Upshaw, by proclaiming league success for steroid policy in a writing posted on *NFL.com*. Later, testifying for Congress, Tagliabue said the NFL did not need outside intervention to prevent steroids from affecting athletes and competition.

Now NFL players rallied in media blitz, on Tags' lead, to counter steroid stigma. At New York Giants practice in East Rutherford, every player interviewed said random urinalysis limited juicing to isolated individuals. "I think they keep you on your toes in the NFL as far as making sure everybody's on an even keel," said linebacker Carlos Emmons, who alluded to rumors of wider use in the past. Testing produced "a level playing field," said linebacker Nick Greisen, adding he would be "blown away" to learn the entire NFL had even a half-dozen steroid users. Center Shaun O'Hara said that without random urinalysis the league would be "a mess" of muscle substances. "It's basically saving the players from themselves," O'Hara said.

Green Bay players backed the commissioner on every point, including the question of outside intervention. "This is not a league driven by steroids," said linebacker Na'il Diggs, who played college football at Ohio State and claimed to have never known a steroid user in football. "The major leagues can handle this on their own. There's no reason to bring paid politicians into this. The economy, that's what [lawmakers] need to be worried about. We have the strictest policy on steroids in the world, probably." Doping critics charged that potential earnings lured an athlete to performance enhancement, but Packers center Mike Flanagan rationalized money to be exactly why one would avoid steroids. "The TV revenue and all the dollars that are coming in… everybody knows this business is a golden egg and everyone's got to protect it," he said.

The NFL suspended 50 to 60 players under its anabolic-steroid policy from 1990 to 2006, among roughly 150,000 random tests. For the few who commented to media, their favorite excuse was either injury rehabilitation or a banned substance was consumed unknowingly through a supplement. At least one player claimed a cortisone steroid caused his positive result. Some admitted their intent was performance enhancement, but they downplayed the effectiveness of anabolic steroids. Virtually every suspended player who commented publicly blamed only himself for his "mistake," while apologizing to team, league and fans. Teammates of a suspended player typically acted surprised, sorry, dumb about doping. Some teammates said they heard rumors of muscle drugs in football, back in college or high school, but not in the NFL.

Retiring players typically said nothing about muscle doping, year after year, and two tied to modern steroid scandals offered little of substance, mostly just hints about forces at work. Romanowski was identified for juicing largely through BALCO proceedings, and Todd Sauerbrun was known as the punter who bought muscle drugs from Dr. Shortt in Carolina.

Sauerbrun found himself out of the league in October 2006, released by Denver after serving a four-game suspension for ephedra, and still wearing the scarlet letter of steroids for the Panthers case. Sauerbrun was disappointed his services apparently were no longer wanted in the NFL, and his agent, David Carter, alleged a blackballing. "I fully expected Todd, the best punter in NFL history, statistically speaking, would be playing [again in the league], and it doesn't look like he is and that bothers me," Canter said.

Romanowski produced a curious autobiography, *Romo: My Life on The Edge: Living Dreams and Slaying Dragons*, in 2005, following the breakout of the BALCO scandal, his positive result for THG, and his retiring from the NFL. In several respects the work was revealing of football insanity, like Romanowski's maniacal on-field personality, his insatiable lust for winning, and his hearty consumption of painkillers and speed. He had a home IV tent, where a favorite substance to mainline was DMSO. Undoubtedly, league officials would have preferred to see a different type of story in print, but the book posed no threat to NFL image, despite billing as an antihero boldly speaking out.

Romanowski's story did not go far enough to provoke NFL contempt or counter-campaign — it crossed no line in a very brief address of his steroid use. In fact, Romanowski's primary co-author was a *league employee*, Adam Schefter, NFL Network analyst and writer for *NFL.com*; in addition, writing credit was afforded Phil Towle, Romo's psychotherapist and performance coach associated with league personnel. The book perfectly negotiated a tolerance zone with the NFL, particularly on muscle doping, allowing nothing about league steroid history, nothing about Tagliabue or Upshaw in the issue, nothing about inherent faults of urinalysis, and nothing about HGH, which Romanowski *later* said he used briefly, during a TV interview promoting the book.

The only steroid discussion was about Romanowski's use, in edited version of the complete story, critics cried. Romanowski recalled he first used anabolic steroids in 2001, the THG obtained through Victor Conte at BALCO. But that was the linebacker's final season in Denver and a few years removed from the Broncos' Super Bowl titles, when Romanowski was highly visible in strength training with team stars. Conte had his own version in an interview with *ESPN The Magazine*, saying Romanoski began using steroids in 1999; other reports had witnesses pegging earlier start dates for the linebacker.

Romo drew CBS praise for "brutal honesty," but San Francisco sportswriter Scott Ostler classified the book "science fiction" and steroid users as cold liars. "Maybe performance-enhancing drugs don't enhance the performance of one's memory. They do seem to shrink your truth gland," Ostler wrote for *The Chronicle*. Regarding apparent story omissions, Ostler asked: "Two years fiddling with 'roids, or a decade-plus on the juice? It's an important distinction. It speaks to Romanowski's football legacy, and to the legitimacy and honesty of the sport."

Jockocrats and Compliant Sportswriters Bolster NFL Image

An NFL weapon for spin control was its foot soldiers infiltrating media, the *Jockocracy*, ex-players turned TV heads and radio voices, dominating talk for massive audiences of game broadcasts and daily shows.

Jock pseudo-reporters had angered journalists since TV football's emergence as pop culture, the game's selling "as psychodrama," observed Lipsyte, who fashioned "Jockocracy" and "jock chic" in the 1970s — terminology Cosell ran with for his regular barbs at televised sports. "My medium, with its over-corruption, knew the sole way to go was to create the Jockocracy," Cosell said in 1985. "We're not positioned in this industry to provide truth anyway. Commissioner Pete Rozelle has exactly what he wants… what he wants is a jock who has ties to the league and a redundant plethora of clichés. They're not journalists or communicators; they're not trained."

The Jockocrats were willing communicators, at least, yammering endlessly for the camera, in studio and on set, just like the locker room. They talked arcane Xs and Os, second-guessed coaches and referees, retold personal feats, and laughed deliriously at inside jokes, each other, themselves. Jockos were washed-up, recognizable names and faces from days of yore on the football field, typically stars from Super Bowls past. They could talk, and TV producers handled the rest. Airtime was filled and golden sponsorships snapped up by advertisers, selling out the inventory of 30- and 60-second spots.

The network Jockocrats were trusted parrots of NFL rhetoric, of course. Having entered television with the league's blessing, they had to maintain league favor for keeping lucrative TV gigs — one was always replaceable by another waiting in line, if needed. A Jocko could rant all he wanted about instant replay, bandannas, slashing gestures, bad calls, vicious hits, and Terrell Owens; in fact, Jockos had to take sides and debate meaningless subjects ad nausea, diverting attention from real problems.

The heavy issues, potential threats to the cash-cow NFL, were avoided by the Jocko. He did not, for example, address the brutality in stark, quantifiable terms, like the widespread suffering among his fellow retirees, the disabled, infirm, and dead. The Jocko did not discuss in-depth the health ramifications of players' enormous physiques, muscular or fatty, that strained body systems and vital organs. He ignored historical, long-term taxpayer debt for subsidizing the NFL, billions carried by cities and states including New Orleans, where millions more were dumped for the dramatic reopening of the Superdome on *Monday Night Football*, amid ongoing disasters following Hurricane Katrina.

An NFL Jockocrat on TV or radio avoided making hot-button issues of doping, especially since he likely knew much himself. A Jocko might be outspoken about an individual user or so-called isolated group of users, but he never alleged a systemic problem that translated into institutional responsibility. An NFL Jocko could have been a user in the past, as a player. He might have spoken up in the past, and still had freedom to blame colleges and high schools for muscle doping in football. Just not the NFL, not in his job, where loyalty to league was assumed, including by the audience who understood this guy was no journalist.

Cris Collinsworth was one who went from college star to Super Bowl receiver to TV booth. And when he made the cushy network job, pulling big bucks for broadcasting games, he provided cover against steroid fire for both the NCAA and NFL. In 1993 Collinsworth, employed by NBC, ridiculed solid book allegations of widespread use at Notre Dame, the network's home team and icon of NCAA football. Ten years later Collinsworth stepped up for the NFL, offering effusive praise for league urinalysis amid damning fallout of the BALCO eruption. "I take great pride in the way [the] NFL has handled the steroids issue," Collinsworth wrote in a posting for *NFL.com*, late 2003. He contended the league combated the problem, achieving competitive fairness, protecting players, and providing positive modeling for kids. Collinsworth, who considered his fluffy commentary to be a "report," concluded "the NFL and the players union should be complimented for what they are doing with steroids."

Jockocrat Glenn Parker, former lineman, came to the NFL fore in spring 2005, as Tagliabue, Upshaw, and other officials were called to Washington for a congressional hearing on drugs. "The NFL does a great job with its testing. It's phenomenal," said Parker, analyst for NFL Network and NBC. "Congress has its own problems from what I can tell from reading the newspapers, to start worrying about steroid use."

The Jockocracy extended to former NFL coaches on television. John Madden, bona fide member, answered a reporter's steroid question by steering focus off football. In baseball players "started to look different — the way the uniforms started fitting — right in front of us," Madden said. "Football guys were always big."

Boom. Most sportswriters held on that basic reasoning, firm or flimsy, and continued framing content in traditional fashion, of NFL drug policy as adequate if not superior. News writers and like-thinking editors accepted the football denial, repackaged it and passed it along to consumers, in circuitry of the spiral.

For most of Tagliabue's reign, the media majority went along with NFL rhetoric on muscle substances — or reflected league silence — and *Sports Illustrated* was conspicuous in the trend. Once the undisputed leader of sports journalism in America, *SI* hardly mentioned football doping from the Alzado confessional of 1991 until the BALCO scandal in 2003, a period when the corporate-owned magazine developed close marketing ties with the NFL.

Sports Illustrated pursued bodybuilders, cyclists, and a female swimmer for steroids in the 1990s, but its do-nothing approach on football was evident in lead gridiron writer Peter King, who came aboard as cynical staffers like Telander and Keteyian were leaving. King largely ignored steroids, growth hormone, and more drugs in the league after Tagliabue took charge. He did pen a 1990 analysis on steroids in the NFL, featuring lineman Bill Fralic's candidness, but the thrust was endorsing Tagliabue's random urinalysis. Then, the next year, King slammed Alzado and other steroid users in a short commentary, relying strictly on league word that everything was under control.

Afterward King basically went to sleep on the issue for more than a decade, finally stirring for the Panthers-Shortt story of 2005. Then his main source for a dubious report was aspiring Jockocrat Tiki Barber, the Giants running back bent for television post-football. King griped some about NFL testing relative to the Carolina situation, particularly the obvious dilemma with HGH, but overall the writer stayed in line with the NFL, even evoking classic rhetoric mimicked by Barber, who told King the Panthers players using steroids represented "a very small percentage" in the league, "a microcosm of our society." King was satisfied. "For now, I'm buying what Tiki's selling," he wrote. "I haven't seen the 'roid excesses, nor have I heard anything but unsubstantiated whispers of them. So until I learn differently, I'm going to consider the Carolina problem an *isolated one* [author's emphasis]."

Many more go-along writers for the NFL and NCAA flourished into the mid-2000s, epitomized by those blasting baseball but praising football for its steroid policy. "One by one, the NFL has cleaned up the league as far as steroids," surmised sportswriter Mike Preston, the *Baltimore Sun*. Preston claimed league policy struck "fear" in players, continuing, "There are still going to be *isolated cases* [author's emphasis]. ... *but the problem is nowhere near as severe as it was in the 1970s and '80s*."

Sycophant football media were confronted by the winter 2006, however, with doping revelations continuing steadily, such as new information on the Panthers, a fresh allegation about growth hormone, and the nandrolone use of Chargers star Shawne Merriman, nailed by a positive test result.

Jon Heyman, a writing counterpart of King at *SI*, represented the magazine's neo-skepticism about football growing throughout mainstream media. Commenting on *SI.com*, Heyman wrote, "One of the NFL's top defensive players, Shawne Merriman, has failed a test for steroids... And all it inspires is a yawn. As long as football fans have their fantasy team, their couch, their Sunday food spread and their office pool (or more serious gambling), they couldn't care less about steroids."

Spiral of Football Denial Mutes Outcry of Resurgent Scandal

The world of football fans in America — led by opinion leaders in politics, business, education and media — always absolved the sport of major ills like drugs, according to criticism converging in media, academia, and science.

Baltimore Sun sports columnist David Steele bemoaned "the country's love of the game remains unconditional, and the NFL smirks its way to the bank." Mike Maniscalco, radio host in Richmond, Virginia, said, "The double standard of steroid use is really getting to me. The way baseball has been bastardized by the fans and media, yet football gets a free pass, is just flat wrong." Shelly Anderson, *Pittsburgh Post-Gazette*, goaded locals in particular: "If we give Bonds an asterisk, do we do the same with stars and teams in other sports? We could start with the NFL and Super Bowls. Wait — Steelers fans might not like that."

The majority of football fans literally refused to fret over muscle doping. Tom Jelke, sports fan in Miami, considered the NFL saturation of society and remarked: "I think the national pastime is baseball, but the national obsession is football. That's what people are excited about." Doping expert Yesalis said fans represented "that great ace in the hole" for football organizers and de facto partner media, on the subject of doping. "Their customers don't give a damn. And when I say 'customers,' it's not just customers of the NFL, but the customers of the sport page, of the radio stations, of the TV networks." Yesalis indicted the sport-media-*fan* complex, wherein everyone, he said, could put up with the occasional exposé on football doping. "But what they won't tolerate is a continuing haranguing, no matter how well done. Their little emperors are not wearing any clothes, and they won't tolerate it."

Public toleration of doping served football in summer 2006, when a cavalcade of negative headlines befell American sports, blighting baseball, cycling, and track while also touching the NFL. Prior to the league's celebrated opening weekend, new details emerged from the Carolinas, more about players, a physician, and prescription drugs for performance enhancement.

The *Charlotte Observer* broke the story on August 27, documenting abuse patterns of steroids and growth hormone by a half-dozen NFL players, drugs obtained from Dr. James Shortt, including Panthers offensive linemen gearing up for a Super Bowl. *Observer* reporter Charles Chandler built the story on court records from the criminal case of Shortt, by now imprisoned on a federal conviction of conspiracy to distribute the drugs illegally.

Nine NFL players had been publicly identified as patients of Shortt, and about nine more, unnamed, were also alleged to have been customers. Yet no client of Short had tested positive in steroid screening by the NFL, which remained steadfast in characterizing the case as insignificant. Union leader Upshaw insisted dopers "get caught" by the NFL, but the clientele list of Shortt, who reportedly instructed athletes for beating steroid urinalysis, attested otherwise.

Following Chandler's story, several sportswriters criticized football, renewing the charge of widespread doping to a public level not seen for decades, since media outcry led to the establishment of urinalysis for steroids.

Jason Whitlock, of the *Kansas City Star*, commented, "If you want to get rid of performance-enhancing drugs in team sports, start punishing the team owners, coaches, universities and high schools that benefit financially from steroid abuse."

"The National Football League is a lovely fantasy," C.W. Nevius wrote in San Francisco. "What no one wants to talk about is that the sport almost certainly has a performance drug problem that makes Barry Bonds look like a Jenny Craig spokesman".

"Even cycling has had its day under the bare light bulb," Gary Peterson observed, *Contra Costa Times*. "But football has, amazingly, managed to fly below the radar. How do you figure that?"

John Ryan, *San Jose Mercury News*: "For some unknown reason, many of us... have been willing to believe the NFL was doing what it could to police performance-enhancing drugs while baseball turned a blind eye."

Football denial had to regroup in a big way, on call once again, and repel attacks on The Spectacle. Football America stated unequivocally to forget drugs. A brand new season stood at kickoff and everyone was ready, from personnel to media and fans.

"The NFL's logo is a shield. Nothing could be more perfect," criticized Dan Brickley, *Arizona Republic*, for the league's Thursday-night opener from Pittsburgh on NBC. "It is a league where fans wear blinders, where players hide under helmets, where the product remains untouched by criticisms that plague other sports. In the NFL, problems just bounce off that shield. And here on the brink of another season, fans have their eyes wide shut all over again."

Once again, controversy was muted about football doping. Viewpoints like Brinkley's were few compared to the media army heralding the gridiron's glorious return in American life. Sportswriters continued in their traditional role of football media, being channeled by the institution they "covered"— and fans cherishing it all.

Reporters hammered reporters for practically everyone's forgetting muscle drugs in the NFL. Thomas Grant Jr., *Times and Democrat*, South Carolina, blasted "habitual" hypocrisy of sportswriters and fans. "Ladies and gentlemen of the sports world, the verdict is in," Grant wrote. "As a collective entity, sports media and fans have been guilty in the first degree." Rick Maese, *Baltimore Sun*, maintained it was "completely hypocritical that Congress, the president, sporting officials and members of the media would go out of their way to scold baseball and be willing to turn a blind eye to football's indiscretions."

Some sportswriters dismissed criticism and defended their profession for coverage of sport doping, including Telander, veteran Chicago scribe. Legendary in the business for historic work on steroids in college football, among other issues, Telander bristled at allegations of incompetence by the sporting press, contending that extensive focus on drugs would amount to media suicide.

Telander repeated sport media's survival mantra, largely unspoken while rigidly maintained: Serving ethics or duty was idealism, but serving fans, consumers, was realism. "People don't go to the sports arena... to be concerned about societal issues," he said. "They go for fun, and entertainment." And sportswriters could not consistently attack the entertainment. "We're the *cheerleaders*," Telander reminded, sarcastic. "We can't keep being the critics. We can't do it. If you're going to cover the Super Bowl, nobody wants to read endless columns [stating] the guys are all on drugs. People don't want to see it."

Anyway, Telander figured, society already understood football required extensive drug use, having been informed for decades by writers like him. Certainly, no citizen required contemporary media's moralizing or probing to understand a football problem existed, particularly for the wealth of information now available electronically. Rather, Telander believed the fact football escaped doping scrutiny reserved for other sports, like baseball, was merely to be expected. "We like what we see. *We like looking at big guys*," he stressed. "There's no statement about drug use; you just assume. The assumption is you hope the players are not like that naturally, that they're loaded to the gills."

Telander himself had assumed the media role of moral force about steroids, investigating football, interpreting consequences for society, offering suggestions for change, yet he begrudged no reporter who would not go as far. Telander believed journalistic duty amounted to informing the public, no more. To moralize on an issue was a reporter's choice, he said, as it was an athlete's decision, ultimately, to illicitly enhance his or her performance.

"You have a duty to yourself," Telander reasoned about journalism, the individual's self-expectation. As for the enterprising journalist pondering a sport-doping investigation, Telander would have offered *good luck*, especially in football. "Ah, you know, I've rung the bell now for 30 years," he reminded.

Then what should be the message from sportswriters, for kids and their parents who aspire for heights in competition such as football?

"I think it's very clear: You say *beware*," Telander said. "Beware what you hope for, beware what you wish for. *Understand* what's going on. The first football game ever played, there were about three or four cheaters, guys who were academically ineligible. So, *that's the American way*. This hand-wringing, sometimes...," Telander paused, agitated. "We just have to stay educated and informed. And if you know you've got a kid who weighs 275 but he's gotta weigh 320, and to do that he's gotta take steroids, then you make your choice.

"And hopefully you make the right choice."

VII. Hope Renewed: Costas Nails NFL About HGH

Bob Costas got back to me, was the way I looked at it, although we hadn't communicated for a decade.

In spring 2005, Congress and the NFL danced around again about steroids, with bipartisan avoidance of evidence for futile testing. Indeed, lawmakers and league officials mutually concluded pro football was largely clean because of random urinalysis. It was a replay of spring 1989 on Capitol Hill, ignorance and apathy for football doping, aided and abetted by politicians.

Football could no longer hide or obscure doping, especially the NFL. Events, information were compounding and going public through Costas and other journalists who would not look away. In the year and a half following the latest congressional show, Costas produced impact HBO reports of muscle doping in the league that indicated systematic abuse, many players on anabolic steroids and human growth hormone. His "Costas Now" report of September 6, 2006, contained players' comments about HGH, stoking the doping fire on the eve of the NFL season and capping a summer of related headlines from several sports.

Meanwhile, a growing number of print columnists were attacking football doping, and they heeded Costas' story, which featured Redskins lineman Jon Jansen and retired NFL lineman Dana Stubblefield. San Diego reporter Tim Sullivan declared, "One look in any NFL locker room would tell you that the league's testing policies are successful primarily as public relations. … Compared to some NFL linemen, Barry Bonds is built like Olive Oyl."

Some media ignored the report of Costas, but far fewer writers were drug-oblivious this season. Even Mike Freeman, an NFL diehard among media, second-guessed his own long-held assumption the league was effective against muscle doping. "We are beginning the celebration of a new NFL season," Freeman wrote on *CBS SportsLine.com*. "As a stone-cold football addict, I will watch every snap and pancake block. Something, though, is different. My favorite sport is taking a credibility hit. This season is the season of drugs and needles and HGH and pimp-like doctors pushing their product. This season-opening celebration is more grim and dark than others in the last few years."

Politicians also felt compelled to revisit football's problem, in response to recent investigative work by Costas and *Charlotte Observer* sportswriter Charles Chandler. "The combination of these reports about the abuse of performance-enhancing drugs in the NFL shows that there are still important lessons to be learned for the league, including how the NFL drug testing program could have failed to detect this use of banned substances," wrote Rep. Henry Waxman of California, co-chair of the government committee monitoring sport doping, in a letter to new NFL commissioner Roger Goodell. "I hope the NFL will make every effort to learn these lessons and apply them to a new and more effective policy to rid the league of performance-enhancing drugs."

With respect to Representative Waxman, to whom I had already forwarded much information, my faith was gone for politicians to do anything constructive about muscle substances in American football. However, my hope was renewed journalists could do something right, including myself, and I could thank Costas for help in the lesson, once again.

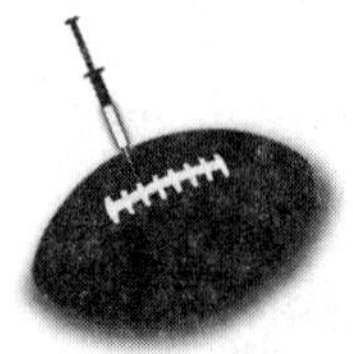

REFERENCES

Alesia, M. (2006, March 30). Colleges pay, public pays $1 billion. *Indianapolis Star* [Online].

Alexander, D. (2005, August 24). Winning ugly. *Los Angeles City Beat* [Online].

Alfano, P. (1983, August 30). CBS's Pan Am balancing act. *New York Times*, p. D20.

Almer, E. (1999, December 2). Bears lose Miller to steroid suspension. *New York Times*, p. D3.

Alzado, L. (1991, July 3). Television interview with Roy Firestone. *ESPN.*

Alzado, L. (1991, July 8). 'I'm sick and I'm scared.' *Sports Illustrated*, p. 20.

Anderson, S. (2006, April 6). No asterisk for Bonds, please. *Pittsburgh Post-Gazette* [Online].

Apathy Danger. (2006, April). Steroid investigation shows danger in apathy. *Northern Star* [Online].

Armour, N. (1999, December 20). Players, teams learn the hard way that supplements aren't so simple. *Associated Press* [Online].

Austen, I. (2006, July 10). Irksome as an athlete, and now as a reporter. *New York Times* [Online].

Balog, T. (2006, August 16). Bucs' Razzano starting over. *Sarasota Herald-Tribune* [Online].

Bamberger, M. (1997, April 14). Under suspicion. *Sports Illustrated*, p. 72.

Bandyopadhyay, S., & Bottone, M. (1997, Spring). Playing to win. *Marketing Management*, p. 1.

Banks, L.J. (2006, October 2). Outspoken Madden lowers the 'Boom!' *Chicago Sun-Times* [Online].

Barnhart, A. (2005, February 1). Chiefs star helps prospect say, 'You're hired!' *Kansas City Star*, p. E1.

Barnhart, A. (2005, February 5). The return to decency? *Kansas City Star*, p. A1.

Barrett, W.M. (1998, January). Greed and hypocrisy in a land of plenty. *USA Today Magazine*, p. 69.

Barringer, F. (1999, May 4). Newspaper industry fails to stem circulation drop. *New York Times*, p. C8.

Bax Suspended. (1990, August 16). Bax suspended Thursday. *Associated Press* [Online].

Bax Test. (1990, May 19). Bax takes drug test, tries to clear name. *St. Louis Post-Dispatch*, p. 2C.

Baxter, K. (2006, July 9). Divided attention. *Miami Herald* [Online].

Bayless, S. (1990). *God's coach*. Simon and Schuster: New York, NY.

Beacham, G. (1999, September 22). Waddy unbowed after completing four-game steroid suspension. *Associated Press* [Online].

Bell, J. (2005, May 16). Castillo's andro use casts cloud over 'model citizen.' *USA Today* [Online].

Benjamin, A. (2006, June 9). Experts concerned HGH is a growing problem. *Boston*

Globe [Online].

Bianchi, M. (2006, September 11). NFL fans prove short memories help in long run. *Orlando Sentinel* [Online].

Bickley, D. (2006, September 7). NFL gets kid-glove treatment from public, Congress. *Arizona Republic* [Online].

Bisher, F. (1991, July 14). Alzado has spoken; will the NFL doing anything about it? *Atlanta Journal and Constitution* [Online].

Blake, S. (2005, April 18). NFL steroid policy draws LT's praise. *New York Post* [Online].

Blaudschun, M. (1993, September 10). Thunder being shaken from Notre Dame sky. *Boston Globe*, p. 82.

Blaudschun, M. (1993, September 17). Holtz has been exposed, now let's call of the dogs. *Boston Globe*, p. 87.

Bohannan, L. (2006, September 10). Steroid furor not evident in NFL fans. *Desert Sun* [Online].

Bonfatti, J.F. (1989, August 30). Bills rookies' dreams sidetracked by steroids. *Associated Press* [Online].

Bosworth, B., & Reilly, R. (1988). *The Boz: Confessions of a modern antihero*. New York, NY: Charter Books.

Boyle, B. (2005, November 5). Revealing Romo. *DenverPost.com* [Online].

Broadcasts Loss. (2001, November 22). Broadcasts become loss leaders. *Kansas City Star*, p. B2.

Brockinton, L. (1997, November 24). Jags help Times-Union become fatter cat. *Mediaweek*.

Brown, B. (1993, September 7). Irish eyes not smiling about book. *USA Today*, p. 1C.

Brunner, B. (2006, August 3). NFL is top dog when it comes to fan interest. *Chronicle-Tribune* [Online].

BSU Program. (2005, August 17). BSU bulks up steroid-testing program. *Idaho Statesman* [Online].

Buchanan, N. (2006, June 1). Steroids threaten athletes beyond professional level. *Guardian*, University of California-San Diego [Online].

Bunch, W. (2006, April 19). Pulitzers confirm a 'dangerous trend.' *Editor & Publisher* [Online].

Burwell, B. (2006, August 29). Now is time for the NFL to receive more scrutiny. *St. Louis Post-Dispatch* [Online].

Caesar, D. (2003, January 31). NFL cements dominance in the ratings in 2002. *St. Louis Post-Dispatch* [Online].

Caesar, D. (2004, November 21). Selling sex & sports. *St. Louis Post-Dispatch*, p. B1.

Campaign Trail. (2004, October 15). On the campaign trail: Condoleezza Rice visits Browns facility. *Kansas City Star*, p. A2.

Canavan, T. (1994, January 5). Eric Moore's lost year. *Associated Press* [Online].

Carey, C. (2004, November 10). New TV deals prove the NFL is considered the best show in sports. *St. Louis Post-Dispatch*, p. D1.

Chad, N. (1986, February 28). Cosell keeps telling it like it is, but his reach shrinks. *Washington Post*, p. C2.

Chaikin, T., & Telander, R. (1988, October 24). The nightmare of steroids. *Sports Illustrated*, p. 82.

Chambers Joins. (2006, November 7). Chambers joins NFL training camp. *BBC Sport* [Online].

Chamoff, L. (2006, July 10). Scandals in sports are nothing new, observers say. *Stamford Advocate* [Online].

Chandler, C. (2005, April 30). Mitchell apologizes for link to steroid investigation. *Charlotte Observer* [Online].

Chandler, C. (2006, August 27). Report is snapshot of doping in the NFL. *Charlotte Observer* [Online].

Chandler, C. (2006, August 30). Congressman 'stunned' about steroids. *Charlotte Observer* [Online].

Chandler, C. (2006, September 8). Lawmaker's letter to NFL chief rejects steroids claim. *Charlotte Observer* [Online].

Chaney, M. (1987, March 20). Big Apple proving to be poisonous place for Dr. K. *Fenton Journal*, p. 4C.

Chaney, M. (1990). SEMO State Athletics timetable 1988-90. *Non-published.*

Chaney, M. (1998, October 2). Big Mac steps up to the plate; steroid awareness steps back. *Kansas City Star*, p. C7.

Chaney, M. (2000, February 24). Yes, athletes are role models. *Kansas City Star*, p. B7.

Chaney, M. (2001). *Sports writers, American football, and anti-sociological bias toward anabolic drug use in the sport.* Warrensburg, MO: Central Missouri State University.

Christ, D. (2006, July 9). Selig vs. Tagliabue (LOE). *Beacon Journal* [Online].

Christopher, H., Jr. (1999, November 18). Lip readers take note of Cunningham's cursing. *Kansas City Star*, p. E4.

Christopher, H., Jr. (2006, July 5). These dreads turn heads. *Kansas City Star*, p. F1.

Chun, L. (2006, May 24). NCAA cracks down on steroid use. *KGMB-TV* [Online].

Cialini, J. (1989, August 29). Eagles lose Solt to steroids, reduce roster. *United Press International* [Online].

Cialini, J. (1989, September 27). NFL reinstates Solt, Douglass, 9 others. *United Press International* [Online].

Coach 'Joking.' (2005, November 30). Coach 'joking' about NU steroid use. *Omaha World-Herald* [Online].

Colleges. (2000, May 14). Tennessee professor says office broken into, phone bugged. *Kansas City Star*, p. C2.

Colleges. (2005, August 10). Rouse suing his former attorney. *Kansas City Star*, p. D2.

Collier, G. (2000, January). The ex-sportswriter. *Columbia Journalism Review 38, 5*, p. 38.

Collinsworth, C. (2003, October 23). The best policy. *NFL.com* [Online].

Colson, B. (1997, September 8). Sports Illustrated's weekly pro and college football columns have doubled in size this season. *Sports Illustrated*, p. 10.

Colson, B. (1999, September 20). Total football. *Sports Illustrated*, p. 14.

Colson, B. (1999, December 13). Taking action. *Sports Illustrated*, p. 17.

Condoleezza Rice. (2006, October 26). Condoleezza Rice interview with Sean Hannity; press release. *United States State Department* [Online].

Condoleezza Sexy. (2005, May 15). Condoleezza Rice's high-heel boots and sexy wardrobe. *Parade*, p. 2.

Conte, V., & Assael, S. (2004, December 13). BALCO owner comes clean. *ESPN The Magazine* [Online].

Cook, F.L., Doppelt, J.C., Ettema, J.S., Gordon, M.T., Leff, D.R., Miller, P., & Protess, D.L. (1991). *The journalism of outrage*. The Guilford Press: New York, NY.

Corallo, M. (2006, August 23). Stop Justice Dept.'s attack on reporters. *New York Daily News* [Online].

Cosell, H. (1985). *I never played the game*. New York, NY: Avon Books.

Costas, B. (1987, March 15). Interview with author, St. Petersburg, FL.

Costas, B. (1992, December 16). Postal correspondence to author.

Couch Potatoes. (2005, December 21). It's official: We're major couch potatoes. *Kansas City Star*, p. D2.

Coughlin, T. (2005, August 10). 'T'-ing off. *Northeastern News* [Online].

Cour, J. (1989, May 10). Knox favors random testing. *Associated Press* [Online].

Courson, S. (2005, August 16). E-mail correspondence to author.

Covitz, R. (2005, April 28). Our steroid policy is working, NFL says. *Kansas City Star*, p. D1.

Covitz, R. (2006, October 3). Football message control. *Kansas City Star*, p. C1.

Covucci, D. (2006, June 14). It's not cheating if it's legal. *Collegiate Times* [Online].

Cowboys Apparel. (2001, June 2). Cowboys break away from NFL on apparel sales. *Kansas City Star*, p. C2.

Cracking Down. (2006, June 28). NFL cracking down on drugs. *Associated Press* [Online].

Cripe, C. (2006, May 24). More steroid tests in Boise State football's future. *Idaho Statesman* [Online].

Crouch Retirement. (2002, September 12). Eric Crouch will announce retirement. *Kansas City Star*, p. D10.

Cunningham, M. (2006, August 9). NFL's steroid policy merits skepticism. *South Florida Sun-Sentinel* [Online].

Dad, Mom. (2005, February 23). Dad, mom aren't as tough on drugs. *Kansas City Star*, p. A4.

Daly, S. (2005, October 25). A betting boom is born. *New York Daily News* [Online].

DeFleur, M.L., & Ball-Rokeach, S.J. (1989). *Theories of mass communication* (5th ed.). New York: Longman.

De Jong, A. (2006, May 9). Money drives college athletics. *Daily Bruin* [Online].

DeMause, N. (1999, November/December). Conflicts of interest prevent tough coverage of sports issues. *www.fair.org*.

Denham, B.E. (1997, August). *Sports Illustrated*, the "War on Drugs," and the Anabolic

Steroid Control Act of 1990. *Journal of Sport & Social Issues 21, 3*, p. 260.
Denham, B.E. (1999). Building the agenda and adjusting the frame: How the dramatic revelations of Lyle Alzado impacted mainstream press coverage of anabolic steroid use. *Sociology of Sport Journal, 16*, p. 1.
Ditrani, V. (2004, December 5). NFL does it right way. *NorthJersey.com* [Online].
Doctor Pleads. (2006, March 7). Doctor pleads guilty in steroid case. *News-Record* [Online].
Dodds Says. (1990, April 4). Dodds says no steroids probe in Texas football. *Associated Press* [Online].
Donohew, L., Helm, D., & Haas, J. (1989). Drugs and (Len) Bias on the sports page. In Lawrence A. Wenner, *Media, Sports, & Society* (p. 225). Newbury Park, CA: Sage Publications.
Douglass Denies. (1989, August 29). Douglass denies steroid use. *United Press International* [Online].
Ducibella, J. (1999, November 5). Making the best of a second chance. *Virginian-Pilot* [Online].
Duke Mulls. (2005, October 21). Duke mulls over steroid allegations. *Duke Chronicle* [Online].
Dvorchak, R. (2005, October 4.) Keeping steroids out of sports no easy task. *Pittsburgh Post-Gazette* [Online].
Eskenazi, G. (1999, November 26). Ferguson's suspension sends the Jets scrambling again. *New York Times*, p. C4.
Eskenazi, G. (1999, December 23). Jets' Ferguson returns after a four-game ban. *New York Times*, p. D4.
Etc. (2000, February 17). Microsoft co-founder Paul Allen is buying The Sporting News. *Kansas City Star*, p. D2.
Etc. (2002, February 13). Fox Sports writes off $909 million in losses. *Kansas City Star*, p. D2.
Etc. (2002, March 1). Reporters must sign agreement on 'Reliant Astrodome.' *Kansas City Star*, p. D2.
Ettema, J.S., & Glasser, T.L. (1988, Summer). Narrative form and moral force: The realization of innocence and guilt through investigative journalism. *Journal of Communication 38*, p. 8.
Ettema, J.S., & Glasser, T.L. (1998). *Custodians of conscience: Investigative journalism and public virtue*. New York: Columbia University Press.
Ettkin, B. (2005, August 12). One pill fans can't swallow. *Times Union* [Online].
Evans, E.S. (1998, April). Media still ignoring stadium boondoggles. *St. Louis Journalism Review, 28, 205*, p. 17.
Eveld, E.M. (2005, April 18). Old ball game is new 'meet' market. *Kansas City Star*, p. D1.
Falcons, Eagles. (2005, September 16). Falcons, Eagles punished for fight. *Kansas City Star*, D11.
Farrey, T. (1991, September 1). Despite its no-nonsense approach, the NFL has

maintained its favored status. *Seattle Times*, p. C1.
Fecteau, A. (1995). NCAA state action. *Seton Hall Journal of Sport Law, 5,* p. 291.
Feinstein, J. (2005). *Next man up*. New York: Little, Brown and Company.
Ferstle, J. (2000). Evolution and politics of drug testing. In Charles E. Yesalis (Ed.), *Anabolic steroids in sports and exercise* (2nd ed., p. 363). Champaign, IL: Human Kinetics Publishers.
Finger, M. (2006, July 19). Not so loud please. *San Antonio Express-News* [Online].
Fitton Says. (1985, December 18). Fitton says he shipped steroids to Cornhuskers. *Associated Press* [Online].
Flanagan, J. (2003, July 27). Kansas City radio stations vie for rights to air NFL playoff games. *Kansas City Star*, p. D2.
Flanagan, J. (2005, April 22). Anchor rejoicing that NBC has NFL again. *Kansas City Star*, p. D2.
Flanagan, J. (2006, October 15). Ex-Knight Pritchard climbing NBA ladder. *Kansas City Star*, p. C2.
Flowers Suspension. (2003, July 27). Broncos safety Flowers gets suspended by NFL. *Kansas City Star*, p. C12.
Freedman, E. (1991, August 5). Judge: MSU violated law by withholding steroid reports. *Detroit News* [Online].
Freeman, M. (1999, September 5). Uneasy lies helmet with Broncos' logo. *New York Times*, p. 8—10.
Freeman, M. (2000, August 27). Drug policy loophole revealed in an appeal. *New York Times*, p. 8—11.
Freeman, M. (2001, October 7). N.F.L. is seeing fewer flaws in testing players for drugs. *New York Times*, p. 8—7.
Freeman, M. (2006, September 8). A look inside the beefed up huddle. *CBS SportsLine.com* [Online].
Friedman, J. (2006, May 31). Bonds puts pressure on sportswriters. *Investor's Business Daily* [Online].
Gano, R. (1989, August 29). Packers tackles suspended for steroid positives. *Associated Press* [Online].
Gano, R. (1997, December 1). Alonzo Spellman returns to Bears. *Associated Press* [Online].
Gano, R. (1999, February 2). Payton has rare liver disease. *Associated Press* [Online].
Gano, R. (1999, December 1). NFL suspends Bears quarterback for drug policy violation. *Associated Press* [Online].
Gantt, D. (1999, December 3). Panthers could learn from Miller's mistake. *Rock Hill Herald* [Online].
Garrison, B. (1993). *Sports reporting* (2nd ed.). Ames, IA: Iowa State University Press.
Garrity, J. (1997, May-June). Jason Whitlock scores in K.C. *Columbia Journalism Review 36, 1*, p. 51.
Gay, N. (1999, October 22). Jervey suspended for steroid use. *San Francisco Chronicle* [Online].

Georgatos, D. (1999, November 23). Jervey completes suspension. *Associated Press* [Online].

George, T. (1989, March 23). Stunning owners, Rozelle says he's retiring. *New York Times*, p. D23.

Gold, A. (2006, August 29). It's just a fantasy. *The Blog* [Online].

Gordon, K. (2002, July 5). Sentiments mixed on ephedrine ban in NFL. *Columbus Dispatch*, p. 6D.

Grant, T., Jr. (2006, October 15). Hypocrisy in sports. *Times and Democrat* [Online].

Gray, R. (2000, January). Laptop quarterback. *American Journalism Review*, p. 16.

Grossman Experimented. (1989, May 17). Grossman experimented with steroids. *Associated Press* [Online].

Hansen, E. (2005, October 22). Steroids atrophy at college level. *South Bend Tribune* [Online].

Hardwig, G. (2006, May 26). Morgan: Don't single out just one or two users. *Naples Daily News* [Online].

Harris, J. (2006, June 13). Mark Fainaru-Wada. *www.truthdig.com* [Online].

Hartman, S. (1993, September 10). Holtz has his backers around these parts. *Minneapolis Star Tribune*, p. 2C.

Hayes, D. (2005, August 23). Online music seller makes deal with three Missouri universities. *Kansas City Star*, p. D10.

Hayes, D. (2005, October 12). Sprint makes a play for NFL fans. *Kansas City Star*, p. C3.

Hayes, D. (2006, September 13). Sprint offers a bigger phone perk. *Kansas City Star*, p. C1.

Hayes, D. (2006, September 29). The clock runs out on Mobile ESPN. *Kansas City Star*, p. C1.

Helitzer, M. (1992). *The dream job: Sports publicity, promotion, and public relations.* Athens, OH: University Sports Press.

Hendricks, M. (1997, May 21). Live sports afflicted by TV morons. *Kansas City Star*, p. C2.

Hendricks, M. (1998, April 3). The result of making sports life and death. *Kansas City Star*, p. C2.

Henry, G. (2005, November 23). Falcons vs. Lions. *FalconInsider.com* [Online].

Herrmann, A. (2000, October 11). Violence not everything — it's only thing. *Chicago Sun-Times*, p. 57.

Heyman, J. (2006, October 24). 'It was pine tar' (cont.). *SI.com* [Online].

Hiestand, M. (2006, July 10). Fox eyes interviews from on-deck circle. *USA Today* [Online].

Hilliard, D. (1994, February). Televised sports and the (anti) sociological imagination. *Journal of Sport & Social Issues*, p. 88.

Hirsch, P.M., & Thompson, T.A. (1994). The stock market as audience: The impact of public ownership on newspapers. In J.S. Ettema & D.C. Whitney (Eds.), *Audiencemaking* (p. 142). Thousand Oaks, CA: Sage Publications.

Hoffman, S. (2005, July 7). The NCAA sets a high bar for drug testing standards. *Iowa State Daily* [Online].

Hohler, B. (2005, April 6). Broad steroid policy pursued. *Boston Globe* [Online].

Holtz Allegedly. (1993, August 31). Holtz allegedly funneled money to former Minnesota player. *Associated Press* [Online].

Holyfield, J. (1991, January 16). Michigan State panel finds no evidence of steroids. *Associated Press* [Online].

Honan, W.H. (2001, January 7). Do big-money sports belong in college? *New York Times*, p. 4A—19.

Houlihan, B. (1991). *The government and politics of sport*. New York: Routledge.

Howard, J. (2002, May 12). NFL and union do the right thing. *Newsday*, p. C11.

Howell, S. (2005, October 24). "A history of violence"...in sports. *Stanford Daily* [Online].

Huebner, B. (1996, December 22). Pro football retains its allure for women. *Boston Globe*, p. D1.

Hyams, J. (2005, June 14). UT strong-arms athletes who test positive. *Nashville City Paper* [Online].

Internet Delivers. (2000, March 24). Internet delivers for NFL expansion team. *Kansas City Star*, p. D2.

Invesco Pays. (2001, January 30). Invesco pays a bundle for Mile High naming rights. *Kansas City Star*, p. C2.

Itule, B.D., & Anderson, D.A. (1987). *News writing and reporting for today's media*. New York: Random House.

Jackson, J. (2005, November 20). Pro sports don't need Congress' help. *Chicago Sun-Times* [Online].

Jacobson, G. (2006, April 27). College coaches 'looking other way.' *Dallas Morning News* [Online].

Janofsky, M. (1986, March 6). Rozelle wants stricter drug plan. *New York Times*, p. B13.

Jenkins, B. (2006, May 27). McGwire and Sosa didn't save baseball in '98 but fans sure enjoyed it. *San Francisco Chronicle* [Online].

Jervey Suspended. (1999, October 22). 49ers' Jervey gets 4-game suspension. *Minneapolis Star Tribune*, p. 9C.

Jets Waived. (1989, September 26). Amoia and Riley waived by Jets. *Associated Press* [Online].

Johnson, T. (2006, September 3). Are sports media more juiced over baseball steroid use? *NewsBusters.org* [Online].

Jorgensen, E. (2005, May 23). Some UCD athletes say they have never been tested. *California Aggie* [Online].

Junkin Positive. (1989, May 7). Junkin tested positive for steroid in 1987. *Associated Press* [Online].

Jurkowitz, M. (2006, April 5). It's time for baseball — and all sports — to be covered just like any other multi-billion-dollar business. *The Phoenix* [Online].

Kaduk, K. (2004, December 6). Gimmicks makes them Super. *Kansas City Star*, p. C8.

Kamran, J. (2006, October 6). Who knows? Who cares? *Columbia Spectator* [Online].

Katz, M. (2006, July 11). Unlike football, baseball's big men keep taking hits. *Dayton Daily News* [Online].

Keisser, B. (2006, February 6). NFL Network scores on league's TV contract power play. *Los Angeles Business Journal* [Online].

Kerkhoff, B. (1999, November 28). Remote Control. *Kansas City Star*, p. C8.

Kerkhoff, B. (2000, May 24). Tube-socked sports. *Kansas City Star*, p. D1.

Kerkhoff, B. (2007, March 15). Digital madness. *Kansas City Star*, p. D1.

Keteyian, A. (1989). *Big Red confidential.* Chicago: Contemporary Books, Inc.

Kettmann, S. (2000, August 20). Time to flush steroids out of baseball. *Springfield News-Leader*, p. 3C.

King Joins. (2006, April 27). Peter King Joins NBC's 'Football Night in America.' *thefutoncritic.com* [Online].

King, P. (1990, July 9). 'We can clean it up.' *Sports Illustrated*, p. 34.

King, P. (1991, August 5). One more lesson. *Sports Illustrated*, p. 15.

King, P. (2005, April 4). Here's how the league can get tougher on steroids. *SI.com* [Online].

King, P. (2005, April 5). MMQB Tuesday Edition. *SI.com* [Online].

King, P. (2005, August 22). Monday Morning Quarterback. *SI.com* [Online].

King, P. (2006, August 28). Monday Morning Quarterback. *SI.com* [Online].

King, P. (2006, September 11). Dawn of a new season. *SI.com* [Online].

King, P. (2006, October 23). Tiki takes on the world. *SI.com* [Online].

King, P. (1999, December 20). The war on steroids. *Sports Illustrated* [Online].

Kjos,, L. (1990, September 24). Brian Sochia rejoins Dolphins. *United Press International* [Online].

Klis, M. (2005, October 14). Romo juiced while a Bronco. *Denver Post*, p. A1.

Knight, B. (2006, April 6). NCAA to extend test for drugs. *El Paso Times* [Online].

Koppett, L. (1994). *Sports illusion, sports reality*. Boston: Houghton Mifflin.

Kramer Says. (1988, October 7). Kramer says drug testing more effective than education. *United Press International* [Online].

Krieger, D. (2006, September 5). NFL avoids going under steroids microscope. *Fort Wayne Journal Gazette* [Online].

Landers, A. (2001, October 2). Son forced into football, he's miserable. *Daily Star-Journal*, p. 2.

Lapchick, R.E. (1986). *Fractured focus.* Lexington, MA: Lexington Books/D.C. Health Co.

Lederman, D. (1991, May 13). Big sports programs are out of control, most say in survey. *Chronicle of Higher Education*, p. A33.

Legwold, J. (2005, May 25). Bowlen says to behave or else. *Rocky Mountain News* [Online].

Legwold, J. (2005, October 13). Romanowski comes clean on steroid use. *Rocky Mountain News* [Online].

Lidz, F. (2006, April 28). Can't shy away from controversy. *SI.com* [Online].

Lie, Deny. (2006, July 31). Lie, deny, alibi, falsify. *Spiegel* [Online].

Limon, I. (2006, April 12). NCAA extends drug testing. *Albuquerque Tribune* [Online].

Lipsyte, R. (1975). *SportsWorld.* New York, NY: Quadrangle Books.

Lipsyte, R. (1999, January 31). Trial balloon has evolved into religion. *New York Times*, p. VIII-17.

Lipsyte, R. (2007, February 2). Telephone interview with author.

Lipsyte, R. (2008, March 13). Telephone interview with author.

Lohf, K. (2005, July 12). ISU athletes are tested for 'street drugs.' *Iowa State Daily* [Online].

Long Admits. (1991, December 4). Steelers guard Long admits using steroids. *Associated Press* [Online].

Long Positive. (1991, July 25). Steelers' Long tested positive for steroids. *United Press International* [Online].

Long Suspended. (1991, November 14). Long suspended four games by NFL. *United Press International* [Online].

Long Used. (1991, December 4). Long admits to steroid use. *United Press International* [Online].

Lowenkron, H. (1996, April 26). Mandarich ready to compete for job. *Associated Press* [Online].

Maese, R. (2005, September 9). For athletes, 'I didn't knowingly' excuse has positively failed believability test. *Baltimore Sun*, p. 1F.

Maese, R. (2006, September 5). Drug testing in NFL has wide-open loopholes. *Baltimore Sun* [Online].

Maniscalco, M. (2006, August 16). Maurice Clarett doesn't have to look far to find out who is responsible for his problems. *Richmond.com* [Online].

Mannie, K. (2004, April 13). Designer steroids. *NaturalStrength.com* [Online].

Mannie, K. (2005, April 25). Time to strike out the steroid mess. *www2.ncaa.org* [Online].

Manoyan, D. (1999, November 2). 'Walter is the best there ever was.' *Milwaukee Journal Sentinel*, p. News-1.

Mann, J. (2004, September 21). The NFL's next move? Casual wear. *Kansas City Star*, p. D6.

Marchiony, J. (1991, July 3). NCAA spokesman, telephone interview with author.

Marcus, S. (2006, January 6). SBU officially starts random drug testing in the spring season. *Newsday* [Online].

Martzke, R. (1993, September 9). Irish receive support from unlikely sources. *USA Today*, p. 3C.

Maske, M. (2006, September 7). Redskins' Jansen says use of HGH is rising. *Washington Post*, p. E1.

Maske, M., & Shapiro, L. (2005, September 8). Leagues ahead of the rest. *Washington Post*, p. E1.

McCallum, J. (2006, October 4). See no evil, hear no evil. *SI.com* [Online].

McCarthy, M. (2005, October 17). Former-players-turned-analysts unsympathetic to Romanowski. *USA Today* [Online].

McCarthy, M. (2005, June 8). More sports leaders turn to political pros at crunch time. *USA Today* [Online].

McChesney, R.W. (1989). Media made sport: A history of sports coverage in the United States. In Lawrence A. Wenner (Ed.), *Media, Sports, & Society*, p. 49. Newbury Park, CA: Sage Publications.

McCleneghan, J.S. (1997, July). The myth makers and wreckers. *Social Science Journal 34, 3*, p. 337.

McCudden, K.A. (2006, September 14). Chiefly feminine. *Kansas City Star*, p. E1.

McDonough, W. (1989, March 23). The Rozelle resignation; colleagues pay tribute. *Boston Globe*, p. 66.

McDonough, W. (1996, April 27). The Patriots knew enough to know better. *Boston Globe*, p. 55.

McMasters, P.K. (2006, October 10). Shooting the messenger is getting popular. *Baxter Bulletin* [Online].

Mellinger, S. (2006, December 24). Some fans need reality check for fantasy football. *Kansas City Star*, p. C1.

Merrill, E. (2005, October 15). Welbourn glad his 'vacation' is finally over. *Kansas City Star*, p. D1.

Menzer, J. (2005, August 13). Walls named in HBO show as former patient of Shortt. *Winston-Salem Journal*, p. C9.

Michener, J.A. (1976). *Sports in America*. New York, NY: Random House.

Miklasz, B. (1996, December 2). Telephone interview with author.

Miklasz, B. (2004, February 4). Only thing 'shocking' about that halftime show is NFL's hypocrisy. *St. Louis Post-Dispatch* [Online].

Miller, R. (1988, October 12). Cooper says two positives 'too many.' *Associated Press* [Online].

Miller Suspended. (1999, December 1). Bears QB Miller suspended for season. *United Press International* [Online].

Moore, J. (1994, November 29). Wycheck suspended by NFL for steroids. *Associated Press* [Online].

Moore Mum. (1993, July 20). Giants' Moore mum about legal trouble. *St. Louis Post-Dispatch*, p. 3C.

Mortensen, C. (2005, April 13). DT prospect Castillo admits steroid use. *ESPN* [Online].

Mossman, J. (1989, May 10). Broncos officials say steroid use low, perhaps non-existent. *Associated Press* [Online].

Mott Denies. (1990, February 21). Jets linebacker Mott denies drug use. *Associated Press* [Online].

Murphy, E.C. (1992, November 14). Sports falls short (LOE). *St. Louis Post-Dispatch*.

Myers, G. (2006, August 30). Upshaw: Player in Panthers steroids scandal was in NFL program. *New York Daily News* [Online].

Names Emerge. (1991, September 1). Names emerge in L.A. steroid case. *Washington Post*, p. D2.

NBC Fiscal. (2002, January 10). NBC opts for fiscal responsibility. *Kansas City Star*, p. D2.

NBC Opts. (2002, January 10). NBC opts for fiscal responsibility. *Kansas City Star*, p. D2.

NCAA Hall. (2000, April 14). NCAA opens Hall of Champions with hoopla, exhortations, and mixed messages. *Chronicle of Higher Education*, p. A69.

NCAA Manual. (1989, March). *1989-90 NCAA manual.* Overland Park, KS: National Collegiate Athletic Association.

NCAA Tests. (2006, July 7). Ups and downs in NCAA drug tests. *Inside Higher Ed* [Online].

Nederpelt, D. (2006, March 23). Bailing on Bonds. *SanFranciscoSentinel.com* [Online].

Neff, C. (1985, December 9). Steroid justice. *Sports Illustrated*, p. 11.

Nevius, C.W. (2006, August 29). The NFL drug problem: Does anyone care? *San Francisco Chronicle* [Online].

Neubert, J. (2005, August 29). Armstrong, Bonds, Palmeiro apart of the latest steroid talk. *Rebel Yell* [Online].

Newton, D. (2005, September 25). Headlines just scratch surface, critic says. *State* [Online].

NFL Gains. (2004, November 9). NFL gains flexibility in new TV deal. *Kansas City Star*, p. C3.

NFL Network. (2006, April 28). NFL Network will rival ESPN on draft day. *USA Today*, p. 3C.

NFL Suspends. (2002, November 15). NFL suspends Peppers. *Kansas City Star*, p. D3.

Nickel, L. (2005, July 4). NFL players defense on steroids. *Milwaukee Journal Sentinel* [Online].

No Probe. (1990, April 3). Texas not expected to probe reported steroid use. *United Press International* [Online].

Noelle-Neuman, E. (1993). *The spiral of silence* (2nd edition). Chicago, IL: University of Chicago Press.

Northwestern President. (1990, March 8). Northwestern president says isolated cases were possible. *Associated Press* [Online].

Not Aware. (1987, January 10). Osborne says he was not aware Steinkuhler, others used steroids. *United Press International* [Online]

Noonan Used. (1987, May 5). Noonan used steroids to regain weight. *Associated Press* [Online].

NPPA Letter. (2006, April 10). NPPA letter to NFL expresses 'extreme disappointment' in sideline vote. *National Press Photographers Association* [Online].

NYT Expanding. (1997, September 14). Newspaper's updated look breaks with journalistic tradition. *Kansas City Star*, p. A11.

O'Brien, R. (1993, September 13). The book. *Sports Illustrated*, p. 15.

O'Hara, M. (1996, April 26). Mandarich tries comeback, looking for a better ending. *Detroit News* [Online].

Oriard, M. (1993). *Reading football: How the popular press created an American spectacle.* Chapel Hill, NC, and London, England: University of North Carolina Press.

Oriard, M. (2001). *King football: Sport & spectacle in the golden age of radio & newsreels, movies & magazines, the weekly & daily press.* Chapel Hill, NC, and London, England: University of North Carolina Press.

Ostler, S. (2005, October 17). Romo's words don't ring true. *San Francisco Chronicle* [Online].

Ostruszka, S. (2006, March 28). Are NIU athletes juicing up? *Northern Star* [Online].

Ostruszka, S. (2006, March 30). Steroids on campus? *Northern Star* [Online].

Padwe, S. (1986, September 27). Symptons of a deeper malaise. *The Nation*, p. 276.

Palladino, E. (1999, December 10). NFL players should avoid dietary supplements. *Westchester Journal News*, p. ARC.

Palladino, E. (2004, December 4). Testing slows use of steroids in NFL. *Asbury Park Press* [Online].

Panthers Like. (2006, August 28). Boy, the Panthers sure do like their steroids. *deadspin.com* [Online].

Passan, J. (2005, August 28). Trading spaces. *Kansas City Star*, p. G1.

Pearlman, J. (2006, June 2). Pee no evil. *Slate.com* [Online].

Pells, E. (2004, January 1). Union finds system to check supplements. *Associated Press* [Online].

Pepper, M. (1997, December 14). Too much sports or too little? *Kansas City Star*, p. B2.

Perloff, A. (2006, March 9). NFL out-does MLB once again. *SI.com* [Online].

Peters, J. (2006, February 22). Athletes to face tougher drug tests. *St. John's Torch* [Online].

Peterson, G. (2006, September 6). NFL clean? Tell the Easter bunny. *Contra Costa Times* [Online].

Pitoniak, S. (2005, January 21). Area doctor fears apathy will crush anti-steroid campaign. *Rochester Democrat and Chronicle* [Online].

Players Advised. (2005, December 3). Players advised on cheating tests. *Kansas City Star*, p. D3.

Pollack, J. (1996, July/August). Sports/Media. *St. Louis Journalism Review*, p. 7.

Posnanski, J. (2006, November 1). Sports still thrill Deford. *Kansas City Star*, p. D1.

Preston, M. (2006, October 24). Likes of Merriman just a speck in cleaner NFL. *Baltimore Sun* [Online].

Price, C. (2006, August 6). Pats' big secret is now out. *www.patsfans.com* [Online].

Pro Football. (2001, July 12). Viacom, AOL Time Warner, SportsLine.com agree on NFL pact. *Kansas City Star*, p. D2.

Prospect Admits. (2005, April 14). Draft prospect admits steroid use. *Kansas City Star*, p. D8.

Protess, D.L., Cook, F.L., Doppelt, J.C., Ettema, J.S., Gordon, M.T., Leff,

D.R., & Miller, P. (1991). *The journalism of outrage: Investigative reporting and agenda-building in America*. New York and London: The Guilford Press.

Rand, J. (1998, October 15). League uniformity. *Kansas City Star*, p. D1.

Rand, J. (1999, October 7). Houston's $700 million buys NFL expansion spot. *Kansas City Star*, p. D1.

Rand, J. (2000, March 28). Internet hot topic for NFL. *Kansas City Star*, p. C1.

Rapoport, R. (2005, August 23). OK, it's only preseason, but NFL off to sorry start. *Chicago Sun-Times* [Online].

Ratto, R. (2006, February 1). NFL, players need to act now to trim weight. *CBS SportsLine.com* [Online].

Ratto, R. (2006, February 4). Tagliabue loosens up — or at least, is less robotic. *San Francisco Chronicle* [Online].

Red, C. (2006, August 31). NFL aims to implement effective test for HGH. *New York Daily News* [Online].

Redskin Suspended. (1994, November 30). Redskin player suspended for steroid use. *New York Times*, p. B19.

Renck, T. (2006, December 29). NFL video game remains hot item in homes all over country. *Pueblo Chieftain* [Online].

Renck, T.E. (2006, June 9). Loophole puts HGH on map. *Denver Post* [Online].

Reusse, P. (1993, September 9). Holtz book a wakeup call only to Rip Van Winkle types. *Minneapolis Star Tribune* [Online].

Richman, H. (2000, August 30). Tigers QB has stress fracture. *Kansas City Star*, p. D4.

Ritter, J.K. (2006, January 31). Foundation examines steroids and recruiting. *Herald-Sun* [Online].

Results 'Steroid.' (2006, August 28). Google search results for 'steroid.' *Google News* [Online].

Roberts, S. (2005, August 26). Truth has been sullied too many times. *New York Times* [Online].

Robinson, Je. (2000, March 13). Fans' joy and agony (LOE). *Kansas City Star*, p. B4.

Robinson, Jo. (2005, October 6). Testing the Ivy League. *Columbia Spectator* [Online].

Rock, S., & Dillon, K. (1997, July 19). Open documents, NCAA urged. *Kansas City Star*, p. C3.

Romanowski, B., Schefter, A., & Towle, P. (2005). *Romo: My life on the edge*. New York, NY: HarperCollins Publishers.

Rookie Suspended. (2005, September 17). Bucs rookie suspended for violating NFL steroid policy. *Associated Press* [Online].

Ryan, J. (2006, August 29). After further review: NFL testing has flaws. *San Jose Mercury News* [Online].

Salwen, M., & Garrison, B. (1994). Survey examines extent of professionalism in sports journalism. *Editor & Publisher*, p. 54.

Sanchez, M. (2006, August 15). Real men value truth and do the right thing. *Kansas City Star*, p. B9.

Sandomir, R. (1998, December 20). For CBS, a difficult balance is found. *New York*

Times, p. SP2.

Saraceno, J. (2005, October 18). Insincerity obvious when Romanowski opens mouth. *USA Today* [Online].

Schlosser, J. (1998, June 1). A league of their own? *Broadcasting & Cable*, p. 8.

School Spending. (2005, May 25). School to up spending to $100K. *Associated Press* [Online].

Schreiner, B. (1986, October 15). Osborne said one or more Cornhuskers used steroids. *Associated Press* [Online].

Scranton, L. (2006, May 17). Scifres awaits Chiefs' decision. *Springfield News-Leader* [Online].

Scruggs, N. (2005, August 6). Off the air. *Star-Telegram* [Online].

Seymour, K.B. (1997, November 24). Jags help 'Times-Union' become fatter cat. *Mediaweek*, p. 16.

Shanahan 'Disappointed.' (2006, July 28). Shanahan 'disappointed' in suspended punter. *Associated Press* [Online].

Shapiro, L. (1999, December 2). Bears QB Miller gets sacked for steroids. *Washington Post*, p. D5.

Sherman, J. (1988, April 28). Cadigan cites reasons for using steroids. *United Press International* [Online].

Sherrington, K. (2005, August 15). Steroid denials flunk test. *Dallas Morning News* [Online].

***SI* Editor.** (1990, August 27). *SI* editor: Magazine is not targeting Notre Dame. *Associated Press* [Online].

Slezak, C. (2005, February 20). Yes, steroid use is bad, but it's time to move on. *Chicago Sun-Times* [Online].

Smith, B. (2005, August 3). Montclair journalist helps state tackle steroid problem. *Montclair Times* [Online].

Smith, H.I. (2002, March 30). It's not news (LOE). *Kansas City Star*, p. B6.

Smith, M. (2006, October 18). Falcons C Lehr our four games for violating steroid policy. *All Headline News* [Online].

Smith Ready. (2003, March 28). Smith ready to run for the Cardinals. *Kansas City Star*, p. D2.

Smith, T.W. (1991, August 18). Troubled Steeler is sitting out while waiting for league ruling. *New York Times*, p. 8—7.

Smother Brothers. (2006, May 20). Smother Brothers. *New York Daily News* [Online].

Sneyd, R. (1990, August 8). Media draw fire at sports ethics conference. *Associated Press* [Online].

Solomon, J. (2002, July 28). No quick fix. *Houston Chronicle*, p. Sports 2—1.

Solt Used. (1989, September 1). Published report says Solt previously used steroids. *United Press International* [Online].

Souhan, J. (2000, September 1). America's game. *Minneapolis Star Tribune*, p. 1C.

Spear, B. (1992, July). Telephone interview with author.

Spellman Says. (1997, November 28). Spellman says he'll return. *Kansas City Star*, p. D4.

Spellman Suspended. (1997, November 24). NFL suspends Spellman for refusing steroids test. *Associated Press* [Online].

Sperber, M. (1999, January 8). The NCAA is haunted by its past. *Chronicle of Higher Education*, p. A76.

Spindler Disputes. (1990, April 24). Spindler disputes positive steroid test. *United Press International* [Online].

Sports Bubble. (2003, August 5). Sports TV bubble pops. *Kansas City Star*, p. D3.

Stafford, D. (2002, December 10). To your conscience be true, professor advises. *Kansas City Star*, p. D22.

Stan Cohen. (2001). Stan Cohen: States of denial: Knowing about atrocities and suffering. *www.lse.ac.uk*

Stapleton, A. (1998, December 24). Pack's Waddy says no on steroids. *Associated Press* [Online].

Steed's Words. (1995, October 27). Steed's words come up a bit short. *Nando.net* [Online].

Steele, D. (2000, October 18). At least Olympics seek fix for drugs. *San Francisco Chronicle*, p. E1.

Steele, D. (2006, October 5). The non-stick league. *Baltimore Sun* [Online].

Stein, M.L. (1998, February 14). Making hay from Super Sunday. *Editor & Publisher*, p. 29.

Steroid Investigation. (1986, August 28). Steroid investigation concerns two Husker football players. *United Press International* [Online].

Stone, L. (2006, April 15). Welcome to the new steroids era. *Seattle Times* [Online].

Strupp, J. (1999, February 6). Super Bowl coverage tackles NFL's biggest. *Editor & Publisher*, p. 10.

Strupp, J. (2006, October 1). Sportswriters say they dropped the ball on steroids in major league sports. *Editor & Publisher* [Online].

Sullivan, T. (2006, September 9). Drug double standard gets NFL off hook with fans. *San Diego Union-Tribune* [Online].

Tammeus, B. (1999, June 6). Newspapers face daunting list of problems. *Kansas City Star*, p. K3.

Teicher, A. (2002, November 7). NFL suspends Chiefs' Bush for using banned substance. *Kansas City Star*, p. D1.

Teicher, A. (2006, March 21). Tagliabue will retire in July. *Kansas City Star*, p. C1.

Telander, R. (1989). *The hundred yard lie*. New York: Simon and Schuster.

Telander, R. (1989, April 24). The big enchilada. *Sports Illustrated*, p. 40.

Telander, R. (2006, August 29). Dear fellow sportswriters, sports columnists, sports editors. *Groupwise e-mail.*

Telander, R. (2006, August 31). Telephone interview with author.

Texas Denies. (1990, April 11). Texas denies steroid use among athletes. *United Press International* [Online].

This Story. (2006, August 27). How we did this story. *Charlotte Observer* [Online].
Tierney, J. (2006, June 27). Soccer lacks the drama that Americans crave. *Kansas City Star*, p. B9.
Timmerman, T. (2003, July 11). Not your father's Sporting News. *St. Louis Post-Dispatch*, p. D1.
Toner, J.L. (2006, September 25). Telephone interview with author.
Uhlenhuth, K. (1998, January 25). Postgame pain. *Kansas City Star*, p. G1.
UNC Policy. (2005, October 6). UNC-Chapel Hill sets steroid policy for athletes. *The Dispatch* [Online].
Union Wants. (1999, December 6). Union wants to talk about changing the NFL drug policy. *Associated Press* [Online].
Uryasz, F. (2006, February 15). Interview with author. Kansas City, MO.
Vaccaro, M. (1997, August 3). Take away games, and most of us would be lost. *Kansas City Star*, p. C20.
Vaccaro, M. (1998, January 22). Changing times, changing channels. *Kansas City Star*, p. D1.
Vacchiano, R. (2004, December 4). Giants back drug tests. *New York Daily News* [Online].
Vacek, R. (1999, April 18). Sports' leaders discuss the state of the games. *Kansas City Star*, p. C7.
Vecsey, G. (1990, December 9). The quarterback who was going to the beach. *New York Times*, p. 8—8.
Vedantam, S. (2006, August 21). Cheating is an awful thing for other people to do. *Washington Post* [Online].
Vint, T. (1989, September 2). Osborne said book isn't all bad. *Associated Press* [Online].
Voy, R. (1991). *Drugs, sport, and politics*. Champaign, IL: Leisure Press.
Walder, B. (2002, June 7). Expose should spur stronger sports coverage. *Newsday*, p. A51.
Walker, D. (2006, January 31). Poll: Commercialism exploits athletes. *Milwaukee Journal Sentinel*, p. C6.
Wenner, L.A. (Ed.). (1989). *Media, sports, & society*. Newbury Park, CA: Sage Publications.
West Suspended. (1999, November 24). Giants' West suspended. *New York Times*, p. D5.
Whannel, G. (1993). Sport and popular culture. *The European Journal of Social Sciences 6*, p. 1.
White, J. (1995, August 17). Turner looking for another Novacek. *Associated Press* [Online].
White, J. (1999, November 3). Speedy Stevens gets start against old team. *Associated Press* [Online].
Whitlock, J. (2001, August 1). Making peace with Peterson. *Kansas City Star*, p. D1.
Whitlock, J. (2006, August 29). Steroid users victim of system. *Kansas City Star*, p. C1.
Whitlock, J. (2006, October 25). Lauding Rogers shameful after ripping Bonds. *AOL*

[Online].

Wieberg, S. (1989, February 10). Sooners tackle adversity. *USA Today*, p. 1C.

Williamson, B. (2006, October 12). Agent believes Sauerbrun receiving raw deal. *Denver Post* [Online].

Wine, S. (1990, August 24). Suspension is isolated case on team, says Shula. *Associated Press* [Online].

Wine, S. (1990, September 25). Sochia says suspension taught lesson. *Associated Press* [Online].

Witz, B. (2006, September 11). L.A. issue might be on back burner. *Los Angeles Daily News* [Online].

Wolper, A. (1997, December 27). Worship on the sports page. *Editor & Publisher*, p. 27.

Wolper, A. (2005, August 9). Reporters lament the steroid secret. *Editor & Publisher* [Online].

Wood, J. (2006, March 18). Journalists missed story (LOE). *Chicago Tribune* [Online].\

Woods, M. (1992, August 5). Innocent until proven guilty — unless a muscular Chinese swimmer. *Florida Today* [Online].

Wyman, T.P. (1990, August 22). Holtz denied report steroids widely used at Notre Dame. *Associated Press* [Online].

Wyshynski, G. (2006, June 9). The steroid gossip game. *SportsFan Magazine* [Online].

Yesalis, C.E., & Cowart, V.S. (1998). *The steroids game.* Champaign, IL: Human Kinetics.

Yesalis, C.E. (2006, September 12). Telephone interview with author.

Chapter 8 [Winning]

Cultural ethos and doping in football

"The better you do, that's what shows. It's not how moral you were in getting there."

Alice Newhall
American teenager, 2002

Loose as America had become in 21st century, the republic chose to impose said morality on *athletes*. Among a society taking advantage of synthetic enhancement, jocks and female counterparts were the ones scrutinized harshly for "values," and role modeling for youth. Common citizenry including children could employ performance-enhancing drugs, or surgical procedures for body image, but athletes had to be "clean" for competition.

Individual athletes accused or known as dopers were subject to public torching, and critics derided the double standard. "Talk about cheating usually has a ring to it, and that ring comes from having a high moral tone. In this, it is fair to say, most people are hypocrites," observed writer Shankar Vedantam, *Washington Post*, for analysis on lying that addressed cultural hypocrisy about sport doping. Vedantam referenced academics and their research corroborating that the large human majority was "open to — and extraordinarily adept at — bending moral rules when it is convenient," he wrote.

Many analysts viewed America's latest moral crisis as the worst, but others saw no "culture war," just a modern, powerful nation shackled by outmoded idealism and mission. Sociologist Wayne Baker believed America struggled to let go Puritan or religious ideology of the past for its real pursuit of individual choices and freedom. Opinion analyst Seth Rosenthal, who conducted polls on U.S. leadership and worker competency, said, "Americans... hold the country in high esteem. Maybe higher than is realistic."

Wherever contemporary values ranked on history's morality meter, the act of breaking rules was accepted, full-throttle, and widespread. "Starting with the debacle of the 2000 Presidential election, the nation has been wracked with an unprecedented run of scandal and bad news which left virtually no facet of American culture and character unsullied," wrote Peter Reuell, for *MetroWest Daily News* of Boston. Syndicated columnist Leonard Pitts, Jr. wondered if cheating was "ever as brazen, as thoroughly rationalized or as high-profile as it is now?" Answering in part, Pitts wrote, "We are witness to a yawning dearth of integrity. And a corresponding death of authenticity."

"Cheaters win all the time," argued James A. Fussell, *Kansas City Star* cultural critic. "They win World Series games and college scholarships. They win big bicycle races and home run titles. The sign six-figure book deals and multimillion-dollar sports contracts and have critically acclaimed movies made about their lives."

"We are not, as a human race, consistently living up to what it seems we could or ought be," opined newsman Marvin Read, *The Pueblo Chieftain*. "We pillage when we get the chance, hoping never to get caught and, when we do, blaming the victims rather than the perpetrators, ourselves."

Being caught, indeed, constituted the sin line for many Americans. Otherwise, an act was not wrongful but simply taking what one could get. A variant situational ethic was judging an action according to laws of the land — anything legal by the courts was therefore moral and just. In addition, for those caught or accused of misdeed, an option was fervent denial against whatever evidence.

"Modern society is inevitably obsessed with excuses," wrote Andrew Petiprin, guest columnist for *The Orlando Sentinel*. "The sanctity of the individual in a democracy requires a system in which we are only as guilty as someone else can prove us to be. As admirable as the ideals of justice are, our emphasis on individual guilt has unfortunately created a society without remorse and without honor."

Throughout society, the dominant rule of competition was clear: Forget "morality" if that stood in way of "achieving" a goal. Human values were facedown in the pit. Certainly, scandal was cancerous for most major institutions of society, exposing greed and deceit. Commerce, government, education, religion, sport, parenting: Each lay exposed of scandalous behavior, riddled with unseemly character and impropriety.

I. Culture Craves Looks, Performance, Youth

Seemingly everyone was buff in 2000s America, at least in media image. Young, old, male, female — culture was inundated by perfection in physique, flawless reflections fed every second by multi-media in multi-dimension, with cyber increasingly the most relevant. Millions of people reacted, believing the muscle ideal, consuming it, coveting it, pursuing it.

Many also shied from working long and hard for a goal. An American penchant was for avoiding tough sacrifice, as though a skill in itself, especially for Baby Boomers. The generation born on TV and air conditioning preferred quick fix long into adulthood, seeking the instant buy, including for looks and performance. Boomers wanted shortcut to sex appeal, sexual prowess, career success, and more conquest, or what was mocked as "effortless perfection my butt" by college columnist Jacqui Detwiler.

All ages embraced synthetic possibilities for perfection, going for testosterone, growth hormone, Rogaine, Viagra, Botox, breast implants, liposuction — and in their sheer hypocrisy for the issue of sport doping. Males and females viewed acquiring artificial looks as healthy lifestyle, but, on the other hand, could chastise athletes for using muscle drugs, calling it "cheating."

American fakeness made compelling rock opera for Canadian performer Jon Mikl Thor, who dramatized narcissism of society. "*Devastation of Musculation* is a terminology I invented to describe our age of steroids and social pressures," Thor said in 2006, to the *Broward-Palm Beach New Times*.

"We're pushed to achieve the impossible every day. You've got the whole Barry Bonds issue. People are doing plastic surgery to get more beautiful. They take steroids to get stronger and more powerful. With all this extremism going on, *Devastation of Musculation* means all this trying to overachieve to the point of killing yourself or destroying yourself."

Thor's theatrics jibed with cries of cultural critics. Meghan Daum, novelist and columnist, wrote Americans "seem to be under some kind of cultural mandate to make ourselves into four-leaf clovers." Dissatisfaction with the natural self was human emotion, but eschewing physiological boundary was strictly modern indulgence, driven by chemical and bio-identical synthesis and plastic surgery and seized upon by Boomers, all grown up as prime consumers for the new millennium. New terms were embraced for enhancement through pharmacy, medical procedure, or combination, such as the following: "wellness medicine," "preventive medicine," "anti-aging," "life extension," "longevity management," "regenerative therapy," and "cosmetic endocrinology." Growing old was "a treatable medical condition," according to believers, with the $50 billion enhancement industry standing in testament, promoted as the *real* fountain of youth, finally. No one could refute the desirable effects of many methods, including synthetic muscle hormones and large false breasts, but neither could anyone speak with certainty on long-term health hazards — or spiritual traps.

Regardless, the breakout business of synthetic self was made for America, had long been in the making. The first of two staple drugs for the craze, testosterone, had reputation as body rejuvenator dating to the ancient Greeks. By 1900, Victorian researchers were crushing bull testes for rough extract or conducting ineffective "glandular therapy," transplanting animal sex glands into humans. Bona fide market for testosterone — and widespread agreement on its potency — was established following synthesis of the anabolic-androgenic hormone in 1935, with pill and injectable forms distributed globally by World War II.

Initial preparations were for treatment of medical conditions such as anemia or late puberty in boys. "Then they began to discover other properties of testosterone, and moved from 'disease' — known abnormality — to making normal better," David J. Rothman observed, historian on medicine, Columbia University. By war's end testosterone was touted for offsetting the aging process, and a headliner proponent was American writer Paul de Kruif, who discussed his daily intake of 20 to 30 milligrams, reporting the drug "caused the human body to synthesize protein... to be able to build the very stuff of its own life."

Medicinal human growth hormone, the other catalyst for anti-aging's boom to come, was introduced by the latter 1950s in precious supply drawn from pituitary glands of cadavers. Doctors prescribed organic HGH to treat dwarfism in children, and limited harvests begat high demand and a black market of bodybuilders, leaving needy medical patients grappling for product.

A young scientist led a breakthrough toward synthetic growth hormone for mass supply, Dr. Herbert Boyer, a biochemist at University of California-San Francisco. In the early 1970s, Boyer collaborated with Stanford geneticist Dr. Stanley Cohen in pioneering the science of recombinant DNA technology, or gene-splicing, *cloning*, to reproduce complex organic substances. Boyer had discovered how to slice a DNA double helix into single strands, while Cohen had employed host bacterium for cell reproduction and cloning, and together they created and cloned a DNA molecule, combining strands of two different substances within one E. coli culture. Boyer and Cohen would become known as the co-fathers of biotechnology.

They soon parted, Cohen remaining in academia while Boyer entered profiteering. In 1976, Boyer joined venture capitalist Robert Swanson to found Genentech, each investing $500, and the handful of company scientists initially focused on reproducing human proteins. Within three years, Genentech cloned somatostatin, insulin, and HGH, and then the company went public, debuting on Wall Street with a soaring stock price. In 1985, Genetench teamed with Eli Lilly Co. to debut marketing of recombinant human growth hormone, or rHGH.

New availability and marketing of HGH coincided with the start of steroid testing throughout major sports, and initially bodybuilders and elite athletes made headlines for illegal or questionable use. But medical interest — and business interest — lay in synthetic growth hormone for more controversial applications. Many adults secured HGH treatment for their shorter children, and *not* parents of the estimated 5,000 to 10,000 youths at risk of permanent dwarfism. The new buyers just wanted their short offspring to be taller, what with studies having confirmed height as an advantage in American quest for riches and social stature. "One man said his son would be a better attorney if his son was taller," said Dr. Rebecca Kirkland, Baylor pediatric endocrinologist, who declined the dad's request for such "off label" use of HGH.

Anti-aging talk exploded around synthetic HGH in the latter 1980s, intriguing adults from layperson to scientist. Studies were underway globally to investigate the varied theories, with some doctors acting as guinea pigs for injections themselves, to discover and experience any benefits. Potential market was obvious, but the legal question was whether normal adults, however old, could be medically designated as *growth-hormone deficient*, a confirmed condition of the prepubescent or child dwarf, for example, whose pituitary gland did not produce enough of the essential protein. "We have long wondered if some aging processes are related to lower growth hormone," said Dr. Robert Blizzard, University of Virginia Medical School. "As we get older, less is secreted into the bloodstream." Blizzard had his doubts about HGH as a preventive for aging, however, after self-experimentation along with other scientists yielded no results to confirm anything.

Other critics were harder on the wonder drug come lately. "There is no real reason to expect this is useful for the obesity side," said Dr. Jules Hirsh, obesity expert, Rockefeller University. "It is conceivably a death hormone instead of a growth hormone," remarked Dr. William Regelson, Medical College of Virginia.

Illicit use of synthetic HGH worried those who saw exploitation by both the black market and unscrupulous physicians. Manufacturers of growth hormone pledged to control stockpiling and distribution, but upwards of 20 percent of the old organic version had been diverted and sold illegally, said one doctor interviewed by the *New York Times*, and thieves recently had hijacked a large shipment of Genentech's synthetic version. Another expert fretted the science cart had come before the horse, in an irrational rush over human growth hormone. "We ought to regard any new drug as ineffective until proven otherwise," said Dr. Gordon Cutler, National Institute of Child Health and Human Development.

Medical prudence, however, was often passé in modern America, especially over drugs designed or said to improve lifestyle. Consumers drove demand for new beauty substances and many physicians were ready to accommodate. Traditional practice of medicine was affected, with more and more practitioners leaving for the boom business of cosmetic substances and procedures.

Human growth hormone was a well-read story in consumer and business news of the late 1980s. Enthusiasts such as clinical researchers touted HGH for bona fide weight loss, among potential "solutions" in the offing. Study findings of the drug's turning fat into lean muscle stoked public attention that was "almost frightening," said endocrinologist Dr. Gilman Grave, National Institute of Child Health and Human Development. Many researchers were hopeful beneficial effects could be proved about HGH, including Dr. Daniel Rudman, Medical College of Wisconsin in Milwaukee. While leading a new, much-anticipated study, Rudman spoke to *The New York Times* at decade's end: "For the first time in history, we have abundant amounts. Medical scientists are looking for additional uses," Rudman said. "Most scientists feel that growth hormone will have important therapeutic uses, but we were really not able to look into this [previously] because of the scarcity of growth hormone."

Soon, Rudman and lab associates made a mainstream splash, completing milestone research on HGH — and inspiring controversy to last decades, over conflicting interpretations of their findings. In the six-month clinical study, injections of synthetic HGH were administered to 21 older men, ranging 61 to 81 in age. Rudman and colleagues monitored effects in the subjects, and the bodies transformed irrefutably. Among measurable changes, lean mass replaced some fat in the men and the epidermal or skin layer gained a reported "youthful thickness."

On July 5, 1990, the *New York Times* went front-page with the stunning news — "Human Growth Hormone Reverses Effects of Aging"— and then continued coverage of research by Rudman and associates. The seeming breakthrough in human quest to defeat aging had arrived, many proclaimed, and world media jumped on the story. "The results are quite amazing," said Dr. Lester Cohn, of the research team. "We're dealing with people with an average age of 70, who for 40 years had been losing muscle mass and mass in internal organs." Moreover, Cohn stated in words to resonate widely, the body clock was turned back "through growth-hormone replacement."

HGH suddenly ranked with the cell phone as revolutionary invention of the moment. "Can you imagine what people will be willing to pay for this stuff?" mused syndicated columnist Richard Reeves. The concept of HGH for anti-aging was out in open, spotlighted if not yet sanctioned, for wide speculation and even some application in America. Early believers easily purchased the drug south of the border, but there was interest in a legal U.S. market, discussed by doctors, politicians, business people, and potential consumers. Previous growth-hormone studies had generated excitement, but now people besieged experts, seeking information and the drug. "I've gotten so many calls and letters," said endocrinologist Dr. Mary Lee Vance, University of Virginia. "They've called me at home — people wanting growth hormone for their parents; lawyers, doctors, wanting me to refer them to physicians who will give it to them."

Vance led criticism of HGH, having authored a cautionary review for the NEJM, about mystery and potential danger surrounding the recombinant hormone, which she called a "double-edged sword." The scientific community largely agreed with Vance, most endocrinologists and gerontologists. Reliable data could only become available through more research, decades' worth, on pituitary mechanism and effects of human deterioration. "Everybody wants a magic wand," said Dr. Fran Kaiser, geriatrics specialist at St. Louis University. "And it would be nice to have one that has no side effects. Growth hormone shows great promise. But it's not a panacea. Its use will probably be for specific problems."

The Rudman findings were "the most dramatic we've seen so far" in growth-hormone research, said Dr. Michael L. Freedman, geriatrician at New York University Medical Center, but he emphasized too much remained unknown. "We have no idea what will happen if we start treating a lot of people with this stuff," Freedman said. "Even if it makes you have more muscle or makes your skin better, if it ends up increasing something in the kidneys or gastrointestinal tract that leads to cancer, that's no good." A large majority of doctors would not condone HGH for anti-aging, said a pioneer in gene cloning, Dr. John Baxter, UC-San Francisco. "Some rich old guys are going to come in asking for growth hormone," he said. "It is premature."

Dr. Rudman, at center of the issue, acknowledged a "positive in all this publicity" to be heightened awareness for need of technological development to benefit the frail elderly. But he was uneasy with fast-growing optimism for HGH as youth serum; he too was fielding many inquiries, from doctors and scientists as well as lay people. "We want to emphasize that there are many aspects of the aging process that aren't going to be influenced by growth hormone," Rudman explained. "This [research finding] is a favorable effect on one aspect of the aging process. Others would require other strategies."

Yet thousands of Americans were convinced, viewing growth hormone, like testosterone, as a potent preventive of aging, a cultural belief, founded or not, bound to spread and endure. Anabolic drug usage for the purpose was hardly novel anyway, and now legions joined the movement, or sought to. An "anti-aging clinic" opened near Cancun, Mexico, in 1993, the El Doral Rejuvenation and Longevity Institute, catering to Americans. Soon the American Academy of Anti-Aging Medicine was founded and membership exploded, buoyed by U.S. physicians leaving behind traditional practice. Emboldened, the anti-agers headed north with their treatments of growth hormone and testosterone.

People ceased trekking to Mexico for the prescription drugs, as doctors and other medical personnel across America — some of dubious repute — began offering anti-aging protocols. For legal foundation, the new practice supposedly treated adult hormone deficiency, a law-specific requirement for prescribing HGH or testosterone in the United States. Hot debate, therefore, focused on proper definition of adult hormone deficiency, a rare condition which many critics of anti-aging charged was being exploited, relative to normal declines through the human life cycle.

Conversely, life cycle was precisely the point for anti-agers, whose general mission was to redefine mortality. Many followers strove to live forever, completely bypassing diminishment and death. Some government researchers shared the enthusiasm, pursuing studies on the concept of hormone-replacement therapy for the elderly and, at times, commenting favorably about possibilities for physical rejuvenation.

One skeptic merely saw greed at work: "The pursuit of the fountain of youth will lead many people not to pay too much attention to the possible downside of the treatment," said Art Caplan, bioethics expert, University of Pennsylvania, "and the pursuit of money will lead many physicians not to pay too much attention to what they may really be doing to their patients." American manufacturers of synthetic HGH reaped golden results, reporting annual sales for the substance at about $2 billion worldwide, about $300 million at home. They remained steadfast in their public warnings about off-label use of the drug, claiming their inventory went strictly to legitimate medical cases, but critics continued to allege a significant amount was steered to uses such as athletics and anti-aging.

By the latter 1990s, adverse side effects of HGH were cited in research literature, including fluid retention, joint pain, and carpal tunnel syndrome. "I won't take this stuff," said Dr. Richard Sprott, former director of the National Institute on Aging. "What hasn't been done is the basic pathology to see what the long-term effects are." Endocrinologists denounced HGH for anti-aging practices. They said only a tiny percentile of the adult population constituted certifiable cases of growth-hormone deficiency, individuals who had the condition as children or those whose pituitary was damaged by accident, cancer, or radiation treatment. [The FDA also approved use for patients with muscle-wasting linked to HIV or AIDS.]

Off-label uses of HGH in anti-aging were illegal, medical officials said, but they believed thousands of doctors and consumers were skirting regulation of the Food, Drug, and Cosmetic Act. "In too many cases, those who... do not need human growth hormone are getting it, and those who truly... need human growth hormone are not getting it," said Dr. Stanley Feld, American Association of Clinical Endocrinologists.

HGH fans scoffed at naysayers and denied they violated law, passing off criticism as typical of stodgy medical establishment. "There is mass disaffection with traditional medicine now. Many doctors are as fed up as the patients," said millionaire John Sperling, 78, founder of the University of Phoenix, as he prepared to open a string of "age-management" clinics in 1999. Commercial outlets covered the nation. Clients paid between $6,000 and $30,000 per year for evaluations and injections of HGH, a drug in vogue among Hollywood types and more cliques of image-conscious people.

For the fashion set in Manhattan, along Park Avenue's "Plastic Surgery Mile," Dr. Adrienne Denese catered to models, musicians, and other professionals, touting benefits such as fat loss, vibrant skin, and increased sexual vitality. "My patients who used to take antidepressants don't take them anymore," Denese told the *New York Times*. "They take HGH and it makes their mood lighter. Even I take it, and I'm more animated. I feel good and I don't take Prozac anymore."

Cleveland clinic owner Dr. Thomas Marosi said HGH was no youth potion, but instead an effective replacement for valid hormone deficiency in virtually every adult of middle age or beyond. "It's sort of like going back to your youth to exercise and eat better," Marosi said. "It buys you back some time that you now have the wisdom to use. Think of it as a gift you might give yourself."

In Chicago, clinic operator Dr. Alan Mintz injested and endorsed multiple hormones, emphasizing "health span" rather than life span. "I'm 60. I function like I'm 45," he said. "I sleep six hours. I keep up endurance-wise with my kids in their 30s. I never get sick. I go to the gym every morning. Sex is much better than five years ago."

New York plastic surgeon Dr. Bruce J. Nadler administered HGH to dozens of patients. The 51-year-old, a competitive bodybuilder, said his life was revitalized by growth-hormone regimen. "Those nagging injuries were healing faster. I was able to work out better. For years, my eating had been an exercise in biochemistry — weighing every gram of protein and watching everything I ate," Nadler said. "Now I… sit down and eat french fries and dessert like I [am] in my 20s without inflating my love handles. It made my body function in a much younger way.

"I'm one of the Baby Boomers. We're the generation that never wants to get old."

Pittsburgh advertising executive Jane Singer concurred: "They're a completely self-absorbed generation," she said of the estimated 77 million Boomers. "They have a sense of entitlement that they're going to stay young and live forever."

II. American Attitude: By Any Means Necessary

A summer morning in St. Louis, football preseason 2003, miserably hot, and sports-talk radio ignited over the issue of performance-enhancing substances. I helped stoke the fire on-air, as guest analyst for "Beyond Ball" on all-sports station KFNS, where show hosts Bryan Burwell and John Maracek had me in studio. We discussed anabolic steroids, growth hormone, and legal supplements, and then solicited phone-ins from listeners. Their calls quickly backed up on hold.

What we heard was startling litmus on American attitude about sport doping. The dominant majority of callers, about a half-dozen, believed synthetic performance enhancement was fine, OK, as long as users employed "safe" substances. Fathers phoned into the show, wanting to know anything their sons could ingest for bulking up, speeding up in sports, just safely, of course. No verifiably safe muscle substance existed, but callers cared little. Nor were they concerned about fair play in team games, whether competition would be school, college, or professional.

It was sad, repeating myself by show's end, telling successive callers I did not recommend any reputed muscle-builder, *nothing*, including creatine, the popular amino acid consumed by millions, especially the young and athletic.

The final call-in was different. Bob, a man about retirement age, did not view sport as vital to the culture. Bob was angry but not with me, my stance, which had come off prudish to the discussion. "All these parents that are calling in, and they want to know how to enhance their kids' performances. ...," Bob said, disgustedly, halting indignantly. "Look, if the kid isn't big enough, strong enough, tall enough, fast enough — do something else. Don't mess with [substances]."

"That's an excellent point!" Burwell jumped in, a *Post-Dispatch* sports columnist unnerved by previous callers despite his decades of covering sports, including pro football.

Conviction surged within Bob the caller. "Do a little weightlifting, running, whatever," he said, voice smoothing out. "And if you can't make in sports, then go learn a trade or go to college and become a B.A. or whatever. But the heck with all this stuff."

Burwell, encouraged, told Bob: "More people oughta' be as mad as you are! Because you're listening to these parents, and it is — it's the *shortcut cycle*."

The show ended. Top of the hour struck, satellite sports took over the air. Microphones off, we three in studio sat silent a few moments, having just staged a public referendum on values in American sport. And the feeling was ill. "Daaamn," I muttered, twangy.

Coming into the show, I knew exactly what to expect in straight question-and-answer with listeners, particularly for discussing various substances, their effects for performance, if any, and potential health hazards. I could have sold that information long ago, of course; people had always wanted how-to from me. By now I had hundreds hours in review of ethics of sport doping, study, and writing focused strictly on the sub-issue of human character, those questions and leads — not to mention plenty of first-person experience, my own misdeeds in perpetuating the problem, multiple roles.

But the experience still caught me off-guard, the radio show's tapping hard into American attitude on winning. I had long known what to expect from organizers of sport as entertainment — a lot of talk, but real commitment to nothing besides victory, profit, by any means necessary. Yet dealing in this vein was unsettling, with the consumer public.

What the hell *was* wrong with this country? The question was traditional cliché in America. However, while previous generations had questioned themselves, they *would* be enraged over social mores of 2000s society. No way would the ancestors have struggled so for the culture to come to this, to *us*.

The business world served up corruption headlines almost daily, making pop vernacular again of "perp walk," with defrocked corporate executives entering courtrooms for the cameras, replacing mobsters of old newsreels. Gretchen Morgenson, *New York Times*, wrote a syndicated column titled "A culture of casual deception" in late 2004. "So this is where we are now in corporate America," Morgenson lamented. "Even in the post-Enron era, some executives still think nothing of misleading investors, analysts and their customers. When they get caught, their companies respond in a way that may provide legal protection but also allows the lie to live."

Evasion, lies made gold storylines for American media — *Scandal!* — taking over human-interest news genre, and politicians starred, naturally, for woeful ethics at every level of government, federal, state, and local. Congressmen, governors, mayors, judges, and police were convicted of criminal acts, among officials, and many more faced allegations of impropriety — including cops for steroid and HGH use and distribution. News reports of shady activity blanketed the land. "Efforts to compromise the integrity of government are much more aggressive because the stakes are so much higher," said ethicist Kirk Hanson. "The election of a friendly city council member or state legislator, or even the insertion of a short sentence into law, can now mean millions to a special interest group."

While reports exposed raw the amorality of public authorities, their sorry behavior was nothing new. Mildly shocking, though, were the exposés of debauchery on part of role models supposedly above reproach, in religion, science, and education. Pastors and priests were accused of crimes, including murder and child molestation, and others stole from religious coffers, such as the secretary who embezzled $356,000 from an Illinois church. Sexual predators were uncloaked among school officials, administrators, teachers, and coaches, female and male, who were caught in relationships or attacks involving juvenile students. School funds were also vulnerable to criminals, like the superintendent caught stealing $844,478 from his rural Missouri district, lost to his gambling habit. Leading research scientists could not resist cheating, their fraudulent studies exposed after publication in reputable journals, and best-selling writers were caught plagiarizing information, manufacturing so-called fact and scenes.

"Regular folks," meanwhile, made a mess of so-called morality too.

Youths certainly took shortcuts, with as many as four in five "teen achievers" admitting they cheated in some form of schoolwork. In another survey, sampling from 4,500 high-school students, researchers found more than half plagiarized information from the Internet. "What's important is getting ahead," Alice Newhall, 17, told CNN reporter Kathy Slobogin in 2002. "The better grades you have, the better school you get into, the better you're going to do in life. And if you learn to cut corners to do that, you're going to be saving yourself time and energy. In the real world that's what's going to be going on." Mike Denny, a senior classmate of Newhall at a high school in Virginia, said he thought cheating was wrong. However, he admitted, "Honor seems like it's a concept of the past."

"Students today find it so much easier to rationalize their cheating," said Donald McCabe, a Rutgers researcher on adolescent cheating. Academic cheating flourished with the Internet, which provided word passages for copying and Web sites for purchasing research papers. Cell phones and other hand-held devices could photograph and send images, such as pages on a test, and also message text with a partner off-site. Computer software could create cheat sheets from a candy wrapper, imprinting test answers on the ingredients label.

Children blamed poor modeling by adults. "I think kids today are looking to adults and society for a moral compass," McCabe said, "and when they see the behavior occurring there, they don't understand why they should be held to a higher standard." Baby Boomers were especially prone to rationalization for stupid choices, in matters such as citizenship, vices, marriage, parenting, family finances, and job.

At work many people did not perform as solid employees, reliable, worthy of pay. More commonly, worker culture espoused snatching everything possible from an employer. People lied on résumés and in interviews to win jobs, or pulled favor from contacts, the overwhelming choice of mode to beat other candidates. "Networking," they called it. Once gainfully employed, Americans lied on expense reports and timecards, stole company items, and used technology for personal reasons, like cruising the Internet. One study found the large majority of American companies were damaged by fraud; *employees* committed most the theft. Employees lied to superiors for skipping work and, when on the job, offered poor service to customers and clients, rude and uncaring. "The bar is so low, service has gotten so bad that today, if it's not terrible, we are relieved," said John DiJulius III, expert on customer service.

Thoughtless, uncaring people infested the culture. We rationalized whatever in order to believe or possess, practicing the *truthiness* of satirist Stephen Colbert, defined as "the quality of preferring concepts or facts one wishes to be true, rather than concepts or facts known to be true."

III. Revisiting, Acknowledging Personal Character

Carrying on a conversation somewhere before this book, with the topic turning to my writing, someone would say, "You oughta write a book about me." I'd wonder why anyone would want private life revealed in public. I didn't anticipate seeing my personal story in book form, and especially for rearing two children who could read.

Writing this book, broaching the topic of doping in football, I had to be honest about my own multiple roles in the problem, as a juicer player, perpetrator coach, ostrich journalist, and drunken fan. Still I put off writing first-person passages, avoiding them, especially for this chapter on ethos of American culture — the foremost factor sustaining football doping. No doubt, I had been and continued to be a person of character lows. This chapter, besides its bombing of American ethics in general, swung the onus on me: What had been my internal values for living? What had influenced me from boyhood to middle age, the 1960s to the New Millennium? How had I been a football player willing to employ muscle drugs, then a writer motivated to address the scourge?

I uncovered and remembered more about me than I cared to, with the trail leading to ethical core of self. I'd collected and boxed the evidence as lifelong packrat: personal records, keepsakes, writings, and other artifacts, like a comb attachment from a blow dryer, 1977. There were memories and mementoes that made me proud for positive deeds, and much to feel rotten about, the misdeeds. I wished I could apologize to several people. Oh, yeah, I had sinned to win, various competitions over time, Boy Scouts to girls to football, and savored most of it.

Sixties Imprints: Assassination, Rock 'n Roll, and the Baptist Church

As I approached four years old, winter 1963-64, two events stormed my consciousness: the assassination of President John F. Kennedy and, no less, America's introduction to The Beatles. Both happenings I witnessed immediately through "electronic media," television and radio, imprinting information through sight and sound before I could read. I'd remember the president's death and The Beatles of equal importance, issues of both national security and pop entertainment. Later, historians generally confirmed my preschool impression: JFK's murder and the Fab Four endured as period quakes.

The 1960s in America were scary, exhilarating, and driven by television, the blossoming mass medium prone to pop-culture overload. My parents didn't exactly go along, as a religious couple committed to rearing children in a home clean, safe, and moral. We brothers never saw Mom and Dad exhibit antisocial behavior in public or private. Our parents didn't curse, didn't touch alcohol, never advocated violence or the breaking of law, and we were constantly reminded in lessons verbal and demonstrated. We were shielded from alcohol, narcotics, and foul language, and monitored for our reading material and consumption of television, radio, and song records. Our parents strictly forbade us to fight — *four boys* — forbade us, in fact, to threaten people in any manner. Our parents mandated we tell truth, good or bad, and accept consequence of our actions, praise or punishment.

In school every day, we Chaney boys were expected to excel in classes and obey our teachers, to avoid any so-called negative behavior. Our father was a school administrator but one wholly committed to colleagues' judgment, not ours, mere boys. Dad clearly stated his rule: "You get in trouble at school, you're in trouble at home." Our family attended First Baptist church throughout the week, seemingly present for every event at the place, including dinner and sermon on Wednesday night. Sundays we made double attendance, morning and evening, for Bible classes and pastor sermons.

Our mother and father were fine role models, yet we sons found trouble and would continue to find it. Undeniably, parents influenced children foremost, positively or negatively, but likewise without doubt, kids acquired attitude and behavior elsewhere — especially through peer interaction and television, communication fronts ever intensifying for youth of the '60s.

As a preschooler I tried to be a good boy, the third son, and through periods I largely met the standards of Baptist doctrine. I believed in honor, honesty, and thoughtfulness for others, compassion. At earliest memory, I judged the world as a close match between good and evil, and wanted to do my part — behave, as the child — to ensure righteousness prevailed in ultimate conflict. I also expected God to protect my family, especially my mother, father, and brothers, in exchange for my being good.

I mostly made A grades for my schoolteachers and typically gave earnest effort in sports, church, Scouts. At home I usually got along with my brothers and respected my parents. I was mostly constructive with my time, per my parents' wishes, and not just to appease them. I *wanted* to be good, honest, productive, and be viewed as such by others. I wanted people's respect, and understood that came with hard work and positive deeds. I dreamt of becoming a writer, for example, as soon as I could read; no other occupation, I thought, could be as fulfilling and honorable.

In alter ego, however, I understood self-gratification through materialism, fun, and I especially enjoyed grandparents who took me dining, bought me toys, and gave me money. In grade school I stepped up negative behavior, seeking mischief or trouble with other kids, using profane language and sneaking cigarettes. I joined some boys at age 11 for my first swig of beer, which tasted terrible. We kept a stash of pornography, confiscated *Playboy* magazines with pictures of naked women. I wanted notoriety, popularity among kids, and saw my way in rebelling, through defying authority like parents and teachers.

My higher instinct — to respect elders, behave, work hard, set a positive example — could crumble instantly against childish insecurities, particularly my desire for attention from other kids. I wanted to look cool, act cool, and peers to buy it.

Big Brother's Tragedy Marks Family

Heartbreak befell my family as I entered junior high, altering our course and shaking beliefs, undoubtedly mine. My oldest brother, Allen, was a talented, lovable, misfortunate youth who struggled in life, for problems rooted in his severe condition of epilepsy, grand mal. Allen suffered terrible seizures in his epilepsy, a disorder of the central nervous system causing misfire of neural charges in the brain.

Allen, seven years older than I, certainly could get down on himself, too easily sometimes, but the world was damned mean to him, and I witnessed much of the cruelty as his alarmed little brother. Allen and his epilepsy first inspired me to stand up for people who needed help and deserved it, against ignorance, callousness. Many kids mistreated Allen, making fun of him, mimicking his violent seizures, rejecting him. They laughed and pointed when, suddenly, he'd stiffen and fall, jerking, drooling, and uttering strange sounds, guttural moans. Youths played pranks involving physical harm to Allen, like bullies who picked fights, knowing he was one Chaney boy ready to throw punches. Then they'd pull in their cronies and gang up, beating him mercilessly. A few adults were no better, humoring themselves at Allen's expense. I witnessed and felt my big brother's pain, wondering how I could save him, dreaming of lifting him up and away from such people.

That would not happen. Allen would not live long, and I *knew*, even so young. I identified his death wish before I turned 10. Beyond his incredible risk-taking — daredevil feats and crashes as an isolated child graduating into, as embittered young man, illegal drinking, drugging, fighting, wrecking vehicles — Allen's gravest obstacle to survival and happiness lay in broken inner spirit. After awhile, I hardly feared Allen wouldn't make it; I practically accepted it. Too often he was despondent, completely down on life, given up, feeling sheer hopelessness. His belief was tough to rebuke, even for loved ones, with the hardships this kid endured.

We tried, refusing to give up. Quicksand was drawing Allen, and we fought to hold on him, especially my devoted parents. Mom and Dad made family priority of their firstborn and his condition, supporting him and battling it since his first seizure at age 4, when he dropped from a high porch onto rocky Ozark ground below, convulsing, bleeding. Mom and Dad propped up Allen's psyche at every opportunity, particularly emphasizing his achievements, and often the growing boy was a trooper, embracing positive thinking and acting on ambition. The teen preferred the nickname "Big Al" when feeling heady, and he had talent.

Allen possessed both physical and mental potential. Pound for pound, he would endure as the strongest and most muscular among four brothers. Allen was a good athlete, outstanding in baseball as a catcher, and fearless in competition. Most importantly, Allen was an A student in school during periods and highly accomplished in music, excelling as a horn player and winning state competition in choir.

Allen's prime passion was the arts, his best way to stand out, allowing him to celebrate and lament life while displaying flair, gift. When arts were the stage Allen just showed off among kids, I always thought, beautifully communicating through acting, singing, concert band, drawing, painting, sculpture, and creative writing. His poetry included a frightening first-person voice courting death, chilling and insightful despite its youth. Darkness did always loom around Allen, inevitably wearing on him and us. When he went down to despair, those times, I could dismiss him in a huff, but my parents stuck by him.

Allen's grand mal episodes were only countered by powerful medication and rigid control of environment. For minimizing seizures, the imperative steps were fitful regular sleep and drug protocol of Phenobarbital. My parents administered the daily structure for Allen without fail, not always easy for them emotionally. They understood Allen's open longing "to just be normal," and it hurt having to contain him so rigidly, including disciplining him for stepping out of the program.

Mom was growing desperate by end of the 1960s, with Allen approaching high-school graduation and increasingly fighting authority and structure. Real trouble followed him now. With his intellect and talent, Allen had potential for independent living as an adult, his dream, yet was evermore resistant to constant routine for health. He was a teenager often missing sleep and optimum timing of meds. He was determined to stay up late some nights and party, even fight. Already hooked on Marlboro cigarettes, Allen had begun to consume alcohol and street narcotics as a loner with dangerous attitude, accepting self-destructive behavior and its painful outcomes.

What was to become of Allen? We brothers had our skepticism, or resignation, but Mom, a homemaker attending college, prayed to God while seeking earthly guidance wherever available, including from the Epilepsy Foundation of America, which she contacted in Washington, D.C. The EFA replied with pamphlets and data sheets, an authoritative overview of epilepsy nationwide. The information was helpful but disheartening, representing a bleak outlook for Allen and young people like him. "References appear in earliest recorded history, though epilepsy is still one of the world's least understood maladies." Surveys indicated almost all Americans knew of epilepsy and a large majority believed in mainstream lifestyle for epileptics, but there was prejudice and more roadblocks. Sufferers comprised about 1 percent of the population, people ranging from mild or temporary cases to the congenital and most severe, such as Allen.

The EFA warned of varied discrimination against epileptics in America, children and adults. One state still outlawed marriage for persons with epilepsy, while 12 condoned sterilization "under certain conditions." Ten disallowed a driver's license. Many epileptic children were denied admission by schools, as were adults by universities. The working class of epilepsy faced major difficulties in holding jobs, including those medically controlled and of normal IQ, the group of most potential, whose rate of unemployment was only one in four. Many epileptics had no chance for obtaining health insurance, auto insurance, or life coverage. Public perceptions about epilepsy generally had risen above dark-age superstition, nightmarish time of abuse for many victims, but opinion surveys revealed ill will held fast in American society. "Though public attitudes toward epilepsy have improved in recent years, a significant number of persons polled still have misconceptions about epilepsy," the EFA concluded.

Allen had much to overcome for reaching normal lifestyle, living independently and possibly marrying, being a father. Sadly, he didn't appear secure for developing the maturity required. Allen the adolescent could angrily defy his prescribed health routine and everyone around him, particularly those trying to help. Family members weren't alone in trying to reach Allen — so did the girl he took to senior prom, proudly driving her in the family Delta 88, his only official date of high school.

Afterward, on a clear night in August 1970, the 18-year-old was thinking of Allen, wishing he were with her. She penned a playful, flowing note in a card he stowed away as keepsake. "Oh, by the way, did you see the moon tonight? (Tonight is Wednesday)," she wrote, continuing:

> The Man in the Moon was so sad. It really was depressing, but rather beautiful anyway. ... I found a quote that I want to pass on to you. It is worded so well, that I hope it will take root in your cynical, skeptical 'rock' of a heart. Here it is — 'It is as absurd to pretend that one cannot love the same woman always as to pretend that a good artist needs several violins to play a piece of music.'
>
> People are lonely because they build walls instead of bridges. Please, dear heart, don't put up any more walls!

The lovely young woman could not save Allen, nor could we family. He kept the walls up awhile longer, until too late. Allen was a college dropout at 19 in November 1972, with little prospects and his epilepsy worsening. He worked for minimum wage pruning trees at a plant nursery, in a new town full of strangers, including several with whom he clashed. He partied many nights, getting hammered, driving fast, and finally totaling his car against a telephone pole. Then he walked the streets, usually alone.

A weekend approached when the family had to leave town, everyone except Allen, possibly, so he and my parents argued again. Allen wanted to stay home, unsupervised, which had already led to seizures and bodily injuries, among problems. My parents wished he would go with us; Mom pleaded. Allen refused, so the rest of us took off Friday afternoon, on a long road trip with my brother Mark's high-school basketball team.

Sunday morning, Mark and the team returned home first. My parents, younger brother Chris, and I had stayed back at my maternal grandmother's. Mark made a frantic phone call from home, and Mom answered. Mark wouldn't tell her much other than Allen had been in an accident, a seizure at home by himself involving a fall into the bathtub. "He hit his head," Mark said. I took the phone but Mark blew me off, refusing to say more. Mark wanted Dad, who was away at the moment with an uncle. "Just tell me where to call Dad!" Mark demanded, and I got the number. I knew the worst had happened.

Minutes later, my uncle's truck drove up and my father got out. Mom, dreadful, rushed to Dad, and he steadied, clutching her by the shoulders. Mom asked about Allen as I watched from a kitchen window. "He's already gone," Dad told her. My mother screamed, slamming into Dad, and I made an announcement inside the house: "Allen's dead." The gathered relatives cried out together as I, the 12-year-old brother, ran out the back door wailing, shaking my fist at God, yelling into blue sky.

"FUCK YOU!" I raged.

IV. College: The Pursuit of Football Hero

During the winter I turned 22, a plodding college student bent on partying and writing terrible fiction, my mother sent letters with love and money. I didn't often visit my parents at home anymore, typically only when I needed something, and she was worried. "Hope everything is going great for you," Mom wrote optimistically, as the new semester began, while enclosing a check for my tuition, books, and extra. "I pray nightly for you and feel the Lord has really great things in store for you. Don't ever forget where your blessings come from."

A month later, approaching my birthday, I'd left my parents hanging as usual. Mom wrote: "Was hoping you would call and let us know about Sunday, but you didn't. Hope we get to come down to be with you on your birthday. You are a man now. My, I can remember the day I had you. You were beautiful and so sweet. We are proud of your work this year and remember we love you."

That letter slashed deep, reading it on a lonely day in Cape Girardeau with actually little good going for myself, February 1982. I'd hyped my present prospects for Mom and Dad, and they were loyal in loving support, but my problems were apparent. Many peer adults were graduating college and starting careers while I floundered along, juvenile still, no direction, taking classes across campus on whim, managing just C grades and facing years yet to complete a degree. I'd talked about *my* great American novel but after a year had only scribbled in circles, without an outline, character sketches or one complete chapter. I'd quit my job as radio jockey to try out for the college football team, only to realize I was ineligible to compete — I lacked enough credit hours the previous year.

So I *felt* Mom's trust, *heard* her voice from a hundred miles away, and I paused, lying down and draping hand over eyes, guilty. I wasted another gray afternoon on the couch, numbed by self-doubt, retreating in sleep. I woke after sundown, the ingrate's resolve steely within, selfish, had been since teen years. Peering out my apartment window at Broadway traffic, bumper-to-bumper in parading headlights, I thought of music, drinking, getting high, and chicks.

I cleaned up, dressed, and strolled a hundred yards behind buildings to The Playdium, a happening Broadway bar across from the football stadium. I lived on as my parents never did, imbibing, smoking, cursing, plotting drunkenly for the opposite sex — and financing indulgence with their money. Next morning, in cycle, I hated myself for it.

Then came spring break, shattering my winter lowdown and negating all blues. My ego burst monstrous in familiar haunt Florida, Fort Lauderdale Beach, as I cruised the strip with new football buddies. We were young, muscular Boomer males on rampage in "Bonedale," where waves of scantily clad coeds highlighted student mobs from everywhere, round the clock. Our gang caroused for everything we could handle short of violent crime.

Triumphantly we returned to Southeast Missouri State University, if not immediately to classes, as gods of party and women in our minds. Male peers revered us, feted us in story, having witnessed our suave in Lauderdale, and more coeds were taking note. Now I ran with the big dogs, football players at top of campus social strata I'd long envisioned for myself, and I was determined to stay in the pack, enjoying pleasures and forgetting graduation or growing up just yet.

I'd missed at football the previous fall, but only for stupidity about scholastic requirements. I'd busted heads on the field but quit against the wishes of coaches, so I vowed to make the team the coming season, to be ready physically, mentally, and academically, and to enjoy life as a football Viking, parties and women.

Walk-On: 'A Thousand Hits to The Game Field'

The freshman recruit and I lined up against each other at scrimmage, and he didn't know what he was preparing to fuck with. I'd make him understand, though, the meanness of college football, emanating through me.

I couldn't fault his misjudgment based on initial impression, especially of me. He'd come here, SEMO State, for a full football scholarship, while my status amounted to shit yet in the program. On surface I was just another walk-on, and the 18-year-old's physique easily exceeded my 6-2, 195-pound frame; I wondered why no big-time school had claimed him. He was muscular, athletic, intelligent, a paper pick for D-I football. The recruit seemed can't-miss for D-II, but I also knew he'd heard it, too often — at least that's the storyline I adopted as personal motivation. The elder at 22, I'd already sized him up and saw cockiness, smugness, before he took note of me among 90 guys at practice.

Sure, I envied coddled scholarship recruits, given every chance to fail while I must succeed at every rung upward. I had to wow coaches to make the team, quickly, and I channeled the goal into thought and emotion of power, pseudo hate for hitting anyone in my way, recruits, starter or All-America. None mattered differently in my personal approach. I psyched myself to waste every bastard, hitting full-speed and face-first, play or drill. I aimed to wear the game uniform and win a scholarship, and knew from previous walk-on experience exactly the requirement: Big, bad dudes stood in my way, and I had to vanquish them in front of coaches. I reminded myself daily: *A thousand hits to the game field, fucker!*

That freshman tight end, lining up with the No. 1 offensive unit and naïve only moments longer, was my beginning.

"Down!" barked the quarterback, offensive linemen taking their three-point stance. The frosh leaned forward at me, meaty right hand planted in turf, his supple body every bit of 6-4, 220. Across the line, I crouched slightly but poised upright, the "meat squad" defensive end. I looked in his eyes, but he was staring at the ground. I knew he was mine.

"Set! Hut... hut... HUT!"

The ball snapped and the kid shot upright, jab-stepped then backpedaled in pass protection, facing me. Immediately I saw the quarterback take a short drop and fire, a quick screen pass away from us, other side of the field, falling incomplete. A whistle blew the play over before I could strike the recruit, and I let up at arm's reach. We trotted along parallel a couple moments, close to each other.

Suddenly, boldly, he made contact long after whistle, reaching up both hands to push me at shoulder pads. I swayed but didn't respond, pointing my eyes past him to where the ball had dropped, signaling in universal language for football: The play was dead. Then he pushed again.

I whipped about in rage, glaring like Damien, Hell boy of filmdom. I instantly dipped hips and attacked him with my facemask, driving into his throat. I saw his startled expression as I struck his chin and rammed upward, lifting and sending him flying to ground on his ass. He got right back up, to his credit, but I knew defeat and humiliation in his eyes. I saw that look: *This shit is crazy.*

Yeah, college football was nuts, but wonderful lunacy for my taste, then and there in life. The kid wasn't into it, and now I understood why big-time schools had passed right over. This prospect didn't *want* football, not after high school, and I'd exposed the fault. His career was done, already. He wanted none of me, nothing of college football. He'd be home by Christmas, leaving the program, his scholarship, and school.

Laying waste to the recruit was a big step for my progress, worth many hits toward that symbolic thousand. The clap of my helmet shot drew everyone's attention.

"Chainsaw!"

"Git'cha some, man!"

"Great fuckin' hit."

I continued smashing SEMO players in practice. The second week, during daily "thud" drill for defensive linemen, I sent two people to the hospital, my target and myself. I put a bull's-eye, facemask stick in the guy's open chest, right under pads where his ribcage came together, and we both went down, he flat on back, gasping, and I rolling off, neck afire. Trainers loaded us into a van for my first trip that fall to the emergency room of Southeast Hospital, where doctors made x-rays. Diagnosis was severely bruised ribs for my teammate and jammed upper spine for me. He was hurting, uncomfortable in any position, but I lay contentedly on a table, wearing collar icepack, buzzed from good painkillers. I relived the hit over and over in mind, hearing cheers of coaches and players.

Not everyone on team was enamored with my guided-missile contact. Some players considered the tactic extreme even for football. In fact, a sizeable majority didn't hit regularly with facemask, although most encouraged it and only a few disapproved enough to bitch at me. These critics classified face-first technique as "spearing," a rules violation established a few years previous defined as hitting with *top* of the head. Their emphasis was colliding with shoulders and no higher on a target than the chest.

The issue affected football, with coaches and players struggling to meet public demand for increased safety. Collision deaths had spiked in frequency following World War II, through technology of hard helmets complete with facemasks. Officials denounced head-to-head contact, representatives of education, government, medicine, and the insurance industry, and new safeguards were implemented. Football went along, grudgingly; for many in the sport, the change was like restricting high speeds from auto racing, unrealistic.

Other insiders scorned head-ramming in football. Michael Oriard, author and former NFL player, criticized "maniac" hitters in his book released as I played college football. "Coaches undoubtedly prefer the players with self-destructive tendencies," Oriard wrote, "and teammates regard them with a certain awe — an admiration not coupled with any desire to emulate them." Oriard noted fans thrilled over "crazy" players, recounting his years on special teams for the Chiefs, when he strove to be "sensible" but ended up ramming one ball-carrier. In kickoff coverage, the frenetic traffic of players funneled Oriard and the return man right at each other, and he exploded face-first into the guy's chest, leveling him. Fans jumped to their feet in exultation, "the biggest ovation of my career," Oriard recalled, but he'd stung nerves in his neck and wouldn't repeat the kamikaze technique. "My body was not available for sacrifices," he wrote

Mine was, at least for time being. While Oriard's neck injury dissuaded him from ramming, I wasn't fazed by jammed vertebrate, and on return to practice, I continued bashing people with my head. No rule strictly forbade face-first contact, and I indulged relentlessly, typically ending practice with pounding headache and seeking trainers for a handful of Tylenol. Consequently, injuries mounted in my neck, shoulders and head; certainly I suffered one concussion, undiagnosed and untreated, causing intense headaches, cold sweats, and sensitivity to light. I practiced on, never letting up for trauma or foe. I had to make the team. This was strictly manhood quest for me, likely my last chance, I figured at my age.

I was passionate about big hits and savored overcoming injury and pain with mind power, any distress: purple-swollen fingers, ripped nails, bloody cuts and abrasions, deeply bruised arms. In morning I'd examine my injuries with wonder, anticipating the afternoon's violence to come. There was a rage inside, likely linked to boyhood, the bullying of Allen and me by other boys, and now I responded to inflict punishment. I daydreamed about blasting dudes on the football field, hitting head-on, envisioning doing so throughout the day, in class, at lunch, grocery line, home, wherever. I pulled up emotion for the coming storm, my vengeance against teammates in practice. Some were friends, though, so I steered conscience to frame self-concept as Football Hero, not maniac, within the traditional themes society likewise utilized to justify the game's very existence, such as Warrior. Laying out guys on the street was violent crime, but that equated to goodness in my vocation, even moral courage. I was a "student-athlete," innocently roaming a football field in educational manner, decking guys. No one cared about my intent to seriously injure peers. After I laid out a guy, drilling through his throat, I didn't want him to get up. I thrilled if he couldn't, as did most everyone around.

I had more strengths than insane contact and toughness; my game included athleticism from soft hands to snap reaction. I consistently scored big plays from defensive end, making quarterback sacks and other tackles for loss, causing fumbles and recovering them, deflecting and intercepting passes. Players, coaches, and trainers began watching for what I'd do next, and one Friday afternoon I lit 'em up, dominating a "Toilet Bowl" scrimmage among we players who didn't dress for games.

I'd entered the scrimmage mentally stoked to "kill people," having consumed two amphetamine pills an hour before, timing the drug for optimum effectiveness at competition. The Toilet Bowl pitted scout-team offense versus defense, my team, and we boasted several bad-asses, guys headed upward like me. Our meat defense often hammered the *first-string* offense, which we faced daily in practice, so on Fridays, with the big boys gone in preparation for the game next day, we annihilated scout opponents.

That Friday we were kicking the scout offense when the game squad and staff arrived to watch, having returned from walk-through at the stadium. The game players wore their shiny jerseys for Saturday, beautiful mesh half-cuts in black with red-and-white letters, stripes, and big white numbers. I watched rows of game players and coaches flop down on the hillside, taking seats above the practice field and having a grand time. They patronized us, jeering, hollering for real action, preferably some ass-kicking. I knew I'd provide it.

Our defense had just stuffed the offense, and two offensive series remained for this Toilet Bowl, set on the dusty lower practice plane. I nullified one possession immediately, on first down at the 50. The offensive huddle broke with tight end heading to our left, lining up wide side of the field.

"Strong left," I called, as strong-side defensive end, and went with the tight end, wide side of the field open to my left. On the snap, the quarterback swung right around to pitch two-handed; the old "student body" toss sweep was coming my way, designed to go around me. I already knew I'd foil the play, with a chance to really wreck it. Bolting through the tight end's weak reach block, I banged him back inside and took the open field.

As the quarterback pitched the ball, I was free and running laterally, already calculating angle on the tailback meant to receive it. The back saw me coming, looking just as the ball hit his hands, and it bounced down, rolling along at his feet. I saw the fumble and the back slowing to stoop for it, defenseless in shuffling along with profile exposed to me. *You're dead, fucker.* I ripped in, knocking him flying out of the way. Falling on the fly myself, I reached back at the ball with hands and feet. Slamming to ground, I recovered that ball mostly with my legs, pulling it up by feet to snatch possession and complete my glittering play.

Everyone cheered wildly for me: coaches, Toilet players, gamers, and female spectators in girlfriends and wives. "God-damn, Chainsaw," said a linebacker in admiration, upon reaching me. "Fuckin' unreal." I wasn't finished. The offense was determined to throw in its final series, but I sacked the quarterback three straight plays, chasing and dropping him every time.

The losses I pinned on the offense made it fourth down and about 40, and coaches ended the scrimmage by rushing on field, whistling and clapping. The whole scene was buzzing over me. The smokin' older girlfriend of an assistant coach followed me from above, her eyes riveted as I left the field stripping off jersey, shoulder pads and undershirt. For a moment I thought the bodacious woman was coming on down. "Incredible!" she offered me from the hilltop, clapping bravo-style, clearly excited. "You were awesome!" Her boyfriend was only a coach now; I was a player.

There would be more women like her, coed and older, for I was headed to the game field where I'd preen and strut. After the scrimmage, some senior players solicited coaches on my behalf, asking them to issue me a uniform. The official word reached me downstairs as I showered.

"Chaney!" a grad assistant called back into the steam, from fringe of the showers, avoiding naked bodies.

"Yeah."

"You're suiting up tomorrow for the game. Call your parents. Now."

"Fuckin' A!" I whooped. Mom and Dad would hear from me tonight, and I didn't even need cash.

Anabolic Steroids: Final Ingredient For Football Stardom

Practice feats aside, I remained vulnerable on the field in college football, particularly as a defensive lineman. My body was good and strong, a superior physique athletic and muscular from genetics nurtured by running and strength training since boyhood. I also consumed food heartily, massively if not healthy, often topping 10,000-calorie intake in a day cycle.

Yet I could not gain weight, once in top shape and practicing football daily. On the contrary, the battle then was to prevent *loss* in weight and strength, the *catabolic* effect or breakdown virtually inevitable for the exerting human body unaided by synthetic drugs. As the season wore on, I fought to maintain just 195 lean and muscular, and knowing I had to get much bigger. Overcoming nagging injury and avoiding serious wounding were other issues.

So I looked to anabolic or tissue-building steroids, readily available. I didn't merely want to become a starter for SEMO State; I strove to excel against our challenging schedule of opponents. Southeast Missouri was member of a competitive state conference in D-II football, but our supreme tests were foes from Division I-AA, including Murray State, Southern Illinois-Carbondale, and Northern Iowa.

Without drugs, I was too lightweight and physically weak to run that gauntlet, not on the defensive line. I had seen guys trot out for SEMO in the starting lineup on opening night, and many were vanquished quickly, beaten out of the lineup by opponents or, worse, maimed and laid out for the surgeon's knife. Huge guys from larger schools were killing us, even our own juicers.

Undeniably, player sizes were on fast-forward in American football, everywhere, and increases were commonly attributed to advances in weightlifting. We players at SEMO felt the pressure, facing teams bigger, stronger, and more athletic throughout our schedule. Hardly anyone believed training alone keyed the arms race. Only the very naive among us didn't understand anabolic steroids were primary reason, even if only about 10 percent of us used the drugs. Many SEMO players lifted weights intensely, variously — there could be no fundamental progression in resistance training, with none left to discover — and we understood our personal plateaus, limitations in strength.

We stood affected by steroid users in the game, exposed directly in field confrontations and indirectly by the perpetual drive to gain size, strength, and speed. Some SEMO guys were in small-college ball because of steroids at the major level, where use had been pervasive for years. I would've tried out at Missouri a couple years before, if big-time football hadn't been awash in hormone-pumped giants, including backs weighing 250 and running 100 yards in 10 seconds. I needed steroids to compete in major college, a bunch of the drugs, and shied away.

Still I headed toward muscle dope, increasingly assuming user profile by developing myself to play college football, and by summer 1982 I seriously considered steroids for walking on at Southeast Missouri. My personal culpability would be explicit, per the illicit use of any drug, but a systemic force was also at work: the steroid problem sweeping football, bound to pervade every college level by decade's end, top to bottom. How many footballers faced steroids before me? Thousands had, with likely millions to follow, as time would demonstrate.

Most summer evenings I trained at the football complex, lifting weights and catching passes with receivers, and there a player encouraged me to try anabolic steroids, one cycle at least. "The shit really works," he said, rebuking establishment propaganda the hormones didn't build muscle. "You'd kick ass."

The footballer told me nothing I didn't understand. Already, huge bodybuilders looked me over in gyms, soliciting me to juice, openly speculating how steroids would fill mass around my large bone structure, particularly the chest, shoulders, and thighs. In addition, I had personal models earlier, including two imposing cops, among the first steroid users I knew. I'd known directly of steroid use in SEMO football and recognized more, minimal but present, among starters in power positions. The large majority of players used amphetamines.

To use steroids myself was greed in one measure, for I could've made the team without them. But I knew I might star, and I resigned to the step reluctantly, like many first-time juicers in football of the period. In that generation of athletes, the majority of us still embraced quaint sport value, the talk of playing fair and square. Stupid, faulty idealism perhaps, but we acquired the sporting mantra rather innately, a veritable American narrative passed from fathers and mothers borne of economic depression and world warfare.

I'd already been around, though, on the street and in athletics, experiencing mostly real-world antithesis to those old stories about wholesomeness, team attitude, individual honor. Plus, I was readying for football's physical world, to lay my body on the line. My ultimate rationale was there all along, underlying, singular, a question with set answer: What's wrong with a prescription drug for college football? I also reasoned internally that as long as I didn't combine or "stack" different steroids, I wasn't abusing anything.

Late July, I paid $35 for a vial of testosterone cypionate from a bodybuilder, 10 milliliters of synthetic male hormone. As instructed, I went to a local pharmacy for needle-syringes to shoot the drug. At home I paused briefly over the materials, bothered most by the needles — emblematic of hard-core drug use to me — then loaded 1 milliliter of testosterone cypionate, 200-milligram strength, and injected a buttock myself.

I felt no effects immediately, but doubling dosage in the second week brought marked strength increase, about 20 pounds on my bench press. For the first time I approached a 300-pound press — a standard increasingly demanded by college coaches — and easily handled multiple reps with 225 on the bar.

The change scared me, understanding basic facts of anabolic steroids. I knew powerful hormones were coursing my bloodstream and attaching to tissue everywhere, muscle fiber including the heart. Hesitating again about juicing, I consulted a friend on the team who opposed the drugs, and he berated me. His persuasion was convincing, really what I wanted to hear, and I ceased the injections, but I didn't throw away the vial.

Homecoming: Making The Team, Debuting in The Big Game

Starting from meat-squad defensive lineman at Labor Day, or nowhere on the SEMO depth chart, I dressed out for our fifth game of the 1982 season, making fast but expected progress toward my goal of becoming a starter and winning a scholarship. By October 18, Monday morning of week eight, my name was posted in lineups for special teams and the upcoming game, Homecoming. I was on kickoff team, punt team, and punt block, and I expected to stand out for hitting and making plays. In addition, I moved up the depth chart to a backup defensive end, meaning I'd practice with the starting defense and likely get some snaps on Saturday in the game.

In team buzz I headlined. Teammates debated whether I'd kick ass in games like in practice, while coaches were convinced I was walk-on magic, a player for immediate help and longer promise. Already coaches discussed with me the possibility of my gaining an extra season of eligibility. I could play two more years by sitting out one college semester, coaches apprised me, and mutually understood was that meant scholarship money for me.

Also understood was the fact I needed size and strength to become a formidable player. "You've got to hit the weightroom, Chaney," I heard constantly from coaches, trainers and teammates. I *was* banging iron through the soreness of contact injuries, practicing more self-discipline for training than most the team. Yet my game had a glaring weakness at defensive end: handling the tight end's base block, his straight-on drive move that defeated me against a guy much bigger and stronger. I thrived with room to charge for ramming attack, needing but a few steps to explode facemask into people of big size, including juicers bearing 25 percent more mass. Head-to-head at the line, however, those big, strong athletes would blast me in base block, driving through my 200 pounds and weaker strength.

So, handy remedy, I'd resumed injections drawn from the steroid vial, emptying the remaining six to seven milliliters of testosterone in two weeks, and approaching Homecoming my football performance was definitely enhanced, with recent intake exceeding a thousand milligrams. The entire week was sensational for me, on and off the field, hitting emotion at full range top to bottom, strutting as Big Man on Campus then suffering precipitous fall.

The football was exhilarating. Autumn's chill helped stay my weight, natural testosterone surged, but the synthetic steroids expanded lean mass noticeably this time, to about 210 and holding. Long-term, the coming year, I planned to juice for two or three strong cycles, stacking multiple steroids for synergistic efficacy, while committing to strength training, conditioning, and nutrition as never before in my life. I planned to play football next season at about 240 while benching 400, squatting 600, and running a 4.8 forty, maybe faster. I was going to destroy fuckers in D-II ball.

My newly growing physique was gear enough for this season, SEMO's remaining games. I felt like a tiger, bursting on anabolic hormone infusion unmatched since puberty. With our rugged non-conference games concluded, we faced only D-II opponents in coming weeks, and no one was going to fuck with me. I always performed better in fall's temperature and angling light, the summer's sun and heat subsided, but the synthetic testosterone jacked vitality of body. I cruised through practices without speed pills, feeling a heightened physical confidence to match effervescent mental will. I raised my personal bar in hustle and focus, including for the most mundane of drills. For scrimmage snaps I was relentless, covering the field wide and long, smashing dudes and making plays. Then I went home feeling strong and no soreness, still ready to run and hit. Even my skin seemed tougher, bearing little marking after heavy contact.

I made another huge play at practice, in front of everyone, four days before Homecoming. Tuesday's practice had the most contact, and the final segment was full-speed scrimmage for about a dozen snaps, the game offense versus the game defense. It was "full go" with the quarterback open for getting hit, which I craved particularly. Lining up at defensive end for my three plays in scrimmage — another mark of my rising roster ranking — I would shine on the first snap.

"Hut… HUT!"

The entire offensive backfield bolted at me, in-sync on a triple-option right, with quarterback leading the run play. He grasped the ball out front two-handed, deciding what to do on his reads of defense, especially me at end. The quarterback declined the first option, faking and drawing back a handoff to the fullback, who steamed by and dove into bodies at scrimmage. The quarterback stepped on outside, encountering me as planned, the defensive end intentionally left unblocked.

My simple assignment, conversely, was to erase the quarterback and force his pitchout, so he couldn't cut and run the ball. My hit obliged the mission, a signature face-first strike that flattened him. Thus the quarterback pitched to the tailback, whose goal was to get outside, around pursuit, and bolt up-field.

But I wasn't out of the play yet. After jabbing the quarterback to turf, I stayed on my feet, cutting outside in perfect time with his pitch. I trapped the tailback as he caught the ball and nailed him on arrival, knocking his head around and grinding his body into ground. Fucker was lucky to keep the ball. It was great sequence by a defensive end, my double kill of the triple option, laying out the quarterback and tackling his pitchman for loss. The field erupted in cheers.

"*Chaaaiin-SAW!*"

Next day was more wallow in glory for me, The Walk-On Who Made Lineup, everyone's feel-good story if not so accurate on the details. I mean, I was *supposed* to perform well at this level, had expected as much from myself — especially on anabolic steroids — but most people enjoyed treating me as the long-shot who'd made it, an old movie cliché, which was fine. Others recognized me as merely a football player hungry to win, succeed. Football was *my* game, since childhood, and it was coming fruition in my life. My amazing tackle during Tuesday scrimmage was further evidence.

Wednesday before practice, a group of coaches and players gathered round a VHS, watching the replay over and over, raving as I passed by for the locker room.

"Chainsaw!" a teammate greeted. "Great play, man."

"Git some more on Saturday, Saw," said another. "Bust some fuckin' heads. We need ya."

Now I was a member of this football team.

Living Football Fantasy: Big Man On and Off Campus

I felt like a fucking king and why not, as dashing Football Hero with hot College Chicks, in this case a car ride south from St. Louis on Interstate 55. Moreover, the ladies were driving for me, as they did last night.

It was Thursday, October 21, 1982, a sunny, lovely harvest afternoon for Missouri countryside — and the day after St. Louis won the World Series, topping Milwaukee in Game Seven at Busch Stadium. The city had celebrated through the night, metro-wide, and I'd done it all, I figured in smug recollection. Tooling along in the back seat, windows down, I regarded myself highly, enjoying breezes and flirting with two smiling coeds up front, chatty and mirthful themselves.

The day before was flurry of events to bolster personal legend, largely only in my mind at this point. After Wednesday football practice in Cape Girardeau, five teammates and I jammed inside a car bound for downtown St. Louis, the World Series, a hundred miles north. None of us had tickets for Game Seven, but we didn't care, aiming instead for the sure party around Busch Stadium, win or lose for the Cardinals.

Bonus factors were in play as we arrived at the stadium around 8:30. First, the 'Birds were ahead after the sixth inning, thanks to a 3-run comeback in the home half on RBIs by Keith Hernandez and "Silent" George Hendrick. If the Cardinals won St. Louis would go crazy! Better yet, team officials threw open gates to the stadium, and we joined waves of fans rushing inside.

We roamed the aisles, cheering the St. Louis to victory as reliever Bruce Sutter closed it, retiring Milwaukee in order over the eighth and ninth innings. Joaquin Andujar got the win, Sutter the save, and manager-executive Whitey Herzog his proper due as baseball genius. And we young males made our way down to the field, where we paraded with the throng for awhile, whooping and hollering, until the attraction wore thin. Finally we headed outside Busch, for the massing party.

Raucous was Seventh Street, a mob scene pressing outside stadium entrances for players and club personnel. Screaming fans extended like ground cover across Seventh and upside of the parking garage, filling in street, bridges, and walkways. Everyone was ecstatic, cheering even stadium cops emerging from the glass doors.

I made my next move, abruptly bidding adieu to my football chums, startling them. "Thanks for the ride, fellas. I'll see you at practice tomorrow in Cape." And I booked, leaving them on the sidewalk, mouths hanging open, wondering what the hell Chainsaw was up to now — exactly as I wanted them to think. This story would really boost my stature among the dudes and ladies at college. I wasn't as bold as putting on, of course, acting as though striking out alone in the big city.

In reality, a good buddy was honcho in Cardinals offices, and a security guard escorted me inside, as usual. Within minutes of abandoning football mates, I was partying inside Busch with local celebrities and Stan Musial, our own baseball great of yore. Stan The Man and I clanked bottles of cold Budweiser, toasting the Redbirds and St. Louis.

Soon more friends arrived outside, amid a chain of limousines encircling the stadium. I left in one of the black stretches, bound for The Landing entertainment district on the riverfront, snorting cocaine from trays passing around.

I ran into familiar women at bars on The Landing, including several from college. The sexy girlfriend of a buddy was quite friendly; I hadn't seen the guy in a year while she looked great, felt great, hugging and kissing me, pressing her ample cleavage. Friends tore us apart and we moved on, promising to catch up later. I had a girlfriend back at school, supposedly, but far from mind this night. I ended up leaving with other young women from college, a shapely pair led by one I always fired on.

And, next day, the chicks drove me back to Cape Girardeau, straight to football practice. Talk of my St. Louis exploits already percolated among the boys, according my little plan, as the two smokin' coeds dropped me off. The one kissed me over the seat as the other hugged, teammates and coaches looking on, envious. I remembered a story about Paul Hornung, grid golden boy, how he once left a team bus to jump in a convertible with two blondes. Dude was like Elvis, and I felt that same machismo, drawing prized male respect, however hollow.

In the locker room, I recalled enough of my night for the guys crowding around.

No sexual act had occurred, but they didn't need to know. And while I didn't kiss and tell on a chick, I still fashioned this tale for tantalizing effect, without specifying or confirming fact of importance. Dudes added detail on their own and I smiled, neither confirming nor denying. Image enhanced, I actually remained timid of casual sex, really still more Magoo inside than McQueen.

Male adulation for my perceived conquest continued into football practice, during team stretch. A young position coach talked me up, too, burnishing my credential, relaying that he'd met women in a bar who wanted me naked. Teammates chimed in, saying the same. Given how everybody talked, females panted for me at every corner.

I rode the Me high into Thursday practice, my ego-boosted virility becoming manifest on the football field in more standout, aggressive play. I was a real player, in lineup for the big game, and my focus for role cranked up in drills and scrimmage situations with authority. Working with the No. 1 defense, I blew up plays and picked off a pass in the backfield. On special units for kickoff, punt, and punt block, I hit hard and fast, proficient in my assignments. I planned on *killing* fuckers Saturday! Hopefully we'd open the game on kickoff, when I'd rush downfield and dive into the return wedge, laying people out. I fantasized launching bodies at the return man, dropping him with the carcasses of blockers.

Despite my manufactured playboy facade, my face for football was genuine, intensely. I was positive of impending success, *knowing* I would star, and almost felt urgency to begin the big game, an unsettling feeling I disregarded as normal. In the past, as a boy on Christmas Eve, I'd fretted the house would burn down before opening presents.

Homecoming, my first appearance in a college game, was two days away.

Imagery in Mind's Eye: Wreaking Havoc on The Football Field

Most the big plays I made in football, I *imagined* them first, carrying them out in mind's eye while reclined on a couch, typically.

"Imagery," the practice of envisioning a task ahead of time, working it through in mind, was perfect mental preparation for success in American football. I utilized imagery commonly as a player, since my turnaround in high school when I read the classic *Out of Their League* by David Meggyesy, a ferocious hitter at linebacker. Football was choreographed in sets or formations, and an athlete could mentally preview dozens of plays away from live competition, including when relaxing at home.

Sometimes I'd be "out" partying, at a bar or crowded house, buzzed, females abound. But I'd fantasize instead about football, making plays like destroying the triple option — or the show-time sequence I put together for real at practice, taking out the quarterback and pitch man in one swoop. Driving down the highway cranking the jams, especially KSHE 95, St. Louis, I could literally get off on my bad football self, thinking what I'd do to people. But preferably I'd find a quiet stationary spot to pause, daydream a few minutes, tipping back, eyes closed — couches in the theatre foyer at college were ideal — and instantly see myself kicking ass on a the football field.

Friday morning, October 22, 1982, I skipped a class to do football imagery at home, on the sofa. The stereo cranked Pink Floyd's *Mettle* album, complementing bong hits of sensimilla for my theatre of the mind. I practically squealed in delight, fat on myself, *my life*, regardless its actual substance and misdirection. Typically I didn't consider the danger zone I navigated, in this case college football. I only wanted payoffs of inflicting the popular violence: manhood rushes, renown, great parties, hot women.

I always enjoyed a Friday, but this one figured huge personally, through the day and onward, culminating with late-night ditching of my girlfriend for a rendezvous with a new chick. All the while, I anticipated, excitement would surround tomorrow, my debut as a SEMO football player *and* starring in a college game. Oh, yeah, I expected to electrify the home crowd tomorrow, including my parents and friends — by scoring a touchdown on special teams. I envisioned it all, going down in mind ahead of time.

Lincoln, the winless team we faced, presented opportunity for our punt-block squad and me in particular, leaving two gaps open on the line in its punt formation. My assignment would be simple when Lincoln punted: I'd spring through a wide-open gap to smash the right "up-back," or a blocker protecting his punter, and thus free my teammate Wayne "Bo" James to block the kick. Bo James would stand as one of the decade's great kick blockers in college football, on way that season to averaging one block per game, 11 total. I was positive he'd get one on Lincoln, with its loose punt formation ripe to exploit. No way would Bo James be stopped; he'd engulf at least one punt Saturday.

And when Bo James blocked that Lincoln punt, I'd be at his side, grabbing the loose football and streaking to the end zone, the SEMO radio man screaming: *Touchdown! MATT CHANEY! The WALK-ON! The former Hillsboro Hawk, making an impact his first college game. His teammates call him Chainsaw...* That's how I planned it, psyching up, watching film of Lincoln, working on the practice field. In a final preparatory step, courtesy of Coach Oakes, I stamped in memory all opposing jersey numbers I'd hit personally, adding other info bits of those behind the facemasks. I was fucking ready.

We had four games to go, small colleges in our conference, and I was utterly convinced I would lead victory in every one, beginning at Homecoming against Lincoln University. What a stage to for my opening! I thrilled at the thought, tingly. Twenty-four hours to go, I'd be a real college football player, finally.

I presumed a lot.

Going Down Hard, Short of The Big Game

I arrived early for practice Friday afternoon, as usual, around 2:30. I always wanted ample time to dress and anticipate football, any session.

But this day I also needed orders for the workout, whether I'd go to the stadium with everyone else on game roster, for walk-through, or stay back for Toilet Bowl scrimmage with the meat squad. I didn't care, and in fact preferred the Toilet Bowl, the chance to do some hitting. Just in case, I carried two amphetamine pills in my pocket, to pop on moment's notice. I stashed more speeders for the Homecoming game.

The head coach left it up to me, Jim Lohr, whom I liked and respected. We agreed I was prepped for special-team assignments to start the game tomorrow. "But you can come on with us to the stadium," Coach Lohr offered.

I hesitated, ambivalent.

"We are a little short of bodies on the D-line for scout team," Coach said, noting injuries and defections had depleted the corps. "They could use you today."

"That's cool," I replied, decisive. "I'll stick around and play the Toilet Bowl." And so I would follow the moment.

I headed downstairs, swallowed amphetamines, got taped and dressed. Returning upstairs to the hallway outside Coach Lohr's office, he pulled me aside for a favor. "Chaney, can you meet a few minutes with those Cub Scouts outside? They're here to watch the scrimmage. Just say hello and answer some questions from the boys."

"Sure!" I savored the chance, recalling my boyhood admiration of big football players; perhaps I could impress the Cub Scouts, teach them something. And they would learn, although nothing of the greetings and small talk I extended in our meeting. The Cubs and den leaders met me on a personal level, which would accentuate, for them, the bad scene to witness shortly.

By 3:10 we scrimmage participants hit the practice field, for stretching and warm-up drills, while buses left the football complex, carrying game squad and coaches across campus to the stadium. Half-past three marked the start of another Toilet Bowl. A student coach placed a football at midfield, whistles blew, and we on the meat squad clapped and hooted. A smattering of spectators cheered up on the hill, led by my fans the Cub Scouts.

The offense broke huddle for the first series, and I lined up across the ball at defensive end. The first play was a run, which we stopped, then the offense went airborne on second down. The quarterback dropped back to pass as his tailback came to block m in, pass protection. The back knew I had to contain the outside on a rush, or not allow the quarterback to loop me, so he set up wide to make me go around him. Before we could hit, the pass whizzed just by my head, on inside field, and I glanced over to see the quarterback just a few feet away.

"Fuck that!" I warned the tailback. "Next time, I'm cuttin' inside your ass and nailin' the quarterback."

He smiled, disbelieving; if I cut inside and allowed the quarterback to escape around me, my mistake would be glaring. But I didn't plan on missing. Next play, another pass, the tailback did the same, flaring out wide to block, herding me around him in a long semi-circle to quarterback.

I didn't cooperate, faking a step up-field but cutting hard inside, flying, completely eluding the block and closing instantly on the quarterback, a right-hander just cocking back his arm, torso exposed to me. I had only two steps in open field, untouched, for a facemask shot to his throat, and he saw me coming.

I didn't make it, falling instead at his feet, as though shot by a sniper.

One step shy of the quarterback, my right foot had suddenly planted and locked the leg at knee to begin hyper-extension, inside-out, the femur head rolling through unnaturally atop the tibia. Stress capability at knee's core exceeded, stretching and tearing tendon that anchored hamstring to the joint, creating slack in the big backside muscle. Then energy unleashed in full-blown hyperextension. My upper body fell forward over the reversing knee — later estimated from film to reach negative 30 degrees, inside-out — throwing my face down to see the joint's violent shredding outside, disintegrating lateral ligament complexes.

The entire second, my most injurious step, resounded as Hercules tearing apart raw chicken. I didn't chip a bone. Everyone within a hundred yards heard that noise and saw me down. Thrashing in the dirt, my body systems shocked, I gasped for air, breaking loose terrible screams and curses. I realized I wouldn't play in the Homecoming game, but my next worry was the Cub Scouts watching me from the hill, their role model — I'd totally fucked up their football experience.

Trainers rushed to me but players moved away, only a couple lingering around to offer encouragement, observe my injury and pain. The trainers heard the tissue explosion but didn't know exactly what happened.

"It's my fuckin' knee!" I told them, moaning, gritting teeth, but calming enough to cease rolling around. Someone pulled off my helmet, and I lay back flat in dirt. "Mu-ther-fuck-er!" I cried, hands over my eyes. "Aw, shit!"

"Hang in there, Chainsaw, hang on, buddy," said Tim Barron, a trainer and friend, disappointed. "Timmy B.," one of my biggest boosters, knew my knee was trashed and I wouldn't play football again for a long time, if ever. His hopes were dashed along with mine. I calmed enough within a minute or so, as the knee pain subsided amazingly. I could even withstand the trainers' bending the joint and poking into tender areas. Then I understood something else was wrong: Rays of pain shot from my toes and foot upward on the lower leg, in front, and the sensations were different, tingling, a numbness, but fiery, electric.

"Aw, fuck, my ankle," I said, grimacing. "I must've broke my fuckin' foot or something."

The trainers removed my cleat, checked the ankle and foot, perplexed: No sign of trauma, nothing seemed amiss. Then one recognized symptoms of a nerve injury he'd heard about, damage around a knee. He instructed that I raise my foot by bending it straight up. I tried, in mind, but the lower leg made no motor response: My toes didn't raise, my foot didn't budge upward, although all other movement was intact. My foot was partially paralyzed!

"That's a bad injury," someone said. "We gotta get him to the hospital."

Timmy B. was already moving, headed for a phone to call Dr. William P. Thorpe, team surgeon, who would ready the ER staff at Southeast Missouri Hospital.

A couple players came to haul me off the field, without stretcher. Draping arms under my shoulders and butt, they lifted me off ground as I gripped the back of their necks, straining in renewed pain and breathlessness. A student trainer led the way, gingerly holding my feet. Onlookers were largely silent, players, coaches, and spectators, save for a few muted words of support and scattered, lighthearted clapping. As soon as

I cleared the field, whistles blew and everyone fired back up, enthusiastic and yapping for football. This sport would outlast us all.

I held on in agony, carried about a hundred yards to the training room, where I was placed on a table and stripped of jersey and shoulder pads. Another injured player was in there, John Overby, "O.B.," an excellent kicker sidelined for the season with torn quadriceps muscle.

Everyone else left, returning to the scrimmage, and I again considered the reality I would miss tomorrow's game, the football season, everything. The injury replayed over and over in mind, its violence and sound. I dreaded surgery and a trying rehabilitation, but I knew that was the prognosis, from what I witnessed. Maybe I would never step on a game field in college. I began to sob, and O.B. squirmed a little at the whirlpool, his bad leg dunked in swirling water. He felt bad for my misfortune. "It's all right, Chainsaw," the injured player assured quietly. "Things will work out."

I cried only seconds, and trainers reappeared led by Tim Barron, fetching a stretcher. My leg was immobilized in an air cast, and within minutes I was delivered to Southeast Missouri Hospital, in central town on a hill over Capaha Park — and my place of residence for the next nine days.

Timmy B. sent the other trainers back to campus and stayed with me in the ER, where leg x-rays opened a series of procedures. Next I was wheeled to a side room and met by several staff, nurses and internists under direction of Dr. Thorpe, head surgeon for athletics at both SEMO State and SIU-Carbondale.

A towering, engaging man, Dr. Thorpe was a rising surgeon in progressive sports medicine, employing state-of-art technology and technique, like tendon grafts to replace knee ligaments, and embracing aggressive rehabilitation for the injured athlete bent on comeback. I was fortunate a sports-med specialist was available in Dr. Thorpe, a former Princeton football player in his first year as our team surgeon.

Outlook was rather optimistic for me that Friday evening, on the part of everyone. I was calm, pleasant, conversing normally outside of having to bend the knee or endure prodding for tender spots. The pain generally wasn't strong, like my jammed neck on previous visit to this ER a month before, and I declined medication. I began to think maybe I wasn't injured severely.

X-rays were negative for a knee fracture, showing neither crack nor chip where the two large leg bones met at joint. The patella or kneecap was in place and undisturbed, signaling the huge tendon was sound as well, and lack of general swelling was another positive. I managed to bend the knee full range "with difficulty," Dr. Thorpe noted later in his report.

The surgeon, relying on x-rays and preliminary external exam, expressed hope the damage might be confined to the lateral or outside ligaments. I was sure the laterals had shredded, from my view, but those ligaments were not so important as the anterior cruciate within the heart of the knee. Dr. Thorpe explained torn lateral ligaments were often fixed by new arthroscopic surgery, the insertion of thin robotic tubes carrying camera and tools. In such procedure, Surgeon and staff watched a TV monitor to operate without scalpel to open wide the joint membrane. Sounded good to me.

The nerve damage worried Dr. Thorpe. It impeded external exam and the paralysis still hadn't subsided in a couple hours post-injury. "There is hypesthesia [sensitivity loss] of the entire foot and lateral calf and weakness of dorsiflexion [raising] of the right great toe," he recorded

I had "drop foot," commonly known. I couldn't budge the foot or toes upward, and numbness radiated through muscle and skin from shinbone into toes. Hard as I'd try mentally to raise that foot, straining and puffing, it was dead, motionless, as were all the toes — the brain could no longer signal throughout the peroneal nerve channel, cut off somewhere around the knee. In best-case scenario, the injury was more superficial than a torn channel, caused by bruising contact.

Lack of sensitivity marked the areas for palsy, of course, although differently than I'd previously imagined of paralysis — the football player's great fear short of mortality. For my introduction to paralysis, the lower leg areas weren't entirely "dead" to sensation or touch, and pain was a discernible although inconsistent, such as shooting hot at times. I couldn't really feel pinpricks in areas, notably webbing of my right big toe, just faint pressure at the surface. Touching the zones myself was strange, a feeling of skin like rubber but pulsing in current.

Dr. Thorpe hoped the paralysis temporary, informing me of the probabilities for recovery, saying the nerve function could restore itself at any time. The nerve damage dictated my admission to the hospital for the weekend, awaiting surgery Monday morning.

The personable surgeon expressed regret I wouldn't play in tomorrow's game, and I appreciated the sentiment. We shared small talk about football and our respective college careers, and I was impressed. We speculated cause of the knee's unwarranted hyperextension, free of contact, and I noted a "sandlot" football injury four years previous, a guy's head-on shot resulting in hyperextension and swelling. Dr. Thorpe figured that a likely culprit, then he bade me farewell until morning, when he'd see me on daily rounds at the hospital. His upbeat nature was infectious for me, very appealing in the situation, and I felt better. I was confident this surgeon was superior and a good guy, being a former college footballer.

I watched big Dr. Thorpe leave my room and pause in the busy hall, to record one of many audio reports on knee exams with me, years to come. Oblivious to others around, big Dr. Thorpe spoke loudly into the hand-held micro-cassette: "This is a 22-year-old SEMO college student admitted with a diagnosis of lateral collateral ligament tear, probably Grade III, [and] superficial peroneal nerve palsy, right lower extremity, from a football accident today. The patient is admitted for observation and bed rest over the weekend with plan for examination under anesthesia on Monday with probable lateral collateral ligament repair and possible peroneal nerve exploration." Dr. Thorpe completed his oral report and bolted into hallway traffic, moving out of my sight.

I called Mom and Dad, informing them I'd injured the knee and wouldn't play in tomorrow's game. I reassured them prognosis was good, even if involving surgery, and they shouldn't travel to Cape until my operation on Monday. They agreed, reluctantly, and I was sure my educator parents took a different mindset to the evening's high-school football game, starring my little brother as quarterback. Mom and Dad didn't necessarily care about football but supported their sons who played. Now I was laid up, and my trial ahead would become theirs.

A hospital bed for the weekend I hadn't planned, but I made the best of it for Friday night. The atmosphere held a sense of novelty, my first night in a hospital, and I ignored any pain or discomfort, instead having fun with the steady flow of visitors, friends. There were cute young nurses around, and the food even tasted good.

I had the room to myself on the top floor, out of way, no army of personnel in the halls, and a little party ensued. My girlfriend dropped in, followed by buddies who snuck beers and a joint. I quaffed Budweiser and got out of bed on one leg, hopping easily to the open window; we smoked dope through a soda straw extended outside, the traffic of Broadway honking below.

The night's elements made for my escapism: the party scam, attention of my girlfriend and friends, good buzz from narcotic substances. I momentarily forgot hurt inside, deep disappointment, for missing my chance to play tomorrow, Homecoming.

V. Self-Pity, Severe Injury

Reality hit early Saturday morning, my first wakeup in a hospital. An older nurse rousted me at 6 o'clock, snapping on lights and barking orders, affirming my existence as hospital patient. She made me sit up in bed and take breakfast on a tray. My injured knee was swollen like a basketball within the air splint, for my moving about last night.

I ate alone, humbly, gazing out the top-floor window at sunup over Cape Girardeau, longing to be out of here. The feeling was self-pity, loss. I could see a beautiful autumn day at hand for town and campus, a football Saturday I'd anticipated, been scheduled for in spotlight, merely 24 hours ago. Now, stuck in that bed, crippled, I only knew I wouldn't take part. It was unfair.

By 7:30 I heard the big parade forming in the park down from hospital hill, marching bands, floats, and more gala. Horns blared, drums beat, tractor engines revved, cars and people hummed about. At 9 o'clock, the parade moved forward in perfect fall weather, headed downtown toward the stadium.

Left behind, gloom onset in the hospital room, my emotion bottomed. After the parade, a good buddy and his fiancé dropped by; I was grateful to see them, but nothing like the host of last night. I couldn't laugh along now, as if everything were fine, and my mood infected theirs. We dwelled on my damaged leg, staring down at it in the bed, discussing it glumly.

"Damn!" said my pal, an alumni football player who'd encouraged my tryout at SEMO. He'd made the trip from St. Louis specifically to see me break out in the Homecoming game. "You would've *jammed* out there today," he said, regrettably. Subdued, the couple said good-bye for returning to the celebration along Broadway, bound for my hangout The Playdium, meeting spot for partying alumni before kickoff at the stadium.

I listened to the game by clock radio, and SEMO led Lincoln 29-27 at halftime. As I'd surmised in scouting Lincoln on film, the opponent literally flaunted chances for guys like me to score — or like me formerly. Our defense chased the Lincoln backfield through breakdowns in the offensive line, sacking the quarterback and tackling running backs for loss. In the third quarter my D-line buddy Tee Thompson drew real blood, firing me up in the hospital bed. A brutish noseguard, Tee hit the quarterback on the Lincoln 10-yard line, causing a fumble he scooped up and returned to the end zone for a touchdown. I whooped in joy and hesitated, selfish. "Dammit!" I said aloud, happy for Tee but sorry for myself, unable to join the fun on defense.

I thought of my touchdown that could've been, my imagery of punt block with body intact, so vivid in mind only the morning before. Hell, I still *knew* Bo James would block a punt with Lincoln's lousy formation, and the urge to be there was forceful inside. I contemplated snatching crutches somewhere and heading uptown to the game. Now I was really dreaming, seeing myself enter the field gloriously on crutches, something in the role of Injured Football Hero Returns, lame but happy, strong, rallying team and fans, one muscular arm around a crutch and the other upraised in victory.

Then it really happened, the touchdown as I envisioned, just without me. Bo James streaked in to block a Lincoln punt and the ball bounced free, toward the SEMO goal line. My replacement on punt-block team, Glenn Edwards, picked up the football and ran 23 yards to score, fans cheering and photogs snapping his picture.

I was shocked, numb in the bed, hearing what I'd wholly expected. "You gotta be SHITTIN' ME!" Angrily I switched off the radio, the pathetic irony twisting my senses into full-blown self-pity, and yelling. "UN-FUCKING-BELIEVABLE!"

Fallen Player Meets Surgeon's Knife, Finally

My day of reckoning, Monday, October 25, after thousands in tackle football: I'd played the game since kindergarten, scoffing at hazard, but now I'd have knee surgery. I still didn't comprehend how serious my condition — no one did — and I'd only complicate matters with a stupid decision.

Wakened to eat in hospital that morning, operation pending, I started to turn back the breakfast tray, recognizing the obvious mistake in the nurse's instructions for my care. I knew the mandate was no liquid or food for me entering surgery, since 10 o'clock last night. But I thought twice, being hungry, and decided to say nothing, opting to slyly consume the full menu of eggs, bacon, toast, juice and coffee.

Forbidden food seemed a good idea, another fun ploy to circumvent bothersome rules of hospital stay — until I met the anesthesiologist before surgery in the operating room. I lay prepped on the table, answering his safeguard list of questions:

"When did you last have something to eat or drink?"

Shit! "Uh...," I paused, searching, "about two hours ago."

"6 a.m.? This morning?"

"Um, yeah."

"What!"

I realized I'd fucked up, just clueless of how so; I had no idea of this man's job. My breakfast fiasco increased risk exponentially for knee surgery, primarily pressuring the anesthesiologist for overseeing my unconscious state, the most dangerous component. His steps had to be calculated, skillful, while administering combinations of powerful chemicals and sedatives along with life-sustaining technology and technique.

Variables could change suddenly while I was "under" in the mask, particularly if my system triggered vomiting from the digestive tract. Muscles of my mouth could spasm, locking it shut, with food clogging my airway of larynx, trachea and lungs. Complete obstruction would lead to quick suffocation, or surgery's dreaded "aspiration death."

The anesthetist's responsibility encompassed three potential minefields in my procedure: to safely induce unconsciousness, to safely maintain my unconsciousness during surgery, and to safely restore consciousness afterward. Normally in non-emergency situations, "elective" surgery was scheduled days in advance, allowing control of the patient's intake of food and beverage. That had been the plan in my case, until I messed it up.

Instead the anesthetist's job was made much tougher to start Monday, and he didn't appreciate it. He'd have to reconfigure intravenous chemicals and monitoring my vital signs. He was pissed at the nursing staff, but me as well. "Weren't you told, informed, that you were not to eat or drink after 10 o'clock last night?" he queried, eyes glaring from the blue mask and cap.

"Well, yeah, but..."

The anesthetist huffed and turned away, continuing his task and finished hearing me. I felt like an idiot, no excuse, and later I'd really regret my foolishness, having to endure effects of emergency anesthesia to my body.

Now, knee surgery.

I lay awake another minute or two, already sedated by Demerol, watching the ceiling, the OR's pace picking up around me. More staff arrived, exchanging morning talk and laughter as they prepped selves and stations. I was ignored as meat slab of the moment, other than by a silent, veiled staffer who snapped up my left forearm to poke an IV needle port into protruding veins.

Dr. Thorpe entered the room, clad and masked in white, unmistakable in his strong physique, voice, and enthusiasm. The surgeon greeted me loudly at the table and reaffirmed hope my injuries could be minimal. "We'll know more soon enough," he said.

The anesthetist placed the heavy front of a rubber mask over my face, gassing me with cool nitrous oxide while simultaneously dropping an IV dose of Pentothal sedative, ultra-short acting. "Count backwards from 10," he said.

Right. I could no longer speak. Room sounds escalated round me, whirring into one big monotone, and I fell comatose.

The anesthetist strapped the full mask around my head and thrust rubber tubing down my throat, my lax body cooperating fully. I was but construction material for surgical personnel, the labor crew working me, prodding, yanking, and positioning, sawing and suturing flesh, drilling and chiseling bone. My injury challenged them, unfortunately, for I'd wrecked the knee, disconnecting much of the tendon, ligaments and muscle that formerly lashed everything together.

Dr. Thorpe immediately understood my injury was major, a knee dislocation. With me asleep he pulled and pushed the joint, side-to-side, front-to-back and reverse, finding serious instability of the ligament structure. Among the four classes of knee ligament, Dr. Thorpe estimated two to three were damaged or destroyed, based on this final external exam.

The knee swung inward like an opening book, for example, no lateral ligaments left to bind the outside. More ominous was "drawer" movement with the knee bent 90 degrees: The tibia's flattop slid out from under the femur about 9 millimeters, a blocky bonehead tracing forward through skin. I had a tear of the anterior cruciate ligament, critical for attaching bones at joint's core. Only in the past decade had surgeons advanced technique for reconstructing a torn ACL, employing tissue graft harvested from patella tendon encasing the kneecap.

The three arthroscope tubes — a camera, a multi-tool head and a water jet — were inserted into my knee briefly. As soon as Dr. Thorpe confirmed a snapped ACL in the monitor view, he ordered removal of the tubes to avoid further fluid buildup. *Then* he picked up scalpel.

The "arthrotomy" or open-incision phase began with an inverted-C, a foot-long cut running upper leg to lower and arcing over the kneecap. This penetrated skin layer, and epidermis separated wide around the propped knee, bent and poking upward. Blood trickles were vacuumed away by a nurse. "It became immediately obvious that the patient had completely avulsed [torn from bone] the entire lateral ligament complex," the doctor later noted. "Accordingly it was felt the lateral structures should first be put back together."

Stapling down muscle tendon, suturing ripped ligaments, drilling tie-off holes in the femur, Dr. Thorpe slowly reformed and reattached the knee's outside complex for stability. The laterals refastened, he rechecked the outside, yanking again for open-book movement but seeing none. Satisfied, he rechecked for drawer movement, knee cocked at 90 degrees. He grabbed around my calf and pulled frontward; the bones had retightened, but the ACL tear still allowed millimeters of tibia head to slide out.

Now Dr. Thorpe focused on the anterior cruciate for repair, requiring him to dig under the patella tendon and kneecap to access the joint's interior. He plunged knife for a second large cut, the "parapatellar incision," roughly following the first but smaller. The tendon was extremely tough, impossible to slice cleanly like skin, so the surgeon sawed it, progressing in a loop around the kneecap. He peeled back the tendon flap and embedded kneecap, exposing the joint marked by big white boneheads.

Dr. Thorpe was heartened by the preserved state of the damaged ACL, one piece, and, remarkably, with chip of femur bone attached at loose end, including blood vessels. "Somewhat surprisingly, some of the vascularity… was intact, and great care was taken to avoid damage." Basically, Dr. Thorpe plugged my original ACL right back into its vacant slot at the femur head, a tight refit he secured with sutures tied at drill holes.

Now I didn't need an ACL reconstruction, which would've violated tendon for making a ligament graft. Two hours before, a thousand suture stitches ago, Dr. Thorpe had encountered a joint like spaghetti, my knee. But he'd put it back together and jerked in every direction to confirm. "There was essentially no instability," he'd dictate.

The peroneal nerve, meanwhile, displayed no improvement. The surgeon soberly measured the bloodied channel. The damaged portion of nerve sheath had separated vertically in shards, caught within super-inversion of knee joint, similar to rope fibers yanked so taut to split. Blood had rushed in, saturating the nerve channel, choking off signals of motor function and sensory.

The operation concluded about 10:30 in the morning. Thorpe sought my parents, but they hadn't arrived. "I will speak to them this afternoon in office concerning the situation," the doctor recorded. "Prognosis is very guarded. This patient [has] significant tear."

I myself didn't get word until mid-afternoon, after I wakened in post-op, heavy headed, groggy, seemingly days since the anesthetist put me under. Because of the intense emergency anesthesia, I felt horrible, lying prone and tasting a petroleum-like chemical that seemed to line my innards from mouth to stomach. Parched, I begged for ice water, despite the nurse's warning I'd vomit. I did so gladly, drinking lustily and regurgitating in a bedpan.

My mother, now on scene, gently apprised me of what was happening. She'd spent time with Dr. Thorpe, liked him, respected his judgment, and relayed his cautious outlook. The injury was much worse than expected, Mom explained, the most complicated knee operation Dr. Thorpe had conducted. He said I would wear a full leg cast for *five to six months*. Moreover, he and consultant neurologists couldn't say when my leg paralysis would heal, if ever. Mom said I may never run again.

I absorbed the verdict, crestfallen, but protested strongly, declaring I would not merely run again: "I'm gonna *play football* again!"

Mom supported me as she could. "We'll see, Matt," she said quietly, atypical of her usual optimism.

The pain was fresh, lasting, searing beneath the blood-soaked surgical cast. I cursed, forgetting my mother momentarily, but she only leapt up to summon a nurse. I'd had Demerol before surgery and I wanted more. For the next five days, I sought a Demerol shot every four hours, round the clock, or I couldn't rest for pain. It felt like burning hot jelly had replaced the knee under plaster.

The surgeon forwarded a report to my coaches in SEMO football, and they were disappointed, for me as well as the team. They wrote me off for playing again, much less being worth a scholarship. Hell, I resigned to forget a scholarship at this point, needing a miracle comeback to merely step back onto a football field. Yet I had to be a real college player, one game at least. Thinking about it, wanting it so badly now, I'd get teary.

On my behalf, an assistant coach contacted the *De Soto Republic* newspaper back home, resulting in the only news report of my college career. "Chaney injured at SEMO," the weekly's headline noted, over its brief account:

> CAPE GIRARDEAU — Matt Chaney, a third-string defensive end for the Southeast Missouri State University Indians, sustained a severe knee injury Friday during a scrimmage, according to Coach Dennis Darnell.
>
> Chaney… underwent surgery on Monday. A long rehabilitation period is expected, said Coach Darnell.
>
> "He did it as bad as you can," said the coach. "The injury involved torn ligaments and cartilage"
>
> The SEMO junior was on the varsity traveling team.
>
> He is the son of Mr. and Mrs. Louis Chaney of Hillsboro.

By my second weekend in hospital, I was a thoroughly humbled young man. My grandmother had always warned "You'll get knocked off your high horse," and I had fallen hard. The major leg injury and corrective procedures taxed my body, but inner spirit had withered as well. I lay bedridden in the room, staring off from TV, watching bloody ooze seep into a glass jar at bedside, through plastic drains sewed into my surgical wound. Notebooks and reading materials piled up in a corner chair, mostly untouched; textbooks were already gone, returned to campus, for my official withdrawal from classes. No way could I finish the semester, hardly able to stay upright on crutches yet.

I was a good patient, attentive and accommodating to medical staff because I wanted to get well; I wanted out of there. I was in bad shape, however, needing constant care. I felt ravaged, having dropped 25 pounds in seven days, mostly muscle, because of the heavy anesthesia of surgery followed by round-the-clock IV injections. Amazingly, only weeks before, I'd injected potent, repeated dosages of testosterone cypionate, but the anabolic hormones still couldn't offset such traumatic breakdown of tissue.

Stomach nausea, headaches, queasiness racked me. First time the nurses pulled me upright for physical therapy, tethering me in a wide leather harness, the leg in heavy cast slipped to strike the floor and I spewed vomit. Many sensations grossed me out following surgery because the drugs skewed senses for food, distorting my smell and taste. I couldn't eat anything, recoiling at sight of a hospital tray, which took an aroma strange, revolting. There was no appetite even for Pagliai's pizza fetched by Mom, from my favorite parlor on Broadway.

I sweated IV liquids incessantly, drenching bed sheets, and peed in a bedpan. I didn't bother struggling on crutches to a toilet; there was no bowel movement. I couldn't shower, and nurses' sponge baths seemed useless to me. Varied scum and stench collected on my skin and in crevices, building since I'd gone down in the football scrimmage. My long hair matted and stunk.

My eighth day in the hospital, Saturday morning, I learned I couldn't leave, again, and I faltered completely. Crying, I turned to someone I hadn't since I could remember: my father. I called Dad, begging him to get me out of this place and bring me home.

Next morning, Dr. Thorpe approved my release and shook my hand. I appreciated him, immensely. He would be a lifelong confidant of mine for the bad leg. By noon I was packed, downstairs and checked out, waiting at the lobby door, watching outside for sign of Mom in the family Oldsmobile. Such anticipation for my mother hadn't changed since boyhood, her rescue from places I'd grown homesick. Yeah, I'd strutted as Big Man on Campus recently, but now I wanted out of this town. I wanted to go home.

The Delta 88 appeared on time, Mom smiling through the sunny windshield glass, and she pulled up under the awning at the outpatient lobby. It was never better to see her arrive in that car, unforgettable.

VI. Coaching Football, Tolerating Steroids

Anabolic steroids washed through football's plane by the 1984 season, small colleges and large. None was immune; no one region, league, team, nor individual could wall out the steroid flood. College football had no more isolation, sanctuary, from the sweep of muscle drugs, with every level irreversibly breached.

The ethos-pharmaceutical tsunami had slammed through, and there I found myself starting out as a college football coach, bobbing around yet on the issue. I was, however, seeing the real picture of steroids in the game: No one, no player, no coach, no administrator, could or would do a damned thing, just like amphetamines. *Fuck it,* I rationalized, the young coach. *Just think of the drugs as a personal choice by athletes and keep your mouth shut, do your job.*

It was time I did something with my future in mind — which now concerned a young woman I fawned over — and college coaching offered possibilities with enough ego gratification for me. The job had only recently become a consideration, after my playing career was unceremoniously finished for the bad leg. I liked the idea of staying in college football, still gaining local visibility somehow.

I'd learned my physical vulnerability the previous two years, accepted the disabling injury, what I lost in strength, athleticism, and leg stability through dislocating the knee and paralyzing the foot. I did make it back to the practice field, after 17 months rehabilitation that included a second surgery, but only for spring football. My knee felt like a wooden hinge, remolded internally by foreign materials, and nerve damage was impossible to overcome. My drop foot was permanent, and to play football again, the entire leg had to be strapped in steel, plastic and tape. Once competing again in football on that foot, its outer third paralyzed running upside the ankle, and it became bloody black from daily sprains, through the toes. For treatment I immersed it in ice water two to three times daily, and for workouts trainers taped the foot and ankle heavily. No surprise, I ran a half-second slower in the 40, or about 5.4 seconds, and lacked fast-twitch step from the right side, reaction and acceleration.

Physical disconnections aside, I also couldn't beat the trauma on my macho psyche for football, the former belief I was indestructible with nothing to fear of male peers. Once back on the field, I had a few big moments, sacking quarterbacks, making hits, stealing the football, but more often I was hesitant, *fearful*, having gone from instigator of football violence to mostly bystander. That was telling of my end in competition. And I re-injured the leg, for my third knee surgery and second under Dr. Thorpe, who had politely opposed my comeback in the first place. At least I managed to avoid steroids this time. Some teammates had literally demanded I juice for the comeback, but I wouldn't until determining whether it was worth it again. It wasn't, not on my crippled leg; I was done as a player, which a barrel of 'roids couldn't change.

Coach Lohr had resigned, and a new coaching staff under Bob Smith was in charge, boasting background and connections in big-time college ball. The roster had been taken over by transfers and recruits, including a significant amount of juicers who spanned most positions, linemen, linebackers, tight ends, and running backs. Big, strong players ruled the new program, definitely under a new attitude, and fights were routine in practice.

I took the sideline as a student coach that fall, 1984, my last resort in football. "Coach Chaney" sounded odd to me — *coaching* seemed a strange role — but I still faced a year's classes to graduate college. I was holding onto football a little longer, having vested my campus identity in the program, and I liked the new staff led by head man "Smitty," former O-line coach at Illinois.

Yet I lacked the passion I'd felt as an able-bodied player, cocky and driven. Football was fading for me, replaced by different desire and motive: love, the person I wanted to marry, desperately. She was Laurie Schoenbaum, a beautiful young woman charming, kind, and athletic, who starred in gymnastics for SEMO.

Nicknamed "The Bomb," Laurie was an exotic, embodying whom I'd sought in a life mate. I couldn't fathom a future without her, but self-improvement on my part was prerequisite for the marriage to occur — and I heard about it from family and close friends. I couldn't deny my failed return to football and lack of dedication for anything else. Losing self-control, I logged horrible grades in school, barely passing, and partied like never before, wasting months and incurring debt. My parents, already through hell with me, were as worried as ever.

Mom and Dad also understood how much I cared for Laurie and a future with her, and she buoyed their hopes. My parents were smitten with Laurie too, praying she would be in my life — but stressing foremost I had to strengthen in character, assuming more personal responsibility. "Matt, you must get out and find a job that you can make yourself a living, honey," Mom wrote. "You've got yourself a wonderful girl who loves you, and I know you love her, too. You must now start thinking about getting something together to start on. You can [go to school], but you could work on the weekends."

I heeded everyone's advice, with Laurie constant in mind, and, at age 24, finally set out in earnest to complete requirements for a college degree. Moreover, I had newfound respect for writing, where I'd shown promise, raw ability. I began serious study of writing and method, capitalizing on reading, my fondest pastime since grade school. Long-term I wanted to write books but immediately concentrated on journalism classes and free-lance writing, seeing opportunity in news media.

I worked hard coaching college football, with necessary focus on my job. I was a grunt on staff but valued, particularly for my varied vocational experience applicable beyond the field, like video photography and promotional writing. I was also street-savvy, a definite asset.

An initial assignment was bus driver during summer camp, ferrying a couple dozen out-of-state "student-athletes" to a courthouse so they could register as Missouri voters — therefore saving thousands of dollars for the football program. As an instant Missouri voter, each transfer or recruit was deemed eligible for an *in-state* football scholarship, rather then the costlier out-of-state benefit. Were we skirting the law at least? Damn right, along with spitting on the NCAA rulebook, great reasons to designate me as driver, the only university representative with the players. Later on, in event of questions raised, I could burn for all's sins — even for alleged dummies at the courthouse — since the official alibi would be, of course, that I alone rounded up the players, commandeered a university vehicle, and carried out the scheme.

Back on campus, I checked further into such unique funding arrangements for athletes, not only football players, and learned many males and females received federal work-study money as substitute for bona fide athletic aid. These athletes didn't hold campus jobs for "work study," in violation of the federal program. I also better understood why campus jobs were so scarce: Much of the federal cash went instead to fraudulent athletic "scholarships." The school recruited athletes for many teams on the pretense of offering bona fide athletic aid or scholarship money, classified in the books as privately donated. Once on campus, however, the athletes were instructed to pick up a monthly check of federal funds at the bursar's office, diverted from real work-study jobs. The seamy practice was commonplace at the college, requiring complicity of personnel outside the athletic department. Moreover, it went on *everywhere* in Missouri, state universities' playing shell games with tax dollars to fund an overly ambitious sports mission.

Impropriety aside, my job was primarily on the field coaching football, which I often enjoyed as much as playing. I oversaw the scout-team offense, largely non-scholarship freshmen and other walk-ons, and I took the position seriously as a former meat-squad player. Undeniably, it was a mental rush to design plays and game plans that proved successful on the field, but I also still bought American mythology of the football coach, that I would *mold men*.

"I'm coaching the young kids, the walk-ons," I wrote my grandmother. "They've got a tough way to go, at the bottom of the ladder. They work harder than anybody in practice, and get beaten up pretty badly by the bigger, older guys. But that's where I started, and I know how it is. I've got some kids with real guts though, and those will definitely make it. I love those kids who work hard, and sometimes I wonder if I did as good a job."

I wasn't content to baby-sit these guys, persuade them to stick around just to serve as bodies for pounding by scholarship players. They deserved a fair shot to make the team too, although none would see the game field this season, and only a few ever. My goal was to be honest with these guys, unlike many coaches. I told them foremost what I knew: "To get off the meat squad and play on game day, you better knock the shit out of people," I told them, "every motherfucker you meet on the practice field — and beginning with the No. 1 defense you face every day out here. Don't even let those fuckers push you around. You blast 'em…

"And to become a starter someday, you must get bigger, faster, stronger. Hit the weightroom, now." I didn't say *Do steroids*, but didn't have to explicitly. Reality was apparent, implicit: Size and strength had become paramount in D-II football, just like higher levels, and juicing could mean competing.

Within two years in SEMO football, emphasis on strength training had accelerated from secondary to priority and the use of anabolic steroids had doubled, to at least 20 percent of players. On the offensive and defensive lines, coaching demand for size and power had increased physiques about 20 pounds per position, with more speed required. To contend for starting position at line, linebacker, tight end, fullback, a guy hardly rated coaches' attention until he bench-pressed at least 300, squatted 450, power-cleaned 225 and ran a respectable 40 time. Then we coaches demanded more from him.

"OF ALL THE THINGS IN FOOTBALL... STRENGTH IS THE EASIEST TO IMPROVE," declared the SEMO player's manual.

Bullshit, unless doing drugs was easy. Many wouldn't bench 300 without steroids, players at SEMO and anywhere else in college football. With no juice, commitment to strength training and nutrition was mostly irrelevant, woefully deficient. Overeating didn't do the trick despite public lies of juiced players, claiming their inhuman gains were due to extra steaks, cheeseburgers, and shakes. Bullshit.

Coaches, players, and trainers understood big gains in size and strength did not happen simply or soon for any ready player — without drugs. Only chemicals could key a second burst of tissue-building hormones in a body beyond puberty, and everyone with a brain in college football understood the fact.

We just didn't discuss it in the open, didn't have to. The dynamics of muscle doping were in place: Players competed in size and power and encouraged each other, directly and indirectly, while coaches kept up the pressure, constant emphasis, including many nationwide who took hand in the problem with players. From D-II up in college ball, every program had to have had at least one coach discussing juicing with players; many programs had at least one coach helping players obtain anabolic steroids.

"GET THE 'BULL BODY,' " the program manual commanded, with more proclamations for the player to abide in weightlifting.

"MENTAL TOUGHNESS."

"INTENSITY."

" MAKE AN UGLY FACE."

"BE A BEHEMOTH."

"ONLY THE STRONG SHALL SURVIVE."

"THE WILL TO WIN."

"DOES ANYONE REMEMBER WHO FINISHED SECOND?"

"WHAT IS YOUR OPPONENT DOING TODAY?"

Players mocked the messages as goofy shit when away from coaches, like on a drinking binge among guys, one to another. *Remember, man, 'The will to win,'* they'd joke. Still a player knew this was gospel, imperative directions for pleasing coaches, gaining game time, and for surviving and thriving through the gauntlet. A player knew many of his teammates and opponents were utilizing anabolic steroids, including gigantic teenagers showing up at every school. In SEMO football, weightlifting records were shattered. Among feats, 10 freshmen benched 300 or more; only a few years previous, fewer upperclassman starters hoisted as much.

I lamented the football trend of increasing doping, but quietly, thinking of self, my prospects in coaching. For this problem and certain havoc, ever growing, I was relieved to no longer play the fucking game. Yet I wouldn't avoid the juice in college football.

Once more I would participate in the problem, act in perpetration, and this time as a coach.

Slippery Slope: A Coach's Hypocrisy and Steroids For A Player

As a student coach in charge of scout-team players, I held certain expectations of myself and was not concerned what other coaches thought. My primary intent was supporting the non-scholarship players, especially in the trenches against the scholarship guys, and that meant trouble.

Contrary to program dogma, I did not believe scout-team individuals existed as meat for the program. Rather, I pursued the ideal that anyone could make the team, and to realize success, I told my players repeatedly: "Beat the shit out of guys ahead of you on the roster, at every opportunity." Staff conflict for me, therefore, quickly came to head at the SEMO complex on a hot Tuesday afternoon in September. The team struggled already, winless in games, and pressure was venting in the week's toughest practice. During "team defense," coaches were screaming at game players, singling them out for everyone's failure thus far.

My guys on scout-team offense caught the brunt, the staff hate passed along by roster players who beat them mercilessly. Cheap shots increased on my guys, encouraged by defensive coaches, until I had my fill of the hyena game. "Fuck those people!" I exploded on my players, pointing to defensive starters and coaches — and drawing their attention from across the line of scrimmage. "Are you gonna let them do that to you!" I screamed. "You better starting hittin' somebody! Smash 'em in the goddamned face!"

My guys, attentive to me, snapped together in a better huddle. I continued, to the amazement of defensive coaches. "They don't give a shit about you! They don't care — "

"NO! NO! NO!" The D-line coach cut me off, bursting into our huddle, waving arms, trailed by the fuming coordinator. "That's BULLSHIT!" He shook his finger in my face, and he was a friend of mine. "Every man is part of this team!" the coach yelled at my guys. "WE CARE ABOUT YOU! That's the goddamn truth!"

My guys were silent, some nodding, and I neither protested the coach nor blamed their reaction. I only hoped none of my players were stupid enough to believe the propaganda. I was told to leave the field, go inside. I sauntered away but stopped outside the offices, turning around to watch the end of practice, arms crossed, scowling in token defiance. Powerless to do more, I had lost the war for the meat squad and knew it.

I'd been broken, at expense of my guys. Next time their necks were on the line,

I'd have to sell them out and side with the coaching staff. Screw the meat squad — Did I really believe that? No, but I was pliable, conceding for dirty duty, and I on a Friday soon I carried out the company mission during a Toilet Bowl scrimmage.

A fight broke out on a run play, between a freshman recruit at fullback and a walk-on defensive tackle, Mike, an upperclassman two years in the program and a friend of mine. My first thought was to remove both players from the scrimmage and send them home for the weekend, my regular policy for fighting in Toilet Bowls. I deplored fighting in football, especially among teammates at practice, in direct contrast with many coaches.

This situation, however, cast me on the razor's edge. I would have to employ favoritism, football politics I detested, and not to benefit my friend. The fighters were separated, but I judged Mike as the only one to eject from play. I *had* to keep the fullback on the field, a prize recruit the ranking coaches had personally placed in this Toilet Bowl. The fullback would soon be added to the game roster and staffers wanted him ready. I heard explicit instructions the kid must play the entire scrimmage, carrying the football and blocking.

I told walk-on Mike to leave the field but said nothing to the recruit. My friend was enraged, wanting to deck me, but no need. The look of betrayal in Mike's eyes struck like a punch. He was a veteran of this program, dedicated as anyone to "team," even if struggling to make the game roster, and he knew exactly what was up and got in my face.

"That's BULLSHIT, Chaney!" Then Mike stormed away for the locker room.

I said nothing, couldn't, to stark truth.

While my lack of fairness for scout-team guys like Mike weighed on me, I would fall further as a coach. Steroid use in the program had doubled at least in the two years since I was juicing as player, but I had managed to mostly stay clear of the drugs during both my comeback attempt and my beginning as coach. No mistaking I was still indirectly involved, having heard players discuss their purchasing and using, along with gossip about many more. Some athletes were obvious for physiques and acute effects like acne and balding. I also heard of one coach's encouragement and advice for select players.

Then, one evening after practice, a practice player I was getting to know approached and asked if I would help him find steroids. "Where can I get a cycle? Just one," he said. The guy was relatively new to the program, and I liked him, trusted him, along with understanding his challenge to make the game roster. He *needed* juice. I knew where to get the shit, from a former player selling a variety of anabolic steroids, but I didn't want to make this deal. I would've rather helped the practice player find a bag of pot, so I and other young coaches could've gotten high.

Smoking marijuana may have been illegal, counterproductive if not self-destructive, but it was likewise a personal decision exclusive of football. I still held to a poster in high school, the athletic director's office: "Get high on sports, not drugs." Muscle dope was different than street narcotics, a dynamic that twisted America hypocritical in its so-called war on drugs, a society busting people for pot while glorifying the sport that most channeled a young male to steroids and now growth hormone. Muscle doping, for me deep down, was *insidious* for football.

Yet I didn't close the door on the football player. I felt hypocritical to deny him steroids, as a former user myself who clearly saw the level of muscle dope on the team. Realistically, he couldn't compete without it, so I deferred for the moment. "Look around some more yourself," I said. "Check with me later if you can't find anything."

He came back the next week. "Com'n, Chainsaw," he pleaded, and I agreed, taking his $40 and heading to get this shit over with. Half-hour later I knocked on the player's dorm door, he answered, and I slipped him the steroid vial.

I left the building, saying nothing to anyone, but now as a football coach who provided anabolic steroids for a player. That reality, I could never depart.

VII. Leaving Football Delusion to Begin Real Life

Nearing end of my first and only season as a coach, I was rejecting the delusional image of college football, specifically the myth about the player as young warrior in righteous passage to manhood, defending the honor of alma mater. Ridiculous.

This was not war for country. College football was no just battle for anything, anyone. Alma mater had problems itself for integrity, and a game of young males' butting heads in armor was nothing resembling education or honor. This game dictated survival and conquest, any way possible. Goodness did not fit the football model, an environment negotiated by violence where a moral fool was subject to assault.

Players and coaches were beholden to football, if strictly to win. Losing simply meant weakness and loss of job. As a rookie coach and ex-player casualty, watching SEMO football suffer defeat week after week, I wrote:

> Losing is real. One must joke at the word, at times, but the force is there; what is but positive, negative force anyway? Football is so much reality that it can stagger you, if you really ponder it.
>
> You win, and everything's OK; you lose, and you must put forth effort to make your *life* successful again. ...
>
> Football is battle, but a struggle for shining satisfaction within our souls. The game is our dreams as players. "It's *the world*," says SEMO running back Marvin Johnson, and he's right. We all pay so much just to put on the pads, we can't possibly consider the price until later. ...
>
> Football can, and usually does, change your life.
>
> Winning *is* everything then.

I was fast losing desire for the sport. Motive waned inside, having lost a knee and my naiveté about player reality, the boyish view of college ball as spiritual journey. Now I considered my role as coach in the charade, grooming young men as attack robots and otherwise disregarding them, harming them, and I knew I'd perpetrated enough shit myself.

I couldn't give up the game easily, however, until two loves stepped in and pulled me away: a young woman and writing. I wanted marriage with her and success as a writer, as my football career fizzled.

Laurie and I met in spring 1983, in the months following my knee blowout. Several of us football players were attempting to stage a house party one Saturday evening, but mostly looking at each other until the women's gymnastics team showed up in short shorts, improving atmosphere dramatically. Laurie and I came together over a proven conversation piece, my plaster cast adorned by signatures and notes I'd scrawled for constant inquiries, like "Knee Surgery" and "Football."

Laurie's approach was innocent enough to me at the beer keg. "What happened to your knee?" she asked, smiling, gymnast's legs bursting from shorts — and I'd just been brooding about 20 weeks in the cast. I took over the conversation from there. Laurie resembled Audrey Hepburn but with ballerina stature, gorgeous in her brown hair, Bambi eyes, fine features, perfect teeth and physique. She possessed the muscle lines of her father, a former pro boxer, hardened through gymnastics training since kindergarten.

I'd been around head-jerking females before, and surface looks weren't critical attraction for me. Laurie's character shone through, captivating me, charging my desire through qualities I could only envy. She was quiet, patient, and caring, a great listener of intelligence, humility and kindness. She was angelic. I was 23, she 19, and we talked the rest of the party, until I "walked" her outside on my crutches, meeting her ride back to campus. We went to dinner a few nights later; within a month, I contemplated marriage for the first time. Moreover, I babbled about Laurie to my parents, who were stunned; previously I rarely mentioned a female. But they were thrilled after meeting Laurie.

I wanted to marry Laurie, raise a family with her. I begged God for her hand, and I persuaded her. At Christmas 1984, I put a diamond engagement ring on her finger. I coached only a couple months longer, until spring, when the program hit budget crunch and we student assistants suffered a pay cut. I was on the recruiting trail 20-plus hours a week, driving all directions in the Midwest, and now paid about $1 an hour. I'd already decided coaching wasn't for me, anyway. "To hell with football," I said, and Laurie supported me enthusiastically.

I resigned and took part-time work as pizza deliveryman, then as bartender. I began writing for publication in earnest, with Laurie's encouragement and help. Using a typewriter, she transferred my stories from handwritten to hard copy for submissions. "I like to read, especially your stuff," she wrote me. "You are an *excellent* writer! You can do it — because you do want it!"

We got married in August 1985, as Laurie graduated college. I graduated the following December, with credit for Laurie's influence, and we moved in with my parents, St. Louis area.

I presumed a decent living ahead in writing, beginning with news media, especially for my desire to seek and publicize truth. I viewed the journalistic mission as serving accuracy and fairness, and I possessed the requirements: guts, work ethic, personal altruism rather than materialism. The good knight was excited within, like bedtime in boyhood, when Grandma read me Disney and Aesop's fables.

I would still meet the dark heart of culture and self, however, the politics of "reality" in America, how truth was subject to broad definition under control of influence, power. I'd learned cynicism toward football and would find news media worthy of about the same regard.

VIII. Suspended Belief: Big Mac Mania

Mark McGwire seemed a wash-up in the early 1990s, just another injury-prone baseball player flaming out after starting flashy, but by 1998 he was *Big Mac*, history's most feted home-run hitter, beloved worldwide.

McGwire's comeback was remarkable, or unreal in common parlance. After bashing 49 home runs as a rookie for Oakland in 1987, his performance deteriorated rapidly through 1991, when he batted .201 with 22 homers and 75 RBIs. Considering retirement, McGwire instead committed to becoming bigger and stronger. Already an avid weightlifter, he was muscular at 6-foot-5, 225 pounds, but he would get huge. He enlisted help, including older brother Jay McGwire, a former pro bodybuilder with experience in "banned bodybuilding drugs" who transformed himself through Christianity, reported Rick Reilly for *SI.*

Next spring, McGwire arrived at training camp packing upwards of 20 pounds new muscle, a chump no more, and cranked 42 dingers that season. Transformation toward superstardom had begun. In 1997 McGwire became baseball's second player after Babe Ruth to accomplish consecutive 50-homer seasons, and he did it around a trade to St. Louis in July. Actually, the move set up his mythical assault on power records to come, reuniting the guardedly private slugger with old confidants from Oakland, Cardinals manager Tony La Russa and conditioning coach Dave McKay, a semi-bodybuilder himself like McGwire. McKay, a training guru and author, was an ex-major leaguer serving as strength coach under La Russa since the Oakland glory days of The Bash Brothers, Jose Canseco and McGwire.

Big Mac was instant legend in baseball-crazed St. Louis after his trade. Despite a slow start at the plate, McGwire finished the season with 58 jacks, tantalizingly close to Roger Maris' single-year record of 61. The storied baseball town was mesmerized, and sportswriters churned out voluminous prose on Big Mac, building this Bunyanesque tale of baseball.

The man was larger than life, literally and figuratively. Finally physically mature at age 34, presumably, McGwire was freakish, a ripped 255 pounds at least. He had six-pack abs at core, 20-inch biceps, huge chest and shoulders, bulging forearms, all riding atop massive legs at thigh and calf. The giant with Popeye arms was even *friendly*, gushed media, a fresh, grinning persona changed for the better, went the popular tales of Big Mac. McGwire was a wonder at the plate, prodigious power, ripping shots of distance and ferocity with no precedence in the game. At no time before had someone hit a baseball like Big Mac, not Ruth, not Aaron, Mantle, nor Maris. Not even the old McGwire himself.

In cookie-cutter Busch Stadium, McGwire's displays were almost comical, evermore audacious as the 1998 season carried on. Busch was a spacious park not known for a batted ball "to carry," but Mac riddled the place high and low with hits. Many Cardinals fans had never seen a ball reach the upper deck, but McGwire swatted lasers there daily in BP and games. On the road he did likewise, mammoth homers in every stadium, generating great excitement. People traveled hundreds of miles to "see McGwire," children in tow, as though pursuing a deity.

Big Mac was indeed god-like, for many Americans at least. Anyone watching was awestruck. "There are power hitters, and then there is Mark McGwire," said veteran Cardinals catcher Tom Pagnozzi. "He's way beyond anybody else in the game." Hall of Fame broadcaster Jack Buck, five decades calling Cardinals games, came to expect a homer every time McGwire swung. The power astonished Buck, like Pagnozzi, especially at Busch. "I stood by that batting cage and looked at some of the spots where he hit those home runs," Buck said, "and I couldn't believe it."

McGwire's feats captured America and increasingly the world, and media magnified personal traits in narratives his fans found endearing. Writer after writer made much of the slugger's crusade against child abuse — the big guy broke into tears at one news conference — and also highlighted his fatherhood, humility, and penny-pinching. He publicly expressed disdain for rising player salaries and stunned the baseball world, foregoing a highly lucrative turn at free agency to instead sign a $30 million extension with the Cardinals, three years. He established a foundation touted to provide millions of dollars for abused children. Fans and media were delighted, Cardinals followers overwhelmed. "I've never seen or heard about St. Louis falling for a player like they've done for his guy," said Brian Bartow, team official. "Not for Musial, not for Gibson, not for Ozzie — nobody."

Skepticism, however, followed McGwire and noticeably heftier players like him. Doping analysts and other close observers believed drugs were commonplace in Major League Baseball, and Big Mac was their presumed Exhibit A. "Steroids have completely changed the game," an anonymous baseball executive told MSNBC. "Guys try to cover it up by saying they're using creatine. Or they're just lifting weights now. Come on. It's a completely different look." Baseball had no testing for steroids, allowing players to inject and ingest drugs with impunity, including the classic dope such as Dianabol, Winstrol V, and Deca-Durabolin. Muscle-bound, pimply batters were on every roster, but McGwire drew most attention, and *SI* writer Tom Verducci asked him about steroid use in March.

"Never," replied McGwire. The athlete did confirm consuming "anything that's legal," meaning dietary supplements. "It sort of boggles my mind when you hear people trying to discredit someone who's had success," he said. "Because a guy enjoys lifting weights and taking care of himself, why do they think that guy is doing something illegal?"

That ethical framework or explanation by McGwire, of hard work and nutrition making for great performance, appeared to remain intact a few months later, when a reporter found a bottle of androstenedione in the slugger's locker at Busch. "Andro" was legal, a dietary supplement sold over counter that was not banned by MLB — or so cried McGwire and his apologists of every walk and creed, millions of Americans and more fans spanning the globe.

There was a problem, critics retorted, because scientific literature since the 1930s identified androstenedione as an anabolic-androgenic steroid, among the first testosterone substances isolated. "There's no debate," said Dr. Charles E. Yesalis, doping expert and historian. The substance was banned as a performance-enhancer by Olympic sports, the NFL and NCAA. "Androstenedione is a steroid, there's no question about it," said Dr. Don Catlin, head of the U.S. Olympic testing laboratory. "It shouldn't be available."

Pilgrimage to See McGwire Battle Sosa, Season's Final Weekend

On the final weekend of baseball season 1998, St. Louis was supercharged despite no playoff hope for the Cardinals. It was World Series atmosphere over one man: Mark McGwire. I drove my wife and kids into the city on Friday evening, September 25, making family pilgrimage to see a mere baseball player.

Big freakin' Mac. Who else, right? Personally, I was sick of the guy, an obvious juicer to me. In fact I was shopping a newspaper commentary that alleged McGwire's season wasn't so magical, just tainted by muscle dope. Market for the piece was tepid so far.

Meanwhile, a friend had called to offer tickets for Saturday's game, and we accepted. My 7-year-old son wanted to see Big Mac, and my wife, and, crap, I did too. This *was* Missouri, after all, center of the world's biggest story of the moment: McGwire versus Sammy Sosa of the Cubs in a heartwarming battle over baseball's new home-run crown, single season. We entered St. Louis at the zenith of Mac mania.

Our timing was in theme, reaching the city's outskirts as Big Mac strode to the plate at Busch Stadium downtown, fifth inning, to face Expos rookie pitcher Shayne Bennett. Forty minutes before, Sosa belted his homer No. 66 in Houston, claiming derby lead of the moment over McGwire, who stood at 65. Cardinals voice Jack Buck had the call on KMOX radio, and I turned it up, the ballpark racket taking over inside our little truck. I hit the gas, driving faster, and on first pitch McGwire sent a high drive toward the left-field foul pole, tape-measure distance, stadium roaring.

The ball landed far gone, upper deck inside Busch, but foul by five feet. The capacity crowd standing in unison, experiencing intense baseball religion, moaned and sighed along with Big Mac, who shrugged near home plate. He was still smarting from a lost homer that week in Milwaukee, when an umpire erroneously ruled a double on a ball that reached the bleachers, and meanwhile Sosa was surging, appearing to be on another hot streak to pass our hero.

Now everyone wondered: Was the hex on Big Mac? The big guy shook his red head, re-gripped his bat and dug in again at the plate, returning his focus to the mound, blinking and squinting to get a bead of aim through contact lenses. McGwire was a homer robot for destroying pitches. Bennett had a new ball, fingering it behind his back on the hill, looking in again to his catcher. The right-hander stretched with a man on base. Fans buzzed but restrained, allowing Mac his precious concentration, although thousands flashed cameras on subsequent pitches by Bennett: a ball outside, a swing and a miss, and another foul off.

I saw everything in mind, scenes throughout the stadium, while driving Highway 40 eastbound into St. Louis. I savored the familiar rhythm of Buck on play-by-play and admittedly loved Cardinals baseball, now with the greatest power hitter in history! I believed McGwire would overtake Sosa in the weekend homer fest, and on next pitch I was positive. Mac swatted Bennett's 1-2 offering for a homer to left, 375 feet and fair, tying Sosa at 66.

I turned to my wife at the passenger's side. "You watch, McGwire could hit *two* dingers tomorrow," I declared. "And if he does, he'll slam two more on Sunday to give him 70 for the season." My prediction wasn't improbable for McGwire, whom I knew enough about as a player. I'd watched him hit 49 homers as a rookie in 1987, when I covered MLB for feature stories and he anchored my offensive lineup for "rotisserie league," to be better known as "fantasy" baseball. Mac knocked three homers one Saturday afternoon and I won $125. McGwire loved daylight for batting and I enjoyed cashing in on him, then.

Now I understood more about McGwire, too much. He had synthetic fuel for performance, which I could grasp, but I resented his outright denial of steroids, for the global icon he'd become. McGwire and those close to him were perpetrating a charade of world proportion, and I wrote the slugger a letter saying as much, noting my own juicing past and declaring he could never keep his doping under wraps. He didn't reply.

The magnitude of denial stunned even me, a seasoned doping critic. I'd observed steroid signs in baseball for years while compiling information on football's problem. Major leaguers were doping in the 1980s when I interviewed several suspects, like a scrawny Cardinals player who added 20 pounds of muscle in only months. Later, when La Russa debuted as St. Louis manager, 1996, I spied juicer suspects at spring training like burly hitters, a model-buff older pitcher, and even a coach, rippling and strutting for females.

I also heard about the new and improved McGwire, still with the Athletics, during dugout scuttlebutt that March in St. Petersburg. Mac was mentioned for developing ungodly muscle and size, producing power at the plate unmatched in baseball history. I noted McGwire was always a big bopper in baseball. "No, now he's fuckin' *huge*," declared the dugout source, whose language I understood to mean McGwire had chemical aid. The next season, after his move to St. Louis, I had no doubt. The dude was as big and strong as a Rams defensive end.

Much information to corroborate McGwire's doping would surface in the future, including his training associates of juicers and gurus. But in 1998 I was convinced for his appearance, power numbers and the steroid "andro," along with general pervasiveness of muscle substances in sport and culture. He was peaking in physique and performance beyond natural capabilities, given his personal history.

La Russa claimed McGwire simply ate well and worked hard in the weightroom, on top of games, an absurd assertion with the specimen Mac notwithstanding. Indeed, a regimen of daily weightlifting in professional baseball would dictate synthetic augmentation for the athlete. And McGwire's leap was ridiculous in power numbers. As a rookie in 1987, he mustered supreme output with one home run every 11.4 at bats, or 49 for the season. His ratio declined markedly into the next decade then skyrocketed back upward, climaxing in 1998 at one homer every 7.3 plate appearances, for a man turning 35.

I tried to go along with Cards fans on Big Mac, bite my tongue, ride the merry bandwagon, and it was fun in moments with friends and family. On a July night at Busch I saw him annihilate two pitches, homers, one a 500-footer into upper-deck seats merely in way of the riser, which would've gone 600. I certainly understood McGwire's use of steroids in modern elite sport, and I respected him as a citizen with humble qualities. I loved his genuine disdain for fame and money's power and laughed at his treatment of sportswriters, the general lot deserving no respect.

However, I couldn't take the baseless excuses for McGwire and his doping, growing daily. I was increasingly insulted by everything I read, saw, and heard, particularly in Missouri. By now I was years into study of documented history of doping in American sport, work spawned by my own user-athlete past, and had discussed the problem with hundreds of eyewitnesses. Yet I was largely alone in public for criticizing Big Mac. Practically everyone ignored my complaints, including journalists I contacted in protest of coverage way overdone in support and glory of the guy.

After McGwire hit No. 62 at Busch to break Roger Maris' record, I watched TV to hopefully enjoy the celebration as a fan, but I became incredulous, seeing masses heap worship, love. The scene was so contrived. America was already versed in the facts of widespread doping in sport, not to mention McGwire's documented use of andro. That night I put my son to bed, saw his little McGwire jersey laid out for school the next morning, then fell asleep feeling ill. I had a dream Mac confessed to everything, and woke at dawn to vomit. My morning reality was Missouri's falling over to kiss Mac's butt. Incessant media streams praised the guy, with news and opinion pages gushing like sports sections. Infuriatingly, clueless writers proclaimed the slugger as Mr. Natural, but he was also credited for saving children, for preserving baseball, and, no exaggeration, for healing a fractured America.

I tried the happy face a final time at Busch Stadium on September 26, Saturday afternoon, as the Cards hosted the Expos with McGwire and Sosa tied at 66 homers. We had our friends' great seats behind home at Busch: me, Laurie, Thomas, 7, and Kate, 3. The stadium was electric in the fourth inning, everyone standing as though for a Series win, when McGwire came up for his second at-bat against Montreal pitcher Dustin Hermanson.

First pitch, McGwire strode and swung. *Crack*! If not looking that instant, I wouldn't have seen the 400-foot laser slash into the left-field stands for his No. 67. *That had to kill somebody*, I thought, then we the capacity crow erupted in cheering, red-clad fans covering the stands. Laurie and Thomas hugged, and I was swept up, teary, joyous again over Big Mac, wallowing more in the hypocrisy.

McGwire stroked his second homer of the day in the seventh, No. 68, and on

Sunday we listened during the drive home to western Missouri, as he bashed two more to end the season with 70. Drugs or no, it was an astounding performance, and I believed Mac's humble quote when he said he amazed even himself.

The culture was ecstatic over McGwire, but I felt schizophrenic, and by Monday morning I was critic again, with a buyer for my commentary titled "Big Mac Steps Up to The Plate; Steroids Awareness Steps Back." My piece was rare in chastising the American hero and culture, and several publications had ignored my submission, but opinion-page editor Rich Hood of the *Kansas City Star* ran it on October 2, with the following lead:

"As St. Louis Cardinals slugger Mark McGwire rewrote home-run records in baseball, much of America saluted him, but the debate over his feats will not disappear.

"It should not."

IX. Baby Boomers Embrace Consumerism, Partying

By the new millennium, America's demographic of Baby Boomer was prime suspect for cultural depravity, in the debate whether rampant personal and institutional irresponsibility was exacting toll on civilization. Anyone could have pointed at me for dereliction of citizenship, this aging Boomer with the common symptoms of financial debt, selfishness in family, narcissistic body consciousness, and aversion to work I refused to tolerate. I also wanted baseless gratification, entertainment, the shindig fueled by alcohol.

Then came time to research and write this book chapter on cultural ethic, its impact on football doping. Extensive study had led me to identify American mores as prime support for the problem in continuum. In previous research and writing, I enjoyed a detachment in the role of third-person analyst of available information, mostly insulated from the problem's molten edges. Always looming, however, was critical analysis of self, my own culpability in football doping. I had worn the mask of virtually every guilty party, athlete to coach, writer, and fan.

In addition, now the country was at war, real conflict, not a damned game with pseudo warriors. National security was at stake, not the pride of some city over its football team. But we still didn't want to know, not about bloody fighting overseas for country, and not about drugs in holy sport.

War had extracted tremendous toll of American soldiers and their loved ones, years into conflict on two fronts, Iraq and Afghanistan, with no end in sight. Many military families felt abandoned by the consumer culture soldiers fought and died for, the 300 million citizens of the self-absorbed USA. "America is not at war. The Marine Corps is at war," stated hard-written scrawl in Iraq, on wall at a U.S. military office in Ramadi.

"America is at the mall."

Indeed the nation's collective conscience was shopping for fulfillment, cheering at the football game, strutting at the gym, singing at church, getting drunk, watching television, idling at the PC. The consumer mind was anywhere but on war, with

September 11 an old rerun, a channel to change every time. The Post-9/11 World did not exist for most Americans.

National security and the plight of U.S. military forces did not fit the general American agenda, or values system, at least not yet. The public priority, and that fragmented into personal sets for millions of individuals, lay removed from war on a ghostly enemy to corner. Practically everyone demonstrated that the pursuit of materialism, gratification, out-ranked thoughtful concern for world chaos.

Critic and author Carolyn Baker observed a nationalistic sense to the consumer ethos. "Individuals in America's sibling society are not bad human beings, nor are they inherently greedy," she wrote, "but they have been enculturated to grow up to be good consumers, which has now become synonymous with good citizenship." Adults were fools about money, averaging a negative balance overall — an American first — by spending in excess of income and accumulating more debt for their shortfall. An AC-Nielsen survey ranked America as No. 1 in the world for citizens who lived paycheck-to-paycheck, despite advantages in employment opportunity, salaries, and benefits.

The modern American adult sensed entitlement to spend, regardless of personal income, leaving critics agape. For Boomers especially, debt was standard "to pay for lifestyles their current incomes can't support," reported Bob Davis, *Wall Street Journal*, who continued:

> They are determined to live better than their parents, seduced by TV shows such as "The O.C." and "Desperate Housewives," which take upper-class life for granted, and bombarded with advertisements for expensive automobiles and big-screen TVs. Financial firms have turned credit for the masses into a huge business, aided by better technology for analyzing credit risks.

Piling debt may have been legal, but a host of observers in myriad issues noted the societal threat. Debt menaced economic stability and threatened national security — foreign investment in U.S. debt and service was enormous, led by the Chinese and Arabs — but it likewise reared ugly on marriages, families. "Overspending is no different than being an alcoholic or drug addict," said Jan Dahlin Geiger, financial planner. "What one person is doing could have a huge negative impact on the couple's finances."

Too many adults just had to be entertained, to consume, worse than children. And marketers knew they wanted lifestyle from their spending, some sense of community. Marketers understood consumers wanted to believe materialism could elevate their existence. Pleasurable diversion was at premium, affordability be damned, and an American majority committed to sport fandom as religion, with football the TV era's favorite call to worship, as expensive to watch as ever.

In Kansas City, for example, many cash-strapped citizens paid extravagant costs for attending NFL games — at publicly owned and funded Arrowhead Stadium. Some, at least, were harming family budgets. "It's crazy," admitted one father, a Chiefs fan paying $88 per end-zone seat, among season-ticket requirements that included full cost for exhibition games. And tickets were just the start of expense for Sundays at

Arrowhead, according to a *Star* analysis headlined "Footing the bill for football."

Besides over-consumption of costly football product, adults followed American tradition to inflict the sport upon their children, undeterred by more than a century's accumulating evidence of dangers. Unwilling boys, as usual, were unfortunate for such parents. "Son Forced Into Football, He's Miserable," read the headline for an advice column. A rational mother had written Ann Landers for help. "He wants to stop playing football," she attested of her 12-year-old, "but every time he mentions it, my husband blows up and calls him a sissy. I'm worn out from trying to get my husband to back off."

In contrast to this concerned woman, many females had grown fanatical as fathers about football. The stereotypical soccer mother aside, Football Mom was a 2000s dynamic, spurring analysts to wonder of broader cultural malaise. "Something deeper seems to be going on today," wrote David S. Awbrey, contributing columnist for *The Star*, "than merely frustrated parents forcing their own dreams onto their children or basking in the reflective fame of trophy-winning offspring. What once were considered merely kids' games have become primary metaphors of modern life."

One observer expressed grave reservations for football culture. Michael Goodwin, *New York Daily News* columnist who played the sport through college, saw crass commercialization and exploitation, at *high-school level*. Goodwin lamented that prep football had gone show-time, televised on ESPN and Fox Sports Net and sold as drama in movies and television. "At the risk of being the skunk at the party, I say the rage is madness…," Goodwin declared. "The seedy glorification is turning a character-building ritual into another disposable commodity. And it is bringing out the worst in some adults."

Americans contributed much to debauchery of sport in their consumer approval for negative consequences such as harm to young people, including their own. Notorious were individuals gone berserk around kid games, even if many fans dared not look. Adult wrongdoing unleashed by so-called youth sports reflected upon the nation in regular headlines. Experts blamed parents and coaches in part for a rise in sport injuries, their pressuring kids to play, and for more indirect influence like character demoralization.

"Adult hooliganism" haunted youth sports, the epitome episode being a hockey dad who beat his son's coach into a coma, as children watched; the victim later died. "With the behavior of so many youth-sports parents spiraling downward, it was only a matter of time before someone was killed," wrote Douglas E. Abrams, a Missouri law professor and youth hockey coach.

For football, consumer values were obvious: Americans wanted thrills from the game, athletic feats juxtaposed with violence, and winning. Anything was acceptable for enhancing the circus, including assaults and drugs, as long as sickening results were not waved at the audience. Fans were "the sports industry's wolf-criers," said David Carter, sports business professor. "They always seem to posture about their displeasure and disgust about athlete behavior and indiscretions, and yet they never materially change their consumption patterns."

The two-headedness was societal psychosis, a projection of blame for massive wrong onto a few individuals. "Sports have emerged as one of the last bastions of morality in American culture," wrote columnist Bob Keisser, *Long Beach Press-Telegram*, continuing:

> Politicians can get re-elected despite previous indiscretions, church priests can cop a plea on child abuse, and CEOs get government protection from bailing on pensions. But if you're a baseball hero and you get caught drinking a steroid cocktail, you're done. That's the opinion at least of those who find it easy to put their morality on others. The issue is anything but that simple.

The issue had spun back onto Mark McGwire, unfortunately for him. He ended up a special icon for doping in America, the fantasy-driven culture that never really wanted to know, becoming the first superstar athlete to fry publicly for artificial augmentation. In an ugly cultural rearing crystallized by McGwire's teary evasion before Congress in 2005, America denounced and defrocked him as hero, culminating in his wholesale rejection by sportswriters voting for the Baseball Hall of Fame. The American majority felt justice was done on McGwire, after evidence and speculation of his doping became so plentiful as to turn everyone's stomach.

Critics decried American hypocrisy on McGwire, the complete waffling of opinion led by media. Hypocrisy folded within the hypocrisy, they charged. While McGwire's former flock skewered him, an NFL superstar and known steroid user, 270-pound linebacker Shawne Merriman, basked in multi-media coverage as his Chargers made the playoffs. Despite Merriman's serving a four-game suspension for nandrolone, which he claimed to have unknowingly ingested, his popularity soared and he made All-Pro.

"That's a double standard," Drew Sharp wrote for the *Detroit Free Press*. "The infiltration of steroids and amphetamines in the NFL merits nothing more condemning than an 'Oh, well' shrug. The mere suspicion of usage in baseball triggers a retaliatory response that could define Hall of Fame voting for the next 10 years." Sharp saw "a viciousness to football the public embraces," in contrast to baseball and its hallowed records. "Football might be America's game, but baseball remains America's treasure," Sharp surmised. "We look at baseball and dream of what we want to be. We look at football and see who we are."

David Fleming, *ESPN The Magazine*, wrote, "[A]s much as we want to think of football as a secular form of religion, no one in this church — not fans, owners or coaches — values character more than conquest."

X. MEETING, APPRECIATING STEVE COURSON

My Ford Taurus climbed the rocky driveway on private property aside a mountain in southwestern Pennsylvania. Large beings emerged from the log cabin ahead to meet me, barking dogs and a man, his arms extending massive from sleeveless shirt. I felt fortunate to be invited.

Two towering black Labradors came to my car door, Rufus and Rachel, brother and sister, wary and sniffing as I opened it. No problem: The 12-year-olds warmed instantly as they smelled and I chattered, picking up scent in the car of my own hounds at home. They recognized me as a dog lover. But while new canine friends impressed me, I was astonished by their man companion, Steve Courson, hanging half out the cabin doorway to eclipse the space. "Matt, how ya doin'?" he sounded in personal introduction, deep voicing barreling across the gravelly yard.

Steve resembled a supreme MMA fighter constructed in rocky blocks and appendages like those arms, bulging in muscle and veins down into wrists and hands. I'd never seen a steroid-free specimen like Steve, who hadn't juiced in 17 years. He was 49, standing 6-2 and weighing 245 with 10 percent body fat, and could bench-press 225 pounds for 40 reps. Hardly any middle-age male could look like this, be as strong.

Steve shook my hand gentlemanly and led with his big head back through the cabin door, into the little kitchen and living room, the Labs and I following. Steve was a widower, with Rufus and Rachel his bosom family, and the dogs had their own couch sections for stretching out. I'd heard Steve spent seven grand for leg surgery on Rufus, money he didn't have.

Sitting down at the square kitchen table, Steve and I were already connecting, having never met but conversing immediately. Our mutual friend Dr. Charles E. "Chuck" Yesalis had predicted our compatibility in bringing us together. And the dogs sensed it. As Steve silenced ESPN-TV with remote, I took the chair with Rufus directly behind me on his sofa. But the big male wouldn't ease down; he sat head up, staring into my back and wanting to nose it, whining slightly. Steve's eyes widened. "I think Rufus wants you to acknowledge him," he said. "He's never done that with anybody."

Honored, I turned to stroke Rufus and chatter good dog talk, and he laid his chin down, content. That moment, I ingratiated myself to Steve Courson. He, of course, had done that for me long ago, speaking out against football doping.

Steve and I sealed our friendship that afternoon, March 7, 2005, through four hours of animated conversation and uproarious laughter, even a few my tears, discussing the impact of football doping on our lives and people we cared about. Steve had played nine years in the NFL while I not an official snap in college, but we shared rich commonalities, particularly for our value responses to the game and doping.

Each of us began a reluctant steroid user in college who eventually accepted the long fight for prevention, despite dim prospects, taking paths in the issue so similar that intersection was practically inevitable. Traversing separate but parallel routes, we'd arrived at the same sobering place, or highly unpopular conclusion: Football was beyond help and blame in itself.

We'd both spent our time searching out the pillars of this thing, muscle doping in American football, dusting away obscurity to connect all culprit parties, not only athletes and organizers, coaches, but also the partner sport media and demanding consumer base, fans. Football was the nation's favorite toy for gratification at whatever price, even harm to our young. Steve and I wished it were simple enough to blame just one group, isolate how to turn back the problem. Impossible, for the complete culture served as enabler. Football doping was just a canary in the coalmine for the American ethos, a much larger issue.

From there forward Steve and I spoke several times weekly by telephone, often daily, between Pennsylvania and Missouri. Our value systems were framed in teachings of religious family backgrounds, although we both no longer attended church, and honesty was paramount for living and serving a democratic America. Lying was no gray area for either of us, just abhorrent and rather apparent when practiced, but we tried to keep sense of humor for the denial. Sammy Sosa at Congress, for example, was classic comedy for us.

Generally, we attacked denial of muscle doping in sport, especially for the young people at stake. In fact, the historically repeating consequences for children and young adults keyed motivation for Steve and I. We wanted to aid fellow players, past, present and future, although I was by now discarding the "role modeling" argument for my persuasion. Steve wasn't. Most adults couldn't care less about ramifications of sport doping for kids, and I couldn't persuade them, but Steve was masterful in the point. He'd vested thousands of hours in study and practice, including speeches and sessions with children across America, mostly on his own dime. No one wanted to disregard or debate the modeling effect with Steve, unless seeking to be corrected or humiliated.

Steve and I gravitated to fairytale sorts of heroes real and mythical, but with the modern twist of anti-heroism. Heroic figures we found in literature, news, and everyday life. We weren't dazzled by celebrity but typically suspicious of it, and looked only for genuine people who sold us on reality, like our mutual friend Chuck Yesalis, whom we admired and trusted.

We both believed we had suffered health problems linked to past lifestyle in football, the injuries, performance drugs, and partying. We had each worked hard in recent years to reclaim a healthy physique, craving again physical fitness for living well, our trusted identity renewal since boyhood.

Material acquisitions we largely shunned, by choice and necessity. Economic conservation was the long-time rule for both of us, particularly as vocal critics of SportsWorld and its inherent dangers for youth. For directly opposing the football institution and its tentacles of power, Steve and I sacrificed financially and took down loved ones with us. We refused to acknowledge society's catch-all apology for football ills: *That's just the way it is.*

To protest wrongs, our patriotic right, Steve and I both lost employment opportunity and more. Speaking honestly, we incurred the wrath of organizations, media, and fans who propped up the football spiral of denial. Steve's price included blackballing to end his NFL career while my livelihood had been adversely affected in journalism, teaching, and God knows what else — most daggers came in the back, such as influential phone callers to my employers. In condemning football ills, I gained enemies I usually couldn't see, only feel.

Yet Steve and I still held fast to football, wanting the best for the game and kids who played. Football was our most powerful experience outside family, highly fundamental in each of our beings. We still loved the sport, although we wouldn't wish it on anyone unwilling. In addition, we assumed a technical role in the denial of doping, by refusing to reveal anyone beside ourselves, including names we could've dropped for lucrative investigations or books. In fairness, we knew the game historically was rife with steroids, growth hormone, and no individuals or teams deserved singling out as *the* problem. "The same cultural mentality exists: Punish the transgressing athlete for responding to his competitive environment," Steve said. "But only if he is dumb enough to get caught or honest enough to be truthful."

We may not have exposed anyone, but we *talked* about users and dirty teams, a favorite pastime for Steve in private. He was disappointed with former teammates and opponents who remained silent, and resentful of those lying in public, downplaying the scourge. "Anyone who can think knows that players are bio-chemical machines, basically killer drones," he said. "I knew back in '82 and '83, when I really started getting into anabolics, that I was a lethal machine at that point, with my parameters of size and speed. On or off the field I could really hurt somebody, and that scared even me. ...

"Now the parameters of size, strength and speed have taken *another* leap. And what other way do we have to explain this? In other words, the evidence is obvious, but there are sycophants and administrators of the sport who still want to use the term 'isolated.' It's the old code, man. It's the conspiracy of silence, the code of dishonor."

Some evasive ex-players remained friends with Steve while making rewarding careers in association with the NFL. One former lineman, wealthy and powerful from football, had always denied his steroid use and the game's epidemic. Steve knew old dopers who now coached, taught school, worked in media, without speaking out. Some wore Christianity on their sleeve, speaking to churches as football heroes without revealing their chemical aid. "Some of my best buddies I'm having a little conflict with. Two of 'em," Steve said. "They're basically sports propagandists, former players. They've become football propagandists, but I am football reality. So we have a problem."

Steve watched former players on television, Jockocrats, who lied and covered for the NFL, including a 40-something retiree rumored to use HGH for cosmetic purpose. "These people are pathetic," Steve said. "They're in the club, you know. They're yes men."

Merril Hoge, ESPN analyst and former Pittsburgh running back, angered Steve on March 25, 2005, when each appeared on the network to address fresh doping allegations surrounding the Steelers teams of Hall of Fame coach Chuck Noll. Former linebacker Jim Haslett had confessed his own steroid use and accused Noll's Steelers of pioneering muscle doping in the league. The recollection contained inaccuracies, but Steve supported Haslett and commended him on ESPN's "Cold Pizza" show.

Hoge followed Steve on camera from a separate hook up, but he disparaged Haslett and vouched for Noll as an anti-steroid crusader. Steve and I talked afterward. "Merril was basically giving the company line, going through how Chuck Noll was always against this, and I'm biting my tongue," Steve said. "I'm thinking: 'Yeah, Merril, but why in 1989, when you were in Pittsburgh, did the Steelers draft Tom Ricketts and Craig Veasey, who had tested positive for steroids, in the first and third rounds? And [there was] Terry Long, who tried to commit suicide after he tested positive. Chuck Noll never knew anything about this, huh? If Chuck Noll were so much against this, then why were all the guys who were taking juice on the field, playing? Why weren't they sitting on the fucking bench? Gimme a break, you can't be that stupid.'

"The lying is just so pathetic, and now it's being shown for how pathetic it really is... The hypocrisy is obviously driven by money."

Courson Renews Faith For Reform in Football Doping

Steve Courson was optimistic in spring 2005, about his life but particularly for anticipating impact change in American football. He saw public maneuvering still ahead, but muscle doping could be controlled at last, the cause he had championed as, Yesalis said, the "point on the spear." The struggle had become Steve Courson, consumed him, almost killed him, but he really saw positive signs. "The boat is turning!" he declared repeatedly, on every news event remotely lending support, his bearish laugh booming. And this year would be Steve's last, unbeknownst to any of us.

Steve was positive Congress would get it right this time, by default at least. Lawmakers would investigate sport doping, determine facts and bring pressure to bear upon pro football, like their political screws already pinching baseball. The resultant cleanup would wash down into the college and prep ranks, Steve figured. He even held faith the NFL could own up to the drug problem and go forward with firm prevention.

We disagreed there. "Football doesn't want that yet, and no time soon," I told Steve, within minutes of our first conversation. My historical research demonstrated politicians were paralyzed to act rightfully, functionally incapable, given their cronies, lobbies, and constituent football fans to appease.

The diplomat, Steve technically agreed before his "but" phase of response. "Let's say, worst-case scenario," he posed, "that the owners and coaches in football just went out of their way to misrepresent the facts to the public, to present fairyland to the people. What are they really guilty of doing here? Giving the public what they'd rather hear anyway.... Don't we prefer the romantic image? Label this as deception, but aren't sports federations and sports media giving us what we'd rather hear?

"That's the way I'm approaching it."

I understood what Steve was saying, or doing. He no longer carried a scorched-earth policy against football organizations, which he correctly deduced were unable to change anything on their own. His updated rhetoric focused on *society* as responsible for remedy, and I agreed in principle. Besides, Steve had gone through hell in personal ramming with the NFL, including his court defeat of the latter 1990s, and now sought amends. The NFL was a fraternity like no other on earth, and Steve wanted back in on some level. I figured he deserved renewed membership, with all the goddamned money floating around.

I'd been around his patch of mountain property, beautiful but humble amid the Laurel Highlands, Allegheny Range. Steve's debt and expenses still outweighed income, especially since he'd given up $18,000 annually in NFL disability by reversing his heart disease through nutrition and conditioning — and pride for doing the right thing. Steve willfully ended aid when most old footballers wouldn't think of it.

Moreover, I was positive in our friendship that Steve wanted re-association with pro football *only* if impact change occurred in doping. He wanted inside footing again foremost to battle drugs, all types, from steroids and HGH to painkillers and speed. His motivation wasn't to enjoy the old boys again, nor money. We didn't quibble on the small stuff, like predicting when that boat really would point in new direction. There was too much to do, working and learning together and always leaning on Chuck in the collaboration.

Steve became more inspired of congressional involvement as March wore on, and we both relished the action of regular doping news. The *San Francisco Chronicle* and *New York Daily News* led media in breaking open baseball through BALCO, exposing names like Barry Bonds, Gary Sheffield, and Jason Giambi, while Jose Canseco's book was a sensation for direct allegations against McGwire, Rafael Palmeiro, and Ivan Rodriguez. In football, BALCO and the Dr. Shortt scandal involving Carolina Panthers players rattled the NFL, while in college an anonymous player told lawmakers of widespread doping in the NCAA, now suffering a few scandals itself, though quietly in media.

Canseco, McGwire, Palmeiro, and Sosa were summoned for testimony on Capitol Hill, among baseball figures like commissioner Bud Selig, and Steve really got fired up. He couldn't fathom anyone's missing major facts anymore. "The thing that puts everyone in a difficult corner, BALCO has really, really turned the tables on this. It's exposed the frailty of drug testing… designer steroids and growth hormone. So the public knows, if you've got any brains whatsoever."

Reckoning was at hand, Steve believed. "In other words, we're trying through chemistry to create super humans, and we've achieved that. But we've achieved it at the level that's starting to scare even ourselves." Politicians had vested self-interest in protecting children, Steve reasoned, because their very own interests were at stake too. "I'm going to watch this baseball hearing with extreme fascination," he said, "because the questions that are asked here and the way they're answered, are going to play a big role in the future of doping. Not just in this country, but the world."

I thought Steve put too much stock in the American governmental process, especially by the House Oversight and Government Reform Committee, which I tagged the "Government Deform Committee." But we tuned in that morning, Steve, Chuck and I, as committee members made face time on national TV, supposedly grilling baseball suspects for steroids.

Chuck and I didn't come away impressed, but Steve saw a tectonic shift in the big picture. "This has now definitely become a social issue," Steve said excitedly in a phone message. "Congress has made it one, because they've done what they've always needed to do, to galvanize, to bring us to this point with the media… when the boat turns in the water.

"Because it's basically now about the kids, which is what it always should've been about. It's heavy, brother."

Faith Denied: Courson Duped For Last Time by Football America

For a final time, Steve Courson felt let down by Football America. Once again he'd trusted the game, government and fans to acknowledge muscle doping and support real reform. But nothing really happened, again. It was same problem with same outcome, inept testing as "solution," a 1980s redux playing out in 2005, with no one of power standing up to address reality.

Steve and I were friends for eight months, had yakked hundreds of hours over the phone, but he sounded different the night of November 1. The dude loved to talk on phone, but Steve seemed tired upon my reaching him at his mother's house in Gettysburg. It was late, past 11 o'clock Eastern when we hooked up for a scheduled interview, and Steve had every reason for weariness.

He'd been on the road in rainy weather all day, speaking with teens, of course, driving his camouflage Jeep to three different schools in central Pennsylvania. He'd also managed stops for a gym workout and a mall walk before landing at his old home to see his mother, Elizabeth Courson, the retired nurse. Steve's father, Iber Courson, was deceased and his brother, Bruce, lived with his family in Massachusetts. Steve's 50th birthday was exactly one month earlier.

Steve was worn out but also hanging was his perpetual issue, drugs in football, where he had come to accept defeat once again. The fact was apparent nothing was changing in doping for football or any sport. Once again he had expected a lot from society only to see disregard, ignorance and apathy. Now he denounced the NFL, again, adding his shame of former Steelers teammates and opponents, middle-aged men who still could not admit their juicing decades ago.

Politicians disgusted Steve, their dog-and-pony shows on doping, and he admitted being "duped" again, like 17 years before. He had gone back to Washington for them, agreeing to testify in their April 2005 hearing on the NFL and performance-enhancing substances, a sorry episode amounting to bootlicking of Paul Tagliabue and Gene Upshaw, symbols of pro football. "Yeah," Steve said, mockingly. "The politicans were saying all the great stuff about what they needed to do for kids, you know. They were saying all the right things." He laughed short then paused. "When I went back [to Congress], I kind of already knew what I was walking into. I was optimistic, though."

"They got us all again," I volunteered.

"Yep. They got us."

But it was time to move forward, keep learning and fighting, as far as Steve was concerned. He was ever-willing on the issue while prospects were brightening in his life: increasing speaking engagements, a fitness-consulting business in percolation, a new book in progress, and a woman he admired and loved, Denise Masciola, girlfriend of three years and retired naval officer. "Twenty years in the Navy!" Steve frequently reminded, discussing "DeeDee." The doping challenge wasn't going anywhere, so Steve wasn't budging, with growing stability at home and more fellow believers at large. "The lie's gotten bigger, that's all," he said. "There are more people out there who know what time it is."

Public enlightenment had always been the realistic quest, and Steve helped carry that spear again, the past year, by dropping his media stonewall to reemerge nationally. He'd written commentaries, provided insight and quotes for constant articles, and appeared on network radio and television. Like olden days, he and Yesalis stood shoulder-to-shoulder on the front line. "Chuck's mission, I know, and the part of my mission that's personal to me, is to shine the light under the rock," Steve said. "You may not be able to change things, but at least people will acknowledge what they're watching and quit kidding themselves.

"I've been in drug education a long time, and I've dealt with addiction myself, so I understand this: When you deal with any addiction, whether it's individual or societal, until you overcome denial you have no chance in fixing the problem."

"Yep," I said.

"In other words, we're still in denial *although* we're getting better."

Steve and I spoke and e-mailed frequently those early days of November. He assisted for my book chapter involving the 1989 Senate hearings and his personal trials of the period, and I helped with his growing manuscript. We discussed the NFL and saw a wreck looming over liabilities such as increasing player sizes and concussions — the Mike Webster estate, family of his late friend, was nearing an historic court victory over the players union. Steve speculated gene doping would infest football, resulting in a rash of health maladies for athletes 400 pounds and higher. In response we continued formulating our own prevention plan for capping sizes of players in concert with other safeguards.

Thursday morning, November 10, my cell phone rang in the basement office. I knew it was Steve but didn't answer immediately because, coincidentally, I was trying to fix word transition into a book passage about him. I called him back in a half-hour, noon Eastern, and his phone rang and rang. My finger poised to end the call when he answered, breathing heavily like he'd run from outside, and our typical spirited conversation ensued. We discussed new information, studies, revelations and gossip, punctuating points with curses and laughter.

He had some stuff he'd just heard from Chuck regarding our pet scrutiny of the genetic wonder theory or myth, at heart of excuses for football's increasing sizes. We noted the Roman Circus Maximus as artifact symbol of today's multi-media football, a topic Steve savored that, in turn, referenced Oriard's brilliant analysis of The Spectacle, discussed again, raved over.

We bitched about censorship of our points in media interviews, including recent cases involving Steve. Reports and commentaries typically ignored specific, fact-based allegations from us while privileging the far-fetched comments from football players and administrators. Steve was derisive toward a former defensive lineman a few years removed as Super Bowl champion, now making media rounds claiming he'd lost 70 pounds of mostly muscle by simply dieting. "Yeah, bullshit," Steve grumbled, and I laughed.

I had to end the call after about 25 minutes, abruptly telling Steve I had errands to run on campus, where I taught classes part-time, and a workout to make.

"You gotta do what you gotta do, man," Steve said, yawning. "I've got to go outside and cut some wood."

Off we went for another five minutes talking wood, the cutting, chopping and burning for heat, our mutual and necessary hobby of wintertime. I rattled about my only "perk," the fireplace downstairs, stoked with flame to wipe out the bone-chilling humidity of my basement. "One of my favorite workouts is just bustin' blocks out back," I said. "I use the maul and bust the shit out of 'em."

Steve said he had some blocks to cut from a tree just uphill from his backdoor. "I've got a new chainsaw, Chainsaw," he joked. "My mom gave it to me for my birthday."

No more talking, however. I insisted I had to go.

"All right," Steve said, slight disappointment. "I'll get back in touch tomorrow or the next day."

We hung up.

Within minutes Steve was 100 yards above his house, in a clearing he was fashioning on a little uneven plane, revving his new chainsaw. Rufus was at his side, naturally, as he sized up a standing dead trunk, limbless, 44-foot tall with 5-foot circumference. A friend experienced in dropping trees was en route to help, but Steve wasn't waiting.

Woodcutting, especially felling trees, ranked as America's most dangerous job, wounding and killing professionals in slaughter fashion. *Loggers deal with tremendous weights when they fell trees and it's not always possible to know exactly where a tree will fall or when*, noted a contemporary news report. *Too, they often work on steep hillsides, in poor weather, and in a hurry.*

People would wonder if Steve understood the danger, especially having Rufus tag along, as though on another hike together over the mountain.

Steve swung the whirring blade, swiping into the tree trunk, severing almost through. Then perhaps the wind shifted, investigators later theorized. I'd always wonder about timing of the moments, circumstances, had I talked longer on the phone with Steve, rather than hurrying off to campus.

The dead tree "kicked back" on Steve and Rufus, falling on them instead of away, 180 degrees opposite as planned, surprising the giant man and dog. They broke for their lives.

Around the hill, a neighbor heard Steve's chainsaw suddenly grind out, quiet, and he rushed to the scene. He found Steve pinned facedown, dying, crushed across the upper back by middle of the tree trunk atop him. Rufus was under Steve's legs, injured but alive, wailing in pain of his dislocated hip but more so, I later liked to think, of his lost companion. Investigators would theorize Steve died in saving Rufus, that he shoved the male Lab out of mortal danger.

News of Steve's fatal accident broke from Pittsburgh media barely 30 minutes after he and I hung up the phone, about as long as our conversation lasted, and reports quickly went national. Throughout America, friends and relatives reacted in sorrowful disbelief: Steve, gone now, after overcoming so much? In Pittsburgh, Steve's girlfriend Denise was shocked to get word from a friend at work. In Missouri, I was informed through e-mail, a news report forwarded by an acquaintance.

In State College, phones were ringing at the home, office, and cellular of Dr. Yesalis. A Pittsburgh reporter provided the detail about Rufus, and Chuck, grieving, could grasp what happened. He'd wondered how that tree killed Steve, so cat-quick and alert, but now he understood. "Those dogs were his pals," Chuck attested. "Hearing the news was like a 500-pound weight hitting me in the stomach. It breaks my heart. [Steve] was one of the most caring, honest, ethical people I've met in my 59 years."

The reporter, Robert Dvorchak, *Post-Gazette* veteran, knew and appreciated both Steve and Chuck. He listened patiently as Chuck tried to explain feelings such as his regret for Steve's hardship, dreams never realized. "He was black-balled by the NFL for speaking out about steroids," Chuck said. "And the only thing that really stuck in his craw — and you can quote me on this — was that he was still very disappointed in his teammates for not talking about the truth about steroids.

"He told the truth all along. He was a man of honesty and integrity in a game that lacks it. I just lost one hell of a friend."

XI. Searching For Heroes, Finding One

As a 1960s youth who loved movies at the theatre, Saturday afternoon matinees, I found a heroic model in the boy Charlie of *Willy Wonka and the Chocolate Factory*. In a climatic scene, Charlie spurned ill-gotten gain by returning the "stolen" Everlasting Gobstopper. I wept in admiration, inspiration. As adult writer, it was no coincidence I focused on human beings of virtue, people famous or obscure who stood tall in character. I always sought heroes, gems among mortals.

I wasn't much interested in material achievements, especially by athletes, not if the package lacked humanism. As a former jock and coach, I understood the selfish star was about exceptional as a rock. American sport harbored endless people with no regard for honesty, fairness, charity, but they were gods through mere statistics for public legend. In sport's higher levels, competitiveness required of victory assured a landscape of heartless small characters. And society worshipped on.

Steve Courson caught my attention 20 years before we met, 1985, for his exposé in *Sports Illustrated* of steroids' permeating pro and college football. His courage stirred me, having left the game myself in part for muscle drugs impossible to avoid. I presumed at the time hundreds of thousands of guys were similarly exposed, minimally, and we'd hear more demand for change. I knew one thing: Everyone was aware in football.

Reinforcements didn't materialize, however. Rare few emerged to cover Steve's back, speak whole and informed truth, and the enemy's return fire smoked him. He took patriotic action and got smacked for it, by heavy hands bent on burying football's drug epidemic. Ex-teammates with gall led the stoning, smearing Steve while hiding their abuse of steroids, amphetamines, or, typically, both — and knowing he still wouldn't sell them out.

Columnist Mary Sanchez, *Kansas City Star*, captured the essence of the earnest people required of a civilization to stand, in her piece titled "Real Men Value Truth

And Do The Right Thing." Sanchez lamented whistleblowers were rare in competitive environs like athletics, governed strictly by powerbrokers who steamrolled the dissenter. "People who break from the masses, who question authority or the decisions of others, are often those lower in stature and rank," she wrote. "Rank and titles are often gained because you know how to follow the rules, written and unwritten. But true leaders are willing to stand up for ethical behavior, even when it would be easier to look the other way."

Once Steve defied football's unwritten rules, his life was hard. Always easy, however, was Steve's striking impression on people he met, and upon many people he didn't, for honesty grounded in thoughtful reasoning, informed intellect. And those he affected ran America's rich gamut of individuals, everyday folk to the most powerful brokers of influence. Steve was unmistakable for his humanity and honor.

Steve was asked to appear before Congress a second time on April 27, 2005, the NFL hearing staged by the House Committee on Government Reform. That morning he slept a few hours in his Jeep at a Virginia rest stop, because he couldn't afford a D.C. hotel room. He woke before daybreak and visited the men's room, where he washed, shaved, brushed teeth, and dressed up A few hours later on Capitol Hill, Steve wore the only suit he had left, an old double-breasted gray tweed from the 1980s, now oversized with torn pocket on one lapel — details that didn't escape investigative reporter T.J. Quinn, *New York Daily News*, who thought the outfit kind of sad.

Then Steve, Quinn would recount, "spoke to members of Congress with a combination of knowledge and perspective that almost no one else before them had shown."

Steve shone before the nation that day, according to the gathered media who reflected journalism's best on sport doping. These reporters understood most of what they heard was spin, misrepresentation, lies, whether from scientists of self-serving agenda or historically evasive officials of American football. Steve impressed them, however, especially his opening statement.

"Integrity fit Courson like a new suit," *The News* headlined over the eulogistic commentary of Quinn, November 13, 2005, who wrote:

> Steve Courson did not need to be defined by his NFL uniform, which he wore proudly for the Pittsburgh Steelers. He didn't need the 295 pounds of artificially built muscle that nearly destroyed his heart. At the age of 50, [testifying before Congress,] he was that most uncommon of men who was more than his most famous moment.

Quinn had also trekked to meet Courson in person during 2005, and I knew the journalist clearly grasped muscle doping in football because he understood Steve, particularly on the mishandling of youth. Quinn concluded:

> When we talked steroids, about the work he has done speaking to high school groups around the United States, he spoke with more respect for young people than most of the experts I've interviewed. "You can't lie to them," he said. "They'll know it. Any group I talk

> to I start by saying, 'Steroids work. They will make you bigger and stronger and faster and you'll feel great.' And then I tell them about the dangers."
>
> He knew the kids would find out for themselves about steroids, and he could teach them more by being straight with them than by scaring them. He knew life was more than a sharp suit, that an honest heart and the truth of his words were all that mattered.

Children gravitated to Steve. At the Head Start near his home in Fayette County, Pennsylvania, Steve taught proper nutrition to tots. "I would like to share with you a side of Steve that most people never had the opportunity to see," recalled Colette Sandzimier, facility director, for memoriam postings on the *Post-Gazette* Web site. "[Picture] Steve Courson, Super Bowl Champion, leading a preschool classroom — he was the 'Kindergarten Cop.' The minute he set foot in the room, the children looked at him in awe, their eyes big as donuts. But they quickly adapted to his large stature and deep voice. The Head Start children *loved* 'Mr. Steve,' and Mr. Steve loved the children.

"Thank you, Steve, for sharing your life with us."

The man touched people of every age, evident with the outpouring of testimonials and dedications in his wake, summarized in November 2006 by girlfriend Denise Masciola. "Steve received much deserved recognition over the past year," she wrote, noting the following: the establishment of a memorial walk at the Uniontown Mall, where seniors remembered Steve's joining and imploring them on circuits for healthy cardiovascular exercise; the naming of a children's exercise room for him at the Head Start, The Steve Courson Activity Zone; the renaming of the county Humane Society in his honor, for his love of animals, especially Rufus, Rachal and Kitty; and recognition by the American Heart Association, for his beating heart disease and obesity to regain phenomenal fitness.

"Not a day goes by that I do not think of Steve," Denise wrote. "I will cherish all the memories we shared together. I thank God for the three years He blessed me with Steve."

After Steve died, Denise and others close to him had difficulty with the question of why, including me. Denise found a book in Steve's cabin while clearing his belongings for a property auction, titled *When God Doesn't Make Sense*, by James Dobson. It helped although her grief remained sharp. Occasionally, friends managed to coax her out for dinner, a few drinks, but her heart and mind weren't in the experience. "I keep looking for Steve," she told me over the phone. "There is no Steve out there." I empathized, searching for another friend and colleague just like him, but there, too, he could never be again.

Steve stood up in defense of endangered athletes for 20 years, the vast majority of whom never thanked him. Many of his incredible acts were documented but many more unknown, and I witnessed an example during his final August.

Pro football called on Steve again, extending rather open arms, but the catch remained: Loyalty to League Required. A former teammate and another NFL official contacted Steve, basically offering passage back into the club. Steve would make top money by ostensibly working as an anti-doping counselor, with his first stop Carolina, the franchise reeling amid exposure of Dr. Shortt, steroids, growth hormone.

Steve discussed the offer with friends, eliciting feedback, and was obviously concerned about Chuck and me, what we thought. My interpretation was different than the league's pitch. I believed the NFL merely wanted his name to endorse its so-called steroid prevention, a signature gloss for the public facade of effectiveness. All Steve had to do was go along now, cease criticizing the league as cunning opponent, and financial security was assured. And Chuck saw it same way.

Neither of us, however, tried to dissuade Steve from his primo opportunity. In fact, we urged him to consider accepting it. "Take the money and run, bro," I said. "You've gone beyond the call in this issue. Now you deserve peace, security." Chuck concurred, telling him: "You live in a fuckin' cabin, Steve. You've done everything. You've been beaten up over this. Just take their fuckin' money."

I just wanted more bucks for Steve than they were offering. He was a PR fortune for the NFL, even if kept in a tower. "You call Taglibue himself to accept," I said. "Tell him your price is $5 million over five years. They've got the cash." Steve still wasn't keen on selling his soul. So, without his asking, I promised the episode was off-record with me: If he worked for the NFL, there would be no criticism from my end.

"All right, man, thanks," he said. "I'll think about it."

Next day, Steve called back the league and declined.

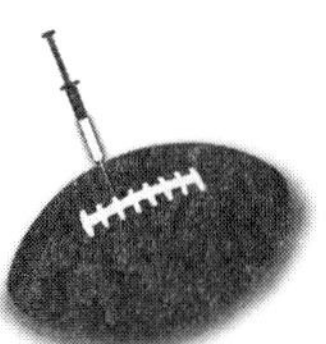

REFERENCES

1983 Roster. (1983). *Southeast Missouri State vs. Northwest Missouri State*, p. 27. Cape Girardeau: Southeast Missouri State University.

1984 Roster. (1984). *Southeast Missouri State University Football*, pp. 38-39. Cape Girardeau: Southeast Missouri State University.

Abrams, D.E. (2000, August 12). Adult hooliganism hurts youth sports. *Kansas City Star*, p. B6.

Against Cheats. (2006, September 30). Shopping around against cheats. *Kansas City Star*, p. B2.

Albach, B. (2005, October 30). An itinerary of nonstop scandals. *Kansas City Star*, p. A5.

Alexander, B. (2006, July 9). A drug's promise (or not) of youth. *Los Angeles Times* [Online].

Angier, N. (1990, July 5). Human growth hormone reverses effects of aging. *New York Times*, p. A1.

Angier, N. (1990, July 6). Growth hormone and the drive for a more youthful state. *New York Times*, p. A9.

Angier, N. (1992, May 20). A male menopause? Jury is still out. *New York Times* [Online].

Armstrong, J. (2007, April 15). Game of deception. *Denver Post* [Online].

Assael, S. (2007). *Steroid nation**. New York, NY: ESPN Books.

Awbrey, D.S. (2000, July 24). The games are meant to be fun. *Kansas City Star*, p. B5.

Bahrke, M.S., & Yesalis, C.E. (Eds.). (2002). *Performance-enhancing substances in sport and exercise*. Champaign, IL: Human Kinetics.

Baker, C. (2007, April 4). Creating a culture of cheerfulness as Rome burns. *Online Journal* [Online].

Balz, D. (2005, August 19). Taft admits ethics violations. *Washington Post*, p. A6.

Barker, J. (2005, November 16). Taking it to his grave. *Baltimore Sun* [Online].

Bavley, A., & Rock, S. (1998, August 29). McGwire's pills. *Kansas City Star*, p. A1.

Benesh, P. (2007, June 11). He's the genius of Genentech. *Investor's Business Daily* [Online].

Berecky, M. (2005, November 11). Courson died trying to save dog. *KDKA-TV*.

Biesk, J. (2006, December 16). Stumbo may face ethics conflict in gubernatorial race. *Associated Press* [Online].

Blakeslee, S. (1987, February 10). Supply of growth hormone brings hope for new uses. *New York Times*, p. C1.

Bridis, T. (2006, September 16). Ohio's Ney admits guilt. *Kansas City Star*, p. A2.

Brown, D. (2007, February 19). Finding our fighters. *Kansas City Star*, p. A1.

Burwell, B., & Maracek, J. (2003, July 23). Beyond ball. *KFNS Radio*, St. Louis.

Campbell, M. (2004, December 23). Freed inmate savors new life. *Kansas City Star*, p. A1.

Canseco, J. (2005). *Juiced.* ReganBooks: Los Angeles, CA.

Chaney Injured. (1982, October 28). Chaney Injured at SEMO. *De Soto Republic*, p. 2.

Chaney, L. (1982, January 11). Postal correspondence to author.
Chaney, L. (1982, February 19). Postal correspondence to author.
Chaney, L. (1984, January 1). Postal correspondence to author.
Chaney, M. (1978, September). Football is stimulated aggression. *Non-published composition.*
Chaney, M. (1984, February). Battle of a wounded knee. *Capaha Arrow.*
Chaney, M. (1984, September 11). An Indian uprising is no myth. *Non-published commentary.*
Chaney, M. (1984, September 17). Postal correspondence to Wilma Githens.
Chaney, M. (1984, October). Losing is real. *Non-published composition.*
Chaney, M. (1998, October 2). Big Mac steps up to the plate; steroids awareness steps back. *Kansas City Star*, p. C7.
Chaney, M. (2005, November 11-16). Road notes. *Non-published.*
Christie, L. (2005, September 23). America's most dangerous jobs. *CNN/Money* [Online].
Chu, K. (2006, April 28). Many marriages today are 'til debt do us part. *USA Today*, p. 1A.
Coach Brawl. (2006, October 22). Youth coach charged after brawl. *Kansas City Star*, p. C2.
Coach Charged. (2000, July 13). Coach is charged with punching umpire. *Kansas City Star*, p. A1.
Coach Sentenced. (2006, October 13). Coach sentenced for beanball. *Kansas City Star*, p. D2.
Coach Shot. (2005, November 27). Texas coach shot by parent pulls himself, team into recovery. *Kansas City Star*, p. C2.
Cohen, R. (2007, January 5). Be honest with fiancée. *Kansas City Star*, p. E12.
Corbett, J. (2005, November 16). On to next hurdle for Manning's Colts. *USA Today* [Online].
Courson, S. (2005, March 7). Interview with author, Farmington, PA.
Courson, S. (2005, March 16). Performance-enhancing drugs are not restricted to sports. *Pittsburgh Post-Gazette* [Online].
Courson, S. (2005, March 16). Telephone interview with author.
Courson, S. (2005, March 19). Telephone message to author.
Courson, S. (2005, March 20). Telephone interview with author.
Courson, S. (2005, March 27). Telephone interview with author.
Courson, S. (2005, April 3). Telephone interview with author.
Courson, S. (2005, April 7). Telephone interview with author.
Courson, S. (2005, May 1). Telephone interview with author.
Courson, S. (2005, May 8). Telephone interview with author.
Courson, S. (2005, May 11). Telephone interview with author.
Courson, S. (2005, May 12). E-mail correspondence to author.
Courson, S. (2005, May 18). E-mail correspondence to author.
Courson, S. (2005, May 23). Telephone interview with author.
Courson, S. (2005, May 26). Telephone interview with author.
Courson, S. (2005, May 30). E-mail correspondence to author.

Courson, S. (2005, June, date unrecorded). Telephone comments to author.

Courson, S. (2005, June 5). E-mail correspondence to author.

Courson, S. (2005, June 7). Telephone interview with author.

Courson, S. (2005, June 26). Telephone interview with author.

Courson, S. (2005, June 30). Telephone interview with author.

Courson, S. (2005, July 20). E-mail correspondence to author.

Courson, S. (2005, July 20). Draft correspondence to former teammate, non-forwarded. [Word file last revised on date].

Courson, S. (2005, August 18). E-mail correspondence to author.

Courson, S. (2005, August 24). E-mail correspondence to author.

Courson, S. (2005, October 2). E-mail correspondence to author.

Courson, S. (2005, November 1). Telephone interview with author.

Courson, Stephen. (2005, November 12). Courson, Stephen P. *Pittsburgh Post-Gazette* [Online].

Crumm, D. (2005, January 30). Scholar insists that a 'culture war' doesn't really exist. *Kansas City Star*, p. A4.

Cupples, T.E. (1982, October 26). Matthew L. Chaney, knee X-ray. *Southeast Missouri Hospital.*

Davis, B. (2005, May 22). Price tag gets higher for living on credit. *Kansas City Star*, p. A1.

Daum, M. (2006, August 8). Bigger breasts, more testosterone. *Los Angeles Times* [Online].

Detwiler, J. (2007, April 18). Effortless perfection my butt. *Duke Chronicle* [Online].

Dvorchak, R. (2005, November 10). Ex-Steeler Steve Courson killed by falling tree. *Pittsburgh Post-Gazette* [Online].

Dvorchak, R., & Lash, C. (2005, November 11). Ex-Steeler Courson dies. *Pittsburgh Post-Gazette* [Online].

Eberhart, J.M. (2006, January 22). In truth, the facts don't seem to matter anymore. *Kansas City Star*, p. G7.

Edington, T. (1976, November 4). Postal correspondence to author.

Edington, T. (1976, November 19). Postal correspondence to author.

Epilepsy Facts. (1967 circa). *Facts about epilepsy and the many groups concerned with its medical and social management.* Washington, DC: Epilepsy Foundation of America.

Epstein, E., & Marinucci, C. (2006, March 3). Governor's ties to fitness lobbying group weigh heavy. *San Francisco Chronicle* [Online].

Etc. (1998, June 25). Youth hockey coach banned for punching teenager. *Kansas City Star*, p. D2.

Ex-governor Admits. (2004, December 24). Ex-governor admits trading clout for gifts. *Kansas City Star*, p. A2.

Ex-Governor Going. (2005, March 20). Ex-governor going to prison. *Kansas City Star*, p. A6.

Fans Brawl. (2006, December 17). Fans brawl at prep hoops game. *Kansas City Star*, p. C3.

Farrey, T. (2006, September 11). The guru of growth. *ESPN The Magazine*, p. 159

Finder, C. (2005, November 16). Courson's legacy is change. *Pittsburgh Post-Gazette* [Online].

Fleming, D. (2007, January 1). Character may not count with Bengals. *ESPN The Magazine* [Online].

Foley Resigns. (2006, September 30). Florida's Foley resigns. *Kansas City Star*, p. A6.

Football, MIAA. (1982, October 24). Lincoln at Southeast Missouri scoreline. *St. Louis Post-Dispatch*, p. 12G.

Football Bet. (2006, November 27). Football bet leads to shooting. *Kansas City Star*, p. C2.

Framed Ex-Cop. (2005, January 25). Framed ex-cop gets millions. *Kansas City Star*, p. A1.

French, R. (2007, February 22). Investigate abuse, denomination urged. *Kansas City Star*, p. A2.

Frey, L.R., Botan, C.H., Friedman, P.G., & Kreps, G.L. (1991). *Investigating communication: An introduction to research methods*. Englewood Cliffs, NJ: Pentice-Hall, Inc.

Fussell, J.A. (2006, November 4). Home of the cheats? *Kansas City Star*, p. E1.

Gebhart, F. (1995, August 14). Antiaging, or just raging? *News World Communications, Inc.* [Online].

Gelfand, L. (1991, September 22). Reader saw danger in words on 'using your helmet.' *Minneapolis Star Tribune*, p. 23A.

Glynn, M. (2006, November 19). Footing the bill for football. *Kansas City Star*, p. D1.

Goodwin, M. (2006, October 23). It's time to turn down the Friday night lights. *Kansas City Star*, p. B9.

Governor Accepted. (2006, May 18). Governor accepted bribe, lobbyist says. *Kansas City Star*, p. A9.

Governor Charged. (2005, August 18). Ohio governor charged. *Kansas City Star*, p. A10.

Governor Convicted. (2006, April 18). Former governor convicted of fraud. *Kansas City Star*, p. A2.

Grathoff, P. (2000, November 27). Violence alters face of sports. *Kansas City Star*, p. C1.

Guilty Plea. (2005, November 22). Plea of guilty points to trail of corruption. *Kansas City Star*, p. A2.

Harr, J. (2005, November 11). Fitness expert touched lives of Fayette residents. *Uniontown Herald Standard.*

Harr, J. (2005, November 22). Walk to honor Courson. *Uniontown Herald Standard* [Online].

Heard, A. (1997, September 28). Technology makes us optimistic. *New York Times*, p. 6-84.

Hicks, R., Westhoff, B., & Wilson, S. (2006, July 13). God of 'musculation'. *Broward-Palm Beach New Times* [Online].

Hoberman, J. (2006, August 21). The doping of everyday life. *Boston Globe* [Online].

Hornung, P., & Silverman, A. (1965). *Football and the single man.* Garden City, NY: Doubleday & Company Inc.

Hoover, T. (2004, August 14). Mix-up gives Blunt tax break. *Kansas City Star*, p. B1.

Hormone Fails. (1996, April 15). Growth hormone fails to reverse effects of aging, researchers say. *New York Times* [Online].

How Neighborly. (2006, October 11). Blagojevich's property tax assessment went up less than 1 percent this year. *Kansas City Star*, p. A2.

Indians Strength. (1984, spring). *Strength of the Indians.* Cape Girardeau: Southeast Missouri State University Football.

Johnson, B. (2006, December 2). Siegelman attorneys say jury tainted. *Biloxi Sun Herald* [Online].

Keisser, B. (2006, December 12). Ease up on the 'Big Mac' attack. *Long Beach Press-Telegram* [Online].

Koch, W. (2006, December 11). Poll: Washington scandals eating away public trust. *USA Today* [Online].

Kolata, G. (1989, December 28). Growth hormone may help adults. *New York Times* [Online].

Kraske, S. (2006, December 31). Major players weren't at a loss for words in 2006. *Kansas City Star*, p. B10.

Landers, A. (2001, October 2). Son forced into football, he's miserable. *Daily Star-Journal*, p. 2.

Lehrman, S. (1992, June). The fountain of youth? Human growth hormone. *Harvard Health Letter* [Online].

Lengel, D. (2007, January 10). The slugger and the scribes. *Guardian* [Online].

Leslie, M. (1998, October 18). The hormone of youth. *Cleveland Plain Dealer Magazine*, p. 14.

Levings, D., & Kraske, S. (2008, February 24). Growing numb to matters of morality? *Kansas City Star*, p. A1.

Lhotka, W.C. (1994, October 23). Refs catch fists, shots over calls. *St. Louis Post-Dispatch*, p. A6.

Lipsyte, R. (1975). *SportsWorld.* Quadrangle/The New York Times Book Company: New York, NY.

Little League bribery. (1999, December 24). Little League bribery alleged. *Kansas City Star*, p. A2.

Man, L. (2005, March 12). Father who punched daughters' coach gets probation. *Kansas City Star*, p. B1.

Margasak, L. (2006, December 9). Foley report issued. *Kansas City Star*, p. A2.

Martinez, M. (2007, June 9). Backers, detractors battle over growth hormone. *Chicago Tribune* [Online].

Masciola, D. (2006, January 7). Telephone interview with author.

Masciola, D. (2006, November). Steve Courson. *Non-published composition.*

Maugh, T.H. II. (1998, October 12). Growth supplement concerns outlined. *Los Angeles Times* [Online].

Mazo, E. (1999, July 6). Graying baby boomers fuel new 'anti-aging market. *Pittsburgh Post-Gazette*, p. F1.

McGwire Clobbers. (1998, September 26). McGwire clobbers 67th, 68th homers to retake lead. *Associated Press* [Online].

McGwire Tied. (1998, September 26). Sosa, McGwire each homer, tied at 66 with 2 games left. *Associated Press* [Online].

McTavish, B. (1999, March 28). Makin' it real. *Kansas City Star*, p. J1.

Montgomery, R. (2006, December 19). Wealth statistics stack up unevenly. *Kansas City Star*, p. A1.

Morgenson, G. (2004, October 14). A culture of casual deception. *Kansas City Star*, p. C3.

Morgenson, G. (2005, January 19). These CEOs wrote the book on hubris. *Kansas City Star*, p. C5.

Morris, M. (2005, May 4). Former judge pleads guilty. *Kansas City Star*, p. A1.

Morris, M. (2005, October 1). Former judge faces prison. *Kansas City Star*, p. A1.

Morris, M., Horsley, L., & Mansur, M. (2007, January 4). Councilwoman charged with mortgage fraud. *Kansas City Star*, p. A1.

Murphy, M. (2007, January 13). The whole truthiness. *Kansas City Star*, p. F4.

National Physicians. (1998, October). National physicians group debunks human growth hormone. *American Association of Clinical Endocrinologists* [Online].

Nossiter, A. (2005, September 30). A dozen officers suspected of looting. *Kansas City Star*, p. A8.

Not Quite. (1990, July 6). Not quite the fountain of youth. *New York Times*, p. A24.

Ochoa, J. (2006, October 4). Lee officers fired for lying about steroid use. *Naples Daily News* [Online].

O'Keeffe, M., Red, C., & Quinn, T.J. (2005, March 13). Hitting the Mark. *New York Daily News* [Online].

Okie, S. (1998, February 24). Can hormones stop aging? *Washington Post*, p. Z12.

Oriard, M. (1982). *The end of autumn*. Doubleday & Company, Inc.: Garden City, New York.

Petiprin, A. (2006, November 25). Pathetic excuses. *Orlando Sentinel* [Online].

Petit, C., & Russell, S. (1990, July 6). 'Youth' therapy unproven, doctors warn. *San Francisco Chronicle*, p. A1.

Pitts, L., Jr. (2006, April 11). Cheating as the cultural norm. *Kansas City Star*, p. B7.

Posnanski, J. (2005, April 18). It's hard to see a hero fall. *Kansas City Star*, p. C1.

Power Abuse. (2000, June 11). An obvious abuse of power by Texas officer. *Kansas City Star*, p. C2.

Quinn, T. (2005, November 13). Integrity fit Courson like a new suit. *New York Daily News* [Online].

Read, M. (2006, June 3). Our leaders: Not what they seem. *Pueblo Chieftan* [Online].

Reeves, R. (1990, July 8). Two significant advances may set off new technological revolution. *Sunday Oregonian*, p. D03.

Reilly, R. (1998, September 7). The good father. *Sports Illustrated*, p. 32.

Reuell, P. (2005, September 18). Five years of troubling news shakes America. *MetroWest Daily News* [Online].

Rizzo, T. (2006, October 11). Ex-police officer sentenced. *Kansas City Star*, p. B5.

Rosener, B. (2008, May 25). Edington, Kalich to be inducted into Hall of Fame. *Daily American Republic*, p. 1B.

Russo, E. (2003, January). The birth of biotechnology. *Nature, 421*, p. 456.

Saltus, R. (1990, August 6). Tinkering with the mechanisms of aging. *Boston Globe*, p. 25.

Saltus, R. (1996, December 8). Youth in a bottle? *Boston Globe Magazine*, p. 12.

Sanchez, M. (2006, August 15). Real men value truth and do the right thing. *Kansas City Star*, p. B9.

Santanam, R. (2005, July 29). Children's coach to stand trial. *Kansas City Star*, p. A10.

Schwartz, L. (2005). McGwire hits his mark. *ESPN.com* [Online].

Sharp, D. (2007, January 13). Double standard given to cheaters. *Detroit Free Press* [Online].

Shinkle, F. (1999, March 25). Keeping up… with the latest health miracles. *St. Louis Post-Dispatch*, p. G1.

Shipley, A. (1998, September 26). Cardinals slugger has answer in St. Louis. *Washington Post*, p. E1.

Simmons, A.M., & Fiore, F. (2006, June 5). Congressman shaped by family's early poverty. *Kansas City Star*, p. A8.

Stafford, D. (2005, June 22). Profligated ways make Americans stand out. *Kansas City Star*, p. C1.

Stafford, D. (2006, April 20). Perp walk patrol is still out. *Kansas City Star*, p. C1.

Stafford, D. (2007, April 22). Money talks, ethics whispers. *Kansas City Star*, p. H1.

Stein, H. (2007, January 13). Writers scrutinize Big Mac and themselves. *New York Times* [Online].

Steinhorn, L., & Holzer, M. (2006, May 7). Are baby boomers the 'greatest'? *Kansas City Star*, p. B7.

Stephen Courson. (2005, November 16). Guest book for Stephen P. Courson. *Pittsburgh Post-Gazette.*

Steroid Parallel. (2007, January 17). Unfair advantage: What is your steroid parallel? *SportingNews.com* [Online].

Testosterone Cypionate. (1977, April). Testosterone cypionate injection U.S.P.

Thomma, S., & Moritz, J. (2005, September 29). House GOP chief indicted. *Kansas City Star*, p. A1.

Thomma, S., & Young, A. (2006, January 4). Lobbyist's plea sends shock wave in capital. *Kansas City Star*, p. A1.

Thompson, L. (1989, July 4). Growth drug gets FDA nod. *Washington Post*, p. Z6.

Thorpe, W.P. (1982, October 22). *Chaney, Matthew L., knee examination.* Cape Girardeau, MO: Southeast Missouri Hospital.

Thorpe, W.P. (1982, October 25). *Chaney, Matthew L., knee operation.* Cape Girardeau, MO: Southeast Missouri Hospital.

Thorpe, W.P. (1982, December 10, to 1985, January 10). *Duboise-McLard, Garry W., medical history, left knee.* Cape Girardeau, MO: St. Francis Hospital.
Thorpe, W.P. (1984, January 26). *McLard, Garry W., knee operation.* Cape Girardeau, MO: St. Francis Hospital.
Three Accused. (2007, January 27). Three accused in sex scandal at school. *Kansas City Star*, p. A2.
Tighe, T. (1990, July 6). Elderly cautioned on hormone. *St. Louis Post-Dispatch*, p. 1C.
Tomkins, R. (1995, January 6). Eli Lilly and Genentech settle dispute. *London Financial Times*, p. 17.
Tufty, D., & Rush, P. (2002, March 30). Is the widespread cheating in our society a moral breakdown? *Kansas City Star*, p. F1.
Unhappy Work. (2002, August 22). Unhappy at work? You're not alone. *Kansas City Star*, p. C8.
Veciana-Suarez, A. (1995, March 11). Kids and sports. *St. Louis Post-Dispatch*, p. D1.
Vedantam, S. (2006, August 21). Cheating is an awful thing for other people to do. *Washington Post*, p. A2.
Vitez, M. (1998, November 8). Group says hormones unlock fountain of youth. *Newark Star-Ledger*, p. 47.
Volland, V. (1994, May 25). Testosterone injections cheat time in study. *St. Louis Post-Dispatch*, p. A1.
Voyles, K. (2006, December 3). At DOC, workers who lie get the ax. *Gainesville Sun* [Online].
Wagar, K. (2004, October 7). Paying tax error is 'right thing to do.' *Kansas City Star*, p. B3.
Weiner, E. (2006, March 30). Baseball buoyant, better than ever. *Orlando Sentinel* [Online].
Wenner, L.A. (Ed.). (1989). *Media, sports, & society.* Newbury Park, CA: Sage Publications.
West, M. (1999, November 2). Aging baby boomers buy time. *Montreal Gazette*, p. F5.
Whalen, J.S. (1955). Emergency paediatric anaesthesia. *Canadian Journal of Anesthesia, 2,* p. 366.
Whannel, G. (1993). Sport and popular culture: The temporary triumph of process over product. *The European Journal of Social Sciences, 6,* (3), p. 341.
Williamson, E. (2006, November 7). America's crisis of confidence. *Kansas City Star*, p. A19.
Wilson, D. (2007, April 15). Aging: Disease or business opportunity? *New York Times* [Online].
Withers, T. (2005, November 21). Youth sports flagged for running out of bounds. *Associated Press* [Online].
Wood, D.B. (2006, June 26). Boot camp for city officials teaches 'a culture of ethics.' *Christian Science Monitor* [Online].
Wrestling Moms. (2000, January 21). Wrestling moms take it to the mat at meet. *Daily Star-Journal*, p. 9.
Yesalis, C. (2008, March 14). Telephone interview with author.

Chapter 9 Circuses: History, summary, 2000 to 2008; The Courson Plan for prevention

> "There's a long, long way to go. But do I see progress? Yeah. And it's very likely that the genie is out of the bottle now. There's probably a critical mass of the public and a critical mass of the sport journalists that have acknowledged testing loopholes. This issue is going to present an increasing challenge for [football]."
>
> **Charles E. Yesalis**
> expert on sport doping, 2006

So, image was deceptive in the modern world, routinely, expectantly. Much was not as it seemed, not so-called morality, not truth, justice, whether for a great civilization or a struggling nation. None moved on ethics, morality, but on power, money, winning by any means necessary. An effective facade was imperative, even if a flimsy see-through. Deniability, evasion need only be plausible in the slightest. "It used to be a badge of honor that you were what you purported to be," wrote Leonard Pitts, Jr., syndicated columnist. "These days, some people think it matters only that you look like what you purport to be. Which is why it has become increasingly difficult to be confident that what you see is, in fact, what you get."

The 2008 Olympiad in China exemplified the circus art form of veiled reality and suspension of belief, "a wonderful and baffling Olympics, all at the same time," wrote Joe Posnanski, the *Kansas City Star* columnist and author. The narratives of Posnanski had changed since the 1990s, when he defended sport shenanigans like "Big Mac," proposing media should ignore athletes' transgressions, focus strictly on "the games," he wrote. Now, from the Beijing Games, Posnanski remarked in jaded writer's perspective, "Nobody is quite sure what's real, what's make-believe, what's inspirational, what's computer-generated, what's a triumph of the human spirit and what's a testament to the capacity of human deception."

In Beijing, Posnanski saw nationalistic exultation in a cheesy Chinese cover for an authoritarian regime, a $45-billion front of imposing architecture, an outlandish stadium ceremony, and feigned friendliness. Yet the lying was universal. Posnanski also saw American swimmers and Jamaican sprinters obliterate world records to rack up medals, creating athletic legends in the process, while officials declared the competitors "clean" — perhaps the Games' biggest catchword. He met a tainted star of the heptathlon, Ukrainian Lyudmila Blonska, who claimed cleanliness of doping after her steroid suspension in the past. When Blonska won silver at Beijing, she took offense to inquiries about possible drug use. "It is very painful to be asked this," Blonska said pitifully through a translator. "I don't think you have to ask it at this moment." Then Blonska tested positive for steroids again and was booted from Beijing, blaming her husband for the transgression.

"It is hard not to be cynical in today's sports world," Posnanski summarized, reflecting growing disenchantment of sports media in particular. So-called sports journalism stood maligned by critics for culpability over doping's half-century in the closet, and media still did not act collectively to investigate issues of sport, including the historically dirty Olympics. Print commentators were principal objectors, griping through opinion pieces the masses did not read, while reporters and TV commentators heaped the stories of sport glory, modern mythology, in multi-media, instantaneous delivery.

Typically, media competed to produce pulp reports and features from Beijing, more than ever, meeting audience demand for drug-free Olympic tales if not athletes. In television, only the Super Bowl rated more valuable than the Olympics for sport content. "Strong feelings of patriotism are continuing to fuel the broad appeal of the Olympics in this country, as past bribery and steroid scandals have done little to diminish the public's enthusiasm for the Games," opined *Brandweek* in 2005, journal for the branding business. "The Olympics has taken its lumps, but for the most part, it's been a pretty stain-free property, unique in its sports and social appeal," said Dr. Paul Swangard, University of Oregon, sports marketing specialist.

The Beijing Games produced the biggest audience numbers yet, with NBC expanding its platform beyond television to capitalize on new content streams through Internet and more conduits. A stain-free Olympics was a matter of opinion at Beijing, but undoubtedly world consumers were worry free, especially in America.

I. Status Quo: Pro Football Denies Muscle Doping

The National Football League faced negative headlines again about muscle doping, as scandal hit many sports through revelations of BALCO, congressional hearings, books, Internet drugs, and doctors like Jim Shortt. League steroid testing finally made a big catch after 16 years of random urinalysis, turning up a nandrolone positive from Shawn Merriman, superstar linebacker of the Chargers. Human growth hormone was pinned on the league in unprecedented fashion, after a lengthy history of use, with an assistant coach turning up among cyber customers for the stuff. Dozens of NFL names ended up exposed, including suspensions for testing, and the league altered posture on the issue within the heightened public awareness. By 2008 the NFL did not brag so much about its steroid testing. A new, younger commissioner was less intimidating than lawyerly Tagliabue, and the league updated its model for rhetoric on muscle drugs, if moderately. Officials allowed more about their limits at prevention, going as far as to acknowledge undetectable growth hormone might pose a problem. They just would never admit the hopelessness for urinalysis.

It was business as usual for the NFL regarding steroids and such, including minor touchup on the anti-doping stance. Revenues counted, remaining golden, stuffing the bank, and enormous players continued roaming the fields. Fifty years after the release of Dianabol, 20 years after synthetic growth hormone, there remained no effective prevention of muscle doping in football, but the public did not care. Football remained the party of choice for millions of fans. Baby Boomers especially took solace in the football circus, customers seeking diversion from war, debt, and dying financial markets. "[T]he NFL is pretty much recession-proof," wrote Pete Alfano, the *Fort Worth Star-Telegram*. "Season tickets are like family heirlooms in some cities and the TV-rights package lines the owners' pockets before a single game is played."

Roger Goodell became the NFL commissioner in 2006, groomed by Tagliabue in-house for the takeover. Goodell, 47, held a prominent family name in New York, as a son of a former U.S. Senator Charles Goodell, and had served as NFL executive vice president and chief operating officer under Tagliabue, overseeing stadium construction and league expansion. Goodell entered the commissioner's office with challenges ahead for the NFL, following a mostly sunny run of 17 years under Tagliabue. Issues on the table for Goodell included player conduct and muscle drugs, both of which Tagliabue had bungled, while problems loomed in owners' infighting, labor unrest, collective-bargaining tension, and a retirees uprising over pension and disability benefits.

Goodell was confronted immediately about HGH, which had been in the NFL for decades, according to former players such as Lyle Alzado, Steve Courson, and Jim Lachey, who reported knowing Chargers players on the drug as a rookie lineman in 1985. As Goodell was named commissioner in August 2006, HGH was linked to NFL players at Carolina and to MLB pitcher Jason Grimsley, and Peter King, *SI* sportswriter, finally got aggressive about doping: "Does the rise of human growth hormone make you worried about the future of the game?" King asked Goodell, apparently the first journalist on topic with the incoming commissioner.

"Yes," Goodell replied, adding he viewed HGH as a credibility threat to the league and a health issue for players.

"Is HGH a big problem right now?" King asked.

Goodell did not answer directly. "It's an area I haven't had much focus on," he said. "But I'll be getting more involved in it." Soon he did, heading into the commissioner's office, when *The Charlotte Observer* and *Costas Now* both hit the league with new allegations of HGH use by NFL players. At Goodell's first press conference, growth hormone was a key question among media, but the commissioner did not go far in discussing it, saying the league had "no indication that we have a significant issue in HGH."

Critics countered that America had many HGH users, untold thousands, particularly in performance roles such as police officers, actors, models, coaches, baseball players — and football players. Recombinant or synthetic human growth hormone was undetectable by testing and readily available from sellers such as personal physicians, online pharmacies, Mexican stores, and home mixers of raw powder. Football players were reported and rumored to patronize "anti-aging" clinics, Internet pharmacies, gurus, and more drug sources legal and illicit. It was disingenuous, said critics like Yesalis, to claim pro football's humongous players could not be significantly involved with HGH, among tissue-building substances.

Gene Upshaw was more candid about the limits of testing, amid the increasing public criticism for management and union over steroids and growth hormone. He repeatedly ridiculed WADA in 2006, correctly labeling its blood sampling technique a farce. During the Grimsley scandal the NFL came under fire to adopt the agency's controversial test for growth hormone. Upshaw opposed blood testing as union executive director, and in concert with WADA critics worldwide, he rejected the agency's claim of a reliable methodology to detect HGH. "The only way to improve the drug program is to improve the science of the testing," Upshaw said. "When that happens, call me." Goodell concurred in the same period: "Right now, HGH doesn't have a reliable test," said the new commissioner.

Within a few days of Goodell's first press conference, Costas' HGH report and accompanying media flare-up had come and gone. The public only cared that the NFL games were underway, and the new season would be another for record revenues. "Welcome to opening weekend of the NFL, where skeletons, scandals, crimes and slimes all are buried and forgotten in the name of America's national passion," wrote Mike Bianchi, the *Orlando Sentinel*, surmising fans would not stop cheering for "rain nor sleet nor massive steroid abuse."

Management, Union Sing From Same Page on Muscle Drugs

Disciplined denial of muscle doping was crafted by the NFL, a legacy of commissioner Tagliabue, who brought management and union together on the issue and other divisive points for an historic run of prosperity. Internal control of information was essential, requiring cooperation of everyone. As Tagliabue approached retirement, a league official gloated about the NFL image, saying, "A lot of people are singing from the same book." For muscle doping, incoming commissioner Goodell needed carryover of company solidarity, and he got it. "I'm really proud of the players and the position they're taking [on the issue]," Goodell said, four months into the job. "The players are indicating they don't want it in the game."

Players soldiered for management, generally appearing oblivious. After Merriman tested positive, some media regularly asked NFL players about drugs, posing intelligent questions on substances like testosterone, anabolic steroids, corticosteroids, growth hormone, clenbuterol, and insulin. Active players and retirees said they knew nothing. Elsewhere, young women were juicing on testosterone patches for flag football, but virtually every NFL player who commented was clean himself, of course, and few professed to know much about anyone else. If anything, a guy said he heard about widespread juicing in prep football and the colleges, or baseball, just not the NFL.

Unnamed players polled by *The New York Daily News* claimed ignorance at circumventing NFL random urinalysis. "I don't see how you can cheat it," said one. "I got to pee right in front of them." They seemed ignorant of the standard undetectable mix for their game, HGH and low-dose testosterone, unlike Panthers players with Dr. Shortt. "That's pretty scientific for someone to go through," a player told *The*

News. "The Panthers didn't win the [2004] Super Bowl. It goes to show cheaters never win."

Players cheered publicly when Goodell and Upshaw announced upgraded testing and tougher penalties at the 2007 Super Bowl. "I like the punishment," said Panthers safety Mike Minter. "You have to make [policy] as hard as possible, and when you start talking about paying back [a portion of bonus money], you're going to get their attention." Colts All-Pro defensive end Dwight Feeney declared: "Cheating has no place in the game." Feeney said he was a natural 6-1, 268 pounds, with speed and athleticism. "It's just about eating the right foods," he said. "And it's not just for pro athletes. It's for everyone. It's called dietary re-engineering."

Rob Tobeck, recently retired lineman, lauded "a very stringent drug policy in the NFL since 1993." Tobeck said he had to weigh about 300 to compete, but he did so by "eating the right foods and not being tempted to take shortcuts." Tobeck isolated Merriman as a user and criticized him, following the lead of All-Pro players Jason Taylor, Dolphins, Champ Bailey, Broncos, and Feeney. Many players were "against" Merriman, Tobeck said. "I think football players may be more active about keeping the sport clean. By contrast, the policy of Major League Baseball is far looser."

The vast majority of retired players stayed in lockstep with the NFL on muscle doping, either indirectly by maintaining silence or directly through endorsement of league testing and policy. In accordance, for example, a series of ex-player autobiographies hit bookshelves in the decade, and while the tomes addressed drugs like painkillers and amphetamines, little or nothing was noted about anabolic steroids, HGH, and pertinent league information. The period from 1990 forward remained largely blank history on doping as far as inside information not released by the league.

A 2009 book by a former lineman apparently would deny steroid abuse in the NFL, given preliminary public comments by author Tony Mandarich. He said he began using steroids during high school in Canada and juiced heavily at Michigan State before stopping in 1989, short of wearing an NFL uniform, after being drafted second overall by the Packers. "The steroid testing in the NFL was random," Mandarich said. "That coupled with all of the allegations of [my] steroid use made me push it away." Mandarich dropped big body weight at Green Bay and was released, but later regained massive size for an O-line comeback with Indianapolis, presumably without drugs.

Like league officials, retirees often mentioned known steroid users deceased, such as Alzado, Courson, and Terry Long. If the dead were a former teammate, culpability for an entire franchise's doping could be projected onto the individual. Former St. Louis Cardinals mentioned Bob Young in that context while old Super Steelers went for Courson, a practice of several when he was alive. In 2008 former Pittsburgh tight end Randy Grossman, a local businessman discussing the Steelers' inordinate amount of deaths among retirees, suggested there would have been "rhyme or reason" to Courson's demise of natural causes, instead of the tragic accident that occurred. Grossman said, "Had Courson died of the medical abuses he indulged in [steroids] at one point in his life, that is something altogether different from having a tree fall on you." Grossman apparently did not mention anyone else with drugs, including known juicers on the death list.

Jockocrat broadcasters on NFL programming were Rozelle's legacy for mass spin, and they supported league efforts in anti-doping, of course. "You can't be independent and dependent at the same time," cracked columnist Ray Ratto, *CBS SportsLine.com*. NBC studio analyst Cris Collinsworth wrote his glowing review of the new commissioner, praising Goodell for the new policy on player conduct. Collinsworth also saluted steroid prevention, depicting a league where players "are saying we don't want to play with or against a guy on steroids, or play with or against a guy who gets arrested all the time." Familiar refrain.

Meanwhile, an NFL broadcast for CBS, Jockocrats preferred forgetting steroids for an interview of Merriman at halftime of a playoff game. Media critics had a field day, with Phil Mushnick writing for *The New York Post*, "While McGwire is a national pariah, studio regulars James Brown, Dan Marino, Shannon Sharpe and Boomer Esiason take turns soft-tossing questions to Merriman, never mentioning that his suspension, this season, was for anabolic steroid use." Mike Ditka stayed in Jockocrat line about performance-enhancing drugs at a press conference in Chicago: "Any guy who uses them is a coward, and he sends a dangerous message to kids," the ESPN analyst said. "I like guys who play the game naturally and don't cheat to get an edge. When I grew up, our only steroid was beer."

Seeking edges was life in the NFL, however, virtually everyone agreed, and players continued to emerge in conjunction with performance-enhancing substances. At least six tested positive for the drug bumantanide in 2008, a masking agent for steroids, and their primary excuse was using it for weight loss. "This is nonsense," countered Sal Marinello, training expert and online columnist for *BlogCritics.org*. Marinello explained bumantanide was a potent diuretic for edema sufferers stricken with heart failure or liver disease, patients with excess water weight from their diseased condition. "Frankly, to assert that anyone would take this drug simply for weight loss, as if it were a matter of losing a few pounds, is an insult to our collective intelligence," Marinello wrote. "Don't be fooled by the weight-loss cover story that is being fed by the league and regurgitated by the media, and don't be duped into thinking that elite athletes took this drug innocently."

Goodell faced stiffer challenges in quieting the doping problem than Tagliabue, whose old presumption of information control was largely incompatible for the modern landscape. A tight lid could not be kept on football doping after 2005, with law authorities and scattered media investigating aggressively, churning up information that flew immediately on the Web and TV.

Among cases, former 49ers and Raiders lineman Dana Stubblefield pleaded guilty of lying to federal agents about his use of substances obtained through the BALCO lab, designer steroid THG and blood-boosting agent erythropoietin, EPO, likely the drug's first documented use in American football. Stubblefield also told *Costas Now* that at least 30 percent of NFL players used growth hormone. At

Tampa, police said Buccaneers receiver David Boston tested positive for gamma-hydroxybutyric acid, GHB, a depressant known as the "date rape" drug, reputed to have anabolic effects. In Pennsylvania, Garrett Reid, 24-year-old son of Eagles coach Andy Reid, was caught with testosterone after a car collision, along with heroin and more drugs.

Speculation surrounded the $10 million fine for a pharmacy in St. Louis, an Express Scripts outlet the government announced "knowingly distributed human growth hormone to certain well-known athletes and entertainers, including a well-known athlete in Massachusetts, knowing that their intended use was athletic performance enhancement." The probe was concluded before the report was made public, and media did not ascertain names. Texans long-snapper Bryan Pittman said PEDs like growth hormone were "a problem" for the NFL, speaking with Jason Friedman of *Ballz* blog in Houston. Pittman estimated "at least forty percent" of players used "some kind of illegal substance." In HBO's *Costas Now* report about growth hormone, Dr. Teresa Denney, Honolulu, said she prescribed HGH and testosterone to perhaps 10 NFL players. Journalists also noted information about anonymous pro players and muscle drugs. When Jason Grimsley was exposed for growth hormone, Bryan Burwell, *St. Louis Post-Dispatch*, posed, "If you think the use of human growth hormone is a big deal in baseball, what on earth do you think would happen in the NFL, if the drug cops showed up tomorrow with a reliable test for HGH?" A few years previous, Burwell reported, a player answered for him: "Mass retirements."

In Goodell's first year as commissioner, investigative writer Tom Farrey analyzed the cultural dilemma of HGH and sport, legalities to morality, for *ESPN The Magazine*. Shaun Assael, another *ESPN Mag* writer and author of the book *Steroid Nation**, also researched the modern American subculture of muscle and substances for image. Farrey and Assael encountered NFL footprints everywhere around the anti-aging industry, individuals from players to physicians.

At modern bodybuilding's world convention, the Arnold Classic in Columbus, Ohio — named for California Governor Schwarzenegger, of course, whose steroid use helped construct his physique leading to film and political stardom — Assael found salespersons hawking a cornucopia of substances. A chiseled 50-something physician had a booth adorned "Human Growth Hormone" in big banner letters. Assael found a legal hookup for synthetic GH in the doctor, who said an NFL punter had already taken advantage, coming back from knee injury.

Former Dolphins running back Abdul-Karim al-Jabbar, NFL touchdown leader in 1997, told Farrey he used HGH as a player for the purpose of regenerating cartilage in a knee. Farrey reported, "Already, athletes are discreetly acquiring hormones to recover from injuries. Some use them to repair tissue and cut recovery time after surgery, others to rebuild joints." Farrey met doctors who prescribed HGH to retired NFL players, special clients seeking restoration of tissue, a better buff, and hopefully an offset for advancing age. Brad Leggett, retired Saints lineman and nutrition marketer, said, "I'm a huge believer in medically supervised use of growth hormone. The aches and pains I had from playing football, I don't have anymore." In a related report, *CNN* quoted a former NFL player who used growth hormone along with his wife. "I noticed in the gym that I was much stronger," said ex-Chiefs lineman Ed Lothamer, 64, business owner and operator in construction equipment. "I had more endurance. My memory was sharper."

In Florida, authorities observed unnamed active players around a pharmacy that doled prescription drugs in off-label fashion, including for performance enhancement, to customers mostly acquired online. The wider investigation focused on cyber dealing and originated from a New York district attorney's office in Albany, reaching into states such as Florida and Alabama. The target network of sellers distributed PEDs to thousands of customers nationwide, a story that broke through *The Albany Times Union* in February 2007. The newspaper reported the investigation was a year old and had uncovered possibly fraudulent Internet prescriptions for anabolic substances "to current and former Major League Baseball players, National Football League players, college athletes, high school coaches, a former Mr. Olympia champion and another leading contender in the bodybuilding competition."

Few names were released initially. First from the NFL was a Steelers physician, Dr. Richard A. Rydze, who had tended to the team on game days as an associate for 21 years. Rydze ordered large quantities of HGH and testosterone by Internet in 2006 — and paid with a personal credit card, which piqued the interest of FDA investigators who traveled to interview him. The $150,000 in wholesale drugs was worth about as much as $1 million retail, authorities estimated, but Rydze said none went to current athletes. Rydze, an internist for the University of Pittsburgh Medical Center, told *Sport Illustrated* he prescribed HGH to a few dozen "elderly" patients through his private practice, including retired football players, for hormone deficiency and tendon repair. The 56-year-old Rydze, a former Olympic diver, said he took patient referrals from another Steelers doctor — the franchise listed six on staff — and team owners were aware of his business outside the team. Rydze was no criminal target, authorities said, and Steelers officials said they were not notified until the initial Albany newspaper report. Franchise president Art Rooney II issued a statement that read in part, "There is no evidence Dr. Rydze prescribed or provided any hormone treatments to any of our players. Dr. Rydze has assured me that this has never happened and will never happen." Three months later, the Steelers dismissed Rydze from staff, without comment by him or team officials.

Additional NFL names were publicized in the probes of prescription performance-enhancing drugs. Patriots safety Rodney Harrison and Cowboys assistant coach Wade Wilson both received HGH from an online pharmacy, reports revealed, and each served a four-game suspension by the league. Former quarterback Tim Couch told *Yahoo! Sports* that he used growth hormone for a comeback attempt, and the online entity also reported Couch filled steroid prescriptions at a Brooklyn drugstore.

Intrigue flared around Cowboys star receiver Terrell Owens and a self-anointed "doctor" in Atlanta, Mack Henry "Hank" Sloan, a naturopath who claimed to treat numerous NFL players year-round utilizing holistic approaches for body recovery. Sloan defended his work in e-mail exchanges with Sal Marinello, *Blogcritics.org* columnist, after the strength trainer ripped the posted regimen for "T.O.," 6-3, 223, in exercise and healing. During an e-mail debate with Marinello, Sloan repeatedly noted insulin-like growth factor 1, or IGF-1, an undetectable PED in off-label use by athletes, and he mentioned human growth hormone. "IGF-1 is extremely beneficial and works very well for healing ligaments, tendon and cartilage," Sloan wrote. "I just recently healed a 60% tear in the ulnar collateral ligament in a Pro Baseball Player using a combination of GH, IGF-1, and [prolotherapy]." Sloan later denied employing substances banned in sport, specifically regarding Owens, during contacts with Marinello and investigative reporter Mike Fish of *ESPN.com*. Owens declined comment, but Lions defensive end Kalimba Edwards acknowledged receiving "prolotherapy injections, liquid vitamins, IVs, anti-inflammatory shots and other non-steroidal injections from Sloan," Fish reported. Georgia authorities investigated Sloan for practicing medicine without a license, after an 8-year-old girl allegedly witnessed his injecting a man in the bare buttocks on a houseboat.

Owens missed an out-of-season steroid test in 2008 and was placed in the NFL's "reasonable cause" program, leaving him subject to increased urinalysis. Owens was not pleased, saying he missed the test because of confusion over phone numbers and had not tested positive in 12 years of random urinalysis by the NFL. "Especially with everything with the steroids and performance-enhancing drugs, for me to be put out there in that light, I think it's just a negative connotation for me," Owens said.

Rumors circulated about player agents' private camps, where prospects were directed in matters from media relations to doping. *New York Daily News* investigative sportswriter Michael O'Keeffe discussed the topic with former Bengals strength coach Kim Wood, reporting, "According to Wood, prospective NFL players attend pre-draft camps run by agents where some trainers and medical personnel school the millionaires-in-waiting on the drugs that will help improve their position in the draft. Wood describes the camps as cult-like facilities where the young men are taught to do whatever it takes to boost their signing bonuses and salaries — and their agents' commissions." The camps were run to brainwash prospects for following their agents like drones. Wood said, "By the time they go through the camp, they are willing to do anything to make the team, including drugs. ... They tell them they can move up in the draft if they lose 15 pounds of fat or make their biceps or pecs bigger. They are taught how to beat drug tests and what drugs are undetectable. They learn how to cycle on and off the drugs. They are taught, 'This is what you have to do to make it in this league.'"

Media rapped league testing, particularly upon scrutiny by the *The New York Daily News*, its rare team of investigative sports reporters and editor Teri Thompson. After the congressional hearings of 2005, the NFL tripled its out-of-season testing of players, but *The NYDN* led media in exposing gaps for urinalysis that allowed undetectable use of muscle substances. The NFL's rigid control of inside information cracked as *The News'* O'Keeffe and T.J. Quinn mined rich information from "drug program agents," urine sample collectors who were embroiled in a multi-million dollar dispute with the league. The DPAs, mostly retired lawmen, detailed two gaps in NFL testing, one directly after the season and one during training camp. Doping experts said players could juice with relative ease in the open periods, especially on low-dose testosterone and steroid pills. Giants running back Tiki Barber affirmed players knew the gaps. "No one told us that. But we don't get tested [then]," he said. "I guess when you look at it from that perspective, it's a pretty big loophole." The NFL denied gaps in testing as described by its DPAs.

Each week during the season, about 10 players per team were chosen randomly for steroid testing, or about 320 of the league's 1,700. About a half-dozen suspensions over steroid policy were announced every year by the NFL in the latter 2000s, not including a number of positive tests overturned in successful appeals by players, undisclosed to the public. *The New York Times* reported the NFL did not test on game days and did not chaperone players when they were unable to quickly provide a urine sample, discrepancies that savvy dopers could exploit. *The San Diego Tribune* noted a lengthy doping period for NFL prospects after college, as long as five months without testing, until they attended the draft combine.

The most damning criticism, however, focused on a fundamental fault in NFL testing, specifically the inability at any time to detect a myriad of substances. "Is there anyone out there with a functioning brain who believes that the sport whose athletes have the most to gain by taking steroids is as clean as it purports to be? Get real," wrote Doug Robinson, the *Deseret Morning News*. "If baseball players and skinny distance runners and tiny cyclists are cheating with performance-enhancing drugs, then it's a sure thing NFL players are doing the stuff." Dr. Don Catlin, UCLA Olympic lab director, acknowledged loopholes in conventional urinalysis while he oversaw NFL testing, aware dopers were not testing positive. "We do have a high false-negative rate," he said in 2006. "I know this, and people should know it. They think testing is a gift to this problem. If you put the right amount of timing and resources into testing, it can be done pretty well. But athletes get fairly sophisticated at beating the tests."

Growth hormone topped the list of public complaints about NFL testing, and likely the doping list for many pro football players. "Because [HGH] is so difficult to test for, it seems to be the product du jour for increasing performance," said Dr. Paul Doering, a University of Florida pharmacology professor and anti-doping official. "It's a drug manufactured to be exactly like what's in the body." Officials of the World Anti-Doping Agency and U.S. Anti-Doping Agency incessantly promoted their blood test for growth hormone, part of their agenda to take over testing for American pro sports, but the Olympic serum screen was ineffective, said experts like Catlin and Charles Yesalis, and could not help the NFL presently.

Pro football insiders stayed their course on muscle doping, denial. Troy Vincent, president of the players union, claimed Major League Baseball had more HGH users than the NFL. "We feel it's not something that's common in our space," Vincent said in 2008, claiming football physiques amounted to genetic wonders en masse. "I'm dealing with 20-year-olds popping with God-given ability," Vincent said. Goodell described NFL steroid testing as the "gold standard" during his annual press conference on the state of the league. On the big question, Goodell said: "I don't think there is a significant amount of HGH use, but I have no factual basis for saying that. I think our athletes are extremely well-trained. I don't think they want HGH or performance-enhancing drugs in the game."

Players echoed Goodell. "We all know what those things can do to your body," said Larry Fitzgerald, Cardinals wideout. "HGH has been shown to increase the size of your head. Well, I don't want my head to get any bigger." Jeremy Shockey, Saints tight end, rebuked the seeming logic that pro football was drug-sodden. "The National Football League has done a great job of regulating and testing," he said. "A lot of sports didn't test until they were forced to test. Football is different. It's unique. People may look at it like football players do use performance-enhancing drugs more than other [sports], but I think it's vice versa. That's just how it is."

Doping rhetoric from pro football was fluffy, often absurd, but players, coaches, and organizers tolerated PEDs in pursuit of winning, financial reward, and security. Straight talk was not considered by the vast majority, according to David Meggyesy, author, former player, and retired western director of the players union. "The league is like, 'We don't want to go to this [topic],'" Meggyesy said in 2008. "And the union is in a difficult spot, because if a player doesn't want [doping] revealed, can you reveal it? No. ... Everybody's scared to death of this thing for different reasons."

II. UNDETECTED: COLLEGE FOOTBALL FLIES UNDER DRUG RADAR

In the debate over college sports of the 2000s, NCAA officials said the critics were wrong about fundamental issues including their mission as well as doping. Granted, football and men's basketball generated billions of dollars for major schools and the NCAA, but the mission remained education, not entertainment, officials said. A player combatant was a student first, athlete second, they said. Granted, century-old problems persisted in football on campus, including mercenary athletes, academic fraud, and violent crime, but "broad-based reform" was in progress, officials said, parroting the catchphrase of NCAA president Myles Brand.

An historic issue wakened for college football, fresh questions about muscle doping. Observers noted giant athletes of the NCAA were obvious like the NFL's. No problem, insisted NCAA officials, because steroid use was practically eliminated through testing and educational awareness. They dismissed most evidence to the contrary as "anecdotal." NCAA officials said to forget critics of college football, especially regarding performance-enhancing substances, because outsiders had no idea what went on. Officials said widespread doping was in the past, despite much larger athletes playing in the present. They proclaimed the only trustworthy evidence came from NCAA testing and anonymous player surveys, as well as in-house data that proclaimed the use of anabolic steroids in football to be about one or two players in a hundred.

In response, critics derided the NCAA and member institutions, saying decades of urinalysis and anti-steroid education had been ineffective, whether performed by school, conference, or national association. Penn State epidemiologist Dr. Charles E. Yesalis complained regularly to college officials, faculty, lawmakers, and media, alleging the NCAA slid by on serious impropriety with PEDs, particularly in football. "None of this is new. It has been a sustained epidemic," Yesalis repeated to Congress in 2005, for a subcommittee reviewing NCAA anti-doping efforts, for his fourth Washington testimony in 17 years. Journalists, doping experts, and some insiders backed Yesalis in his central charge of systemic muscle doping in college football, unabated, and events and allegations kept occurring nationwide in support of his testimony.

"If teenage girls are taking steroids just to look good to their awkward suitors, what are the odds that a few of our comic-booked sized NCAA favorites are gassed?" wrote John McMullen, *AgainstTheLine.com*, continuing:

> Common sense says pretty good but you wouldn't know it by the number who have been snared by the system. When one famous study says up to 7 percent of middle school girls say they have used steroids and the NCAA says 1 percent tested positive, what does that tell you about its policy? Since the '70s, football players have grown in ways that evolution and competent eating habits can't fully explain. The players aren't just bigger; they are faster, stronger and quicker.

An array of anabolic substances remained accessible to college players, and coaches were still accused of direct involvement with steroids, including distribution. At least one assistant coach provided steroids and encouragement to players at San Diego State, according to allegations published by *The Union-Tribune*. Reporter Brent Schrotenboer confirmed years of steroid use in SDSU football during interviews with former players. One former coach was named for involvement, while court documents filed in a lawsuit raised the question about a second. Current and former Aztec players said anabolic steroids were readily available to them, especially for the easy local drive to Mexico, minutes away. "Hell, we went to San Diego State," said Kyle Turley, NFL lineman and former Aztec. "You could just drive across the border and do it in the restroom of the pharmacy where you pick it up." Turley told Schrotenboer he did not juice but knew users in the program during the 1990s. "I don't know of any coach who necessarily would encourage it, but coaches know about steroid use," Turley said. "They know the benefits of it."

San Diego State rarely tested athletes for steroids, relying instead on NCAA visits for random screenings, typically once annually. Eighteen football players and eight other athletes were summoned for testing, and NCAA contracted collectors closely watched them provide urine samples. Two SDSU linemen tested positive in 1995 and a quarterback in 2002. The university downplayed concern of a problem during the coach allegations of 2005, with current football staff and athletic officials mostly declining comment. *Union-Tribune* columnist Ed Graney called for an independent investigation, but the school did not heed. "Of course this is an issue that's always a concern, especially when it appears kids are using steroids at a younger and younger ages," said associate athletic director Kevin Klintworth. "But since 1997 our testing for steroids, coupled with the annual random NCAA tests, have produced just two positive results." Yesalis was not swayed. "There is an unbelievable level of deniability in these cases," Yesalis told Graney, ripping colleges for their predictable, historic response to football doping. "The [denial] gets to the point of being silly, but it's not silly. This stuff hurts kids."

On the East Coast, meanwhile, NCAA investigators established their first major violation for steroids in an athletic program, the shaky football program at Savannah State. The small university was attempting a move into Division I athletics but failing for win-loss records, fund-raising, and rules compliance, according to reports by Noell Barnidge, *The Savannah Morning News*, as well as findings by the NCAA. Barnidge interviewed a wide range of sources including football players, coaches, university officials and athletic boosters. His series profiled a significant event in gridiron doping, although overshadowed at the time by the BALCO story.

In November 2004, NCAA representatives visiting Savannah State were tipped off that an assistant coach dispensed steroids to football players. NCAA Enforcement was already familiar with Savannah State athletics, having slapped major violations on the department a few years before, and an investigation opened immediately on campus. Assistant coach Jerome Pope allegedly distributed anabolic steroids to players up until a recorded conversation was provided to NCAA officials. The previous summer, football coaches were informed about Pope, steroids, and more rules violations, but head coach Richard Basil made no move, even as a player tested positive for steroids in an NCAA urinalysis. Pope remained in his duties coaching wide receivers and directing strength training.

Pope, a former SSU player who had not graduated, was interviewed once by an NCAA investigator, then Basil fired him and he left Savannah and was out of contact. NCAA Enforcement and SSU officials interviewed players, and about a dozen left the team. Barnidge talked to seven former players on their exit from Savannah and broke the story in December. "[The NCAA probe] is all about the steroids," said Zach Wilson, former freshman quarterback. "Jerome Pope's name came out of everybody's mouth. I have so many sources that could vouch for that. … Being my first college football experience, it's a hard pill to swallow. Is college football really like this? It can't be this awful and corrupt." The player who made the secret tape told Barnidge: "I was injured and [Pope] told me that steroids would help me heal faster. I didn't know what to do. … Pope offered me injected steroids during the season. Over the summer, during summer workouts, he offered a lot of us [Dianabol], which are steroid pills. I never took them. I never took any steroids."

The NCAA found several major violations in SSU football, including illicit practices, recruiting violations, and unethical conduct for Pope's steroid dealing. He was barred from coaching in the association for seven years without a "show cause" hearing, and Basil resigned. Savannah State University, guilty of lack of institutional control and unethical conduct, was placed on probation for three years.

Police reports involving college football players and the occasional coach increased during the 2000s. Michigan athletics strength instructor Rondell Biggs, a former UM defensive end, was charged with possession of anabolic steroids after police found 10 stanozolol pills in his car during a traffic stop. Biggs, 24, pleaded not guilty to the charge, and the Michigan athletic department suspended him from his job. Biggs told police an acquaintance gave him the steroids and he thought the pills were for weight loss.

Louisiana State suspended fullback Shawn Jordan for his arrest by U.S. Customs; agents found steroid vials in his car at the Texas/Mexico border. Brandon Catanese, a safety at Oregon State, pleaded no contest to steroid possession and served 18 months probation while finishing his playing career. Corvallis Police had found a steroids vial in his apartment, and he admitted ownership. At Appalachian State, Jonathan Ray, a walk-on defensive lineman, was dismissed from the team after police found drugs in his home. He was later charged with steroids possession. Police in Martin, Tennessee, found drugs and needle syringes at the apartment of two offensive linemen for UT-Martin. Kyle Wisniewski, offensive guard, left the football team and pleaded guilty to misdemeanor possession of steroids, cocaine, and marijuana. He received a suspended sentence and fine. Adam Hansen, offensive tackle, "filed a judicial review and was fined $400 on two misdemeanor charges," a report stated, and rejoined the football team.

In the Ivy League, two players at Dartmouth were indicted on drug charges that included steroid possession and left the team. Former safety Steven DeMarco pleaded guilty to misdemeanor possession of steroids, oxycodone, and marijuana, and was sentenced to 60 days in jail, probation, community service, and fines. Former tight end Sheanon Summers pleaded guilty to misdemeanor possession of drugs that court records indicated were steroids and marijuana, and he was sentenced to community service and fines. A third player tied to the case, former receiver Eric Testan, admitted drug possession, reportedly cocaine, and served three days in jail of a six-month suspended sentence.

University of Maine linebacker Stephen Cooper, named New England's top collegiate defensive player in 2002, continued to play after his arrest for steroid possession during a traffic stop. After state police informed the university, Cooper appeared in four games that included playoff rounds of NCAA Division I-AA. He pleaded guilty to misdemeanor steroid possession and was named an All-America for the second straight year. Cooper entered the NFL and tested positive as a Chargers linebacker in 2007, reportedly for ephedra.

Controversy erupted at the U.S. Air Force Academy in 2004, with the exposure of steroid users among cadets that included football players and a cheerleader. The drugs originated from Mexico and from elsewhere. Air Force linebacker Overton Spence, Jr. admitted obtaining an anabolic steroid, methandrostenolone, from a former teammate, saying he thought the substance was legal. He and Matthew Ward, an Air Force running back who also admitted possessing the steroid, were exonerated of charges brought in military court. Spence remained with the team while Ward left the academy, reportedly for academic reasons. Cheerleader Jonathan Belkowitz was found guilty of lying to investigators about steroids and dismissed from the academy according to reports.

A quarterback recruit for Mississippi was arrested for steroids, and his scholarship was rescinded. Jared Foster later pleaded guilty of selling steroids to a police informant and was sentenced to five years in prison and a $5,000 fine. Foster's jail sentence would be suspended if he finished a state "boot camp-style program" of about six to eight months, reported the *Jackson Clarion-Ledger*. Foster had a previous run-in with the law that reportedly involved steroids during high school. He was instrumental in helping Gulf Coast Community College to a national co-championship in 2007, and an official at the junior college hoped the athlete would get another chance in football.

Violent incidents involving college football players and steroids were reported during the 2000s. Police said three Delaware football players on a mission to steal steroids were arrested after an armed robbery at the apartment of a fourth player. All were dismissed from the football team. The three charged later pleaded guilty: former Blue Hens linebacker Demetrice Alexander and former running back Danny Jones, each for possession of a firearm during the commission of a felony, two counts of second-degree robbery, one count of wearing a disguise during a felony, and two counts of second-degree conspiracy. Former defensive back Jeffrey Robinson was charged with first-degree robbery, two counts of second-degree robbery, and two counts of second-degree conspiracy.

A tragedy involved football players at Arizona State, where the Sun Devils running back Loren Wade shot and killed former teammate Brandon Falkner in a dispute over a female soccer player, authorities said. Wade provided a urine sample the night of the pistol shooting that was positive for several anabolic steroids, said Jennifer Valdez, toxicologist for the Scottsdale Police Department. A jury found Wade guilty of second-degree murder, and he was sentenced to 20 years in prison.

Small colleges in the NCAA were just as susceptible to the use of banned substances by football players. St. Anselm College captain Derek DiMartino was arrested after pellet gunshots from a dormitory window struck three teen skateboarders. Police found HCG in the possession of DiMartino, human chorionic gonadotropin, which could be used to counteract effects of steroid cycling. DiMartino pleaded guilty to felony reckless conduct and was sentenced to 90 days in jail. Elsewhere, in Menomonie, Wisconsin, police recovered steroids, HCG, and street drugs during the arrests of football players for UW-Stout, a Division III school. The team's former leading tackler at linebacker, Luke Steffen, later pleaded guilty to steroid possession and maintaining a drug-trafficking place. He was sentenced to 10 days in jail, community service, and probation. Former linebacker Nicholas OrRico faced felony and misdemeanor charges for marijuana.

Everywhere, officials denied institutional culpability in steroid cases of college football, whether involving player or coach. Those claiming innocence ranged from coaches and athletic directors to faculty, deans, and chancellors. When at least three

Air Force players were implicated for steroid use, coach Fisher DeBerry blamed only them. "It's like a lot of other coaches," DeBerry said. "[Players] made the decision to use." Texas Tech self-reported a violation in providing banned supplements to athletes, including the product "Testosterone Booster," but officials suggested the problem lay with nutrition specialist Aaron Shelley, who was fired. At LSU, the school hosting an elite football program loaded with enormous athletes, coach Les Miles classified Jordan's steroid possession as the proverbial "isolated" incident. Another coach of the Southeastern Conference, Houston Nutt, had steroid allegations in his program at Arkansas, and later he had to boot an initial recruit at Mississippi, Foster, for his legal problems. "It's a shame," Nutt said. "But we're trying to build a football program and that's stuff we can't tolerate." In New Hampshire, "Dartmouth College athletic officials say steroid and substance abuse is not rampant among athletes despite the... arrests of three [players] on drug charges," reported *The Associated Press*.

An Arizona State committee found Sun Devils football did not mishandle Wade, the convicted killer, citing only "errors in judgment" on the part of coach Dirk Koetter and former athletic director Gene Smith, who had moved up to the same job at Ohio State. Wade, a blue-chip running back, passed drug tests and perpetrated troubling acts, including verbal threats against females, before murdering a former teammate and testing positive for steroids in police urinalysis.

At Delaware, the official statement concerning armed robbery for steroids by football players exonerated the institution and its football program and placed responsibility directly on those individuals perpetrating the act. Delaware football coach K.C. Keeler suggested testing caught other users at the I-AA school, but Yesalis disagreed, citing undetectable substances and more techniques for false-negative results by juicers. "If somebody told me one of these drug-testing guys closed these loopholes of how to grow [players] the size we see even in Division II and III ball, I'd shut up," Yesalis said.

At the Division III University of Wisconsin-Stout, officials had to acknowledge problems after a rash of player arrests for narcotics, including steroids, along with positive tests for street drugs and amphetamine in the program. The football coach and athletic director resigned, the NCAA instituted "pilot" random testing for D-III, and Stout officials insisted trouble was in the past. "We don't want to be an embarrassment, and we're not going to be," said Chancellor Charles Sorenson.

Tighter police enforcement of anti-steroid laws propelled the decade's rate of reports on anabolic steroids and college football players. Meanwhile, steroid revelations hit schools large and small in allegations and confessions, along with scattered leaks of positive-test cases, normally non-published. NCAA and university officials cited student privacy and other laws for withholding information, but media reported use or allegations in football programs in schools such as Arkansas, USC, Hawaii, Central Connecticut State, BYU, UNLV, Utah, Portland State, New Mexico, Air Force, Navy, Sam Houston State, Nebraska, Iowa State, and Oberlin College. In a 2007 *Salt Lake Tribune* survey of schools hosting the top-tier football programs, six of the 119 athletic departments representing NCAA Division I-A reported an athlete testing positive under steroid policies of recent years: Idaho, Texas, Iowa, Tennessee, East Carolina, and Oklahoma. A Michigan official before Congress reported a positive result for an athlete.

A faint outcry arose over the U.S. Naval Academy, where news of positive steroid tests among football players emerged long after the fact. *The Baltimore Sun* revealed academy administrators learned in February 2005 that two football players had tested positive for the supplement androstenediol, recently classified as an illegal steroid, during NCAA random urinalysis. A Navy criminal probe found five more football players had used androstenediol, but no formal charges resulted. Officials waited two months to test the additional five, and all results were negative for steroids.

The two midshipmen nabbed by the NCAA were ineligible for the 2005 season, but school officials allowed the other five to compete. The matter remained quiet almost two years, right under the noses of steroid-hunting politicians in Washington, until *The Sun* broke the story in November 2006. "It was a serious thing when it happened, but it's a non-story [now]," said Navy football coach Paul Johnson, who suggested no use of anabolic steroids. Experts and more critics disagreed, including pols, and campus complaints of football favoritism arose since none of the tainted athletes faced court martial or harsh discipline, but no further action was taken.

Sun columnist John Eisenberg believed big-time NCAA football had it easier for muscle doping than any other sport. "We're inundated with roaring headlines about athletes using performance-enhancing drugs in the major leagues, the NFL, the Olympics, the Tour de France and even high school sports, but what about college football? There's barely a whisper, much less a roar," Eisenberg wrote. Yesalis concurred, although he declined to appear at yet another D.C. hearing involving college sports and performance-enhancing substances. "The NCAA has been allowed to skate on this deal," Yesalis said.

Police linked unnamed college athletes and coaches to Internet pharmacies selling prescription PEDs without doctor exams, and Sandra Worth, head athletic trainer at the University of Michigan, told Congress another school's anti-drug counselors discovered parents provided steroids for two athletes who tested positive. "In both cases, the parents believed their children had an outside chance of playing professionally," Worth testified. An anonymous football player alleged systemic doping in his program, speaking with Jim Swanson of *The Prince George Citizen*. The player, a Canadian competing for a U.S. university, said alumni and boosters financed a team steroid program directed by coaches. "I'd say about 90 percent of the guys did it, and the other guys got cut or didn't see the field in games," the player said. "My initial reaction was 'see you later,' but I also loved football and I wanted to play. I thought about it back and forth, and I [juiced]. My roommate didn't do it and he went from being a starter to third string." In Nebraska, prosecutors listed 13 current and former Cornhusker football players as potential witnesses in a steroids case involving steroid trafficking, but none was called to testify.

Former Arkansas lineman Josh Melton confirmed steroids in college football during an interview with *Arkansas Razorback Sports Network*. "Arkansas is no different than any other college in the country. If you want [steroids], you can find them," stated Melton, who last played in 2002. "The Internet has also made access to steroids and other 'performance enhancers' much easier. … The only 'solution' to the problem will be to test every player, weekly." Former BYU lineman Jason Scukanec alleged muscle doping in Cougars football and more D-I programs of the West, during comments published by *The Portland Tribune* and the *Deseret Morning News*. Scukanec said some players beat testing by employing undetectable doses of "steroids, human growth hormone, insulin or what have you." He said juiced players beat tests on short notice with a liquid known as "pink" to clear the body. "Whatever test they have, someone will find a way around it. Once that happens, you don't think information is shared?" Scukanec personally injected a friend at BYU, a program he characterized as "temperate" for PEDs compared to many, and he disavowed use himself. "It's common knowledge of who uses and who doesn't. This is a close-knit group that uses, and they often times get it from the same supplier," Scukanec said.

Former players confirmed their steroid use in college during the 1980s and 1990s, like actor-wrestler Dwayne "The Rock" Johnson at U-Miami and the controversial Tony Mandarich, back in the news while promoting his autobiography. Following years of denial, Mandarich finally admitted he used anabolic steroids for Michigan State in the late 1980s, confirming public suspicion since the time. He passed all drug tests. After Mandarich had left MSU for an ill-fated NFL career, the university community denied allegations of steroids on winning football teams under Coach George Perles. In 2008, Perles said Mandarich's confession "surprised" him. Perles was retired and serving on the MSU board of trustees. Regarding old allegations of steroids on his teams, Perles said, "There was nothing there."

Another former college coach could not leave behind steroids talk, Tom Osborne, who retired from Nebraska in 1997 after three national championships in four years. Elected to Congress, Rep. Osborne helped lead the passage of the 2004 steroid law restricting testosterone supplements and prohormones, but rather quietly given his football past. Instead, Osborne loudly championed anti-alcohol causes in Washington, declaring drinking a much greater threat than steroids for young people. He was largely absent from the Capitol Hill fixation on PEDs, but he did appear briefly for the 2005 baseball hearing, apparently at the behest of House Republican colleague Tom Davis of Virginia, chair of the Committee on Government Reform. Again, Osborne said little, refraining until formally recognized at a microphone by Davis. He talked a minute or two, focused primarily on thanking parents in attendance for bringing attention to steroids, then left. *Washington Post* pundit Thomas Boswell panned Osborne, writing, "And it was amusing to hear an ex-Nebraska coach, now in Congress, make pious noises about steroids. Nebraska linemen can lift TRACTORS. In fact, some of them are bigger than tractors. Okay, I know it's all the farm work. That could be the answer."

A former college player appeared before a Senate Caucus in 2004, having recently completed a four-year career in Division I football. Testifying as a "hidden" or anonymous witness for the public record, John Doe said, "When first arriving at a program like this, the temptation to use steroids is great because of the surrounding players who quite obviously have used drugs to gain physical strength." The athlete said he did not juice, but he knew of at least seven players who bought steroids from a dealer teammate. "Many of these players played significant time in games and most were starters on either offense or defense," John Doe said. "There could easily be other players using steroids that I was not aware of during my career, and in hindsight it becomes very probable that several other people on the team used steroids without many people knowing." The team was aware of juicing "on other big-time Division I programs," said John Doe, who argued that conventional anti-doping efforts were ineffective. "You may be asking yourself how these players get around the NCAA random drug testing policy," he addressed the committee. "This policy is rather weak, however, and fairly predictable with the drug tests falling in roughly the same window of time each year. The NCAA claims to be protecting the health and safety of college athletes but in my opinion has very little pull on the illegal use of drugs in college athletics."

The NCAA dismissed empirical evidence such as public allegations of insiders like Scukanec and John Doe. Such information was "anecdotal," said NCAA people like testing contractor Frank Uryasz, with his lucrative, private business of urinalysis built around annual work for the association. Uryasz collected more than $4 million annually for contracting NCAA random urinalysis, in addition to his educational programs for conferences and schools. Uryasz formerly directed NCAA Sciences. During a 2006 interview, Uryasz contended his testing, combined with anti-steroid education, had turned back juicing in NCAA football from a highpoint in the 1980s — about 10 percent of players, officials said — to a contemporary rate of about 1 to 3 percent, according to urinalysis results and an anonymous player survey. Uryasz said the main preventive factor in his anti-doping was an athlete's fear of being caught.

Critics ripped the rationale of Uryasz, calling his NCAA statistics highly erroneous. Current and former NCAA football players laughed in private, and medical experts like Yesalis scoffed in public. Uryasz could hardly argue with a straight face, so he emphasized "trend evidence" to claim a dramatic decrease in muscle doping for NCAA football through his testing — but he still utilized the in-house numbers. All told in the 2000s, Uryasz and his employee collectors, along with his chemical technicians and out-sourcing to the UCLA lab, would reap a few hundred steroid positives from college football in Divisions I and II. They would conduct tens of thousands of tests to randomly sample roughly 20 percent of football players. Based on annual numbers of college players, if each man averaged about two football seasons then roughly 200,000 competed during the decade.

Dr. Don Catlin's criticism of conventional testing was significant — he was the patent engineer of testing instrumentation and directed the UCLA lab that analyzed NCAA samples for Uryasz and other contractors. Catlin was open about the limitations of conventional anti-doping methods employed by the NCAA, urinalysis technology and processing, especially to catch muscle substances. Catlin maintained a "false-positive" result was impossible for an innocent athlete, but he said an untold amount of dopers were evading proper results by the screening. "There are lots and lots and lots of false negatives, that's the problem," Catlin told *The Michigan Daily* campus newspaper in 2005. "The only way you can operate without false positives is to have false negatives. There are a lot of those, yes. We don't know how many."

Catlin noted substances and techniques to circumvent tests, saying the universal motive lay in winning and money, and college sports was no exception. Regarding undetectable designer steroids, Catlin said, "We don't know which ones the clandestine chemists are making or using. So we need somebody to tell us, which doesn't happen very often, or we need the government to go bust somebody like they did in BALCO." In separate comments via e-mail correspondence, Catlin stated, "I once calculated that I could make 2,000 unique new steroids in the anabolic family." A college strength coach echoed his concern about undetectable steroids, Ken Mannie, Michigan State, who stated, "The drug 'designers' are very well-versed on the mechanisms of the current testing technology and have the bioengineering expertise necessary to fool the system." Doping gurus were not "college kids delving in bathtub chemistry," Mannie wrote for *NaturalStrength.com*. "Individuals with serious scientific acumen are on a mission to produce the perfect performance-enhancing drugs — ones that build muscle and are invisible."

Online, how-to information for doping and beating NCAA tests made for regular chat in steroid forums. Many posts were from self-described college athletes, led by football players, with the vast majority of postings decidedly legitimate based on acumen in the topic. Intelligent and motivated, the college athletes discussed anabolic steroids, prohormones, HGH, drug sources, protocols, off-season tests, and more information, all focused on doping effectively and without detection. Sometimes athletes from high schools joined doping discussions with the big guys.

Irregularities or negligence in handling prescription drugs were found in athletic departments, including anabolic steroids ordered by a longtime physician for the University of Washington. The doctor, dismissed from UW duties, reportedly admitted dispensing medication like painkillers to softball players without medical exams. He also ordered testosterone gel which he said was for himself. *The Seattle Post-Intelligencer* reported the physician improperly prescribed "thousands of doses of banned substances and other drugs to athletes and staff members." Apparently no impropriety tied the physician to Huskies football, but an internal probe unearthed players of the past who said they acquired steroids from practitioners. In NCAA baseball of the 2000s, meanwhile, athletes and coaches alleged widespread steroid use. The witnesses represented various schools, including Duke and Barry University. These voices derided the lackluster administrative concern for doping in the sport that was picked apart at the pro level. Apparently the NCAA did not randomly test a single baseball player during at least one calendar year of the decade.

Male cheerleaders were linked to anabolic steroids by author Kate Torgovnick, informed of use at NCAA schools. Police, meanwhile, made steroid arrests among the general student body at Rowan, Central Florida, and Alabama. Elsewhere, college media reported that suspected and confirmed juicers crowded weight rooms frequented by students. Bars hosted body contests and other stimulating competition that ran on scantily clad physiques shaped by chemicals, male and female. Adderall and Ritalin scripts covered campuses, employed illicitly as off-label stimulants by students and faculty. Muscle substances were easy to obtain at virtually any university in America, according to a chorus of athletes, coaches, general students, and other observers. A federal office documented the simplicity of ordering online. "Our investigators easily obtained anabolic steroids without a prescription through the Internet," summarized the U.S. Government Accountability Office, reporting to the Committee on Government Reform.

Nevertheless, the NCAA and members maintained muscle doping was isolated, static among football players — their central theme for almost 30 years. As usual, society heard and went along with the relatively few objections, but one congressman had enough by March 2005, Rep. Joe Barton of Texas, who chaired the House Committee on Energy and Commerce. Barton, a former prep football player, blasted NCAA officials for proprietary mincing of words under oath in Washington. "You know...," Barton said at the hearing, sarcastic, "I am tired of people sticking their heads in the sand, and saying, 'I don't know how come that kid gained 50 pounds and improved his 40-yard dash two-tenths of a second. I just know he can do it. Go get them, Tiger.' [That] doesn't happen naturally. I lifted weights until I was blue in the face in high school, and gained five pounds. ... I am fed up. I don't want bureaucratic answers. I don't want gobbledygook. I don't want it [to be] the next person's problem. It is [an NCAA] problem, and the professional representatives... it is their problem. And if you don't clean it up, we are going to try to clean it up for you."

While most media still recited NCAA information about anabolic steroids and "student-athletes," or continued to just ignore the issue, some journalists were critical of prevention efforts in analysis and commentary. "In practice, the NCAA's testing is spotty, at best," reported Alan Judd, *Atlanta Journal-Constitution*. Alaina Zanin, student columnist and athlete, observed the public generally misunderstood "there are ways to circumvent the system" in both college and pro anti-doping. "This stems from several different reasons including lack of testing, inability to test for new products, and denial that it is even going on," Zanin wrote for *Murray State News*.

Many administrators presumed that testing foil HGH was beyond affordability for college athletes, but forum postings and media reports portrayed it differently, and Uryasz acknowledged the drug was used in NCAA sports. At Penn State, *Collegian* reporter Emily Davis located an athlete curious about growth hormone, John Cremo, who aspired to make the football team as a 5-9, 225-pound walk-on. "I want to be bigger than everyone," he said. "I would consider taking growth hormones if they were legal, but I would definitely talk to a doctor first to get the correct doses. I wouldn't do anything to hurt myself."

College officials bragged about "institutional" testing, or in-house screenings by schools, as a solid layer of deterrence. Critics charged ineptitude and obfuscation, however, such as at Michigan and Kansas, which did not discuss positive marijuana readings for football stars until reported before drafts through NFL officials. Michael

C. Lewis and Nate Carlisle, the *Salt Lake Tribune*, shredded the murky front around institutional drug testing in their 2007 report titled "Broken college system lets drug cheats slip through the cracks." Lewis and Carlisle outlined the foggy landscape of institutional testing and policy in the NCAA, providing a clear descriptions based on information gleaned from a survey submitted to every major football school. The journalists found fault, concluding:

> While many colleges and universities spend considerable amounts of time, money and energy on institutional drug-testing programs ostensibly meant to keep the competition fair and the athletes healthy, a *Salt Lake Tribune* investigation found vast inconsistencies, curious practices and uncertain accountability in the way the nation's major schools at the top-tier Division I-A level administer their programs.

Lewis and Carlisle discovered problems for institutional testing in areas such as the number of athletes tested, list of banned substances, testing quality, and the consequences for positive results. Some officials contested the findings, notably testing contractor Uryasz in Kansas City. Uryasz wrote a letter to the newspaper defending his urinalysis industry and the NCAA. The name of Uryasz's testing business was Center for Drug Free Sport.

NCAA President Bobs and Weaves about Muscle Doping

NCAA president Myles Brand discussed sport doping on television and on Capitol Hill in February 2008, when PBS host Tavis Smiley challenged him on topics that included the health of athletes and drug abuse. Brand, 65, was a former philosophy professor and president of Indiana University, touted as the "academic" NCAA president during his move to the association in 2002. Brand's familiar NCAA platform was "reform," like his three predecessors, with his stated mission to re-instill educational values. The mantra was recycled cliché, stressing academics before athletics and so forth. "The time when athletes pretended to be students, that day is over," Brand proclaimed boldly. He said pro sports were "entertainment," but not NCAA football and men's basketball. The rhetoric sounded ludicrous to critics, including academic experts in sports economy and public language, but the official talk was essential in one critical regard: Congressional members served notice that Brand's NCAA was under scrutiny as a non-profit organization enjoying tax-exempt status. Big-time football and men's basketball generated billions in tax-free revenue for the NCAA, member conferences, and institutions, but college sports had to promote education and amateurism to be considered non-profit.

Brand told Congress that NCAA anti-drug education, testing, and tough sanctions "have resulted in a very serious decline" for PED use by athletes. Politicians asked few questions, but Smiley got Brand one-on-one and pushed the official to further explain his talking points. Smiley balked when Brand purported the NFL was entertainment while the NCAA was "education," and the official backtracked. "There is a lot wrong with college sports," Brand conceded, "and some of it is even getting worse, rather than better, so there are problems." Brand added that "systemic problems" existed.

Drugs, however, were no such problem, Brand told Smiley. "We started testing in '86. We have the strictest testing rules out there, including the professional leagues," Brand said. "You're caught once, you're out for a year. You're caught twice, you can't participate in college sports ever again." Brand did not mention wide inconsistencies in institutional testing and penalty enforcement, nor did he note the appeal process allowing athletes to negate positive results by then adhering to the NCAA random testing policy. For Smiley and Congress, Brand spoke of "independent" and "transparent" testing without acknowledging the stonewalling of drug information, or that university and former NCAA personnel actually worked in the chain of command for sample handling. Brand did not detail gaping loopholes in testing nor mention crime, NCAA violations, and juicing that involved football players, coaches, and more systemic influences. He revealed nothing of the circumstances surrounding the scant positive steroid results turned up in NCAA football, and no one asked. Brand was not pressed about HGH, IGF-1, fast-clearing testosterone, and more undetectable tissue substances employed by college football players, nor did he not broach the subject.

Smiley did steer Brand into discussing football's mammoth sizes, 300-pound players in high schools and colleges, many qualifying as obese. Drug-pumped and -driven specimens of football were obvious now to every sort of public-opinion voice surrounding the game, athletes, coaches, organizers, doctors, politicians, media, and paying fans. The macabre evidence, the grotesque sizes of football players from teens to men, was "absolutely horrendous," Brand affirmed. "It's very dangerous for them, and it's a terrible precedent to set." the NCAA president spun for Smiley while at the same time contending that the college sports association was not to blame. Brand even absolved college athletes, basically passing responsibility for football's increasing sizes down a level in the sport. "It's so short-sighted of those parents," Brand asserted, "and that's who I blame, not the young kids as much — parents and the coaches. Those high school coaches or junior high coaches, I blame them. So short-sighted that the only thing that counts is winning. Your health counts, your integrity counts. To ruin your life so that you'll have a chance to play Division I football just doesn't make any sense in the world, and I'm glad those kinds of stories are coming out."

In fact, winning and football were paramount in the NCAA. A month after Brand's D.C. visit with the politicians and Smiley, a college senior became the next large player to succumb. The NCAA president, insulated again in Indianapolis, apparently did not comment on this story. Heath Benedict was a promising line prospect leaving tiny Newberry College for the NFL, a 6-6, 330-pound athlete who ran 40 yards in about 5 seconds flat — but he died of natural causes at age 24, alone at home in Jacksonville, Florida, in late March 2008.

Details trickled out about the athlete's health and possible drug use during his transition from college football to the cusp of the NFL, his dream. Ian Begley of *The New York Daily News* reviewed the Benedict case for a larger analysis of PEDs and heart-related mortality among athletes. One study had concluded a young athlete died about every three days of a sudden cardiac complication in America, but experts were certain of little. "The circumstances surrounding most of these deaths have been confounding," Begley reported, "and doctors have struggled to explain why so many seemingly healthy young people have been dying at such an alarming rate. They cite unpredictable abnormalities, and, with frequent resignation, the lack of research into finding a link between all of these incidents."

In Benedict's case, the medical examiner ruled the cause of death was an enlarged heart likely stopped by cardiac dysrhythmia, irregular beating. The decomposing body was found on a couch, clad in gym shorts and lying under a blanket. Nearby, according to reports, were a needle-syringe, two bottles of liquid labeled "L-Dex" and "L-Via," and a bottle of bacteriostatic water. The Jacksonville medical examiner's office noted "small red marks" on Benedict's left forearm, presumably needle punctures, but no testing was performed on the substances. Jesse Giles, deputy chief medical examiner, wrote, "The role, if any, of anabolic steroid or other similar drug/preparation use… is unknown and beyond the scope of this office." Investigators learned Benedict might have used liquid Viagra, which the "L-Via" could represent, while *The News* found athletes employed the drug in competition for quick delivery of oxygen, nutrients, and other drugs into the bloodstream. Begley reported "L-Dex" was a slang term for liquid Arimidex, a drug for treating breast cancer that juicers employed to "cycle off" synthetic steroids, to reduce estrogen levels and restart natural testosterone. Bacteriostatic water, meanwhile, could be mixed with HGH for injection. Benedict's father, Ed, told *ESPN.com* he did not believe his late son used anabolic steroids, noting the autopsy was negative for traces of such drugs.

Begley interviewed a range of doctors about heart-related deaths in sports, and opinions varied on whether PEDs play a role in the growing trend. Some practically recoiled at the suggestion, citing lack of clinical research, or negative autopsy results, but the arguments were "gibberish," said Dr. Gary Wadler, NYU associate professor of medicine, expert on PEDs, and a board member of the World Anti-Doping Agency. Wadler told Begley that many in medicine refuse to consider the potential impact of steroids, HGH, amphetamines, and other synthetics on the state of modern health. The substances often are not detectable in autopsies. "People say you can't really prove a [drugs-death connection] because there's no tell-tale 100 percent sign that people can point to," Wadler said. "They say you're just scaring people when you bring it up." A faculty colleague of Wadler agreed that concern is warranted within the medical community. "I think it's something that absolutely should be looked into, but I don't think we're looking at it as a problem," said Dr. Todd Schlifstein, assistant professor, NYU School of Medicine.

For the game enveloping young lives like Heath Benedict, the public's ignoring of potential problems is standard especially where college football is concerned. "Americans like their collegiate football and basketball just the way it is…," observed

Aaron Steinberg of *Reason Magazine*. Childs Walker, the *Baltimore Sun*, wrote, "Though steroid suspicions have become prevalent in pro sports, it's not clear that the public is ready to turn the same scrutiny on college athletes." Luke Andrews, the *Oregon Daily Emerald*, observed, "The NCAA — even with hundreds of athletes at each of its more than 1,000 member institutions — has seemingly gone unscathed during this turbulent period of drug-use allegations."

At Michigan State, columnist Drew Robert Winter decried society's passion for games and athletes while remaining disinterested in matters "that make a real difference to the public." Winter wrote for *The State News*, "Every weekend in bars, fraternity houses and stadiums, millions of Americans become overjoyed, irate or depressed about droves of steroid-laden strangers sweating their way to artificial glory." In contrast, some student commentators reflect a thoughtlessness for collegiate sports. "I don't care if Ivy athletes do drugs," opined Kamran Obscura for *The Columbia Spectator*. "It just doesn't make a difference to me."

III. Football Physiques: Smoking Gun, Health Menace

There existed no evidence of systemic muscle doping in American football — so said insiders, media, and fans. That was the basic public excuse during the problem's first 50 years. Approaching 2010, America continued to avoid potentially painful reform over drugs in football, preferring instead to gorge on the nationalistic blood sport as it stood. Indeed, on the eve of the recent presidential election, *ESPN* aired the final public interviews of candidates Obama and McCain at halftime during *Monday Night Football*, with Chris Berman posing the questions.

The smoking-gun evidence, meanwhile, remained right in the face of America, had for decades, at least since the 1980s when juiced specimens abounded. Now the old juiced bodies were unremarkable. Unnaturally large sizes of players are obvious at every level of football, viewed on television or in-person at the stadium. As Steve Courson maintained publicly for 20 years, he once toted around bagfuls of steroids in Pittsburgh, but no one had to peek inside for grasping reality. People need only see his build and that of others in football to understand the picture. "One of the reasons I was always open with my steroid use was because it was so apparent with my physique, and I thought it foolish to try to hide something so obvious, legal and tacitly condoned," Courson wrote to a former teammate in the summer of 2005, in correspondence never delivered. Courson continued:

> Take it from someone who admitted the truth long before society accepted it as so. Today, since speaking in front of Congress [again] and in my changed walk in life since my NFL days, I have been

> treated with more respect by the public than when I played. The public appreciates honesty at this point anyway; look at Mark McGwire and how pathetic he was. He would have fared better if he had just said he was entertaining the public, trying to save baseball and made a mistake. It's not like people can't figure this out, end of story.
>
> The local media knows what time it is with these drugs. I have perceived this... through their comments for a while. Currently, as of recent events, the media has decided to report this more openly and accurately. Part of that locally I believe is related to Mike Webster's death. BALCO had a lot to do with the change in reporting.
>
> After two trips to Washington I am definitely disheartened, but not surprised by the incredible (myth, image, fantasy, lie or synonym thereof) that NFL management continues to spin on this situation. It has reinforced my views as a person.

Many voices backed Courson about increasing sizes and juice in football, led by athletes active and retired from multiple sports, along with coaches, weightlifters, trainers, sports organizers, medical experts, media, politicians, adult fans, and schoolchildren. "When you talk about the NFL, what's the first thing you say? Guys who played in the 1970s would be a joke on the football field today," said Curt Schilling, baseball pitcher. Hard data founded the argument, weight statistics and comparisons spanning football during the age of pharmaceutical and bio-identical drugs. Among numbers, the starting offensive line of the 1958 NFL champion Colts averaged about 240 pounds while O-line starters for the 2007 Giants, Super Bowl champions, averaged about 6-5 in height and 314 on scales. The line's runt was center Shaun O'Hara, 6-3, 306.

Evidence suggested a concentrated wave of huge physiques first hit the NFL during the 1970s, and by the late 1990s the league had 200 players weighing 300 pounds or more. That number doubled the next decade, approaching the year 2010, with about 350 players of at least 300 pounds on game rosters and more than 500 in training camps. An additional 100 players hovered near the 300-pound mark. A *Scripps Howard* review found the average NFL body weights had increased 10 percent since 1985, before the start of steroid testing, to a 2006 average of 248 pounds. The average for offensive tackles jumped from 281 pounds to 318. "When I played, a 300-pounder was a freak," said Art Kehoe, Dolphins associate head coach and former NFL lineman. "Today, if you don't weigh 300 pounds, you are a freak."

For major-college football, 300-pounders were the majority among starting offensive linemen in 2008, and the size was consistent on rosters across Division II of the NCAA. At the prep level, top-recruited offensive linemen typically hit 300 on the scales — the online rating service *Superprep.com* often listed a dozen or more players at that weight among its top 40 prospects nationally.

Obesity contributed, particularly in teen players, but numerous witnesses and qualified observers said the 2000s football environment — still stuck on "bigger, stronger" — remained mostly about performance-enhancing drugs. Dr. Yesalis, the epidemiologist, strength coach, and weightlifter, repeatedly remarked God had not "changed the recipe" for humans, always citing additional material evidence of an embedded epidemic. Testing was invalid and football's documented timeline of muscle continually hardened. Organizers now acknowledged they were wrong about the 1980s, for example. Yes, they conceded in official consensus, the problem was in fact widespread during that decade. Confirmed history alone rendered anyone's claim of cleanup as illogical, given time's unfettered progression in performance that constantly placed current players as the largest and most athletic ever.

Nonetheless, the vast majority of active athletes, coaches, and organizers stayed with dubious excuses. They said gigantic physiques were due primarily to strength training and eating. "Fat" athletes had taken over the game, shoving aside muscled juicers, according to a company line voiced by NFL commissioner Paul Tagliabue, testifying under oath for the U.S. House Committee on Government Reform in 2005. "I think it's nonsense...," Tagliabue said of allegations about PEDs and sizes. "Today we have a young man who's 6-feet-6 and 268 pounds playing quarterback. Are we to conclude that he's using steroids? I don't like to smear people in that fashion."

Focusing on 300-pounders, Taglibue contended drugs made "athletes lean and sculpted" — like that quarterback he failed to fully describe as such — and declared "high body fat" beset the league's largest players. The 300-pounders "tend to be the antithesis of the sculpted, lean athlete," Tagliabue testified. The commissioner maintained contemporary players simply lifted much harder and ate much more than erstwhile specimens — who trained rigorously, consumed massive calories, and abused anabolic steroids but were significantly smaller than present-day behemoths.

The same essential testimony, if poorly enunciated, was heard from Dr. John Lombardo, Tagliabue's trusted NFL medical advisor on anabolic substances. "It's called morbid obesity," Lombardo asserted on the question of sizes, in perhaps his clearest statement. "If we have a problem in the NFL, it's the same problem we have with the youth and with society in general." A heavy man himself, Lombardo said football had transformed but drugs were no major factor, citing his tenure that began as a team doctor for high schools, continued as the Ohio State team physician in the 1970s and '80s, then carried through 15 years under Tagliabue with the NFL. Dr. Lombardo, remarking often non-scientifically or imprecisely, said, "I watched the linemen change from lean, fast people to people who were fairly big, fairly heavy, extremely heavy, somewhat obese, because the nature of the game changed," according to the government transcript.

Committee minority chairman Rep. Henry Waxman was not convinced fat athletes en masse were dominating modern pro football. Unnamed sources told the congressman that many players evaded NFL testing. Waxman listened to Lombardo about sizes then redirected questioning to the physician, specifically asking, "Is this just a natural phenomenon or is this the use of drugs? We don't see 300-pound roly poly players. We see 300-pound pretty strong, muscular players. So the number of football players that are much larger than the past is clear."

Lombardo replied, per transcript: "I'm not so certain that you see the 300-pound muscular players as much as you would think as much as the 300-pound roly poly players. I think we need to look at the body fat level of the players, and either one of us would be deemed to be correct on that. But I do think that's a potential, whether it's drug use or whether it's the nature of the game. If it is, like I said, these previous players arrive in the league at 300 pounds, they don't come in the league and then become 300 pounds. As far as the percentage of the people who use drugs, I think anybody's estimate is what I call the 'guesstimates' of people, because they have no idea what the percentage of drug use is in the league, and I would never hazard a guess as to what the percentage of drug use is in the league."

Gene Upshaw backed Lombardo — generally speaking — and Tagliabue during the union chief's testimony at the hearing. Upshaw likewise dismissed muscle doping as the key factor for sizes, saying random urinalysis was a certain preventive of that scenario. If anything, Upshaw said, colleges and high schools produced unhealthy football players. "They come to us the size that we get them," he testified.

In the same period, however, a 300-pound NFL player dropped dead at the age of 23: 49ers lineman Thomas Herrion, whose autopsy showed an enlarged heart and artery blockage. In addition, publicized studies found systemic hazards in league body weights. Within this context, management spoke differently than when testifying for Congress. Here the NFL contended that fat or unhealthiness *was not the* primary reason for player weights alarmingly in excess of healthy standards set by the universal Body Mass Index. Now officials contended the NFL primarily featured muscled specimens with low body fat, so the league could argue BMI standards were an invalid application for its athletes.

League medical liaison Dr. Elliot Pellman said the question of obesity among players still had to be answered by research. The league was commissioning its own studies. "There's a 1-in-200,000 chance that an individual the age of Mr. Herrion will suffer a sudden death," Pellman said. "It happens, and no one knows why it happens." Pellman said obesity was a *cultural* problem, not football's. Officials dismissed a study, based on the BMI, concluding that virtually all NFL players were overweight or obese. Bears nutritionist Julie Burns said NFL players were abnormally muscular humans. Taglibue said, "We have athletes that are fitter than most people in society, bigger than most people in society, and doing things that are different and more demanding than many people in society." PEDs, meanwhile, did not apply.

"Huh?" remarked Sam Donnellon, the *Philadelphia Daily News*, on mixed messages from the league. Basically, official football answers on increasing sizes followed that "fat" athletes were the foremost reason, not drugs; however, if criticism focused on obesity, not doping, then the players were portrayed as muscular and healthy, possessing uncommon physiology. NFL and NCAA rhetoric alike reasoned that modern players gained incredible mass without stuff like steroids, HGH, IGF-1, clenbuterol, and GHB. The necessary presumption held that substances readily available and potent were undesirable, obsolete for modern players.

Impossible, critics responded collectively, a growing legion of insider witnesses and close observers of football, including media, athletes, coaches, and doctors. They rejected official word on drugs from painkillers to amphetamines, anabolic steroids, and HGH. "Can it really be true that the NFL, with more than 300 players who weigh more than 300 pounds each, really has no drug problem?" dismissed Dave Perkins, *Toronto Star* columnist. "Where's the proof — other than the NFL saying it has no drug problem?" Sal Marinello always chortled at football drug rhetoric, contending the NFL and colleges were an historic haven for widespread PEDs. The strength guru wrote for *BlogCritics.org* that "off-the-field training, nutrition and legal modes of supplementation cannot be given credit for the ever-growing NCAA and NFL players." Several mainstream writers were cynical, such as Donnellon in Philadelphia, Paul Zimmerman, *Sports Illustrated*, Carol Slezak, the *Chicago Sun-Times*, Filip Bondy, the *New York Daily News*, and John Eisenberg, the *Baltimore Sun*, who wrote, "A wise doctor who knows about steroids once told me to trust my eyes above all when trying to detect abuse because, as he put it, lifting weights can only do so much. Well, my eyes are telling me that college football, like the pros, has more than its share of juicers."

Dave DePew, personal trainer and nutritionist, told *The San Diego Union-Tribune* he was turned off by pro athletes and PEDs, through with consulting for them. "Steroids will definitely help you, and I think most athletes know that," DePew said. "The unfortunate reality is that most of these athletes will take advantage if they know they're not going to get caught." Player agent David Caravantes said pro football wanted "guys who look like Tarzan and don't play like Jane." The late Lyle Alzado contended the NFL could have few genetic wonders packing extraordinary muscle at any size without dope, perhaps a percentile among a thousand bodies. Charles Yesalis extended Alzado's observation to include absurd sizes in college and prep football, and many agreed. "I think it's escalated even more, and the pressure on kids playing football, it's there," said David Meggyesy, 1960s NFL linebacker and retired union official. "If the steroids are there, they're going to do it."

"You can see all the signs," said Bill Curry, a coach and former NFL center, in 2008. "You gain 40 pounds over the summer, there's something wrong with that. All of a sudden you can't get your headgear on, and your jaws are doubling in size, and I'm callin' ya in and we're gonna do a test." Curry used anabolic steroids to make the NFL in 1965. In his day he saw 300-pounder players genuinely fat, but none could compete. "We just murdered 'em," said Curry, who peaked in weight at about 245. "You could keep them on the ground all day; that's where they wanted to be anyhow. They didn't want to run to the ball."

Fat was a factor for the largest modern players, Curry said, but he still saw drug use for their sustained speed and athleticism. More big bodies of the NFL astounded Curry, the many hundreds ranging from 250 to 300 pounds with tremendous strength, speed, agility, and minimal body fat. Summing up, Curry said, "Now you got guys that are cut-up 300 pounds, and then you got [athletes] that are 400 pounds who are obese, and they're out there in the heat and cold, and they're gonna die. When I watch an NFL game now, I find myself — I would love to just enjoy the football, but

I start worrying about [jersey] number 76. He's gonna die. Soon. He might die in this game, while I'm watching him. I know what he's been doing, and it breaks my heart."

"People want to see gladiators, and you just don't get that way by eating your fruits and vegetables," said Linden King, former Raiders linebacker and self-confirmed steroid user of the 1970s and '80s. Former NFL safety Bruce Laird, who retired in 1982, said there was "no question" drugs impacted contemporary sizes of players, whom he believed faced health risks in the present and future. "You know those guys aren't doing it on peanut butter, and beer, and whatever," said Laird, a leader in the retirees' cause for improved disability and pension benefits. Former defensive tackle Charlie Krueger said he saw anabolic steroids sweeping the NFL as he left in the early 1970s. Krueger was convinced muscle doping drove modern football, especially for requirements in size, strength, and athletic ability. "There are many large, large people in [pro] football, college football, and some in *high school* football," he said in 2008. "And they must be [juicing]. ... I'm glad I was gone before this stuff invaded because you would be forced to use it or lose your job."

Athleticism had hiked up along with sizes, impressing Krueger and many retirees to the point of intimidation. "They're up, they're ready, and they have those huge arms out there," Krueger said, erstwhile 49ers end and tackle at 240 to 255 pounds. "They're big, they can run... I'm glad I'm not exposed to that." Retired players and coaches expressed awe without addressing the question of PEDs. Former Giants quarterback Phil Simms was sympathetic of contemporary players like his son, Chris, a battered NFL quarterback. "The size of players today is unbelievable," Simms said. "I'm glad I played when I did. I wouldn't want to play now. They're too big for me." Former Cowboys coach Jimmy Johnson said, "Years ago a 340-pounder was a fat slob, plain and simple. Now he does not have much excess flab. These guys are working year-round to be fit, not just two weeks before training camp." Former linemen Mark Schlereth, a TV analyst like Simms and Johnson, dropped massive weight following his NFL career. "Muscles and bodies continue to grow and outperform the past generations," Schlereth said. "However, the connective joint tissues are the same since the dawn of time, so something must give."

A current official was pragmatic amid debate over Herrion and health. "Is it good or bad that the league is so big? It doesn't matter, because the players are not going to get smaller," said Giants GM Ernie Accorsi. "If anything, they are going to get bigger. Colleges are loaded with 300-pound linemen." A coach conceded PEDs were at least a factor. "I think part of this size thing happened because of steroids, the need to be bigger and stronger to compete with guys on the stuff," said Joe Bugel, Redskins line coach.

Science, Health, and The Increasing Sizes in Football

No scientific research focused on anabolic substances for football mass and performance, but some literature was pertinent. A pair of English researchers concluded modern athletes had likely reached physiological and mental limits for setting records in running. Their review of data found evidence of a "natural" plateau in speed and endurance for unaided human performance. "The results, of course, assume that athletes in the future do not benefit from scientific engineering or drug use," said professor Alan Nevill, co-author of the 2005 report that appeared in the journal *Medicine & Science in Sports & Exercise*. In America, studies indicated the average physical growth of citizenry had peaked following an industrial-age spurt attributed to advances in technology and nutrition. "Basically, since about the 1960s, there has been very little increase in the height of children or of the [U.S.] population in general," said Robert Kuczmarski, National Center for Health Statistics.

For questions about huge players, football people loved to employ the term "genetic wonder." Historically, organizers, coaches, trainers, and players liberally claimed human anomalies explained the game's incredible sizes en masse, not widespread drug abuse. Meanwhile, medical literature hardly referenced the alleged phenomenon of genetic wonder, and apparently no finding suggested a wave of human freaks had saturated sports. Gene research did offer possibilities like a specific mutation identified in mammals, with human examples among a minute number known of all species. "Scattered throughout the mammalian menagerie are a few super-muscular freaks," Emily Singer reported for *Technology Review*, "double-muscled cows more ripped than any bodybuilder; racing dogs too burly to run; sheep praised for their massively muscled buttocks; and even one small German boy, born in 2000 with muscles twice the size of those of a normal newborn."

Researchers found the mutation disabled a gene normally producing myostatin, a protein that regulated muscle growth, and the certifiable result was phenomenal mass. The German boy was humanity's first documented case, and an American boy was confirmed for the genetic mutation in 2005. A Johns Hopkins expert, Dr. Kathryn R. Wagner, qualified the condition as so rare that an accurate number among humans was likely beyond estimate. Obviously, such specimens did not widely populate America, much less football.

While science offered no support for football's theory of genetic wonder, a 1996 study published by *The Journal of Medicine* was firm that anabolic steroids could explain substantial gains in size and strength. Dr. Shalender Bhasin led the research, an endocrinologist specializing in testosterone deficiency and synthetic replacement in aging men. The team's primary scientific conclusion, finally corroborating years of anecdotal information about juicing, stated, "Supraphysiologic doses of testosterone, especially when combined with strength training, increase fat-free mass and muscle size in normal men." Forty-three men were randomly assigned to four control groups with standardized nutritional intake for 10 weeks: those receiving placebo injections while performing weightlifting; those receiving placebo injections without strength training; those receiving weekly, 600-mg injections of testosterone enanthate while lifting weights; and those receiving the testosterone injections without training.

The group lifting weights while receiving testosterone produced results far greater than the others, gaining an average 13.5 pounds of lean mass while increasing maximum lifts in bench press, 22 percent, and squat, 38 percent. In addition, the testosterone group without exercise gained more lean mass than the group lifting with placebo, and the former also produced relative equal strength data after the trial period.

Overall, valid scientific study on muscle doping was lacking, but a wealth of research supported increased health risks of football because of large bodies. Public debate on football brutality, the game's traditional issue, reemerged during the 2000s through concerns funneling back to physiques, including orthopedic injury, brain concussion, and physiological malady linked to excessive weight. Media examined topics like obesity and sudden cardiac death of young athletes, along with NFL retirees' body maiming, painkiller addiction, cortisone damage, and more disabling setbacks. The issue of healthcare topped the personal agenda of practically every American, and many NFL retirees banded together in complaints against the union administration of the fund for pensions and disability. Press analysis of health issues in football — including size statistics compiled by *Scripps Howard*, *Newsday*, and *The Palm Beach Post* — stimulated public discussion of medical information and witness opinion, so much that politicians dove in to stage a hearing on the disability issue in pro football.

Medical personnel said public focus on increasing sizes was overdue. "Football players have gotten so huge that it has become dangerous from a health standpoint," said Dr. David Bindleglass, orthopedic surgeon and former college player. "No one in the world loves the game of football more than I do, but it concerns me that players seem to get bigger and bigger, and intrinsically, there has to be some natural limit to it. … Rationally, you have to look at this and wonder where it's going." Cardiac surgeon Dr. Arthur "Archie" Roberts was an All-American quarterback at Columbia who later played three years in the NFL. "There's no question that the super-sizing that's occurred in the NFL, college and high school [levels] the last 30 years has tipped the scales in a negative way," Roberts said. "It means there is a serious alert for a health imbalance."

Dr. Joyce Harp, the University of North Carolina, led a study team that concluded more than one in four NFL players in 2003 qualified for class 2 obesity on the BMI, according to height and weight. About three percent of players approached 400 pounds, ranking them class 3 obese. The NFL labeled the conclusions invalid because its players were unique specimens of the human race, but no independent scientists objected to the research. Harp remarked, "I don't know what's going on in the minds of trainers, coaches or other people who drive what happens in the NFL, but clearly there's something going on when they have these guys getting so big."

A veteran player indicated something was up about steroids, if not injuries, while airing gripes at the league in 2008. Redskins cornerback Fred Smoot was mad about player fines over uniform attire. "I think they're worried about all the wrong [stuff]," Fred Smoot told Dan Steinberg of *washingtonpost.com*. "If you really want to do something, stop everybody from using steroids that's using steroids, instead of worrying about how the hell I'm dressed when I walk out there and play. You know what I'm saying? Worry about stuff that count, like people getting paralyzed."

Steroid comments like Smoot's remained exceptional, vague as his was, for the negative cast on the system. Active and retired players typically praised the system for drug prevention or said nothing in public, for longstanding reasons rooted in money and ego. "Everything is so undercover, and so hush-hush. Nobody wants to admit they were on it," said John D. Fair, historian and author. Fair, an amateur power-lifter, uncovered rare written evidence of Dianabol distribution and use, for his steroid history surrounding York Barbell, Dr. John Ziegler, and U.S. Olympic lifters like Lou Riecke, who was later strength coach of the Steelers under Chuck Noll. Even juicers of the distant past "want to make you believe that their gains were natural, by hard work and mental effort, that kind of thing," Fair said. "And there usually are no records kept in this."

In the controversy over NFL disabilities, opposing parties avoided mention of anabolic steroids and growth hormone. Despite the contemptuous discussion and allegations — sordid details like debilitating injuries, painkillers, amphetamines, dangerous weights, fraud, and personal bankruptcy — the topic of muscle doping slid by quietly. "That has not been part of the argument. No one's really brought that up," said Ron Mix, Hall of Fame lineman and an attorney in worker's compensation. "I got a feeling that's part of the equation. ... Just increased size by itself is an extra strain on the entire system, the skeletal system, the joints, and also the various organs. I mean, you have to be clinically overweight just to play [NFL] football now. That's a requirement. Just about every position, the guys weigh far more than what physicians say is the ideal weight for them."

Meggyesy said muscle doping was bound by silence in the league, "but there's a whole range of issues around injuries, and the elephants in the living room are performance-enhancing steroids." The retired player had a monetary interest for denying doping, such as healthcare and disability coverage, Meggyesy said, while management would not admit anything that left the league vulnerable. "It comes back to liability," he said. "It all comes back to who is responsible."

IV. Juicing Among Preps: 'Not In Our School'

As the high schools of America were drawn into national debate on anabolic steroids, prep coaches and officials maintained that use was minimal. Politicians and media expressed outrage, proclaiming that kids mattered while denouncing pro athletes as poor role models. Studies concluded teens used steroids, and kids said the drugs were accessible and becoming more popular, for enhancing looks as well as athletic performance. Critics called for tighter laws, steroid testing in schools, and funding for anti-steroid education. "The thing that is most scary...," said a government health official, "is the kids do it for what society would view as very positive values, winning and success."

That was the 1980s. Decades later, Dr. Charles E. Yesalis was amused with America acting as if the scourge were new, teen use of muscle hormones in pursuit of athletic stardom, ego fulfillment, and sex. Indeed, Yesalis helped pioneer studies on teens and steroids back in the '80s, when he heard the same denial he was hearing in the new millennium, from schools across the country: *There may be a problem elsewhere, but not here.* "It's always somebody else's kid. It's always somebody else's school," Yesalis said in 2005. For Yesalis, high-school representatives hardly differed from college and pro officials in their shirking of responsibility. "If I had $100 for every time a high school principal or coach said to me during the past 27 years, 'Doc, it's a problem, but not in our school,' I'd have a Ferrari sitting in my driveway," Yesalis told *The Houston Chronicle.*

Of the 16,000 plus football programs nationwide, perhaps there existed an American high school with never a juicing football player — improbable concept, said one expert — but apparently a significant portion had users. Nurturing circumstances for a national problem in prep football included a parental mindset for winning and performance enhancement, coaches who looked the other way, the lack of any impact prevention, and the accessibility of anabolic substances from steroids to HGH and supplements. Moreover, the football ideology of "bigger, stronger" ruled in continuum, predating steroids, the dangerous size obsession implanted for players at the prep level.

At least one prep coach considered gene doping by 2008. Media stories were fanning interest for genetic therapy's possible applications in athletics, and a prominent researcher, Dr. H. Lee Sweeney, the University of Pennsylvania, reported contact from a football coach at a high school. The coach wanted his players to try gene doping, the reputed cutting edge for muscle building, even if some experiments killed humans and lab animals. The coach "wanted to know if we could make enough serum to inject his whole football team," Sweeney told *Discover Magazine.* "He wanted them to be bigger and stronger and come back from injuries faster, and he thought those were good things." Sweeney declined, informing the coach his proposition was illegal and potentially dangerous.

Teens were familiar with anabolic steroids. Studies had long found steroid use at high schools, and news media disseminated reports of police busts and other information. After the BALCO story broke in 2003, authorities, media, and common citizens were increasingly vigilant about steroids. High schoolers were using for football, wrestling, baseball, and track and field. Some football programs hosted multiple teen juicers down to junior varsity, according to school confirmations and witness allegations. A former cheerleader recounted purchasing steroids from football players at her high school, telling media she sought toned abdominal muscles at 17.

News of juicing preps generated from Florida, Georgia, Virginia, Pennsylvania, New Jersey, New York, Connecticut, Illinois, Kansas, Louisiana, Texas, Arizona, Utah, California, and more states. The teen athletes mostly used steroids, but also growth hormone, experts said. In some instances football coaches and parents were identified as illicit sources of the drugs. In other cases, no reported links to teens, criminal charges for steroids and HGH were filed against coaches, teachers, and a district board president.

Parents regularly pestered pediatrician Dr. Bernie Griesemer in Missouri, seeking HGH prescriptions for athletic offspring, and he was publicized as a *critic* of such doping. "Everybody thinks they are going to retire on their children's sports incomes," Griesemer told *The New York Daily News*. In Dallas, athletic trainer Ken Locker knew of an 18-year-old football player who tested positive for steroids as a college freshman. "The parents admitted giving it to him," Locker told *The Morning News*. "They wanted him to get a scholarship." Only one prep football player in 17 would play in the NCAA, but many parents sought scholarships for their sons. One study found about 10 percent of parents polled knew of PED use by a prep athlete.

Often the pushy parents knew little about anabolic substances, never understanding they might channel children to drug use, said psychologist Dr. Robin Kowalski, Clemson University. "I'm not sure how many parents really sit down and think. Parents know there are some kids that use [steroids], but it's certainly not their kids." Football coach George Gatto, Bristol, Pennsylvania, said, "The expectations of parents are sometimes false. We would all like to think that our kids are going to play for Penn State or Michigan, but the reality is that it's only a small of amount of kids who can play at that level."

Prep players grasped their limits for advancing in football, measuring themselves against predator physiques they observed roaming college fields. "When colleges are coming around, everyone just wants to get bigger and better, especially now," said Lucas Cox, senior running back at Red Land High in Pennsylvania, who continued, "You see linemen in college that are over 300 pounds and you see linebackers that are 280 pounds. So everyone tries to get as jacked as they can." Kevin Perez, 275-pound lineman, was a blue-chip recruit at Miami Killian in Florida. "Looking at the college rosters forces you to gain weight," Perez said. "You go to the camps and see how big everybody is. I realized a 250-pounder wouldn't get recruited by a top Division I school." A coach acknowledged football's unreal standards, higher up the ladder. "Colleges like linemen that are 6-6, 300 pounds," said Derek Long, Westlake High in Texas. "They like running backs that run a 4.4 or 4.3 [40]. Not all of us have those physical attributes."

Some prep players attempted to eat their way into college football, but the necessary body package combined size, strength, and athleticism. Drugs offered little help for poor natural specimens, but good athletes could capitalize. "If a coach or someone offers them to you, there's a real temptation to do it to take yourself to the next level," Brad Artis, Canal Winchester running back, told *The Eagle-Gazette* in Lancaster, Ohio. "You see how fast and strong people get by doing it." Don Matheney, defensive lineman, said he did not use steroids but understood the forces at work, and the physiques of high school were intimidating enough. "I don't know if it's as much the guys on TV as it is seeing the guys you're competing against," he said. "You feel a little threatened, so some players take things to get an edge."

Former football players urged parents to heed threats of youth sports from steroids to injuries. Kansas City columnist Jason Whitlock, a large man and former college player, suggested other endeavors for kids. "I wouldn't criticize any parent who directs a child to stay away from organized sports," Whitlock wrote for *The Star*.

Former NFL lineman Brent Boyd testified about concussions before Congress in 2007. Suffering from vertigo linked to multiple head traumas in football, Boyd, 50, was reclusive and depressed, confining himself inside on a couch, "hiding from the world," reported *The New York Daily News*. "Right now…," Boyd said, "I would tell any parent don't let your kid play football."

V. Forget It: Football Fans, Most Media Don't Care

Football fans were psychologically incapable of facilitating change in football. Americans would not protest or fall disinterested in football, unless drugs were removed and mere mortals made to compete. Fans were enticed by winning at all costs and drugged-up supermen to stage the play, spill blood. Americans wanted their football, revered cultural tradition, regardless the costs. "You're talking about some powerful forces," ex-49ers lineman Charlie Krueger said in 1989, speaking of football injuries and the abuse of pharmaceuticals. "The only people who can change this is the fan, and the fan doesn't give a damn. The fans don't care, as long as they get their game. The owners put out a product, and the people want that product." In decades following Krueger's comment, market demand for the NFL only ramped up.

During the 2000s, several popular sports enjoyed retail immunity for issues such as drugs, injuries, and thuggish behavior by athletes, including abuse against women and children. The American public hardly blinked over a succession of sports stars exposed for performance-enhancing substances, other than to devour sensational details. By the end of President Bush's second term, a wealth of press coverage established that athletes relied on anabolic steroids, growth hormone, insulin, blood-boosting EPO, amphetamine and cousins, painkillers, and more to compete in football, baseball, track and field, cycling, and other sports. So-called isolated doping was rendered impossible, not only for sport but for the culture at-large.

Genuine outrage against doping athletes was not discernible. Grandstanding by politicians did not count nor did the booing of Barry Bonds. The mass popularity of sports continued to be measured in huge revenue and audience numbers. "Fan sensibilities have not been offended as much as they've been anesthetized," wrote William C. Rhoden, *New York Times*.

Sports columnists critiqued public apathy over sports doping. Veteran sportswriter Art Spander did not detect "the slightest bit of interest" among fans. Another long-time scribe, Jim Donaldson, *Providence Journal*, wrote, "Foremost among the things I've learned in more than 30 years of covering sports is that when values are in competition with winning, values almost always lose."

"If there was ever any doubt that athletes are made of Teflon, as long as they perform, the last few years have proved the point," wrote Gwen Knapp, *San Francisco Chronicle*. "They can be charged with rape, exposed as dopers or accused of beating their wives by their own children over 911calls, and their fans will rally behind them. Often, the adoration just grows stronger, because their heroes have been victimized by the media, or vindictive spouses, or calculating bimbos, or the French."

"Baseball fans don't care whether Bonds did or did not use steroids. *They don't care*," stressed Bob Kravitz, *Indianapolis Star*. "The things the media care about, the things Congress professes to care about, are of no concern to the multitudes who pay to watch Bonds hit baseballs."

Football, observers noted, had it much easier than baseball and individuals such as Bonds and McGwire. "I'm not saying it's wrong for baseball to come under attack," said Mark Fainaru-Wada, investigative reporter and co-author of *Game of Shadows*. "I think the question is whether football's gotten the attention it's deserved." Hank Steinbrenner, Yankees senior vice president, did not understand how football escaped doping scrutiny that dogged baseball. "I don't like baseball being singled out," Steinbrenner said. "Everybody that knows sport knows football is tailor-made for performance-enhancing drugs. I don't know how they managed to skate by. It irritates me. Don't tell me it's not more prevalent. The number in football is at least twice as many. Look at the speed and size of those players." Football fans did notice the game's increasing sizes, but only to marvel. They preferred not to see anything amiss. "Steroid scandals? After the 2004 Carolina Panthers went to the Super Bowl, it was revealed that several of their players had taken steroids," wrote Bruce Arthur, of *The National Post* in Canada. "But that became nothing more than a blip."

"Nothing in sports seduces Americans the way the National Football League does," wrote Michael Wilbon, *Washington Post*, continuing:

> The games have become a national sporting prescription, able to divert attention from just about everything that ails athletic competition, from Barry Bonds to Tim Donaghy to Michael Vick. … If it seems as if the NFL is bigger, better, smarter and more relevant, that's only because it is. People don't want to hear, particularly, that a Rodney Harrison has been suspended for HGH, or that an assistant coach, Wade Wilson, has been suspended. If a baseball player uses a performance-enhancing substance, he's a bum and a national disgrace; if a pro football player does it, he's just trying to, you know, get an edge, be all that he can be.

"It's a gladiator sport," said Todd Boyd, sport sociologist at USC. "People may give a certain amount of slack to football players because there's this unspoken sense that, in order to play the game well, you need an edge. That's what people want in a football player. Someone who's crazy and mean." Football players were "99.4 percent disposable," surmised Adam Gold, blogger. "Other than the true superstar players and the guys that hang around for an extended period of time, the players are interchangeable and completely expendable." Jim Souhan, *Minneapolis Star Tribune*, observed that "football combines two of the most powerful and popular aspects of modern American life: violence and TV." Some football fans were not concerned enough to act against doping. Dave Pell, self-described "NFL addict," wrote in an online post:

> I don't want to sound preachy here. But this is a game that is all about rage and violence. We are all sitting in front of the tube waiting for that perfect crushing and violent blow. And if we don't get it there, we flip on the Playstation and direct animated versions of our favorite players to crash into each other.
>
> Should players take steroids? Of course not. But pretending that the biggest health problem facing NFL players is roids is like holding hearings on the sport of boxing to determine if the corner stools are ergonomically correct.

Most fans wanted "good" football stories, the happy stuff, and media accommodated, following the Golden Press rule for making fans part of benign, trivial coverage. In turn, most media relished football and avoided stories about steroids and HGH. "Tailgating, and all the fanfare that goes with it, is one of the reasons I love college football," wrote Lya Wodraska, the *Salt Lake Tribune*. "But enough about my thoughts; we at *The Tribune* want to know what yours are." Wodraska continued:

> How is it that one sport can have so many reasons for loving it? Is it the tailgating? All the hoopla that surrounds the sport like the school band, the raucous student sections or the pranks pulled before big rivalry games? Don't forget that glorious run of bowl games at the end of the year. ... There are personal elements, too, like family allegiances and that old college sweatshirt that is faded, stained and threadbare but that you just can't bear to throw away. Doing so would seem like tossing away all those memories of post-game frat parties or countless Saturdays spent yelling at the TV.

Writing of the 2007 college team at Utah — where 1970s school officials distributed steroids to athletes and the late Thomas Herrion starred in 2003 — Wodraska asserted that playing football for the Utes was "a refreshing ideal in today's talk of steroids and contract holdouts, isn't it?"

Some critics in media saw social ramifications for over-indulgence in football mythology, but fans fired back. When the *Kansas City Star* columnist Jason Whitlock called steroid users "victims" of drug-sodden sport systems, reader Craig Davis responded in a letter to the editor. "As it is plainly evident, a person is a victim only when acted upon by a force outside of his control...," Davis wrote. "We don't care about cheating drug users. Steroid users choose to use, and as such, we have no sympathy whatsoever for them."

Whitlock, former college player, had writer allies in empathy for juicing athletes — and in criticism for ostrich fans and media. "We live in a culture that artificially manufactures superheroes, while at the same time wants to be told quick morality tales. It has an insatiable appetite for both," wrote author Laura Robinson, former Canadian rowing and cycling champion, for *The Ottawa Citizen*. Fans "must watch because they need men, who, thanks to performance-enhancing drugs are nearly as artificial as someone who comes from the planet of Krypton, to perform modern parables." Fans demanded "their heroes," said author David Wallechinsky. "They don't want a drug scandal. They want to look the other way."

VI. Football Liability: Game Issues, Real-World Threats

By 2008, I was impressed American football continued to get away with butchery, even killing. Like me, many former players saw through the football mythology, understood The Spectacle, the power of denial for issues that impacted the health of athletes. Popular sentiment held football as essential for American life, right? Yeah, we older guys heard that. What amazed us in the Post-9/11 world was how America continued to pick up the medical expense for football, to pay for the harm done young players and former athletes in their retirement. There were millions of us. Didn't America understand mere football profiteers — including the "nonprofit" NCAA and powerful athletic departments — continued to pass enormous healthcare costs to the public?

Clearly this country didn't mind footing the bill for stadiums, arenas, and practice facilities, paying billions in construction and renovation along with ongoing maintenance and security. Over the 21st century, the sport-entertainment domain would cost Americans billions just in loan interest and debt service — for capital borrowed and spent within the first decade. What the public didn't realized, apparently, was the fact *we all* paid for football's ravenous consumption of the vital talent commodity, the bodies of players — and for as long as they lived.

Society paid the lion's share for football casualties, short-term and long-term, in healthcare costs and insurance premiums. Costs compounded annually with hundreds of thousands of fresh injuries, leaving many young people with qualified disablements. Medical insurance for colleges and high schools paid some immediate coverage, but school and athletic officials often shifted costs to the injured individuals and their families. Barring death or catastrophic injury, a player assumed full healthcare costs once no longer listed on a school's game roster, whether by choice, graduation, or other medical condition. Future medical coverage and payments related to football were the individual's burden.

Every year, the nation's school districts collectively racked up a fortune in injury costs, and college football churned out its enormous medical expenses, incurred at the thousand or so institutions hosting their blood sport. Even major colleges liked to dodge medical expenses. "In fact, the NCAA, which reaps billions from the efforts of 'student-athletes,' somehow maintains its status as a nonprofit organization (with all the accompanying tax loopholes)," Wayne M. Barrett wrote for *USA Today Magazine*. "Yet, the NCAA doesn't adequately insure its athletes..."

The NFL was hardly better. Barring catastrophic maiming, retirees were responsible for their medical care until death, and many couldn't afford adequate coverage, especially among generations predating 1977 in the league. The atrocious physical condition of NFL retirees was thoroughly documented, mass orthopedic injuries, and accumulating research focused on concerns such as concussions. The disability and pension issue of NFL retirees blew up in 2006 and would continue for years, apparently, with public sentiment growing against management and the union.

"The richest sports league in America can't take care of its own," observed Gwen Knapp, *San Francisco Chronicle*, citing the case of 1970s lineman Conrad Dobler, in his 50s and facing a myriad of challenges in health and finances along with his wife, a paralysis victim. The league wasn't any help. "The way Dobler sees it, the NFL often dumps its medical problems on an unsuspecting public, either through social services or higher insurance costs for a player's future employer," Knapp wrote. Dobler said, "You see how they get the money for their stadiums. … They're always saying, 'Hey, let's get the public for some more.'" Charlie Krueger, former 49ers lineman, said, "Part of the cost of playing football is physical damage. The NFL has been able to get away with monumental monetary advantages without paying for it."

Surely the general public understood modern football was dangerous as ever. Every American saw vicious collisions of pro and college up close and repeatedly on video, supported by hard data of sizes, speeds, and casualties. Contact death had not occurred for decades in mass-marketed, entertainment football, the 32 NFL franchises and 70 or so big-name schools — each a valued brand name of American football — but disabling injury was common in the variety of shattered bones and ripped knees, tendons, and shoulders. The tragic cases included brain traumas and crippling paralysis, with the latter much less frequent but more publicized. "The health consequences of high-impact sports is not just an issue for old timers. Increasing numbers of present-day players are reckoning with the short- and long-term consequences of concussions and cranial trauma," wrote Dave Zirin, cultural critic on sport, for *The Nation*. "This is partly because there is far more research and awareness about concussive injury. But the game is changing: Players today are bigger, stronger and faster then even ten years ago."

The reality of football destruction and death had been quashed, minimized, disinfected to the extent it rolled by out of sight save for the relative few witnesses to genuine horror. Victims of serious injury and their families endured terrible tragedy of American football. If the game indeed taught positive values to untold young athletes, it should have, because the other side was much darker than commonly portrayed.

The game outright killed 1,006 players during the 77 years through 2007, for example, including at least one girl, and led to deaths of 683 more players, including of heatstroke and cardiac arrest, according to statistics of the National Center for Catastrophic Sports Injury Research, University of North Carolina-Chapel Hill. In addition, the center reported 278 catastrophic incidents classified as cervical-cord injuries, affecting the region of spinal column to brain. Many victims did not recover fully from damages in motor and neural function, and I could vouch for other types of paralysis the center did not track. My right foot remained 90 percent "dropped" with paralysis of a nerve shredded at the knee in 1982, sustained playing college football. In the same season, the Catastrophic Injury Center logged 11 cases of cervical-cord injury.

Raw data, stark as it may be, was not the full story, though. To paraphrase the butcher Joseph Stalin, from his staff briefing on fine propaganda, the public viewed 5,000 deaths as a statistic but one victim's story as tragic. Maybe that was why the media routinely reduced football deaths to the few lines of a brief report, and the game and fans demanded it that way.

When I was a newspaper sportswriter, I penned a column titled "A Player Dies Quietly in Football America," recounting a college player's collapse in Georgia. The local prep coach complained to my editor. He said I made it difficult to recruit kids to play, and he was correct. I liked the coach, even understood him to a point. He certainly took as much precaution for the heat as possible with his team, while also properly conditioning players for the trying task of competing. My point was the game could never be safe enough, regardless of anyone's good intent, and I was a messenger, not a recruiter. Elsewhere, I was agape in seeing researchers, doctors, claim the game could be made "safe" through rules enforcement or technology. Impossible!

Regarding football horror stories, the Stalin rule applied: More detail on victims altered the response. Even the cold, calculated annual report of the Catastrophic Injury Center could chill the blood with its additional notes on cases nationwide. The research encompassed all types of football, pro, college, prep, sandlot, and youth leagues, with financial grants and statistics contributed by the NCAA, the National Federation of State High School Associations, and the American Football Coaches Association. The 2007 report covered football involving about 1.8 million participants, including 1.5 million at junior and senior highs and 75,000 in college football.

In 2007 there were four direct deaths in football, nine indirect deaths, and eight injuries of the cervical cord. Less impersonal details were found in the report's case descriptions, including the following on non-fatal injuries:

> A 17-year-old high school football player was injured… while being tackled in a game. The helmet of the tackler hit the ball carrier under the facemask and drove his head back. He had a fracture of CV-5 and had surgery… At the present time recovery is incomplete. A 16-year-old… had a collision with a teammate while rushing the passer. He is quadriplegic. A 17-year-old… was hit in the head by the knee of the ball carrier. He was [5-6] and weighed 140 lbs. Recovery is incomplete. A 16-year-old… was a ball carrier fighting for extra yards when he was hit by another tackler from the front. He had surgery and recovery is incomplete. He is presently in a rehabilitation center. … A 16-year-old high school football player was injured… Contact was head-to-head with the tackler. He collapsed after the game… The injury was subdural hematoma with surgery and incomplete recovery. A 17-year-old… was involved in a number of hits during the game and it was not possible to say which hit caused the injury… diagnosed as

a bleed in the brain. The player had surgery and was in rehabilitation.

The football year's four direct fatalities involved collisions, per the definition, and death was not immediate in three cases. Indirect deaths involved various circumstances attributed to football. Samples of case reports included the following:

> A 14-year-old middle school football player was injured while tackling… was diagnosed with a brain injury. After two weeks in a medically induced coma he died… An 18-year-old high school senior [6-5, 275]… was being tackled at the time of the injury. Contact was made by the helmet of the tackler. Injury was diagnosed as internal, with damage to the spleen and small intestine. The athlete died [a month after injury]. A 13-year-old… was injured while being tackled from behind with a blow to the head. The injury was diagnosed as an acute subdural hematoma. … The athlete died [a day later]. A 25-year-old World Indoor Football League football player was injured… a helmet-to-helmet tackle. He was [6-1] and weighed 180 lbs. … Injury was diagnosed as a brain injury and he was dead on arrival at the hospital. …
>
> A 17-year-old collapsed at practice… and died [a week later]. He was running laps at the time and cause of death was heart related. He did not have a physical exam before the season. A 16-year-old… received blunt trauma to the knee during practice… He died of a blood clot that broke loose to the lungs, [a] "pulmonary thrombi emboli." A 17-year-old… collapsed at practice… and died at the hospital the same day. Cause of death was diagnosed as heatstroke. The player was [6-4] and 290 lbs., and the temperature was 100 degrees. … A 19-year-old college freshman football player collapsed and died during a team workout… He was [5-11] and weighed 210 lbs. He was working with weights at the time, and cause of death was heart related.

Beyond cases of direct and indirect fatalities, at least three more deaths were reported around football in 2007: a 14-year-old with a torn aorta; a 17-year-old who died in his sleep; and a teen player who died playing touch football following a team lifting session, caused by an aortic aneurysm, according to the Catastrophic Injury Center.

I saw several problems affecting the future business of football, including for the vaunted NFL, whose fans consumed anything, and I wasn't alone. "The fact that the public may not care isn't the issue and doesn't change the facts and indications that the NFL is sitting on a powder keg," observed Sal Marinello, *BlogCritics.org*. Franchises and doctors had already been sued for abuse of pain-killing pills and shots, a well-publicized discussion for 40 years. In 2008, Patriots offensive tackle Nicholas Kaczur was charged with misdemeanor possession of oxycodone pills, part of a larger investigation, and Giants tackle Shane Olivea said he kicked a painkiller habit after intervention by loved ones. "Seeing my family [gathered] in my living room… seeing how hurt they were and the pain I had caused them was pretty humbling and gut wrenching," Olivea told reporters. Hero quarterback Brett Favre was documented with a painkiller addiction back in the 1990s, and I thought it impossible for him to continue through the next decade without the stuff. "I don't think anyone comes with 'no baggage,'" Favre said in 2006. "And I'd be the first to say that I had my share of troubles and addictions…" The next season, Favre endured shoulder and elbow injuries in his throwing arm, saying he could "shoot up and still play."

I would always remember Dolphins great Jake Scott, rebel model of mine for rejecting the bullshit of football. Scott told coaches to kiss his ass from high school to the NFL, particularly Don Shula. Scott was the MVP of Super Bowl VI — with two pickoffs to secure victory over the Redskins and literally hand Shula his 17-0 season — but he disappeared from the game after retirement, ignoring media queries and Dolphins functions. "There is an odd nobility to the man with his back to the parade," Greg Cote, *Miami Herald*, characterized in 2006. Football disobedience likely cost Scott his deserved place at Canton and certainly his spot on the Miami roster in 1976, for refusing a team doctor who wanted to inject him with xylocaine during an exhibition game. Scott played the second half without drugs, but Shula suspended him for insubordination and traded him to Washington. Painkillers were problematic in NCAA football as well as the NFL, yet officials liked to blame player addiction on society.

The plague of brain concussions was a certifiable legal nightmare for the NFL, given the union's court defeat by the family of the late Mike Webster. The estate finally prevailed at the U.S. Court of Appeals, Fourth Circuit, a 3-0 decision in December 2006, and collected $1.5 to $2 million in retroactive disability benefits, interest, and costs. There were more Mike Websters out there. Battered bodies were evident among retirees, garishly displayed at team reunions and other public gatherings, when young and middle-aged men hobbled and jerked about on replacement parts. A few guys motored by wheelchair. "It's an orthopedic surgeon's dream," union official Miki Yaras-Davis said of such a sight in 1995. "[Retirees] all have the crab-like walk, and it's hard to believe they were once these feared gladiators. Forty-year-old players are having the same problems as 80-year-old men." In 2002, veteran Raiders lineman Trace Armstrong met many retirees as president of the players association, "and some of these guys don't look so good," he said. "Young men, onetime great athletes, but they don't move around so well." Armstrong, himself facing retirement, had 16 surgeries by his latter 30s.

The obesity issue of players loomed for the game as a whole. There were already lawsuits, notably for NFL heatstroke fatality Korey Stringer, the enormous Vikings tackle who succumbed in training camp. Research doctors and other medical experts collectively reviewed thousands of football specimens, teens to middle-aged men, and generally concluded risks were apparent, including for cardiac disease leading to complications like enlarged heart syndrome.

Heatstroke continued to kill in football, mainly kids, despite the game's horrific record of four deaths in a week during August 2001, including Stringer. Everyone in football vowed to forever avoid this *completely preventable* condition but the promise fell broken. In 2006 five players died of heatstroke, for example, ages 11-17. For cardiac death, meanwhile, researchers corroborated alarming rates of fatalities among athletes, all ages and types.

Nonetheless, as football continued with its grotesque sizes, a few researchers overlooked the obvious health risks, proposing the NFL had genetic wunderkinds immune to problems universally documented. As far as I was concerned, those scientists played a political game, pursuing crackpot theses for publicity if not prostituting their credentials for special interests. Many observers were incredulous, including sports columnist Ron Kantowski, the *Las Vegas Sun*, whose physician instructed him to lose weight at 6-1, 200 pounds. Herrion had dropped dead at 6-3, 310 pounds, yet football folks and scattered doctors defended the NFL. "Thus, it boggles the mind there exists an occupation where a man only two inches taller than me but some 110 pounds heavier is considered physically fit. Or, at least, physically normal," Kantowski wrote.

Big people in football were widely associated with anabolic substances and danger, not surprisingly. Eyesight and common sense constituted enough study for the assumption. "Evolved Reality is this: It's starting to feel like a significant segment of the NFL is on drugs," observed Chuck Klosterman for *ESPN The Magazine*. A Chicago physician, Dr. Terry Simpson, saw evidence of malpractice in examining and treating former players of the NFL, damage left by cortisone and xylocaine injections of the past, and he expected disablement rates to increase because of muscle doping and sizes. "Steroids contribute to the overall injury patterns," Simpson told *The New York Daily News*.

Steve Courson had little doubt sizes and drugs contributed to health maladies, such as the cardiomyopathy he worked for years to overcome. "I believe the NFL is a prisoner to [its] own public relations myth," Courson wrote in 2005, continuing:

> They try to sell the image of a "crusader" like purity of sport image, when reality is so different. Large amounts of money automatically make it "mercenary" in purpose and invite corruption. ... The level of deception and exploitation that the NFL requires to do business still amazes me. Today, at least the players are better compensated for their compromises. This is particularly true in the area of performance-enhancing substances. The coercive aspect of this and the system's refusal to acknowledge that obvious fact speaks volumes for the level of control that it employs.

Active players themselves acted oblivious, befuddling outsiders as intended. Despite the evidence of a doping epidemic, players would outright deny it, and in turn the public wondered why so many would unite in a flimsy lie. Many retirees were prone to acknowledging a problem, but they didn't say much. "The guys that we knew... were doing it, we would never say anything about them," said Bruce Laird, former safety. "It's just locker room stuff." Self-acknowledged steroid user Bill Curry, who juiced decades ago, believed players and coaches were ashamed of drug abuse. "It's hard to come clean on it if you did if for a long time. It's easy to come clean in my little story [of brief use]. That's like a Sunday School story," Curry said, adding "no coach can look me in the eye and say, 'Well, gee, I didn't know [a player] was doing it.' " Curry noted monetary concerns hindered open talk. "Sadly, as in the case of most human experience, it's going to take maybe a series of disasters that are obvious. ... We don't do anything until there's a disaster, until everybody feels it. And when everybody *feels* it, then we'll do something that's very, very serious, but not until."

Money was definitely the impetus for denial by many juicers past and present, along with the league and union administration, according to numerous insiders. Silence or denial was "a self-interest thing," said Meggyesy, who didn't use steroids as a player but knew juicers as a union official. "Look, you go to apply for a medical claim or disability, and you can be denied this claim because you used steroids. You know how insurance companies are. For Christ's sake, any reason you can provide them to *not* cover you..." In 2004, Giants center Shaun O'Hara echoed Meggyesy as he denied steroid use to inquiring media. "How can we ask someone to insure us if we're doing something harmful to ourselves? The insurance companies would never do that," O'Hara said.

Insurance carriers in the U.S. market struggled mightily in the 2000s, with liquid capital always subject to wipeout by global events such as terrorism, war, natural disaster, and collapsing economy. American football felt the heat too, long overdue, despite the nationalistic sport's appeal to the insurance industry as sort of a loss leader. Football could still acquire coverage for medical and liability, but premium and deductible rates skyrocketed for sports overall during the decade of disaster, as they should have. American football was increasingly exposed and defeated in civil suits — or predisposed to settle — for its inherent hazards and casualties.

Coaches, trainers, and other personnel gambled on, despite knowing they stood legally vulnerable in potential injury situations involving athletes and even fans — especially at the prep and college levels. On the matter of concussions, for example, NFL commissioner Roger Goodell suggested football's lower levels had more to worry about, and he was correct. For sheer numbers of football participants and lack of resources, fertile litigious conditions existed over unavoidable shortcomings at school districts and colleges, such as inadequate health screening and medical support, and insiders knew it. Kids understood it. Injury "waivers" for football, signed by parents and athletes, were mostly legal ploy anywhere in America. What taxpayers didn't get, they paid too, especially in the event of an athlete's death or catastrophic injury, which meant a huge deductible, as high as six figures, and more costs not covered by insurance.

The insurance industry closely monitored the issue of PEDs in American football, and had since the 1980s, when carriers began dropping the sport for steroid abuse and injuries reported by media. In 2007, as Texas mandated worthless $6 million random testing for prep sports, one high school required parents of football players to sign a "Steroid Dangers Acknowledgement form."

Moving forward in the young century, the institutions of insurance, healthcare, and education were all cash-strapped while the legal peril grew in litigious America. Already, insurers had dropped coverage on numerous hazardous activities at schools and colleges, from rope climbing in PE class to pyramid building by cheerleaders. Football had slid by thus far, likely since it was institutionalized in schools and culture, but this was a money issue, after all. Forces were converging beyond the game's control, even the all-powerful NFL's, and it was anyone's mistake to presume football could roll forward in its present form.

Football reform lay dead ahead for absurd injury and illness — and financial costs — requiring the reversing of drug use and player sizes, particularly for colleges and high schools. The monetary costs alone would mandate change, if not real concern for young people, and the courts, insurance, and healthcare would carry it out, if football wouldn't of its own volition. Approaching 2010 in America, with a scary, tough world coming down to roost atop our heads, deflating our formerly insulated cocoon of consumerism and pleasure, the sane choices to make about football began with the athletes, coaches, and other officials.

VII. Perspective, Proposal: Limit Sizes, Improve Health

The reality was obvious: American football was beset by muscle doping and related systemic problems at all levels by the 2000s, professional, collegiate, and secondary school. The primary evidence was increasing sizes, the documented history of anabolic drugs in football (steroids from about 1960 followed by human growth hormone, clenbuterol, GHB, IGF-1, and more), and the inability to produce a valid system of testing. Football's widespread problem of the past was confirmed even by present-day officials, rendering illogical their claim of effective prevention, given the environment's humongous athletes with various body frames weighing in at 250 pounds and up at all levels of play.

Urinalysis, the standard theoretical option for combating doping in football's vast domain, was proven a failure for detection and practicality. Steroid testing, either random or scheduled, would flunk as a grade-school chemistry project, with no chance of meeting its objective because of loopholes. The null hypothesis prevailed: Urinalysis could not prevent doping in football, although incessantly promoted by the sport's doctors, employee scientists, and other associates of the game. The entire player population, preps to pros, could juice with impunity through undetectable steroids, HGH, and more tissue-building substances. Even the NFL, easily the game's most controlled and resourceful environment for battling doping, could not prevent systemic use among its 1,700 athletes and personnel such as coaches.

Invalid urinalysis, random or scheduled, was exploited through huge loopholes. The technology was limited for detecting substances, and the relative few players subject to testing understood calendar gaps of the process for employing patent steroids. "Fear" of testing was marginal among users, trumped heavily by their confidence and motive for evading detection. The technology was utterly useless at the college and prep levels for its detection faults, lack of funding, and logistical barriers. In 50 states and the District of Columbia, college football had thousands of players at about 1,000 institutions while 1.5 million comprised prep football, scattered among more than 15,000 districts. The average cost of a steroid test was about $100, and a positive result could lead to court litigation, given the cultural factor of sports-minded parents bent on winning.

In addition, so-called Olympic testing was no answer for American football, despite incessant hype from officials of WADA, USADA, the USOC, and IOC. Expert critics lined up globally, detailing insurmountable loopholes in the conventional testing of Olympic athletes, and a primary engineer of the technology agreed, Dr. Don Catlin. "I don't think we've done anything that really ameliorates the problem; we've just pushed it into different areas," Catlin said, noting that athletes and clandestine chemists always found substances and techniques to defeat screening. Dr. Yesalis believed designer steroids, invisible to screening, keyed many false-negative results for dopers. "You don't know the hot drug, nor do I," Yesalis said in 2006. "When we find out about stuff, they've already gone on to the next one. Growth hormone's use in athletics is as big a surprise as the Army Jeep. … The real secret stuff is new designer drugs." Designer steroids were associated with notorious gurus and superstar athletes, but the drugs could reach any person through over-the-counter supplements, according to investigative reports by Amy Shipley of *The Washington Post.*

The NFL and NCAA, conducting a thin ploy amid the hot steroid politics of the 2000s, promised to begin effective year-round testing, which they originally claimed to do in 1990. "I'm not sure anyone has worked out the logistics yet, but they are supposed to be doing year-round testing," trainer Dave Binder, the University of New Mexico, said in 2006. "They called it year-round in the past, but this is really it." Anonymous NCAA football players, however, stated they knew of no testing in their programs during summer break. Regardless, off-season or out-of-competition testing had proved impractical for anti-doping in Olympic sports and cycling, primarily for excessive costs, logistical impossibilities, and privacy issues. "No-notice out-of-competition tests are easily dodged despite the rules," wrote Robert Weiner, former White House drug policy spokesman, and Cael Pulitzer, sports policy analyst, in their co-commentary for *The Seattle Post-Intelligencer.*

A greater impracticality for prevention in football was proposed blood testing, including "bio-marking" a body's physiology for doping signs such as fluxing levels in proteins and testosterone. Among challenges, serum analysis in America would require heavy funding, qualified personnel, and likely litigation. Moreover, experts worldwide ridiculed WADA's purported HGH blood test, calling it questionable science. Since the 2004 Olympics, thousands of HGH tests had failed to produce one positive result. Independent experts also questioned the experiment of bio-marking practiced sparingly by the USADA and on a wider basis in cycling.

Meanwhile, bio-identical substances, stem cell therapy, and gene transfer technology — or "gene doping" in sports parlance — promised a new wave of undetectable doping for athletes. Gene doping might have hit sports as early as 2005, a German court case revealed, when a track coach tried to purchase Repoxygen, the gene-therapy drug for boosting red blood cells in anemic patients by manufacturing extra EPO. Athletes and coaches worldwide contacted Dr. H. Lee Sweeney at Penn University, inquiring about gene transfer he employed to create "super mice" with bulging muscles and incredible performance. Scientists engineered hybrid animals such as cows with disease immunity, salmon with rapid growth, and eco-friendly pigs that produced low-phosphorus manure. "Some athletes will want to use gene doping to create super-strong muscles. Some will want to increase the supply of red blood cells so they have greater stamina," said bio-ethicist Thomas Murray, president of The Hastings Center.

The process entailed the needle insertion of a plasmid composed of a virus and a gene — such as a gene for fast-twist muscle development — into a host's particular muscle group. The virus carried the new gene through cellular walls for proper uptake. Sweeney doubted gene transfer could be detected by anti-doping in sports, but WADA claimed its scientists were making progress. A muscle biopsy would probably be the only way of finding the telltale transport virus. Sweeney planned to introduce a commercial product for dogs in 2009, gene therapy to treat muscle wasting or immobility, and he anticipated that calls from the sports world would increase. "I think the real threat is from scientists and clinicians who decide they want to make money off the athletes to make this available," Sweeney told *The London Telegraph*.

More experimental substances and techniques enticed athletes and associates. "I think there's a whole new horizon for anabolic therapies, and the potential for abuse will be exceedingly high," said Dr. William Evans, the University of Arkansas. SARMS, or selective androgen receptor modulators, locked into steroid receptors of specific muscle groups to foster growth, and myostatin inhibitors blocked the protein that halted expansion of muscle. Prior to the Beijing Olympics, *Sciencentral.com* reported substances reputed to be myostatin inhibitors were sold in China, Korea, and online. Sweeney found that injecting IGF-1 into target areas stimulated specific muscles, and an injectible "HGH releaser" was on the market, Sermorelin, said to stimulate the pituitary gland for secreting more of the hormone. "MK-677," a similar substance, stimulated production of HGH and IGF-1 in older adults. Resveratrol was another prospect for performance enhancement in athletes, as a drug said to boost endurance and lifespan in mice and rats.

So, with the undeniable failure of conventional testing, what could be done about muscle doping in American football?

The historic argument of game abolishment lingered in citizens like M.E. Davis in Missouri, angered by Stringer's unnecessary death of heatstroke. "It calls attention to the stupidity, callousness, inhumanity and cupidity of the 'game' of football and all who promote it," Davis wrote to *The Post-Dispatch*. Abolishing football wasn't widely discussed, but in the wake of BALCO's exposure many media and policymakers believed Congress should handle the drug problem for sports. However, politicians accomplished nothing in years of wasted time, expense, and misinformation. Public patience had diminished for federal investigations into scattered individuals, even superstar athletes like Barry Bonds and Roger Clemens.

Law agencies did make progress in combating PEDs during the 2000s, but they were incapable of tackling the problem alone. Many police personnel were juicers themselves, with hundreds exposed for purchasing, distributing, or using anabolic steroids and growth hormone. In addition, the notion of teaming law enforcement with sports organizers to share information and bust athletes was badly misguided, given Constitutional rights and the potential for abuse by athletic organizations with historic, ongoing complicity in doping.

The overall hypocrisy and ineptitude of traditional anti-doping policies and programs led to the increasing public call for "legalizing" synthetic performance enhancement in American sports. The argument completely aligned with the culture's prevalent value for success through virtually any means necessary, or true American ethos, and it certainly merited discussion for leagues comprised strictly of adult athletes. In addition, pro sports like the NFL already *allowed* anabolic drug use for select athletes, although mostly unknown to the public. The "therapeutic use exemption" in policy sanctioned tissue-building substances for diabetes and other medical conditions, including dubious "hormone deficiency" problems that doctors legally "diagnosed' in younger men without pituitary or testicular damage. Moreover, the simple brutality of football at the pro and college levels mandated the use of painkillers and anabolic drugs, if not stimulants, yet only athletes remained at a punitive risk for exposure.

Throwing open the barn door to PED use at the prep level was untenable, however.

The Courson Plan: Hope for Immediate Prevention, Longer Success

The Courson Plan for the immediate prevention and future control of muscle doping in football was rather simple by composition, largely drawn from the elements of the *marketplace of ideas*. I was forever fond that the Courson Plan evolved in American fashion. The marketplace of ideas was the great Colonial vision for public debate, including the hearing of falsehoods. With rhetoric in the open, everyone could arrive at sound conclusions. The Courson Plan perfectly demonstrated the practice of democracy.

For eight months Steve and I mulled together ideas reported for possible prevention, and we added a few ideas ourselves. We framed a common theory in agreement, although unwritten at the time of his death, basing it on the reduction of player sizes. We capped the weights in a reasonable, equitable manner, especially for the high schools and colleges. Our big disclaimer was the method could never make football safe, much less fully eradicate doping, but it would undoubtedly improve the environment, especially for youth, at least until better ideas came long.

Given the quantifiable data of football sizes in 2008, The Courson Plan would turn back body weights while very likely reducing risks of drug use, obesity, and physical danger in competition. At least one writer was thinking in the same general approach, although separate from us: Sam Donnellon of *The Philadelphia Daily News*, who specifically noted the BMI for possible use. Several writers of the decade, including Dan O'Neill of *The Post-Dispatch*, called for size limits in general.

Steve and I also agreed on certain components of traditional anti-doping that were compatible in their proper forms. We advocated that police should enforce the law where applicable and that anti-doping education continue based on earnest, straight talk — absent of scare tactics about known health risks and without presenting juicer suspects as so-called role models for abstinence, specifically NFL players and otherwise abnormally large athletes. We endorsed public and private funding for research and development of effective anti-doping strategies, from new testing to educational upgrades. We endorsed sound, vigilant medical precautions and care around football participation, including heart screening for every player as part of a thorough and regular checkup. Without these precautionary policies, a school, college, or pro franchise should not host the dangerous sport.

Based on our personal experiences and through decades of study, Steve and I believed anabolic substances contributed to health problems that struck each of us in the near and long term. He was almost certain that the incredible size and exertion he maintained for football contributed to his heart condition, and I believed potent injections of testosterone contributed to the hyper-extending and shredding of my right knee. Like our friend and collaborator Chuck Yesalis, we were convinced performance-enhancing substances were the foremost reason for the ridiculous sizes of football players beginning in the 1960s. In turn, founded on what we experienced and acquired, we believed that football sizes posed a national health menace for young males. After Steve's death, for example, an Iowa State study determined 9 percent of Iowa prep linemen were obese by BMI standards. Such dangerous health conditions of adolescents could not be tolerated by a civil society for its institutionalized, nationalistic sport.

Therefore, The Courson Plan proposed football participation based on a BMI application. It began with establishing a baseline weight for every individual frame by height. Independent experts could debate limitations for the BMI regarding muscular or low-fat physiques, but allowable percentages of weight above one's baseline — such as 189 pounds on a 6-1 frame for maximum normal — could account for discrepancies. For example, Steve was about 6-2, 230 entering college as a true genetic wonder or ultra-elite specimen fully strength-trained and athletic. He would have to employ chemicals to grow good mass from 230, where he possessed abdominal muscles and probably less than 10 percent body fat — yet he qualified as overweight on the BMI with a high risk for complications. The maximum normal or baseline weight at 6-2 was 194 pounds, with 243 the marker for entering the qualified obesity level on the scale.

That marker weight for entering obesity in Steve's case — or a half pound from exactly 25 per above his normal maximum under BMI — represented a sound cutoff for the weight of any 6-2 specimen in high school football. Colleges might set a 30 percent maximum above a body frame's baseline, and the NFL could adopt a maximum of 35 to 40 percent above baseline, or no more than about 272 pounds on a 6-2 frame. A player could not compete weighing above these standards at any level, and close monitoring of one's weight loss for meeting eligibility would be imperative. Obviously, a player could still juice under these guidelines, but another player could compete without drugs. In addition, a triple-pronged reduction could be realized in lowering rates of drug use, obesity, and field casualties.

"People wonder why athletes take the risk [of doping], but the risk is going out on the football field in the first place," Steve said about a month before his death, during an interview with Robert Dvorchak, *The Pittsburgh Post-Gazette*. "Even if you're not taking them, steroids have had a profound impact on sports. Some juiced-up beast is trying to blast you out of the stadium. Athletes didn't invent this stuff. We opened Pandora's box. We're still trying to figure out how to close it. It's bottomless. It's impossible to eliminate them. Let's accept it's inevitable. But don't put athletes on a moral pedestal when it's an absolute joke. Don't speak of purity and ideals. There's too much money invested in performance."

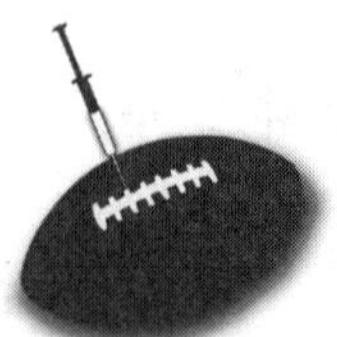

REFERENCES

The author files many items in addition to works cited.

A Crackdown. (1991, August 17). Finally, a crackdown on steroid trafficking. *St. Louis Post-Dispatch.*

Ability, Excel. (2002, March 7). Ability to excel in free-agent derby is key for Rams. *St. Louis Post-Dispatch* [Online].

About Deca? (2006, December 10). What can i do about deca? *forums.steroid.com.*

Abrahamson, A. (2005, November 3). New test for steroids is devised. *Los Angeles Times* [Online].

Acee, K. (2007, January 15). Goodell backs strengthened steroids ban. *San Diego Union-Tribune* [Online}

Achenbach, J. (2006, April 16). Back then, players cheated discreetly. *Kansas City Star Magazine*, p. 10.

AD Resigning. (2007). UW-Stout AD resigning in wake of drug cases, tests. *The Associated Press* [Online].

Adams, B. (2005, August 5). Summer sweat on Cal campus. *San Francisco Chronicle* [Online].

Adderall. (2008, April 10). Adderall: Questionable benefit, definite risk. *New York Daily News* [Online].

Adler, E. (2001, November 26). They might be giants? *Kansas City Star*, p. E1.

Adler, E. (2007, April 8). Break grip of obesity, youngsters are urged. *Kansas City Star*, p. A1.

Adler, J. (2004 December 20). Toxic strength. *Newsweek*, p. 45.

Admitting Steroids. (1991, August 19). Former Washington State tackle admitting he used steroids. *The Associated Press* [Online].

Aichele, M. (2007, April 17). Dream genes *Walrus Magazine* [Online].

Air Force Coach. (2004, July 24). Air Force coach says players admit steroid mistake. *The Associated Press* [Online].

Alanis, M. (2006, June 3). Drug tests catch few students; none are positive for steroids. *Dallas Morning News* [Online].

Aldridge, D. (2007, October 11). Is anybody honest these days? *Philadelphia Inquirer* [Online].

Alexander, B. (2005, July). The awful truth about drugs in sports. *Outside Magazine* [Online].

Alexander, J. (2007, May 29). Rare condition gives boy incredible strength. *Muskegon Chronicle* [Online].

Alfano, P. (2008, October 28). Goodell's get-tough campaign not intimidating anybody. *Fort Worth Star-Telegram* [Online].

Alipour, S. (2008, October 3). A candid conversation with Tony Mandarich. *ESPN.com* [Online].

Allen, K. (1990, December 26). Bowl-bound athletes faced expanded drug testing. *USA Today*, p. 6C.

Allen, M. (2008, May 13). Interview with President Bush. *Politico.com* [Online].

Almond, E. (1995, January 23). Drug testing in NFL under a microscope. *Seattle Times*, p. Sports-1.

Almond, E. (1996, September 29). A world of hurt. *Seattle Times*, p. D1.

Almond, E. (2007, May 26). Truth serum. *San Jose Mercury News* [Online].

Altman, L.K. (1988, November 20). New 'Breakfast of Champions.' *New York Times*, p. 1—1.

Alzado, L. (1991, July 3). Television interview with host Roy Firestone [transcript]. *ESPN.*

Alzado, L. (1991, July 8). 'I'm sick and I'm scared.' Sp*orts Illustrated*, p. 20.

Anderson, D. (1986, November 30). X factor in N.F.L. violence. *New York Times*, p. 5—1.

Anderson, R. (2005, August 25). Expanding concerns. *Roanoke Times* [Online].

Andrews, L. (2006, June 9). Steroid prevention the NCAA way. *Oregon Daily Emerald* [Online].

Anti-Doping Tests. (2008, May 27). Scientists to investigate anti-doping tests on Everest climb. *Medical Laboratory World* [Online].

Apathy Danger. (2006, April). Steroid investigation shows danger in apathy. *Northern Star* [Online].

Araton, H. (2001, August 2). Culture of extremes and extreme heat collide. *New York Times* [Online].

Archer, T., & Watkins, C. (2008, June 9). Dallas Cowboys' Owens in NFL's 'reasonable cause' drug-testing program. *Dallas Morning News* [Online].

Arizona State Probe. (2005, July 25). Arizona State probes cites no violations in handling of Wade. *The Associated Press* [Online].

Armstrong, J. (2007, April 15). Game of deception. *Denver Post* [Online]

Around League. (2007, September 10). Blitz package. *Kansas City Star*, p. C11.

Arthur, B. (2007, September 6). In their own league. *Canada National Post* [Online].

Assael, S. (2007). *Steroid Nation**. New York, NY: ESPN Books.

Assael, S. (2007, March 26). Business as usual. *ESPN The Magazine*, p. 98.

'Athlete Passport.' (2007, October 16). 'Athlete passport' could help cut doping in sports, official says. *The Associated Press* [Online].

Atlas, D. (2008, February 5). Teens using steroids cheat themselves and their health. *Dallas Morning News* [Online].

Avila, J., Tribolet, B., Pearle, L., & Michels, S. (2008, February 20). Girls and steroids: Anything to be thin. *ABC News* [Online].

Babb, C. (1992, January 5). Telephone interview with author.

Babwin, D. (2001, August 8). Wheeler's parents want answers. *The Associated Press* [Online].

Badger, E. (2008, June 11). NCAA hopes to thwart academic blitz. *Miller-McCune.com* [Online].

Baker, M. (2008, July 24). High school coaches blames steroids on commercial gyms and personal trainers. *Mesomorphosis.com* [Online].

Baker, S. (2007, February 13). LTE: High school athletes. *Kansas City Star*, p. B10.

Ban Testing. (2008, October 20). Ban on drug testing won't serve athletes. *News Tribune* [Online].

Ban Urged. (2008, March 29). FDA, DEA urged to ban andro sales. *The Associated Press* [Online].

Banks, L.J. (2005, September 28). Ditka on 'roids: Cowards use them. *Chicago Sun-Times* [Online].

Barker, J. (2006, July 28). With deep roots, cheating grows, soils perception *Baltimore Sun* [Online].

Barnas, J. (2005, March 23). CMU duo research drugs' allure, danger. *Detroit Free Press* [Online].

Barnes, D. (2006, January 28). Labs one step behind designer steroids that pop in, out of use. *Edmonton Journal* [Online].

Barnes, M. (1989, January 10). Track & Field Notebook. *United Press International* [Online].

Barnhouse, W. (2007, August 17). Razorbacks must move past turmoil. *Fort Worth Star-Telegram* [Online].

Barnidge, N. (2004, December 9). SSU football program under NCAA investigation. *Savannah Morning News* [Online].

Barnidge, N. (2004, December 10). SSU president acknowledges NCAA investigation for alleged steroid use. *Savannah Morning News* [Online].

Barnidge, N. (2004, December 11). SSU athletics, a program divided. *Savannah Morning News* [Online].

Barnidge, N. (2005, February 10). SSU releases list of football players who asked to be released from their scholarships. *Savannah Morning News* [Online].

Barrett, W.M. (1998, January). Greed and hypocrisy in a land of plenty. *USA Today Magazine*, p. 69.

Baseball Responds. (2008, January 18). Major League Baseball responds to WADA. *MLB.com* [Online].

Battista, J. (2006, September 6). N.F.L. is willing to consider stronger drug-testing program. *New York Times* [Online].

Baum, B. (2005, June 25). Track chief hails Congress in drug fight. *The Associated Press* [Online].

Bavley, A. (1998, June 10). Athletes missing thorough screening. *Kansas City Star*, p. C1.

Be Legal. (2005, December 16). Doping in sport should be legal, claim experts. *DeHavilland* [Online].

Be Sure. (2006, December 25). How can I be sure what i'm getting is real? *forums.steroid.com.*

Begley, I. (2008, June 28). *News* examines relationship between steroids and heart-related deaths. *New York Daily News* [Online].

Behar, M. (2008, August 5). Will gene therapy destroy sports? *Discover Magazine* [Online].
Bell, J., & Corbett, J. (2008, March 28). Dark days ahead? NFL meetings set serious tone. *USA Today* [Online].
Bell, T. (2006, October 8). IHSA drug tests likely this year. *Chicago Sun-Times* [Online].
Benjamin, A. (2006, June 9). Experts concerned HGH is a growing problem. *Boston Globe* [Online].
Berkow, I. (2001, August 5). In plain talk, there is an explanation for Stringer's death. *New York Times* [Online].
Bernstein, Joe. (2008, November 17). Missed drug tests put two footballers in danger of ban. *Daily Mail* [Online].
Bernstein, Josh. (2008, May 1). Juiced in the valley. *www.abc15.com* [Online].
Better Sex. (2008, September 22). All News: Survey 30% of U.S. men say sex is better after NFL team wins. *ESPN The Magazine*, p. 43.
Bevitz, R. (2006, April 20). Former UTM player pleads guilty to drug charges. *Jackson Sun* [Online].
Bhasin, S.; Storer, T.W.; Berman, N.; Callegari, C.; Clevenger, B.; Phillips, J.; Bunnell, T.J.; Tricker, R. ; Shirazi, A.; & Casaburi, R. (1996). The effects of supraphysiological doses of testosterone on muscle size and strength in normal men. *New England Journal of Medicine*, p. 1.
Bianchi, M. (2006, September 11). NFL fans prove short memories help in long run. *Orlando Sentinel* [Online].
Bigger Better. (1996, October 19). Bigger is better. *Kansas City Star*, p. D5.
Bigger, Stronger. (2007, February 7). Bigger, stronger faster: Recruiting pressure drives some to steroids. *KXAN-TV* [Online].
Biggs, Michigan. (2008, August 7). Rondell Biggs, steroids and Michigan. *Ann Arbor News* [Online].
Bishop, G. (2005, October 11). Steroids issue offers no room in middle. *Seattle Times*, p. D7.
Black, B. (1989, June 22). Utah athletic director thrilled Gadd's acquitted of charges. *The Associated Press* [Online].
Blood Doping. (2007, September 24). How to really stop blood doping in sports. *Canadian Broadcasting Company* [Online].
Blood Sample. (1991, April 17). Olympics consider blood sample testing of athletes. *Daily American Republic*, p. 3B.
Blood Work. (2006, December 26). blood work results. *forums.steroid.com* [Online].
Bodybuilder Busted. (2007, March 14). Pro bodybuilder busted. *Home News Tribune* [Online].
Bonds Represents. (2007, August 14). Bonds represents American values. *Tonawanda News* [Online].
Bondy, F. (2008, January 31). Surrounded by cookie monsters. *New York Daily News* [Online].
Bondy, S. (2007, October 3). Football's weight limits preventing Lodi boy from playing games he loves. *Herald News* [Online].

Bonk, T. (2005, August 23). Doctor: NFL exams far exceed standards. *Los Angeles Times* [Online].
Bonner, M.F. (208, September 18). Ex-QB Foster enters drug plea. *Jackson Clarion Ledger* [Online].
Booked That? (2007, January 12). Who booked that slot? *Wilton Villager* [Online].
Borges, R. (2007, February 3). Goodell takes safe approach. *Boston Globe* [Online].
Borzilleri, M. (2004, September 17). Air Force player found not guilty in steroid case. *Colorado Springs Gazette* [Online].
Boswell, T. (2005, March 18). Columnist Thomas Boswell chats with readers about hearings. *washingtonpost.com* [Online].
Bouchette, E. (2007, March 1). Probe touches Steelers doctor. *Pittsburgh Post-Gazette* [Online].
Bouchette, E. (2007, June 15). Steelers drop longtime MD. *Pittsburgh Post-Gazette* [Online].
Bouchette, E. (2008, November 12). Should steroids be allowed? *post-gazette.com* [Online].
Bowman, L. (2005, October 26). Sales of human growth hormone widespread, study finds. *Scripps Howard News Service* [Online].
Bowman, L. (2006, January 31). Living large: Why it's not necessarily good for us. *Scripps Howard News Service* [Online].
Brainard, C. (2007, August 8). To juice or not to juice? Journalists float the idea of legalizing sports doping. *Columbia Journalism Review* [Online].
Brand Looking. (2004, June 7). Brand looking to integrate athletics within universities. *Sports Business Daily* [Online].
Brand's Association. (2006, May 3). Brand's association: NCAA president discusses ideas. *Sports Business Daily* [Online].
Brennan, C. (2008, November 20). Obama whiffs on his first call on sports front. *USA Today* [Online].
Brisendine, S. (2004, July 19). Reform, politics will be ongoing hot topic in NCAA. *The Associated Press* [Online].
Broad, M. (2007, April 3). In the spotlight: Michael Broad. *Sun-Sentinel* [Online].
Brubaker, B. (1994, May 22). At Navy, conflicting missions. *Washington Post*, p. A1.
Bruscas, A. (2003, October 24). UW scandal stuns NCAA's expert. *Seattle Post-Intelligencer* [Online].
Buckley, T. (1988, August 30). Insurance at a premium. *St. Petersburg Times*, p. Football-4.
Buckley, T. (1988, September 3). Insurance becomes big part of the game in Florida football. *St. Petersburg Times*, p. City Times-6.
Bulked Up. (2005, November 30). Bulking up: The dope on steroids. *Free Lance-Star* [Online].
Burned Records. (2003, July 19). Northwestern doctor burned medical records. *Kansas City Star*, p. D2.
Burwell, B. (1993, August 6). Leagues deserves praise for rethinking drug policy. *USA Today*, p. 7C.

Burwell, B. (2006, June 9). Ordinary player rattles baseball. *St. Louis Post-Dispatch* [Online].

Burwell, B. (2006, August 29). Now is time for the NFL to receive more scrutiny. *St. Louis Post-Dispatch* [Online].

Burwell, B. (2007, February 2). NFL's cold-hearted stance regarding its vets is deplorable. *St. Louis Post-Dispatch* [Online].

Buscema, D. (2005, August 23). NFL perception doesn't match steroids reality. *Times Herald-Record* [Online].

Bustos, J. (2008, September 23). Student avoids jail on steroid charges. *saukvalley.com* [Online].

Buyanovsky, D. (2008, April 17). Gym is only welcome to muscleheads. *Hurricane* [Online].

Byrne, J., & Smith, T. (2002, May 13). Oberlin College students bring light to steroid use. *Oberlin Review* [Online].

Cane, M. (2005, October 20). High school football players bigger than ever. *Everett Herald* [Online].

Cantu, R. (2007, April 20). Athletes, administrators on steroid testing bill: Where's the juice? *Austin American-Statesman* [Online].

Caplan, A. (2005, August 14). Why does it matter how an athlete wins? *News Journal* [Online].

Cardiac Deaths. (2001, March 2). Cardiac deaths up among young. *Kansas City Star*, p. A7.

Carey, B. (2002, August 3). Doctors debate risks of doping, but no one has enough data to really know. *Los Angeles Times* [in *Montreal Gazette*, p. G12].

Carpenter, L. (2007, June 20). Compromise reigns at summit on concussions. *Washington Post*, p. E1.

Casey, T. (2003, November 13). Weighing game: Prep football players literally becoming big men on campus, with more tipping the scales near 300 pounds. *Sacramento Bee*, p. C1.

Catastrophic Medical. (2008, August). Catastrophic medical & disability insurance plan. *Missouri State High School Activities Association Journal*, p. 6.

Catlin, D. (2005, May 24). Testimony, Committee on Commerce, Science and Transportation, U.S. Senate. Washington, DC [Online].

Catlin, D. (2007, February 15). Telephone interview with author.

Catlin, D. (2008, October 28). E-mail correspondence to author.

Caucus on International Narcotics Control, U.S. Senate. (2004, July 13). *The abuse of anabolic substances and their precursors by adolescent and amateur athletes* [S. Hrg. No. 108-814]. Washington, D.C.: U.S. Government Printing Office.

Chait, J. (2007, July 18). Machine helps find your body mass index. *Tribune-Star* [Online].

Chandler, C. (2006, August 27). Report is snapshot of doping in NFL. *Charlotte Observer* [Online].

Chandler, C. (2007, January 21). Agency: HGH kits coming in 2007. *Charlotte Observer* [Online].

Chandler, C. (2007, January 27). Minter: Steroids policy sends a strong message. *Charlotte Observer* [Online].

Chandler, C. (2007, March 25). Upshaw digs in: No positive test, no action. *Charlotte Observer* [Online].

Chandler, L. (1996, October 17). McNairy continues to use steroids, and NFL dreams closer to coming true. *Charlotte Observer* [Online].

Chaney, M. (2007, July 12). Prep football coaches. E-mail correspondence.

Chass, M. (2007, May 12). Mum is the word in steroid inquiry. *New York Times* [Online].

Cheaters Prosper? (2007, November 5). Do cheaters prosper? Always. *Los Angeles Loyolan* [Online].

Cheer Bans. (2006, August/September). Cheer bans continue. *Athletic Management Magazine* [Online].

Cheng, M. (2008, November 13). Rates of paranoia slowly increasing. *Kansas City Star*, p. A7.

Chest Kill. (1998, June 18). Light blow to chest an kill, study finds. *Kansas City Star*, p. A7.

Christianson, E. (2006, May 19). Savannah State University Infractions case Handled Through Summary Disposition. Indiapolis, IN: National Collegiate Athletic Association [Online].

Christie, J. (2007, October 17). WADA comes under fire from former French sport minister. *Toronto Globe and Mail* [Online].

Christl, C. (1998, August 16). NFL's big boys. *Milwaukee Journal Sentinel*, p. Sports-1.

Christou, F. (2007, February 22). Interview, Dr. Paul Strauss, Agency for Cycling Ethics. *Pro Cycling News* [Online].

Chu, J. (2008, June 16). Making old muscle young. *Technology Review* [Online].

Clay, D. (2006, July 4). Teen son's death leads his parents to warn of steroids. *NewsOk.com* [Online].

Clement, S. (2007, September 13). Cornell sprint football steeped in tradition. *Cornell Daily Sun* [Online].

Coaches Say. (1988, October 19). Coaches say nine Big Ten schools test for steroids. *The Associated Press* [Online].

Coakley, E. (2005, October 1). UNC center helps ex-athletes cope with aches and pains. *Herald-Sun* [Online].

Coffey, W. (2005, April 24). Hand that rocked the cradle. *New York Daily News* [Online].

Coffey, W. (2007, March 25). A body to die for. *New York Daily News* [Online].

Coffey, W. (2007, December 16). Teens' big worry: For high school athletes, steroids still the rage. *New York Daily News* [Online].

Cohen, H. (1985, January 13). Parade's All-America High School Football Team. *Parade*, p. 15.

Colarusso, L.M. (2004, September 27). Second academy steroid case opens can of worms. *Air Force Times* [Online].

Colleges. (2006, April 18). Colleges. *Kansas City Star*, p. C3.

Cole, J. (2006, February 26). Latest case could put NFL policy to the test. *Miami Herald* [Online].

Colleges. (2005, March 20). Myles Brand steadfast about academic reform. *Kansas City Star*, p. D2.

Collinsworth, C. (2007, April 11). Goodell's decisions show his strength. *nbcsports.msnbc.com* [Online].

Colston, C. (2006, June 28). Hassles, indignities come with NFL drug testing. *USA Today* [Online].

Coming Clean. (1986, November 5). Coming clean about steroids. *New York Times*, p. D24.

Commissioner Goodell. (2008, February 1). NFL commissioner Roger Goodell, Super Bowl XLII news conference, Phoenix, Arizona. *49ers.com* [Online].

Committee on Energy and Commerce, U.S. House of Representatives. (2005, March 10). *Steroid in sports: Cheating the system and gambling your health* (H. Hrg. No. 109-65). Washington, D.C.: U.S. Government Printing Office.

Committee on Government Reform, U.S. House of Representatives. (2005, March 17). *Restoring faith in America's pastime: Evaluating Major League Baseball's efforts to eradicate steroid use.* (Serial No. 109-21). Washington, D.C.: U.S. Government Printing Office.

Committee on Government Reform, U.S. House of Representatives. (2005, April 27). *Steroid Use in Sports, Part II: Examining the National Football League's Policy on Anabolic Steroids and Related Substances* (Serial No. 109-21). Washington, D.C.: U.S. Government Printing Office.

Committee on the Judiciary, U.S. House of Representatives. (2004, July 20). *Good Samaritan Volunteer Firefighter Assistance Act of 2003, the Nonprofit Athletic Organization Protection Act of 2003, and the Volunteer Pilot Organization Protection Act.* (Serial No. 108-107). Washington, DC: Committee on the Judiciary.

Concussions Unreported. (2004, June 16). Concussions in college often go unreported. *Kansas City Star*, p. D2.

Condotta, B. (2005, January 22). UW head trainer on leave for falsifying medical records. *Seattle Times*, p. D5.

Connolly, C. (2008, November 30). U.S. 'Not getting what we pay for': Many experts say health-care systems inefficient, wasteful. *Washington Post*, p. A1.

Conte, V. (2008, August 18). Conte: World Anti-Doping Agency needs to beef up offseason steroid testing. *New York Daily News* [Online].

Cook, B. (2006, June 9). Consider ending drug policies in sports. *msnbc.com* [Online].

Cook, R. (2005, May 3). New steroids plan won't get past Fehr. *Pittsburgh Post-Gazette* [Online].

Cormier, A. (2006, October 1). Simms' case highlights NFL doctors' dilemma. *Sarasota Herald Tribune* [Online].

Cote, G. (2006, August 30). No question Scott should be honored. *Miami Herald* [Online].

Couch, G. (2001, August 24). Experts foresee legal wrangling. *Chicago Sun-Times* [Online].
Couch, G. (2005, August 22). Sports culture becoming something that isn't healthy. *Chicago Sun-Times* [Online].
Cougars Positive. (1991, June 15). Bailey: He and four other Cougars positive for steroids. *The Associated Press* [Online].
Coughlin, T. (2005, August 10). 'T'-ing off. *Northeastern News* [Online].
Courchesne, S. (2005, December 4). Hard forged by controversy. *Hartford Courant* [Online].
Courson, S. (2004). Childhood obesity: An ominous foreshadow of the future? Farmington, PA.
Courson, S. (2005, March 7). Interview with author, Farmington, PA.
Courson, S. (2005, March 20). Telephone interview with author.
Courson, S. (2005, March 27). Telephone interview with author.
Courson, S. (2005, April 3). Telephone interview with author.
Courson, S. (2005, May 1). Telephone interview with author.
Courson, S. (2005, May 8). Telephone interview with author.
Courson, S. (2005, May 11). Telephone interview with author.
Courson, S. (2005, May 12). E-mail correspondence to author.
Courson, S. (2005, May 18). E-mail correspondence to author.
Courson, S. (2005, May 23). Telephone interview with author.
Courson, S. (2005, May 26). Telephone interview with author.
Courson, S. (2005, June 7). Telephone interview with author.
Courson, S. (2005, June 22). Telephone interview with author.
Courson, S. (2005, June 30). Telephone interview with author.
Courson, S. (2005, July 8). Super-size me, please. Non-published media commentary.
Courson, S. (2005, July 10). E-mail correspondence to author.
Courson, S. (2005, July 17). E-mail correspondence to author.
Courson, S. (2005, July 20). Correspondence to former teammate, non-forwarded.
Courson, S. (2005, November 1). Telephone interview with author.
Coury, J. (2007, October 6). Steroids in college world going under radar. *Universal Journal* [Online].
Covitz, R. (2005, April 28). Our steroid policy is working, NFL says. *Kansas City Star*, p. D1.
Covitz, R. (2007, May 6). Character issue is costly in draft. *Kansas City Star*, p. D6.
Covitz, R. (2007, October 7). Providing hope. *Kansas City Star*, p. EXTRA3.
Covitz, R. (2008, April 9). Talib reportedly tested positive. *Kansas City Star*, p. D3.
Covucci, D. (2006, June 14). It's not cheating if it's legal. *Collegiate Times* [Online].
Cranmer, J., Caliendo, H. (2005, November 29). Poisoned for pride: Despite side effects, steroid use increases among students. *OU Daily* [Online].
Creglow, Z. (2008, March 24). Drug tests coming for athletes. *Galesburg Register-Mail* [Online].
Crisp, E. (2008, January 30). Former MCHS QB released on bond in steroid case. *Jackson Clarion Ledger* [Online].

Curry, B. (2008, June 7). Telephone interview with author.
Cycling Needs. (2007, November 3). Just what cycling needs. *Kansas City Star*, p. D2.
Cyphers, L. (2008, October 6). Can athletes prove they're clean? In a word, no. *ESPN The Magazine*, p. 18.
Dahlberg, T. (2008, October 28). Steroids in the NFL, but no steroid scandals. *The Associated Press* [Online].
Daly, D. (2005, October 18). Rules are not made to be broken. *Washington Times* [Online].
Dangerous Football? (2007, August 17). How dangerous is high school football? *ScienceDaily.com* [Online].
Dartmouth Steroids. (2004, June 27). Despite arrests, steroids said not in excess at Dartmouth. *The Associated Press* [Online].
Davis, C. (2006, September 3). LTE: Steroid users aren't victims. *Kansas City Star*, p. C3.
Davis, E. (2007, April 24). Illegal hormone use remains undetectable. *Collegian* [Online].
Davis, M. (2007, November 14). Former ASU football player arrested. *Watauga Democrat* [Online].
Davis, M.E. (2001, August 10). LTE: Summer heat can be deadly. *St. Louis Post-Dispatch* [Online].
de Jong, A. (2006, May 9). Money drives college athletics. *Daily Bruin* [Online].
DeArmond, M. (2007, March 14). Life eclipses football at MU. *Kansas City Star*, p. D6.
Death Lesson. (2005, August 22). Player's death is lesson for NFL. *Central Florida Future* [Online].
Debunking Myths. (2007, March 21). Debunking some health myths. *Kansas City Star*, p. F12.
Defends Steroids. (2000, January 21). Ex-top athlete defends use of anabolic steroids. *Montreal Gazette* [Online].
DeFrank, F. (2006, June 28). Student steroid law lacks teeth. *Macomb Daily* [Online].
Delaware Players. (2006, September 15). Delaware football players plead guilty in steroids theft. *The Associated Press* [Online].
Deny Truth. (2001, August 5). Why NFL, fans deny the truth behind death. *St. Louis Post-Dispatch* [Online].
Detecting Designer. (2006, November 20). Detecting designer steroids. *Chemical Science* [Online].
Detection Easier. (2005, October 12). Steroid drug detection made easier. *Independent Online* [Online].
Dexheimer, E. (2005, May 26). Flexing his muscle. *Denver Westword* [Online].
Ditrani, V. (2004, December 5). NFL does it right way. *NorthJersey.com* [Online].
Donaldson, J. (2007, July 10). Our values don't hold any worth. *Providence Journal* [Online].
Donnellon, S. (2005, May 1). Steroid use? Fat chance. *Philadelphia Daily News* [Online].

Donnellon, S. (2005, August 23). What's so wrong if the NFL got smaller? *Philadelphia Daily News* [Online].

Doping Organized. (2008, December 2). 'Doping is organized along mafia lines': Interview with Dick Pound. *Spiegel Online.*

Dorney, K. (2005, October 6). Mandatory steroid testing for all. *Scout.com* [Online].

Dorsey, V.L. (1990, January 31). Prep coaches worry about alcohol. *USA Today*, p. 1C.

Dreessen, J. (2008, February 28). Steroids in the NFL? No chance, local player tells Rotary. *Fort Morgan County Times* [Online].

Drehs, W. (2007, August 8). Future of cheating might rest in our own cells. *ESPN.com* [Online].

Dropped Ball. (2006, November 21). Who dropped this ball? *Baltimore Sun* [Online].

Drug Testing. (2008, March 5). Drug Testing. *ncaa.org* [Online].

Dubner, S.J. (2008, May 30). The Guinness Book of World Records. *freakonomics.blogs.nytimes.com* [Online].

Duck Tests. (2005, August 15). Some former Huskers say a tackle dummy could duck drug tests. *Nebraska StatePaper.com* [Online].

Duke Mulls. (2005, October 21). Duke mulls over steroid regulations. *Duke Chronicle* [Online].

Dunham, W. (1987, January 31). NFL injuries rise, insurers get tough. *United Press International* [Online].

Dvorchak, R. (2005, April 3). $135 million jury award forces new look at high cost of sports and drinking. *Pittsburgh Post-Gazette* [Online].

Dvorchak, R. (2005, October 2). Steroids in sports: Experiment turns epidemic. *Pittsburgh Post-Gazette* [Online].

Dvorchak, R. (2005, October 3). Steroids in sports: Officials bungled steroid regulation from the start. *Pittsburgh Post-Gazette* [Online].

Dvorchak, R. (2005, October 4). Steroids in sports: Keeping steroids out of sports no easy task. *Pittsburgh Post-Gazette* [Online].

Dvorchak, R. (2005, October 5). Steroids in sports: Good uses for steroids overshadowed by bad. *Pittsburgh Post-Gazette* [Online].

Dvorchak, R. (2005, October 7). Bob Dvorchak chat transcript. *post-gazette.com* [Online].

Dwyre, B. (2001, October 26). A special report on medical precautions in high school football: How safe is it? *Los Angeles Times*, p. 4—1.

Eason, N. (2008, August 25). It's getting down to cut time in the NFL. *vindy.com* [Online].

Easterbrook, G. (2007, August 13). Numbing problem in the NFL. *ESPN.com* [Online].

Edison, J. (2005, August 11). Collets continue crusade against performance-enhancing drugs. *Pioneer Press* [Online].

Eggers, K. (2005, April 19). NCAA athletes on the juice? *Portland Tribune* [Online].

Eggers, K. (2005, April 19). Possession led to OSU safety's arrest. *Portland Tribune* [Online].

Eilek, R. (2007, February 19). Latest gang chapter shameful. *North County Times* [Online].
Eisenbath, M. (1992, November 24). Stress on sports hurts teens. *St. Louis Post-Dispatch*, p. 1A.
Eisenberg, J. (2006, November 18). NCAA, fans stay blind to steroids in football. *Baltimore Sun* [Online].
Ellis, E. (2007, April 11). Griffin resigns schools post. *Shore Line Times* [Online].
Encina, E.A. (2007, December 16). Report costly, not valuable. *St. Petersburg Times* [Online].
Engber, D. (2006, June 8). Why is HGH so hard to detect? *Slate.com* [Online].
Engber, D. (2007, August 6). What if doping were legal? *Slate.com* [Online].
Enough Grandstanding. (2005, August 8). Enough grandstanding on steroids. *Nashua Telegraph* [Online].
Erectile Drug. (2006, January 10). NFL drops erectile drug deals. *sportbusiness.com* [Online].
Every Athlete. (1989, March 23). Doctor said almost every athlete took steroids. *The Associated Press* [Online].
Excessive Weight. (2005, December 5). Excessive weight loss, gain dangerous for young athletes. *Kansas City Star*, p. A9.
Ex-USF Player. (2007, February 28). Ex-USF player dies from injury. *Sun-Sentinel* [Online].
Fainaru-Wada, M. (2008, January 18). Former NFL lineman pleads guilty to lying to feds. *ESPN.com* [Online].
Fainaru-Wada, M., & Quinn, T.J. (2008, May 22). How U.S. sports measiure up to the 'gold standard' of testing. *ESPN.com* [Online].
Fainaru-Wada, M., & Williams, L. (2006, December 24). Steroids scandal: The BALCO legacy. *San Francisco Chronicle* [Online].
Fair, J.D. (1999). *Muscletown USA*. University Park, PA: The Pennsylvania State University Press.
Fair, J.D. (2008, June 2). Telephone interview with author.
Family Mourns. (2008, May 20). Family mourns as cause of death remains unknown. *KOLN/KGIN-TV* [Online].
Farley, G. (2008, October 12). Cooper's success in NFL isn't a surprise in Maine. *Brockton Enterprise* [Online].
Farmer, S. (2005, April 28). NFL: We can handle this. *Los Angeles Times* [Online].
Farmer, S., & Wharton, D. (2002, January 29). Weight matters. *Los Angeles Times*, p. 4—1.
Farmer, S., & Wharton, D. (2007, February 9). Bullet proof. *Los Angeles Times* [Online].
Farner, K. (2007, February 10). Performance enhancers not just a pro sports problem. *Independent Mail* [Online].
Farrey, T. (2000, December 7). Mouse beats cat in NCAA testing. *ESPN.com* [Online].
Farrey, T. (2006, September 11). The guru of Growth. *ESPN The Magazine*, p. 158.

Farrey, T. (2007, January 29). The case for HGH. *ESPN The Magazine*, p. 48.
Favre Doubts. (2006, September 20). Favre doubts he'd be traded midseason. *NFL.com* [Online].
FDA Change. (2007, June 1). Hellman calls for FDA change. *Inside Endocrine Practice* [Online].
FDA Teeth. (2007, May 10). Senate passes bill to give FDA bigger teeth. *Medical News Today* [Online].
Feeley, J. (2008, August 15). Cheats of strength: 10 next-gen Olympic doping methods. *Wired* [Online].
Felony Possession. (2006, May 19). Felony possession. *Baker County Standard* [Online].
Female Athletes. (2005, July 5). Girls' game: Young female athletes do steroids, too. *Pittsburgh Post-Gazette* [Online].
Fermoso, J. (2008, October 22). What Facebook and steroid use have in common. *Wired* [Online].
Fernandez, B. (2008, January 27). Parental pressure may contribute to youth steroid usage. *Greeley Tribune* [Online].
Fialkov, H. (2006, December 30). Rough hit costs Thomas $7,500. *Sun-Sentinel* [Online].
Fight Club. (2007, April 16). 'Fight Club' member gets 6 years in state prison. *San Diego Union-Tribune* [Online].
Final Bill. (2007, April 11). Memorial head coach waiting for final bill. *Victoria Advocate* [Online].
Finder, C. (2005, March 19). PSU steroids expert laughs at testimony. *Pittsburgh Post-Gazette* [Online].
Finder, C. (2006, December 14). Appeals panel gives Websters win in disability case. *Pittsburgh Post-Gazette* [Online].
Fine, A. (2007, December 27). Weighing in on performance-enhancing drugs. *Cleveland Jewish News* [Online].
Firm Settles. (2006, December 21). Drugs firm settles with athlete doping victims. *Expatica* [Online].
Fish, M. (1991, September 29). Steroid stigma affects even retired players. *Atlanta Journal and Constitution*, p. F1.
Fish, M. (2002, October 15). A new boss in Indy. *CNNSI.com* [Online].
Fish, M. (2005, December 2). 'Cream' of the flop. *ESPN.com* [Online].
Fish, M. (2007, January 25). 'Doctor' treating T.O., others is under investigation. *ESPN.com* [Online].
Fisher, M. (2005, July 11). Waters, steroids and a slippery slope. *TheRanchReport.com/Scout.com* [Online].
Fitzpatrick, F. (2001, January 14). Death stalks athletes. *Milwaukee Journal Sentinel*, p. 1C.
Fleming, D. (2008, August 27). What I did on my summer vacation. *ESPN.com* [Online].

Fleming, D. (2008, September 16). Cleaning up the cutting room floor with Jeremy Shockey. *ESPN.com* [Online].

Flitter, A. (2008, April 22). UNH officials sa steroids are a nationwide concern, but not widespread in Durham. *The New Hampshire* [Online].

Foley, R.J. (2007, February 8). UW-Stout to begin drug testing after football players' steroid bust. *The Associated Press* [Online].

Football. (2006, May 17). Football. *Kansas City Star*, p. D2.

For Football. (2003, October). He started taking steroids for football. *AnabolicSteroids.com* [Online].

For Parents. (2007, February 5). Tips for parents. *Columbia State* [Online].

Forbes, G. (1999, December 10). Suspensions prompt union meeting on drugs. *USA Today*, p. 8C.

Former Huskers. (2005, August 10). Two current players, 11 former Huskers listed as witnesses. *The Associated Press* [Online].

Former Teacher. (2006, October 22). Former teacher gets one year for steroids. *15WMTV* [Online].

Fort Worth Students. (1986, April 27). Fort Worth area high school students admit using steroids. *United Press International* [Online].

Friedman, J. (2007, September 10). Sex, drugs and rock & roll in the NFL: Long snaps with Bryan Pittman. *blogs.houstonpress.com/ballz* [Online].

Friesen, P. (2007, June 5). CFL gave legendary QB a chance when others wouldn't. *slam.canoe.ca* [Online].

Funk, A. (2006, September 6). Another insurance option? *training-conditioning.com* [Online].

Gallagher, C. (2006, March 15). Steroid use affects many college sports. *Cavalier Daily* [Online].

Gallagher, D. (2007, February 14). Former Prosper, Celina running back charged with steroids possession. *McKinney Courier-Gazette* [Online].

Gallegos, A. (2007, May 18). The Landis Hearing: Day 5—A lawyer's view. *VeloNews.com* [Online].

Galli, M. (2006, May/June). On a pass and a prayer. *Christianity Today* [Online].

Gamecock Fan. (2007, October 17). Gamecock fan obsessed with man-children. *Columbia Free Times* [Online].

Gamerman, E. (2005, November 27). High schools use sophisticated tools to detect, prevent injuries. *Wall Street Journal* [in *Chicago Sun-Times*, p. A6].

Gammage, J. (2006, May 30). Incentives vs. ethics. *Philadelphia Inquirer* [Online].

Garafolo, M. (2008, July 28). Olivea happy NY Giants gave him a second chance. *Star-Ledger* [Online].

Gardner, A. (2005, August 21). Texarkana is no stranger to 'juice.' *Texarkana Gazette* [Online].

Gauper, B. (2000, January 30). Go, tourist, go to Packerland. *Kansas City Star*, p. H1.

Gavin, R. (2007, June 18). DA: Narcotics cop received steroids. *Albany Times Union* [Online].

Gavin, R. (2007, June 21). Soares: Albany detective who ordered steroids was allowed to stay on drug case. *Albany Times Union* [Online].
Gay, N. (2007, November 30). Changing of the guard. *San Francisco Chronicle* [Online].
Gene Abuse. (2006, November 30). Gene abuse in sport 'detectable.' *BBC News* [Online].
GHB Positive. (2007, September 10). Police say Bucs WR Boston tested positive for GHB. *USA Today* [Online].
Giants Roster. (2007). New York Giants Roster. *nyg.scout.com* [Online].
Gilbert, M. (2007, June 19). Pharmacy board to aid UT probe. *Toledo Blade* [Online].
Gillen, H. (2008, March 28). Few problems with steroids for high school students, coaches say. *Capital News Service* [Online].
Girls Use. (2005, June 15). Girls use the juice, too. *The Associated Press* [Online].
Glauber, B. (2005, September 25). Growing concerns. *Newsday*, p. B6.
Glauber, B. (2006, September 7). Goodell focuses on HGH issue. *Newsday* [Online].
Glazer, J. (2005, April 6). Steroid 'experts' need to open eyes wider. *FOXSports.com* [Online].
Glines, J. (2008, June 26). Syracuse High School football players admit to burglary spree, police say. *kutv.com* [Online].
Gold, A. (2006, August 29). It's just a fantasy. *850/620 The Buzz* [Online].
Goldaper, S., & Cavanaugh, J. (1988, October 3). Sport imitates art. *New York Times*, p.C2.
Goldberg, D. (2006, August 8). NFL chooses Goodell to succeed Tagliabue. *The Associated Press* [Online].
Goldberg, K. (2007, August 30). Prep football players bigger than ever. *Times Herald-Record* [Online].
Goodman, E. (2007, May 25). Fuzzy line divides technology and talent. *Boston Globe* [in *Record Searchlight*, Online].
Gordon, K. (2002, July 5). Sentiments mixed on ephedrine ban in NFL. *Columbus Dispatch*, p. 6D.
Graham, K. (2007, September 20). For giving boy steroids, man gets 15 months. *St. Petersburg Times* [Online].
Gramza, J. (2006, July 18). Weightlifting death risk. *ScienCentral.com* [Online].
Gramza, J. (2008, April 8). Muscle drug injuries. *ScienCentral.com* [Online].
Graney, E. (2005, April 20). School must take strong action to determine extent of problem. *San Diego Union-Tribune* [Online].
Gregorian, V. (2008, January 24). The high school high road. *St. Louis Post-Dispatch* [Online].
Gregory, A. (2005, October 4). Hilton looks back, but focuses on the future. *Bristol Herald Courier* [Online].
Greifner, L. (2007, March 28). N.J. steroid testing gets attention in other states. *Education Week* [Online].
Gridiron Granny. (2003, May 16). 'Gridiron Granny' tackles the spotlight. *Kansas City Star*, p. D2.

Grinczel, S. (2008, October 1). Perles surprised by Mandarich's steroid use. *mlive.com* [Online].

Grossfeld, S. (2008, February 18). When cheers turn to depression. *Boston Globe* [Online].

Grossman, D. (1986, October 16). Metro has bumper crop of beefy football stars. *Toronto Star*, p. H14.

Grossmith, P. (2006, January 4). Former St. A football captain headed to jail. *Manchester Union Leader* [Online].

Growing Problem. (2007, January 24). A growing problem. *Kansas City Star*, p. D2.

Growth Chart. (2005, September 11). Off the growth chart. *Lexington Herald-Leader* [Online].

Guilbeau, G. (2005, May 19). LSU player suspended following steroid arrest. *USA Today* [Online].

Habib, H. (2008, August 4). Cheating athletes turn to gene doping. *Palm Beach Post* [Online].

Hack, D. (2006, December 14). Former Steeler's family wins disability ruling. *New York Times* [Online].

Hage, J. (2006, August 30). Retired math teacher charged with four felonies. *Chippewa Valley Newspapers* [Online].

Hall, John. (2006, July 17). Jurors hear final jailhouse tapes in shooting trial. *North County Times* [Online].

Hall, John. (2006, July 25). Accused says he kept race views from students. *North County Times* [Online].

Hall, Joseph. (2005, August 28). Cheating athletes know the tricks. *Toronto Star* [Online].

Hanna, J. (2004, September 4). KU, media face off over records. *Kansas City Star*, p. B3.

Hanson, A. (2008, April 9). Players tested for drugs six times per year. *Central Arkansas Echo* [Online].

Hardy, D. (2007, October 18). Former Penn-Delco school officials arrested. *Philadelphia Inquirer* [Online].

Hargrove, T. (2006, January 31). Heavy NFL players twice as likely to die before 50. *Scripps Howard News Service* [Online].

Hargrove, T. (2007, January 31). Is NFL on diet? Smallest teams make Super Bowl. *Scripps Howard News Service* [Online].

Harmon, D. (2005, April 20). Ex-Coug tells of steroids at Y. *Deseret Morning News* [Online].

Harness Resigns. (2008, January 9). Harness resigns, board questions severance benefits. *Dunn County News* [Online].

Hart, S. (2008, March 2). WADA rethinks hormone test. *London Telegraph* [Online].

Hart, S. (2008, November 15). Drug cheats may benefit from animal test. *London Telegraph* [Online].

Hasen, J. (1989, February 1). Commentator says track and field yet to recover from Ben Johnson. *United Press International* [Online].

Hawaii Tests. (2007, August 20). Former Hawaii WR: NCAA drug tests 'not random. *The Associated Press* [Online].

Hayes, N. (2006, June 13). A joint solution to stop cheaters. *Contra Costa Times* [Online].

Heart Defects. (2008, November 12). Heart defects found in 5 Russian hockey players. *The Associated Press* [Online].

Hegarty, M. (2005, August 22). $3 million effort is aimed at developing new exams for detection. *Daily Racing Form* [Online].

Heilemann, J. (2006, April 10). Let juice loose. *New York Magazine* [Online].

Hellerman, C. (2007, April 11). Human growth hormone use rises, but is it legal? *CNN.com* [Online].

Helliker, K., & Kranhold, K. (2005, June 23). Signs of heart defects in young athletes ignored. *Wall Street Journal* [in *Pittsburgh Post-Gazette*, Online].

Henderson, J. (2007, January 18). Athlete's sudden death stuns USF. *Tampa Tribune* [Online].

Henderson, J. (2007, December 28). Whatever it takes to stay in the game. *Tampa Tribune* [Online].

Herman, J. (2005, October 20). Muscle bustin' for steroids. Does it pay off? *Michigan Daily* [Online].

Heuser, J. (2008, August 13). Lawyer: Ex-UM player Biggs innocent of steroid charge. *Ann Arbor News* [Online].

HGH Continues. (2007, November 29). HGH continues to stump anti-doping forces. *The Associated Press* [Online].

HGH Detectable? (2006, November 16). HGH Detectable? *forums.steroid.com* [Online].

Hicklin, S. (2008, September 12). Only one player in the state failed steroid testing program. *South Florida Sun-Sentinel* [Online].

Hightower, K., Limon, I, & Hoppes, L. (2008, April 11). UCF players, coach differ over football player's death. *Orlando Sentinel* [Online].

Hiltzik, M.A. (2007, May 31). Landis case succeeds in exposing faults. *Los Angeles Times* [Online].

Hobby, D. (2007, July 23). 'Roid rage. *WALB-TV* [Online].

Hofmann, R. (2002, June 23). Testing won't shrink players. *Philadelphia Daily News*, p. Sports-1.

Hofmann, R. (2005, August 25). Weight limits the NFL can live with. *Philadelphia Daily News* [in *Centre Daily*, Online].

Hogs Buzz. (2007, August 8). Las Cronicas returns to ruin Hogs buzz. *everydayshouldbesaturday.com* [Online].

Hohler, B. (2005, July 22). Ex-Barry University baseball player says he witnessed steroid use. *Boston Globe* [Online].

Hohler, B. (2007, July 22). Living in a downward spiral. *Boston Globe* [Online].

Hopkins, J. (2006, December 13). Chesapeake police drop steroid charges against former coach. *Hampton Roads News* [Online].

Hormone Pusher? (2007, September 28). Is Pfizer's Pharmacia & Upjohn the unnamed growth hormone drug pusher? *Corporate Crime Reporter* [Online].

Howard, J. (2002, May 12). NFL and union do the right thing. *Newsday* [Online].

Huff, D. (1985, July 7). Drugs in the high schools. *Washington Post* [Online].

Huff, D., & Berkowitz, S. (1987, January 5). Athletes' medical care may be inadequate. *Washington Post*, p. C3.

Human, K. (2006, January 18). Cutting-edge alternatives to steroids helping cutting horses. *Denver Post* [Online].

Hunter, W. (2007, May 4). Police probe possible steroid use at O'Hara. *KYW-TV* [Online].

Hyde, D. (2002, December 29). The strange journey of Jake Scott. *South Florida Sun-Sentinel* [in *Kansas City Star*, p. C8].

Insurance Halts. (1986, November 21). Insurance firm halts new football policies. *United Press International* [Online].

Insurers Balk. (2004, August 22). Insurers balk at big coverage areas. *Kansas City Star*, p. A12.

Investigational GH. (2008, November 12). Investigational GH drug increased muscle mass in older adults. *Endocrine Today* [Online].

Isikoff M. (1990, September 8). HHS says teen steroid use appears to be spreading. *Washington Post*, p. A1.

Israelsen, S. (2007, February 21). '06 Lehi shooting victim arrested. *Deseret Morning News* [Online].

ITF Player. (2005, November 10). ITF player tracking. *Australian Herald Sun* [Online].

Jackson, D. (2008, May 8). Where the candidates stand on sports issues. *USA Today* [Online].

Jacobson, T. (2004, August 3). Cadet's steroid purchase detailed. *Colorado Springs Gazette* [Online].

Jacobson, T. (2004, September 2). AFA football player cleared in steroid case. *Colorado Springs Gazette* [Online].

Janofsky, M. (1986, December 2). Dowhower gone as Colts' coach. *New York Times*, p. B9.

Jeansonne, J. (2004, December 5). No learning from history. *Hartford Courant* [Online].

Jenkins, J. (2006, January 1). Who pays the bills? Former players frequently face financial pain. *Sacremento Bee*, p. C7.

Jenkins, S. (2007, October 12). There's a legal remedy to the doping issue. *Washington Post*, p. E1.

Jennings, J. (2004, August 27). Pro football is brief, but life is eternal, says Derry pastor. *Blairsville Dispatch* [Online].

Jensen, M. (2006, December 2). A common goal. *Philadelphia Inquirer* [Online].

John Doe. (2004, July 13). John Doe, hidden witness, college athlete, NCAA Division I football team. *The abuse of anabolic steroids and their precursors by adolescent and amateur athletes*. Washington, D.C.: U.S. Government Printing Office.

Johnson, A. (2005, October 2). Bulking up, right vs. wrong. *Carlisle Sentinel* [Online].

Johnston, J. (2002, July 20). Worth dying for? Questions abound a year after four football players died in the heat. *Tampa Tribune*, p. Sports-1.

Jones, G., & Jacobson, G. (2005, February???). Coach knows value of hard work, patience. *Dallas Morning News* [Online].

Jones, G. & Jacobson, G. (2005, February??). Signals missed or ignored. *Dallas Morning News* [Online].

Jones, G. & Jacobson, G. (2005, February??). Whispers from the weight room. *Dallas Morning News* [Online].

Jones, G. & Jacobson, G. (2005, February??). Signals missed or ignored. *Dallas Morning News* [Online].

Jones, G. & Jacobson, G. (2005, June 5). A life undone by doping. *Dallas Morning News* [Online].

Jones, L. (2006, June 16). Stopping HGH use among athletes difficult. *Palm Beach Post* [Online].

Josh Melton. (2006, April 24). ARSN interview: Josh Melton. *Arkansas Razorback Sports Network* [Online].

Joyner, K.C. (2008, June 2). Line of fire. *ESPN The Magazine*, p. 78.

Judd, A. (2008, May 6). College drug testing varies by school. *Atlanta Journal-Constitution* [Online].

Judge Tells. (2005, October 14). Judge tells lawsuit parties to 'work it out.' *nbc5i.com* [Online].

Kallestad, B. (2008, March 14). Tests: Steroid abuse rare in Fla. high schools. *The Associated Press* [Online].

Kamm, G. (2008, June 17). Autopsy: Enlarged heart killed NFL draft prospect, but possible drugs were nearby. *First Coast News* [Online].

Kamran, J. (2005, October 6). Who knows? Who cares? *Columbia Spectator* [Online].

Kantowski, R. (2005, August 22). Herrion's death brings up weighty issue in NFL. *Las Vegas Sun* [Online].

Karash, J.A. (2003, September 23). Sticker shock: The rising cost of health-care insurance sends employers, workers staggering. *Kansas City Star*, p. D1.

Kanaby, R.F. (2008, February 27). Testimony of Robert F. Kanaby, executive director, National Federation of State High School Associations. In Subcommittee on Commerce, Trade and Consumer Protection, U.S. House of Representatives, *Drugs in sports: Compromising the health of athletes and undermining the integrity of competition.* [Online].

Kay, J. (2005, April 22). She's a grade-school teacher by day, a linebacker at night. *St. Louis Post-Dispatch*, p. D3.

Keteyian, A. (1998, August). Mass deception: Athletes using body-enhancement drugs. *Sport*, p. 26.

Kelley, T. (2007, March 14). New Jersey suburb stunned by 15 arrests in latest drug raid. *New York Times* [Online].

Keegan, T. (2008, November 14). Ex-NFL chief Tagliabue full of surprises. *Lawrence Journal-World* [Online].

Keeling, T. (2006, January 19). Big enough. *ASU Web Devil* [Online].
Keidan, B. (2000, December 31). Fans don't deserve to be honored. *Pittsburgh Post-Gazette*, p. D2.
Kelly, M. (2005, January 7). Three '05s settle drug charges. *The Dartmouth* [Online].
Kelly, R. (2006, March 31). Hillsboro High students are upset over decision on dismissals. *St. Louis Post-Dispatch* [Online].
Kelso, P. (2005, October 26). Taylor fights dope testing plan. *Guardian* [Online].
Kindred, D. (2001, August 12). Bodies so powerful, yet so vulnerable. *The Sporting News* [Online].
Kindred, D. (2001, September 17). A sea change in thinking is in order. *The Sporting News*, p. 72.
Kindred, D. (2005, July 25). Of lasers, scalpels and steroids. *The Sporting News* [Online].
King, P. (2006, August 28). Monday Morning QB. *SI.com* [Online].
King, P. (2008, June 9). The cautionary tale of Jason Peter. *SI.com* [Online].
Kinkead, L.D., & Romboy, D. (2005, October 30). Chasing glory: Football is an all-consuming passion and dream for many young Utahns. *Deseret Morning News* [Online].
Klein, G. (2006, August 2). USC player has positive steroid test. *Los Angeles Times* [Online].
Klitzing, M. (2006, November 7). A closer look at the NFL's efforts to catch steroid users. *North County Times* [Online].
Klosterman, C. (2007, March 26). Why we look. *ESPN The Magazine*, p. 90.
Knapp, G. (2001, August 12). Drug policies can be paradoxical. *San Francisco Chronicle*, p. D11.
Knapp, G. (2005, November 6). Race sponsor's product sends wrong message. *San Francisco Chronicle* [Online].
Knapp, G. (2007, June 17). Outside help should embarrass the NFL. *San Francisco Chronicle* [Online].
Knee Injuries. (2008, May 23). High school knee injuries by sport and gender. *ScienceDaily.com*.
Kolata, G. (2008, April 30). Some athletes' genes provide license to outwit testing. *New York Times*, p. D1.
Korte, S. (2007, February 25). Former Flyers back Nash is dead at 24. *Belleville News-Democrat* [Online].
Korth, J. (2006, January 29). XL means Xtra large. *St. Petersburg Times* [Online].
Kotowski, J. (2007, September 25). Arrests focused on steroid suppliers. *Bakersfield Californian* [Online].
Kovner, J. (2005, November 8). An Rx for testosterone on Websites. *Hartford Courant*, p. A1.
Kovner, J., & Doyle, P. (2005, November 7). Wrestling the octopus. *Hartford Courant* [Online].
Kravitz, B. (2007, July 4). Embrace the monster. *Indianapolis Star* [Online].
Kremer, R. (2007, January 10). Unsure how this works. *Joliet Herald News* [Online].
Krueger, C. (2008, June 11). Telephone interview with author.

Lab Technician. (2007, May 18). Lab technician denies leak. *Herald Sun* [Online].
Lacy, E. (2008, October 2). Mandarich wants to help others, not hurt MSU. *Detroit News* [Online].
Laird, B. (2008, June 5). Telephone interview with author.
Lamy, M. (2008, November 6). The Big Interview: Don Catlin. *Cycling Weekly* [Online].
Large, Retired. (2008, November 11). Football players: Staying active may lower health risks for large, retired athletes. *Science Daily* [Oline].
Latane, L. II. (2005, October 19). Student says coach gave him steroids. *Richmond Times-Dispatch* [Online].
Lazerus, M. (2007, July 12). Football coaches unsure if there's a steroid problem. *Gary Post-Tribune* [Online].
League Steps. (2007, August 14). League outlines steps taken to address concussions. *ESPN.com* [Online].
LeBlanc, C. (2005, October 10). Few U.S. physicians face steroid charges. *Columbia State* [Online].
LeBlanc, C. (2005, November 3). Are steroids muscling their way into youth sports? *Columbia State* [Online].
Lederman, D. (1991, March 6). Bill would penalize officials who urge athletes to use steroids. *Chronicle of Higher Education* [Online].
Lee, M. (2007, January 12). Putting sports in perspective. *Kansas City Star*, p. B10.
Leinonen, A. (2006, May 12). *Novel mass spectrometric analysis methods for anabolic androgenic steroids in sports drug testing*. Helsinki, Finland: University of Helsinki.
Lesmerises, D. (2006, July 30). Insurance program in place for injuries such as Gentry's. *Cleveland Plain Dealer* [Online].
Lesnick, G. (2004, August 27). Steroid abuse. *KRT Campus* [Online].
Lesnick, G. (2004, September 8). Steroid problem not just for the pros anymore. *KRT Campus* [Online].
Levine, B. (2006, October 30). Dean Taylor: Getting athletes back in the game. *Duke University News* [Online].
Levingston, S. (2006, February 5). NFL players smash-mouth ball when it comes to branding. *Washington Post*, p. A7.
Lewis, M.C., & Carlisle, N. (2007, November 18). Broken college system lets drug cheats slip through the cracks. *Salt Lake Tribune* [Online].
Liebross, R.L. (2007, January 14). LTE: Proof of steroid use not needed. *New York Times* [Online].
Lieser, J. (2008, October 13). Dolphins anti-steroid program at Boca Raton. *Palm Beach Post* [Online].
Limon, I. (2006, April 12). NCAA extends drug testing: Long defends program's 8-year streak without a positive. *Albuquerque Tribune* [Online].
Linden, M. (2007, September 26). NCAA steroid testing comes to Castleton. *Castleton Spartan* [Online].
Lindey, J. (2007, July 26). Q&A, Ramussen whereabouts. *Boulder Report* [Online].
Lipsyte, R. (1999, January 31). Trial balloon has evolved into religion. *New York Times*, p. 8—17.

Lipyste, R. (2007, January 28). Celebrating the Judeo-Lombardi Era. *Tomsdispatch.com* [Online].
Lipsyte, R. (2007, February 1). Not a Super fan? *USA Today* [Online].
Lipsyte, R. (2007, February 2). Telephone interview with author.
Lipsyte, R. (2008, March 13). Telephone interview with author.
Litke, J. (1989, September 28). Maurice Douglass made a bad decision. *The Associated Press* [Online].
Litke, J. (2005, October 21). NFL needs more than dress code. *The Associated Press* [Online].
Litke, J. (2007, March 2). Players feeling different heat. *The Associated Press* [Online].
Llosa, F., & Wertheim, L.J. (2007, March 12). Rx for trouble: Inside the steroid ring. *Sports Illustrated* [Online].
Lombardi, J. (2006, January 26). School nurses urged to look for signs of substance abuse. *White Plains Journal News* [Online].
Lombardo, N. (2006, May 15). For some, bigger isn't always better. *Oakland Press* [Online].
Longman, J. (1995, April 9). U.S.O.C. experts call drug testing a failure. *New York Times*, p. S11.
Longman, J. (1998, December 26). Unbelievable performances. *New York Times*, p. A1.
Longman, J. (2001, August 4). Supplements deserve scrutiny. *New York Times*, p. D1.
Looney, D.S. (1987, September 14). The best. *Sports Illustrated*, p. 55.
Lopez, J. (2006, November 10). Pre-1977 NFL players fight for better pension. *BlackAthlete Sports Network* [Online].
Lord, C. (2007, October 16). Don says it ain't so but fans the flame. *SwimNews.com* [Online].
Louv, R. (2006, October 31). How business can spread morality. *San Diego Union-Tribune* [Online].
Louwagie, P., & Seifert, K. (2003, April 26). Stringer claims against Vikings dismissed. *Minneapolis Star Tribune*, p. 1A.
Lovelace, S. (2007, December 19). Carrying a heavy burden. *Baltimore Sun* [Online].
Low, C. (2005, September 15). Heavy hitters on Vols line risking health. *Nashville Tennessean* [Online].
Luder, B. (2001, January 22). NOT just fun & games. *Kansas City Star*, p. C1.
Lumpkin, J.J. (2005, September 9). FDA advisers give backing to inhaled form of insulin. *Kansas City Star*, p. A1.
Lyon, A. (2006, February 9). Tucson teens juicing with 'roids. *KVOA TV* [Online].
Lyons, B.J. (2007, February 28). A Web of easy steroids. *Albany Times Union* [Online].
Lyons, S.P. (2001, November 25). School safety: Bill proposes CPR certification for coaches. *Boston Globe*, p. Globe West-1.
Mabin, B. (2006, March 1). No Huskers charged as steroid case ends. *Lincoln Journal Star* [Online].
MacKinnon, J. (2007, September 12). Everett's injury latest in long list of devastating hits. *Edmonton Journal* [Online].

Macur, J. (2007, October 24). Cycling Union takes leap in fight against doping. *New York Times* [Online].

Macur, J. (2008, November 14). Teams' antidoping company shuts down. *New York Times* [Online].

Macur, J. (2008, November 29). Born to run? Little ones get test for sports gene. *New York Times* [Online].

Mahon, R.L. (2005, October 9). Obesity and death on the gridiron. *St. Louis Post-Dispatch*, p. B3.

Mannie, K. (2004, April 13). Designer steroids: Ugly and dangerous. *NaturalStrength.com* [Online].

Mannie, K. (2005, April 25). Time to strike out the steroid mess. *NCAA News Online* [Online].

Marchione, M. (2008, April 12). 'Alarming' peek at kids' arteries. *Kansas City Star*, p. A7.

Marinello, S. (2006, May 25). IGF-1. *Blogcritics.org* [Online].

Marinello, S. (2006, July 25). How are athletes recovering so quickly from major surgeries? *Blogcritics.org* [Online].

Marinello, S. (2007, March 14). A steroid scandal hits a suburban New Jersey high school. *Blogcritics.org* [Online].

Marinello, S. (2008, October 26). The NFL's drug problem rears its ugly head, again. *Blogcritics.org* [Online].

Marot, M. (2007, February 3). Freeney pushing others to find right diet. *The Associated Press* [Online].

Marshall, Janette. (2008, November 16). Waisting away: You and your BMI index. *London Telegraph* [Online].

Marshall, John. (2001, September 9). High school pre-participation examinations beginning to come under growing scrutiny. *Chicago Sun-Times*, p. 106.

Martin, B. (2004, July 13). Bill Martin, athletic director, University of Michigan. *The abuse of anabolic steroids and their precursors by adolescent and amateur athletes.* Caucus on International Narcotics Control, U.S. Senate. Washington, D.C.: U.S. Government Printing Office.

Martinez, A. (2007, April 13). Roid rage: Anger over doping spurs Legislature to push for more drug testing. *McAllen Monitor* [Online].

Maske, M. (2006, June 10). NFL questions effectiveness of blood testing for hormone. *Washington Post*, p. E2.

Maske, M. (2006, September 7). Upshaw is okay with steroid policy. *Washington Post*, p. E9.

Maske, M. (2006, September 7). Redskins' Jansen says use of HGH is rising. *Washington Post*, p. E1.

Maske, M., & Shapiro, L. (2005, August 25). NFL is soul-searching after Herrion's death. *Washington Post*, p. E1.

Matthews, W. (2005, August 24). NFL's obesity a ticking time bomb. *Newsday* [Online].

Matthews, W. (2006, August 6). It's naïve not to believe that cheaters have won. *Newsday* [Online].
Mavreles, T. (2005, August 21). The steroids revolution. *McAllen Monitor* [Online].
Mavreles, T. (2005, August 22). Donna football sparks talk of steroid use from outsiders. *McAllen Monitor* [Online].
Mayo, D. (2008, November 4). To next leaders: Changes needed in sports. *Grand Rapids Press* [Online].
McCarthy, M. (2007, January 7). Romo's blunder bound to live in sports-TV infamy. *USA Today* [Online].
McCloskey, J. (2005, July 2). Here, there, everywhere? Not in my school … *Houston Chronicle* [Online].
McConnaughey, J. (2007, May 31). NFL study links concussions, depression. *The Associated Press* [Online].
McMahon, C. (2008, November 6). Newmarket teen charged three times in three months on host of charges. *Foster's Daily Democrat* [Online].
McManamon, P. (2007, August 7). NFL: Tucker says banned substance part of treatment. *Akron Beacon Journal* [Online].
McMullen, J. (2005, September 13). The NCAA and steroids. *AgainstTheLine.com.*
McNulty, R. (2007, July 9). The truth be told, we're all at the root of escalating problem. *Scripps Howard News Service* [Online].
Meggyesy, D. (2008, June 7). Telephone interview with author.
Mellinger, S. (2000, November 6). Pressure to perform. *Kansas City Star*, p. C1.
Mellinger, S. (2005, December 5). For Chiefs, Broncos fans, rivalry is spelled with RVs. *Kansas City Star*, p. A1.
Mellinger, S. (2006, September 15). Big offensive linemen having a major impact. *Kansas City Star*, p. D12.
Mellinger, S. (2007, January 7). Up in arms on steroids. *Kansas City Star*, p. A1.
Mero, T. (2005, October 15). Survey shows widespread use of supplements among local football players. *Lodi News-Sentinel* [Online].
Mesce, D. (1990, September 7). Adolescents risking harm to build muscles with steroids. *The Associated Press* [Online].
Metabolic Syndrome. (2005, May 7). Metabolic syndrome is costly. *The Associated Press* [Online].
Metz, S. (2006, December 1). Madison Central quarterback gets five-year reprieve. *Jackson Clarion-Ledger* [Online].
Meyer, E., & Wallace, J. (2005, September 3). Wadsworth steroid scare still puzzle. *Akron Beacon Journal* [Online].
Michener, J. (1976). *Sports in America*. New York: Random House.
Mihoces, G. (2002, July 19). Dealing with deadly sin. *USA Today*, p. 3C.
Miklasz, B. (2004, December 4). We can't place much stock in Bonds' credibility. *St. Louis Post-Dispatch* [Online].
Miller, L.J. (2007, January 14). LTE: Winning equals big money. *New York Times* [Online].

Molinaro, B. (2007, September 4). Discovery of HGH use won't spoil football, nor should it. *Virginian-Pilot* [Online].

Montgomery, R. (2005, May 17). The battle over weight. *Kansas City Star*, p. A1.

Montgomery, R. (2008, August 3). A China we've never seen. *Kansas City Star*, p. A1.

Montini, E.J. (2006, July 9). Steroid grandfather still physically and mentally muscular. *Arizona Republic* [Online].

Montone, K.R. (2007, September 25). Huge steroid bust snares 9 in region. *Scranton Times-Tribune* [Online].

Montone, K.R. (2007, September 26). Steroid ring based in Pittston area. *Scranton Times-Tribune* [Online].

Moore, D.L. (2005, May 4). School tackles alarming subject: Steroid use. *USA Today* [Online].

Moore, G. (2006, December 8). Will an asthma medication keep Hollis Thomas off the field? *BlackAthlete Sports Network* [Online].

Moore, K., & Troy, R. (2005, September 11). Steroids? Not around us, athletes claim. *Indianapolis Star* [Online].

More 'Fight Club.' (2007, February 18). More 'Fight Club' constituents arrested. *North County Times* [Online].

Morley, G., & Borodin, B. (1999, May 14). Are drugs really bad? Steroid ban branded as hypocrisy. *Wellington Evening Post*, p. 21.

Mosier, J. (2005, October 15). Judge rules woman can sue coach for slander. *Dallas Morning News* [Online].

Mott, S. (2006, January 24). The 'switching hour' for drug cheats is upon us. *London Telegraph* [Online].

Mott, S. (2008, January 20). Drug runners. *Sydney Morning Herald* [Online].

Mouse Cloned. (2008, November 5). Mouse cloned from frozen tissue. *Kansas City Star*, p. A4.

Move On. (2006, October 4). Time to move on. *SI.com* [Online].

Mnookin, S. (2007, May 6). When to hang it up. *New York Times* [in *Boston Globe*, Online].

Mu, E. (2005, December 15). Bioethicist, sports CEO debate drug use. *Daily Princetonian* [Online].

Mueller, F.O., & Cantu, R.C. (2008). *Annual survey of catastrophic football injuries.* Chapel Hill, NC: National Center for Catastrophic Sports Injury Research.

Mueller, F.O., & Colgate, B. (2008, February). *Annual survey of football injury research.* Chapel Hill, NC: National Center for Catastrophic Sports Injury Research.

Mundell, E.J. (2005, March 1). Supersized in the NFL. *Healthday* [Online].

Murphy, R.G. (2006, August 27). Tour de France's testosterone flap shines new light on Boston's expert in hormone's surprising, softer side. *Boston Globe City Weekly*, p. 1.

Murray, K., & Barker, J. (2007, June 7). NFL, union called to Congress. *Baltimore Sun* [Online].

Muscle Genes. (2005, December 30). Study finds genes that 'fine-tune' muscle development process. *Newswise* [Online].

Mushnick, P. (2007, January 12). A week of steroids, slip-ups and kiosks. *New York Post* [Online].
Myers, G. (2002, July 21). Feeling, heat, NFL makes changes. *New York Daily News*, p. 68.
Myers, G. (2005, August 27). NFL has BIG problem. *New York Daily News* [Online].
Myers, G. (2006, September 3). Put to the test. *New York Daily News* [Online].
Myers, G. (2006, September 7). Goodell: HGH not NFL issue. *New York Daily News* [Online].
Myers, G. (2008, February 1). Gene Upshaw threatens strike. *New York Daily News* [Online].
National Ring. (2005, June 23). Police arrest 3 in what may be national steroid ring. *TheOmahaChannel.com* [Online].
NBA Fat. (2005, March 9). Half the NFL is fat, according to BMI. *Kansas City Star*, p. D2.
NCAA Composition. (2008, October 27). Composition and sport sponsorship of the NCAA. *ncaa.org* [Online].
NCAA Summer. (2007, May 5). NCAA summer drug testing. *forums.steroid.com* [Online].
NCAA Tax. (2006, November 11). Brand defends NCAA tax status. *Kansas City Star*, p. D2.
NCAA Test. (2006, May 3). NCAA drug test. *forums.steroid.com* [Online].
NCAA Testing. (2008, October 31). NCAA drug-testing results 2005-06 and 2006-07. *2008 NCAA Executive Committee Supplement No. 13*. Indianapolis, IN: National Collegiate Athletic Association.
Nelson, G. (1989, June 11). Courts are needed to ease players' pain. *St. Louis Post-Dispatch*, p. 1D.
Nevill, A., & Whyte, G. (2005, October). Abstract: Are there limits to running world records? *Medicine & Science in Sports & Exercise*, p. 1785.
New Drugs. (2007, January 28). Critical new drugs won't be made here. *Kalamazoo Gazette* [Online].
Newell, K. (2006, May 1). Policy matters: Sports insurance for coaches and athletes. *Coach and Athletic Director* [Online].
Next Frontier. (2006, August 8). The next frontier of sports doping. *CBS News* [Online].
NFL Agent. (2007, March 1). Local NFL agent weighs in on steroid probe. *WTAE TV* [Online].
NFL Cardiac. (2007, March 14). Weight of NFL players to be part of cardiac study. *The Associated Press* [Online].
NFL Offseason. (2005, April 26). NFL tripling offseason steroid tests. *The Associated Press* [Online].
N.F.L. Sets. (2008, October 8). N.F.L. sets an active example on fitness. *Wilmington Star News* [Online].
NFL Super-Sized. (2005, March 2). NFL over super-sized, study finds. *Kansas City Star*, p. D2.

NFL WADA. (2005, April 27). NFL leaders bash idea of adopting WADA doping standards. *Agence France Presse* [Online].

Nice Acting. (2007, August 23). 'A nice job of acting.' *Kansas City Star*, p. D5.

Nickel, L. (2005, July 4). NFL plays defense on steroids. *Milwaukee Journal Sentinel* [Online].

Nissley, E.L. (2007, October 12). Four in 'Raw Deal' admit guilt. *Scranton Times-Tribune* [Online].

N.J. High Schooler. (2007, September 12). Random screenings show one N.J. high schooler using steroids. *The Associated Press* [Online].

Obert, R. (2008, October 14). Q&A: NFL pariah Tony Mandarich. *Arizona Republic* [Online].

Obesity Numbers. (2005, August 24). Obesity by the numbers. *Baton Rouge Advocate* [Online].

Obesity Problem? (2005, March 1). Does the NFL have an obesity problem? *The Associated Press* [Online].

O'Brien, K. (2008, October 5). High school players are bigger than ever. *Boston Globe* [Online].

O'Connor, I. (2007, February 3). Battered bodies a symbol of NFL. *Bergen??? Record* [Online].

Offensive Linewoman. (2006, October 29). Offensive linewoman. *Kansas City Star*, p. C2.

O'Keefe, K. (2007). Spartan Football 2007: Paperwork needed for football eligibility. *Seven Lakes High School summer football schedule and camp information*. Seven Lakes, TX.

O'Keeffe, M. (2008, April 27). Agents' secrets exposed. *New York Daily News* [Online].

O'Keeffe, M. (2008, May 10). Specialists teaming with Gridiron Greats to offer care for ex-NFL players. *New York Daily News* [Online].

O'Keeffe, M. (2008, June 4). Patriots lineman Nicholas Kaczur turns informant in painkiller plot. *New York Daily News* [Online].

O'Keeffe, M., & Quinn, T.J. (2005, December 25). Beating the heat. *New York Daily News* [Online].

O'Keeffe, M., & Quinn, T.J. (2006, October 29). Drug agents under fire. *New York Daily News* [Online].

O'Keeffe, M., & Quinn, T.J. (2007, March 6). Fake doc juices up. *New York Daily News* [Online].

O'Keeffe, M., & Quinn, T.J. (2007, March 11). IRS ruling on drug agents could cost League millions. *New York Daily News* [Online].

Ole Miss Recruit. (2008, January 29). Ole Miss QB recruit kicked off team for selling steroids. *ESPN.com* [Online].

Olson, B. (2006, November 16). Navy coach's claim disputed. *Baltimore Sun* [Online].

Olson, B., & Barker, J. (2006, November 18). Academy admits to delay in drug tests. *Baltimore Sun* [Online].

Olympic Sponsor? (2005, November 7). So you want to be an Olympic sponsor? *Brandweek* [Online].

Olympics' Insurance. (2004, April 28). Olympics' insurance covers terror, disaster. *Kansas City Star*, p. D2.
Olympics Loved. (1999, November 28). Poll: Despite scandals, Olympics still loved. *Albany Times Union*, p. C2.
O'Neill, D. (2001, August 12). Football shouldn't be a killing sport. *St. Louis Post-Dispatch* [Online].
Opar, A. (2008, September 16). Beasts of bioengineering. *Plenty Magazine* [Online].
Orsborn, T. (2007, April 12). Local officials don't see major steroid problem. *San Antonio Express-News* [Online].
Osterwell, N. (2007, April 16). AACE: Human growth hormone is no fountain of youth. *MedPage Today* [Online].
Ostler, S. (2001, September 9). The big, the bad and the biggest. *San Francisco Chronicle Magazine*, p. 16.
Ostruszka, S. (2006, March 28). Are NIU athletes juicing up? *Northern Star* [Online].
Ostruszka, S. (2006, March 30). Steroids on campus? *Northern Star* [Online].
Owens, D.E. (2006, May 9). Bigger athletes redefine 'healthy.' *Kansas City Star*, p. E7.
Owens Frustrated. (2008, June 11). Cowboys WR Terrell Owens frustrated about extra drug testing. *The Associated Press* [Online].
Pace, J. (2006, July 24). New heat guidelines to be released. *Tampa Tribune* [Online].
Palladino, E. (2004, December 4). Testing slows use of steroids in NFL. *Asbury Park Press* [Online].
Paralyzed Athletes. (2000, January 25). Paralyzed athletes. *Kansas City Star*, p. C4.
Pardo, S. (2008, October 21). Injury waivers challenged. *Detroit News* [Online].
Parents Want. (2008, November 17). For high school doping, parents want school intervention, low penalties. *University of Michigan News* [Online].
Parr, D. (2005, September 27). The legal steroid. *Daily Iowan* [Online].
Passan, J. (2007, September 12). At the letters: Ankiel angst. *Yahoo! Sports* [Online].
Paul, D. (2008, January 20). Test to trap Olympic cheats. *Sunday Express* [Online].
Pearson, H. (2007, January 2). Boost in mystery muscle creates endurance mice. *news@nature.com* [Online].
Pell, D. (2005, April 27). Pumping up the NFL's steroid policies. *davenetics.com* [Online].
Pells, E. (2007, February 4). Image problem plagues NFL. *The Associated Press* [Online].
Perez, A. (2007, September 26). Using sports sto relieve the stresses of being a student. *Cornell Daily Sun* [Online].
Perez, A.J. (2008, May 28). New hurdle for HGH detection. *USA Today* [Online].
Perez, A.J. (2008, August 27). NFL earmarks $1.4 million for serious anti-steroid message to youths. *USA Today* [Online].
Perez, A.J. (2008, October 24). New law allows Website hosts to just say no to drugs. *USA Today* [Online].
Perez, T. (2005, August 28). LTE: Donna-bashing needs to stop. *McAllen Monitor* [Online].
Perkins, D. (2005, August 23). NFL drug pitch a scam. *Toronto Star* [Online].

Perls, T.T., Reisman, N.R., & Olshansky, S.J. (2005, October 26). Growth hormone illegal for off-label anti-aging use. *Medical Research News* [Online].

Person, J. (2005, May 5). Erving's fathers: Son, Johnson passed drug tests. *Columbia State* [Online].

Peter, J. (2007, September 18). Documents: Animal drugs offered. *Yahoo! Sports* [Online].

Peter, J. (2007, October 3). Couch banned. *Yahoo! Sports* [Online].

Peters, K. (1989, January 11). Scott says track singled out for steroid use. *The Associated Press* [Online].

Petersen, A. (2008, May 26). Legal obstacles prevent Iowa from testing athletes. *Quad-City Times* [Online].

Phillips, J. (2007, February 20). Go Huskers, and forget all else. *Kansas City Star*, p. E7.

Pitoniak, S. (2005, January 21). Area doctor fears apathy will crush anti-steroid campaign. *Rochester Democrat and Chronicle* [Online].

Pitts, Leonard Jr. (2004, December 14). Seeking authenticity among brazen fakes. *Kansas City Star*, p. B7.

Plaschke, B. (2001, August 5). It's time to start turning up the heat on demanding, tough-guy coaches. *Los Angeles Times* [Online].

Player Dies. (2008, October 2). High school football player dies from MRSA. *Central Florida News 13* [Online].

Players Positive. (2008, October 24). McAllister, Smith, Grant, Texans' Pittman among players testing positive. *ESPN.com* [Online].

Plea Deal. (2007, April 11). DA: Plea deal in works for UW-Stout football players accused in drug case. *The Associated Press* [Online].

Poms, M. (2007, September 25). Hypocrisy rules in sports media. *William and Mary Flat Hat* [Online].

Porter, T. (2007, March 1). NFL players in front of yet another police force: Themselves. *Canton Repository* [Online].

Posnanski, J. (1997, August 10). What happened to the fun and games? *Kansas City Star*, p. D1.

Posnanski, J. (1999, June 9). Buzz continues to follow McGwire. *Kansas City Star*, p. D1.

Posnanski, J. (2003, November 18). Steroids just feel too good. *Kansas City Star*, p. C1.

Posnanski, J. (2004, August 24). If we got robbed, we'd cry, too. *Kansas City Star*, p. C2.

Posnanski, J. (2005, April 18). It's hard to see a hero fall. *Kansas City Star*, p. C1.

Posnanski, J. (2007, September 16). Who cheats? Actually, who doesn't? *Kansas City Star*, p. C1.

Posnanski, J. (2008, August 21). He's the mon! *Kansas City Star*, p. D1.

Posnanski, J. (2008, August 24). Call them the Games that transcended reality. *Kansas City Star*, p. A1.

Powell, J. (2005, May 23). Steroids concern baseball coaches: College players not tested regularly. *East Carolina University News* [Online].

Powers, E. (2006, August 31). Drug prevention promises. *Inside Higher Ed* [Online].

Prep Coma. (2008, September 17). Prep player in coma. *Kansas City Star*, p. D2.

Preston, M. (1995, January 4). NFL can provide riches—and risks. *Baltimore Sun*, p. C9.

Prison Term. (2007, August 24). 20-year prison term for ex-ASU RB convicted of 2nd-degree murder. *The Associated Press* [Online].

Pro Bowl. (2007, February 5). No positive tests in next Pro Bowl. *Philadelphia Inquirer* [Online].

Probe Expands. (2007, October 20). Steroid probe expands here. *Staten Island Advance* [Online].

Problem HGH. (2008, February 20). NFLPA's Vincent: NFL doesn't have a big problem with HGH. *The Associated Press* [Online].

Professor Concerned. (2007, January 8). TAMUCC professor concerned over growing steroid use. *KRIS TV* [Online].

Pugmire, J. (2007, March 9). UCI promises to get tough on doping with new program. *The Associated Press* [Online].

Pugmire, L. (2001, August 6). Programs might face higher tolls without trainers. *Los Angeles Times* [Online].

Purpura, D. (2005, August 14). The trickle-down effect. *Lancaster Eagle-Gazette* [Online].

Quinn, T.J. (2006, June 11). A brave new world. *New York Daily News* [Online].

Quinn, T.J. (2006, November 19). NFL testers step up fight. *New York Daily News* [Online].

Quinn, T.J. (2007, April 15). Source: Bonds explored exemption after failed test. *New York Daily News* [Online].

Quinn, T.J. (2007, September 14). Catlin expects new HGH test by next Olympics. *New York Daily News* [Online].

Quinn, T.J. (2007, September 17). Common defense of HGH must be challenged. *New York Daily News* [Online].

Quinn, T.J., & O'Keeffe, M. (2006, November 12). League may have credibility gap: NFL drug agents insist steroid testing can be exploited. *New York Daily News* [Online].

Quinn, T.J., & O'Keeffe, M. (2007, April 15). NFL runs reverse on p-men. *New York Daily News* [Online].

Quinn, T.J., O'Keeffe, M., & Red, C. (2007, February 28). Dozens tied to 'roid sting. *New York Daily News* [Online].

Raiders Lose. (2004, December 2). Raiders lose Wheatley. *Kansas City Star*, p. D9.

Rains, B.J. (2008, November 14). Former NFL commissioner speaks at KU. *Kansan* [Online].

Randle, S. (2008, September 30). Steroid suspects still being sought. *Lafayette Daily Advertiser* [Online].

Random Testing. (2007, April 12). Random drug testing approved for Hanover Park High. *Newark Star-Ledger* [Online].

Ratto, R. (2006, February 1). NFL, players need to act now to trim weight. *CBS SportsLine.com* [Online].

Ratto, R. (2006, August 23). Don't bite the hand—or, in other words, 'Well, duh!' *CBS SportsLine.com* [Online].

Redhage, J. (2007, May 19). Wade had steroids in his system night of slaying, hearing told. *East Valley/Scottsdale Tribune* [Online].

Redwood Toxicology. (2007, June 4). Redwood Toxicology Laboratory announces steroid testing. *Business Wire* [Online].

Reed, T. (2006, February 5). Any time can be test time. *Akron Beacon Journal* [Online].

Reinberg, S. (2005, December 13). Anabolic steroids might be addictive. *HealthCentral* [Online].

Reinwald, P. (1988, October 1). Most area high school football coaches favor drug testing. *St. Petersburg Times*, p. 1C.

Reiss, M. (2007, October 4). Harrison is past any talk of his suspension. *Boston Globe* [Online].

Reiter, B. (2007, July 17). Happy together. *Kansas City Star*, p. C1.

Reminick, J. (1989, February 12). The steroid subculture. *New York Times*, p. 12LI—10.

Renck, T.E. (2006, June 9). Loophole puts HGH on map. *Denver Post* [Online].

Reston, M. (2007, February 21). Parents bristle at 'Fight Club' prosecutions. *Los Angeles Times* [Online].

Reynolds, G. (2007, June 3). Outlaw DNA. *New York Times* [Online].

Rhoden, W.C. (2007, May 26). Steroids not enough to keep fans away. *New York Times*, p. D5.

Ribadeneira, D. (1988, October 31). The quick fix. *Boston Globe*, p. 39.

Riboli, E. (2008, November 13). 'Love handles' raise death risk. *BBC News* [Online].

Roberts, S. (2007, April 8). Cheating is a fundamental. *New York Times* [in *Austin American-Statesman*, Online].

Robertson, L. (2006, January 1). NFL faces weighty issues with super-sized players. *Knight Ridder Newspapers* [Online].

Robinson, D. (2008, January 9). Memo to myself: Sports need help. *Deseret Morning News* [Online].

Robinson, L. (2006, June 7). Comics morality for grownups. *Ottawa Citizen* [Online].

Rogue Pharmacies. (2008, November 18). Rogue Internet pharmacies on the run. *LegitScript* [Online].

Roebuck, J., & Osborne, J. (2007, February 1). Donna bus driver, P.E. coach arrested on drug charges. *McAllen Monitor* [Online].

Romboy, D. (2007, October 27). Painkillers, the dark side of sports. *Deseret Morning News* [Online].

Rosenblatt, S., & Saad, N. (2008, May 30). Irvine high school shaken after death of football player, 15. *Los Angeles Times* [Online].

Rosenthal, K. (2006, March 12). Schilling not surprised by steroid scandal. *The Sporting News* [Online].

Ross, S. (2005, November 9). World records will not continue to rise. *sport.scotsman.com* [Online].
Roth, L. (2005, August 28). Super-sized Bills are worried, too. *Rochester Democrat and Chronicle* [Online].
Ruckno, H. (2007, September 26). News of steroid use discouraging, not surprising to area school officials. *Wilkes-Barre Citizens Voice* [Online].
Ryan, J. (2005, March 24). Alcohol is a much bigger problem than steroids. *San Francisco Chronicle* [Online].
Sagan, N. (2007, September 17). Legal 'roids, better pads may be in NFL's future. *msnbc.com* [Online].
Samson, D. (2003, February 7). Schools can use these lifesavers. *Kansas City Star*, p. D1.
Sandalow, M. (2005, June 16). Many teenage girls abuse steroids, lawmakers told. *San Francisco Chronicle* [Online].
Sanders, L. (2007, February 25). Muscle-bound. *New York Times* [Online].
Sanghavi, D. (2007, October 2). Detecting doping in sports. *New York Times* [in *Boston Globe*, Online].
Sanginiti, T., & Besso, M. (2006, March 8). Illegal steroid use hard to detect. *New Castle News Journal* [Online].
Sanginiti, T., Tresolini, K., & Williams, L. (2007, March 7). 3 UD football players arrested in robbery. *New Castle News Journal* [Online].
Saunders, M. (2002, July 26). Fatalities in heat on rise: Supplements could be cause of deaths. *Cleveland Plain Dealer*, p. D1.
Sceifo, J., & Johnson, D. (2005, March 7). Texas, football and juice. *Newsweek* [Online].
Schaller, J. (2007, August 20). Air Force athletes face multiple drug tests by the academy. *Colorado Springs Gazette* [Online].
Schamber, D., & Pruett, G. (2007, July 13). BCHS steroid use under investigation. *Orange Leader* [Online].
Scharf, G. (2005, July 22). We've lost sight of what's important. *Californian* [Online].
Scheyer Accused. (2004, January 6). Scheyer accused of prescribing without exam. *ESPN.com* [Online].
Schoettle, A. (2006, April 3). Brand balances big bucks and books. *Indianapolis Business Journal* [Online].
Schlosser, G. (2008, June 26). Man charged for selling steroids to undercover drug agent. *West Central Tribune* [Online].
Schmidt, K. (2007, October 14). Steroids: Take one for the team. *Los Angeles Times* [Online].
Schmidt, M.S. (2006, December 7). Football officials dispute Thomas's drug defense. *New York Times* [Online].
Schmidt, M.S. (2007, March 1). Steelers deny players received doctor's drugs. *New York Times* [Online].
Schmidt, M.S. (2007, September 19). Company agrees to a fine over shipments of H.G.H. *New York Times* [Online].

Schmidt, M.S. (2007, December 11). Doping experts find loopholes beyond baseball. *New York Times* [Online].

Schoffner, C. (1989, October 5). Schultz says tougher testing alone won't solve problem. *The Associated Press* [Online].

School Injuries. (2006, November 30). High school sports injuries. *ConsumerReports.org* [Online].

Schools Advised. (2002, August 29). Schools advised to 'proceed with caution' when testing students for drugs. *The Associated Press* [Online].

Schrotenboer, B. (2005, January 22). Accusation is latest in Ohton's legal fight. *San Diego Union-Tribune* [Online].

Schrotenboer, B. (2005, January 28). Aztecs have submitted fewest samples in MWC. *San Diego Union-Tribune* [Online].

Schrotenboer, B. (2005, April 20). Former offensive line coach Baldwin denies claims made by former players. *San Diego Union-Tribune* [Online].

Schrotenboer, B. (2008, September 21). '89 suspensions signaled new era. *San Diego Union-Tribune* [Online].

Schrotenboer, B. (2008, September 21). Why less outrage over drugs in the NFL? *San Diego Union-Tribune* [Online].

Schulte, D. (2008, April 24). Steroid inquiry widens to teen athletes. *Tulsa World* [Online].

Schulz, N. (2005, December 1). The great escape. *Tech Central Station* [Online].

Schwarz, A. (2007, June 15). Lineman, dead at 36, sheds light on brain injuries. *New York Times* [Online].

Sensitive Test. (2008, March 7). New sensitive steroid test for athletes uses oil exploration technique. *ScienceDaily* [Online].

Shaikin, B. (2008, January 17). Anti-doping agency boss blasts baseball. *Los Angeles Times* [Online].

Shelton State. (2007, April 14). UA, Shelton State students arrested in drug probes. *Ledger-Enquirer* [Online].

Sheridan, P. (2006, June 9). With HGH, cheaters stay one step ahead. *Philadelphia Inquirer* [in *Centre Daily Times*, Online].

Shipley, A. (1999, September 24). Drugs: A family tradition? *Washington Post*, p. B2.

Shipley, A. (2002, December 6). New steroids sold over counter. *Washington Post*, p. A1.

Shipley, A. (2005, October 30). Latest steroid batch slips under the radar. *Washington Post* [in *Fort Wayne Journal Gazette*, Online].

Shipley, A. (2005, November 30). Steroids detected in dietary tablets. *Washington Post*, p. E1.

Shipley, A. (2007, March 2). A wider front in doping battle. *Washington Post*, p. A1.

Shipley, A. (2007, May 15). Sports leagues team up to battle drugs. *Washington Post*, p. A1.

Shipley, A. (2008, August 24). Straight dope remains elusive. *Washington Post*, p. D1.

Shorten Lives. (1988, June 27). Careers may shorten lives, say NFL players. *St. Petersburg Times*, p. 1C.

Sikahema, V. (2007, March 15). Vai's view: Sly and steroids. *NBC10.com* [Online].

Silverstein, T. (1996, May 18). How did Packers' Favre get his painkillers? *Milwaukee Journal Sentinel* [in *St. Louis Post-Dispatch*].

Silvestrini, E. (2008, January 7). Dad who gave son steroids is given 6-year prison term. *Tampa Tribune* [Online].

Simms Start. (2004, October 7). Simms to get start for Tampa. *Kansas City Star*, p. D3.

Singer, E. (2007, October 18). Mimicking the massively muscular. *Technology Review* [Online].

Singer, E. (2007, October 26). Next-Generation sports doping. *Technology Review* [Online].

Singer, E. (2008, August 13). How to catch Olympic cheats. *Technology Review* [Online].

Singer, N. (2006, August 10). Does testosterone build a better athlete? *New York Times* [Online].

Singer, S., & Doris, T. (2007, March 25). Steroid use among teens troubles Web investigators. *Palm Beach Post* [Online].

Sirtris Drug. (2007, November 29). Sirtris drug may fight diseases of age. *Bloomberg News* [Online].

Slezak, C. (2002, June 12). Just a 'roid herring. *Chicago Sun-Times*, p. 151.

Slezak, C. (2005, May 1). Steroid hearings a waste of everyone's time, money. *Chicago Sun-Times* [Online].

Small Doses. (1991, September 3). Small doses of steroids negligible, says review. *USA Today*, p. 11C.

Smith, D. (2007, June 4). Sports cheats' game of delusion with growth hormone. *Sydney Morning Herald* [Online].

Smith, J. (2007, April 13). 11 students arrested in drug sting. *Tuscaloosa News* [Online].

Snyder, M. (2008, April 12). How Mario Manningham failed drug tests, yet played for U-M. *Detroit Free Press* [Online].

Son Guilty. (2007, July 27). Son of Eagles coach guilty. *Waterloo Record* [Online].

Sonksen, P. (2008, January 18). E-mail correspondence to group, author.

Sorensen, T. (2005, August 28). For fans, steroids more boring than the PAT. *Charlotte Observer* [in *Columbia State*, Online].

Souhan, J. (2000, September 1). America's game. *Minneapolis Star Tribune*, p. 1C.

Spivey, J. (2008, April 9). Athletic department drug testing not up to par. *Central Arkansas Echo* [Online].

Sperber, M. (2005, January 20). Myles to go at the NCAA. *Insider Higher Ed* [Online].

Sports Injuries. (2006, September 28). Safer gear slashes high-school sports injuries. *The Associated Press* [Online].

Spoto, M. (2008, February 6). Teacher among 5 arrested on drug charges. *Newark Star-Ledger* [Online].

Sprint Football. (2007, September 27). Ivy League rules against Olympian Cheek playing sprint football. *USA Today* [Online].

Squibbs, N. (2006, November 30). Steroid tests results come back for Kofa athletes. *Yuma Sun* [Online].

Stadium Insurance. (2002, August 28). Stadium insurance increasing. *Kansas City Star*, p. D2.

Stamford, B. (1994, November 9). Body shop. *Gannett News Service* [Online].

Standout Pleads. (2006, December 17). Grid standout pleads guilty. *The Associated Press* [Online].

Stark, C. (2005, October 17). Time to reflect on SHSU's football season. *Huntsville Item* [Online].

Steele, D. (2002, September 1). Adding insult to injury. *San Francisco Chronicle*, p. D1.

Steele, D. (2007, October 10). Honesty not the best policy for cheating athletes. *Baltimore Sun* [Online].

Stein, J. (2007, June 17). Big games for toddlers. *Los Angeles Times* [in *Kansas City Star*, p. D8].

Stein, J. (2008, April 7). Normal but fat. *Los Angeles Times*, p. F2.

Steinberg, D. (2008, November 7). Ryan Clark, Sean Taylor tributes and the NFL. *washingtonpost.com* [Online].

Steinbrenner Says. (2008, February 18). Hank Steinbrenner says football has bigger steroid problem than baseball. *The Associated Press* [Online].

Stenson, J. (2008, March 3). Users say they'd take drugs to excel even if it shortejned their lives. *msnbc.com* [Online].

Stephens, M. (2005, May 6). Many coaches view proposed regulations as added burden. *San Francisco Chronicle* [Online].

Steroid Cleanse. (2006, December 8). Steroid Cleanse question. *forums.steroid.com* [Online].

Steroid Parallel? (2007, January 17). Unfair advantage: What is YOUR steroid parallel? *sportingnews.com* [Online].

Steroid Possession. (2002, December 11). College football: Steroid possession not seen as issue. *New York Times* [Online].

Steroid Pushers. (2007, August 15). P in the steroid pushers. *Palm Beach Post* [Online].

Steroids Death. (1989, January 11). Football player's death attributed to steroids. *United Press International* [Online].

Steroids Here. (2007, September 26). Steroids are here. *Newsday* [Online].

Stevens, S. (2003, November). Drug test. *Outside Magazine* [Online].

Stilger, V.G., & Yesalis, C.E. (1999, April). Abstract: Anabolic-androgenic steroid use among high school football players. *Journal of Community Health*, p. 131.

Stocks, D. (2008, October 11). 'America's Most Wanted' fugitive caught in central Phoenix. *KNXV TV* [Online].

Straka, M. (2007, August 14). Grrr! Our steroid nation. *Fox News* [Online].

Straub, B. (2006, January 31). Number of 300-pounders increasing on prep teams. *Scripps Howard News Service* [Online].

Strauss, J. (2006, March 17). A year after the steroid hearings, tremors persist. *St. Louis Post-Dispatch* [Online].

Student Charged. (2007, September 5). Student charged with possessing steroids.

Greensboro News & Record [Online].

Students Arrested. (2007, April 26). 5 students at Rowan arrested in drug case. *Courier-Post* [Online].

Subcommittee on Commerce, Trade, and Consumer Protection, U.S. House of Representatives. (2008, February 27). *Drugs in sports: Compromising the health of athletes and undermining the integrity of competition.* Webcast [Online].

Suggs, W. (1999, September 24). A smaller NAIA looks for ways to better serve remaining members. *Chronicle of Higher Education*, p. A57.

Sumers, B. (2007, August 7). High schools try to tackle the heat. *St. Louis Post-Dispatch* [Online].

Suspended Husker. (2005, August 11). Suspended Husker listed as witness in steroid case. *The Associated Press* [Online].

Svare, B. (2007, March 11). Big dopes. *Albany Times Union* [Online].

Swanson, J. (2007, December 27). Athletes use steroids. *Prince George Citizen* [Online].

Swatek, G. (2006, October 30). Football less affected by steroids cases. *Evening Sun* [Online].

Swezey, C. (2006, November 16). Navy discloses failed drug tests. *Washington Post*, p. E5.

Swift, E.M. (2006, January 9). What went wrong in Winthrop? *Sports Illustrated* [Online].

Tagliabue Problems? (2006, August 13). Pro-Con: Did Paul Tagliabue leave the NFL with any major problems? *Kansas City Star*, p. C15.

Taylor, J. (2006, June 15). Medina solidifies position on drugs. *Bandera Bulletin* [Online].

Taylor, J.J. (2007, June 3). Bulking up steroids policy not enough. *Dallas Morning News* [Online].

Teacher Sentenced. (2008, July 21). Ore. Teacher sentenced for giving kids painkillers. *KOMO TV* [Online].

T/E Ratio. (2006, November 19). T/E ratio or ester tested??? *forums.steroid.com* [Online].

Team Mom. (2007, January 2). 'Team mom' supports Buckeyes. *Kansas City Star*, p. C3.

Teel, D. (2007, September 5). He's big, full of potential. *Newport News Daily Press* [Online].

Teen Attitudes. (2008, March 11). Survey: Teen attitudes on 'roids, HGH. *SI.com* [Online].

Teen Found. (2007, April 25). Police: Teen found on UCF property with AK-47. *WKMG TV* [Online].

Teenagers Steroids. (1988, December 17). Teenagers on steroids. *Washington Post*, p. A18.

Teicher, A. (2006, October 22). One huge hit. *Kansas City Star*, p. Extra1.

Teicher, A. (2008, September 28). Cutler has matured into strong leader. *Kansas City Star*, p. Extra3.

Telander, R. (2001, August 21). Courting disaster at NU. *Chicago Sun-Times* [Online].

Telander, R. (2001, October 10). NU points the finger. *Chicago Sun-Times* [Online].

Telander, R. (2001, November 21). Stringer's lasting legacy. *Chicago Sun-Times* [Online].

Telander, R. (2006, January 15). Steroid debate can be tackled another day. *Chicago Sun-Times*, p. 3.

test e. (2007, August 31). test e and cyp? *forums.steroid.com* [Online].

Test Tutorial. (2006). Beat a urine test tutorial. *UreaSample.com* [Online].

Testing Faked. (2006, February 23). Study suggests IOC testing for erythropoietin is faked. *Doping Journal* [Online].

Testing Intensify. (2007, January 25). Drug testing to intensify. *Kansas City Star*, p. D7.

Testosterone Testing. (2007, January 4). Doc testing Testosterone levels. *forums.steroid.com* [Online].

Texas Tech Admits. (2005, February 28). Texas Tech admits breaking NCAA rule. *Kansas City Star*, p. C3.

Thelen, S.L. (2007, October 11). Ethicist: Why steroid use is bad for sports. *Michigan Daily* [Online].

Thomas, B. (2006, October 2). Congress' letter to the NCAA. *USA Today* [Online].

Thompson, T., O'Keeffe, M., & Vinton, N. (2008, March 15). Houston-area gyms part of drug culture beyond sports scope. *New York Daily News* [Online].

Thorne, N. (2007, March 27). Would you juice if you could? *Yale Daily News* [Online].

Tight End Paralyzed. (2007, September 11). Bills tight end likely paralyzed. *Kansas City Star*, p. C3.

Tobeck Defends. (2007, April 4). Rob Tobeck, All Pro center, defends NFL drug policy as strictest in all of professional sports. *bigbuttradio.com* [Online].

Tolen, T. (2005, August 5). Former football star on probation. *Ann Arbor News* [Online].

Toner Alleges. (1987, July 3). Toner alleges more than half of major college players use steroids. *The Associated Press* [Online].

Toner, J. (2006, September 25). Telephone interview with author.

Torgovnick, K. (2008). Reading guide: Cheer! Inside the secret world of college cheerleaders. *SimonSays.com* [Online].

Torres, K. (2007, May 14). Bill would provide injury insurance for jockeys. *Occupational Hazards* [Online].

Tougher Policy. (2007, January). Freeney: NFL needs even tougher steroid policy. *The Associated Press* [Online].

Tren E System? (2006, September 25). How long does Tren E stay in system? *forums.steroid.com* [Online].

Tresolini, K. (2006, March 12). UD dealing with off-field problems. *New Castle News Journal* [Online].

Tsiovkh, L. (2007, November 20). High schools should test athletes for steroid use. *Kansas City Star*, p. B7.

Tucker, R. (2008, February 19). Pressure of pro days, combine drive some to steroids. *SI.com* [Online].

Tufaro, G. (2006, May 16). Steroid plan not applauded by everyone. *Courier News* [Online].

Tyagi, A., & Quillen, W.S. (2007, April 10). Young and steroids—a deadly combination. *ABC News* [Online].

Ubha, R. (2005, December 16). Drugs should be permitted in sports, professors say. *Bloomberg News* [Online].

Ueberroth Strategy. (2007, April 26). Ueberroth wants new anti-doping strategy. *The Associated Press* [Online].

UNC Study. (2002, July 25). UNC Study: Heat-Related deaths steadily rising. *Newsday*, p. A57.

Urine Test. (2008, January 31). Upshaw: Players to accept urine, not blood, HGH test. *The Associated Press* [Online].

Uryasz, F. (2006, February 15). Interview with author. Kansas City, MO.

Uryasz, F. (2007, December 16). NCAA diligent in drug testing. *Salt Lake Tribune* [Online].

U.S. GAO. (2005, November 3). Anabolic steroids are easily purchased without a prescription and present significant challenges to law enforcement officials. *GAO report to Committee on Government Reform, House of Representatives*. Washington, DC: U.S. Government Accountability Office.

U.S. Obesity. (2007, November 29). U.S. obesity rates seem to be leveling off, study indicates. *The Associated Press* [Online].

Usiak, D. (1989, May 18). State Senate panel told of steroid problem. *United Press International* [Online].

UW-Stout Player. (2007, August 6). Former UW-Stout football player convicted in drug case. *The Associated Press* [Online].

Vanasco, J. (2006, September 30). Tough girls, soft hearts. *houstonvoice.com* [Online].

Vecsey, G. (1987, December 6). A gain for civil rights. *New York Times*, p. 2—1.

Vecsey, G. (1988, July 27). Cantaloupe for the N.F.L. *New York Times*, p. A22.

Vecsey, G. (1991, July 29). The guard who took rat poison. *New York Times*, p. C9.

Vecsey, G. (2008, January 27). Same chemicals, different reactions. *New York Times* [Online].

Verdict Expected. (2004, September 1). Verdict expected in steroid case of ex-AFA linebacker. *Denver Post* [Online].

Victory, J. (2005, October 18). Undetectable steroids easy to get online. *ABC News* [Online].

Vinton, N. (2008, September 29). Anti-Doping expert talks to News about Lance Armstrong's testing program. *New York Daily News* [Online].

Vinton, N. (2008, November 10). Major League Baseball won't have HGH test in the near future. *New York Daily News* [Online].

Voepel, M. (2002, August 21). Head games: Schools trying to understand effects of concussions. *Kansas City Star*, p. D1.

WADA's Credibility. (2007, January 21). Upshaw tells newspaper he doubts WADA's credibility. *ESPN.com* [Online].

Wagh, M. (2007, May). Gene therapy for Fido. *The Scientist* [Online].

Walker, C. (2006, December 10). NCAA tests so few athletes, schools are left to fill gap. *Baltimore Sun* [Online].

Walker, T. (2007, September 12). Always out in front? Keeping up with drug cheats. *The Independent* [Online].

Waller, S. (2008, July 1). Message to avoid steroids getting out, coaches say. *Abilene Reporter-News* [Online].

Walsh, C. (2007, February 17). Bigger steps needed to end steroid use. *Tuscaloosa News* [Online].

Ward, B. (2005, November 20). This just in—Athletes cheat, and always will. *Minneapolis Star Tribune* [Online].

Watson, G. (2008, September 22). Ball State's Love OK after spinal fracture, but career likely over. *ESPN.com* [Online].

Webby, S. (2005, June 6). Unconventional stance. *San Jose Mercury News* [Online].

Weiner, E. (2005, May 31). Make crackdown on steroids real. *Orlando Sentinel* [Online].

Weiner, R., & Pulitzer, C. (2006, February 10). Loopholes in Olympics drug policy big enough to ski through. *Seattle Post-Intelligencer* [Online].

Weir, T. (2004, December 8). Do the fans care? *USA Today* [Online].

Weisman, J. (2007, January). Football, the drug? *Baseball Toaster* [Online].

Weisman, L. (2008, August 21). NFL mourns Gene Upshaw, the architect of free agency. *USA Today* [Online].

Wereschagin, M. (2007, March 1). Steelers doctor not target, Rooney says. *Pittsburgh Tribune-Review* [Online].

Weller, R. (2004, September 1). Cadet found innocent. *The Associated Press* [Online].

Whicker, M. (2005, May 2). Steroids overshadowed by other woes in NFL. *Orange County Register.*

Whitehouse, R. (2007, August 8). We're equally to blame for game's steroid era. *Sun Journal* [Online].

Whitlock, J. (2002, May 30). Steroids have ruined athletics. *Kansas City Star*, p. D1.

Wilbon, M. (2007, September 5). It's the most wonderful time of the year. *Washington Post*, p. H5.

Williams, B.Y. (2006, September 21). High school team under investigation. *Kansas City Star*, p. B2.

Williams, P. (2008, November 6). Straight talk is the best deterrent to steroid use. *Washington Post*, p. G12.

Williamson, B. (2008, May 1). Fun-loving Benedict was considered prime draft prospect. *ESPN.com* [Online].

Winning Prescription. (2007, May 30). Winning prescription. *Bangor Daily News* [Online].

Winter, D.R. (2007, June 14). Athletic priorities. *State News* [Online].

Wise, M. (2005, August 23). Living large, dying young. *Washington Post*, p. E1.

Wodraska, L. (2007, August 12). So many reasons to love football. *Salt Lake Tribune* [Online].

Wood, G. (2005, June 15). Muscular prep athletes fight steroid allegations. *Olympian* [Online].

Woolsey, G. (2008, January 6). For Giants' Strahan, steroids bust worst crime. *Indianapolis Star* [Online].

Worker Hid. (2008, November 7). Drug center worker hid failed tests. *Kansas City Star*, p. A6.
World Tallest. (2007, June 19). New study says Americans no longer the tallest in the world. *ABC News* [Online].
Wright, W. (2008, July 25). Steroids testing not worth the time. *New Braunfels Herald-Zeitung* [Online].
Wulderk, L. (2007, March 8). U of M research shows link between sports, unhealthy weight control and steroid use in teens. *University of Minnesota News* [Online].
Yanda, S. (2007, October 4). Olympic star's steroid use causes doubt regarding collegiate athletic ethics. *Marquette Tribune* [Online].
Yeransian, L. (2006, January 14). HGH threat: Works like steroids but undetectable. *ABC News* [Online].
Yesalis, C.E. (2005, March 10). Statement of Charles E. Yesalis. In Committee on Energy and Commerce, U.S. House of Representatives. *Steroid in sports: Cheating the system and gambling your health* (H. Hrg. No. 109-65). Washington, D.C.: U.S. Government Printing Office.
Yesalis, C.E. (2005, April 19). Letter correspondence to Marsha Blackburn. In Committee on Energy and Commerce, U.S. House of Representatives. (2005, March 10). *Steroid in sports: Cheating the system and gambling your health* (H. Hrg. No. 109-65). Washington, D.C.: U.S. Government Printing Office.
Yesalis, C.E. (2006, February 17). Telephone interview with author.
Yesalis, C.E. (2006, September 12). Telephone interview with author.
Yesalis, Charles. (2006, June 22). Interview with Charles Yesalis. *Fredericksburg Free Lance-Star* [Online].
Youngmisuk, O. (2007, June 11). Former players say enduring pain, concussions not worth it. *New York Daily News* [Online].
Zagoria, A. (2005, October 9). Testing resolve. *Bergen Herald News* [Online].
Zanin, A. (2008, August 29). The new generation. *Murray State News* [Online].
Zeigler, M. (2004, August 8). Growing pains. *San Diego Union-Tribune* [Online].
Zeigler, M. (2008, March 7). Cheaters can prosper on drugs at NFL tryout. *San Diego Union-Tribune* [Online].
Ziegler, M. (2008, November 11). Drug rules 'not enforced.' *Sporting Life* [Online].
Zillgitt, J. (2008, April 22). Pipeline to the NFL? *USA Today* [Online].
Zimmerman, P. (1997, November 24). Bronkosaurus. *Sports Illustrated*, p. 38.
Zimmerman, P. (2008, October 3). QB debate, rankings fallout, more. *SI.com* [Online].
Zirin, D. (2006, August 27). The long odds of success on the gridiron. *Los Angeles Times* [Online].
Zirin, D. (2007, June 27). High impact: What football owes its players. *The Nation* [Online].
Zubeck, P. (2005, March 1). AFA cadet gets light sentence in steroid case. *Colorado Springs Gazette* [Online].